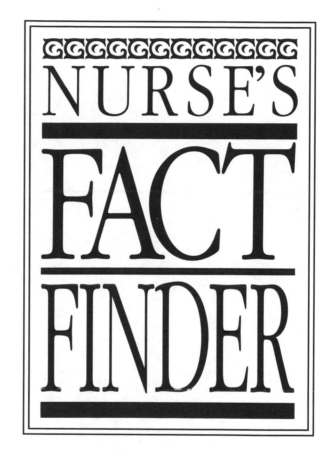

NURSE'S
FACT
FINDER

From the publisher of *Nursing* Magazine

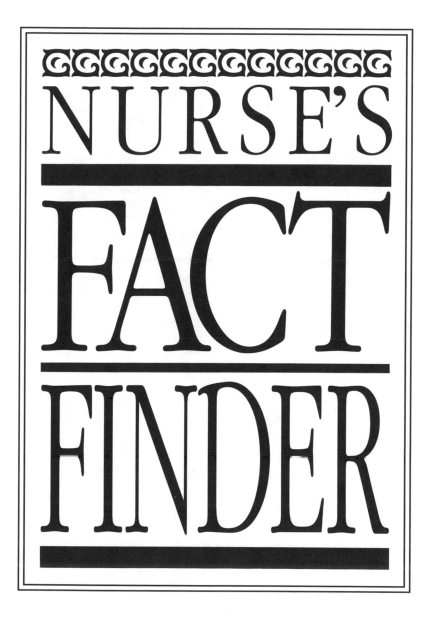

NURSE'S
FACT
FINDER

Springhouse Corporation
Springhouse, Pennsylvania

Staff

Executive Director, Editorial
Stanley Loeb

Editorial Director
Matthew Cahill

Clinical Director
Barbara F. McVan, RN

Art Director
John Hubbard

Drug Information Editor
George J. Blake, RPh, MS

Clinical Editor
Julie N. Tackenberg, RN, MA, CNRN

Editors
Stephen Daly (senior editor), Kate Cassidy, Peter H. Johnson, Michael Shaw, Jean Wallace

Copy Editors
Jane V. Cray (supervisory copy editor), Amy P. Jirsa

Editorial Assistants
Maree DeRosa, Beverly Lane, Mary Madden

Designers
Stephanie Peters (associate art director), Jacalyn Bove Facciolo (book designer), Maryanne Buschini, Darcy Feralio, Linda Franklin, Stellar Visions, Lesley Weissman-Cook

Art Production
Robert Perry (manager), Heather Bernhardt, Anna Brindisi, Donald Knauss, Robert Wieder

Illustrators
Jack Freas, Jean Gardner, John Gist, Robert Jackson, Robert Jones, Judy Newhouse, Robert Newman, Dennis Schofield, Emilie Snyder

Typography
David Kosten (director), Diane Paluba (manager), Liz Bergman, Joyce Rossi Biletz, Kathy Macfarlane, Phyllis Marron, Robin Rantz, Valerie Rosenberger

Manufacturing
Deborah Meiris (manager), T.A. Landis, Jennifer Suter

Production Coordination
Aline Miller (manager), Joy Dickenson, Colleen M. Hayman

Indexer
Barbara Hodgson

Library of Congress Cataloging-in-Publication Data

Nurse's FactFinder/from the editors of Nursing magazine.
   p.   cm.
  Includes bibliographical references.
  Includes index.
  1. Nursing—Handbooks, manuals, etc. I. Springhouse Corporation.
   [DNLM: 1. Nursing. 2. Nursing Care. 3. Nursing Process.   WY 100 N9716]
RT51.N84 1991
610.73—dc20
DNLM/DLC   90-10119
ISBN 0-87434-308-9   CIP

NURF-020791   ISBN-0-87434-308-9

Contents

PART III: Patient management

PART IV: Professional development

Foreword

In today's health care environment, with policies and procedures constantly changing, nurses face greater challenges than ever, their work more complicated and demanding than it was only a few years ago. What's more, to keep pace with scientific and technologic advances, nurses need an expanding knowledge base, sound clinical skills, and familiarity with their professional rights, responsibilities, and risks.

To meet these needs and keep abreast of the latest trends in health care, nurses need accurate, up-to-date, readily available information on a wide range of topics. Fortunately, *Nurse's FactFinder,* a new reference from the publisher of *Nursing* Magazine, provides just that.

The book is divided into four parts: Nursing Snapshots, Clinical Skills, Patient Management, and Professional Development. The first part, Nursing Snapshots, gives an overview of the nursing profession. Besides tracing the profession's history, it provides demographics on where nurses work, what salaries they earn, and what fringe benefits they value most. The chapter also forecasts nursing employment prospects and discusses candidly what nurses like—and dislike—most about their jobs.

The second part of the book, Chapters 2 through 9, focuses on clinical skills. Chapter 2 contains, among many other topics, tips and guidelines for a successful patient interview, an illustrated guide to performing a complete physical examination, a chart detailing the significance of abnormal heart sounds, and a thorough anatomic atlas. Next, Chapter 3 provides a complete, up-to-date list of nursing diagnoses and definitions.

Chapter 4 covers diagnostic procedures as well, with outlines for more than 100 laboratory tests, normal and abnormal findings, and the significance of abnormal findings. Chapter 5 provides a step-by-step approach to interpreting ECGs, with illustrations of common and lethal dysrhythmias, their etiologic factors, and their treatment. What's more, the chapter provides helpful advice on marking an ECG strip, positioning chest leads, and troubleshooting ECG artifacts. It describes and shows how drugs and electrolyte imbalances affect ECG waveforms.

Chapter 6 explains how to recognize and respond to life-threatening illnesses and profiles 100 common and uncommon disorders. It provides the outlook on acquired immunodeficiency syndrome (AIDS) and details the necessary precautions for preventing transmission of the causative human immunodeficiency virus (HIV). Next, Chapter 7 includes surgical patient care—from preoperative care to management of postoperative complications. What's more, it summarizes therapeutic alternatives to common surgeries, explains dietary regimens, and gives guidance on helping your patients steer clear of unproven remedies.

Chapter 8, an in-depth look at drug therapy, gives you specific guidelines for administering drugs safely, one of the most critical aspects of nursing. It includes drug compatibility charts, dangerous drug interactions, additive-containing drugs, and instructions on what to do if a patient has an adverse reaction to medication.

Chapter 9 teaches you how to react in emergency situations, how to prioritize, and how to conduct an emergency assessment. You'll quickly and correctly respond to anaphylaxis, shock, rape, potential suicides, and other crises.

The third part of *Nurse's FactFinder*, Chapters 10 through 15, centers on patient management, showing you the subtleties in securing the trust of your patients and their families, and in meeting the special needs of pregnant, pediatric, and elderly patients. It also supplies you with techniques for improving your patient-teaching skills.

The final part of the book, Chapters 16 through 19, concerns professional development. Designed to help refine your interpersonal skills and ensure success on the job, it covers such practical matters as evaluating educational programs, writing a winning résumé, preparing for important job interviews, weighing benefits packages, and adjusting to a new job. It also gives you cogent advice on career advancement, resolving disagreements with your boss, handling stress, and managing job-related legal and professional problems.

With all this and more, *Nurse's FactFinder* is a timely, thorough, and easy to follow reference. It's an invaluable resource for nurses in the 1990s — one that you won't want to be without.

Linda Teplitz, RN, MSN, CCRN
Instructor, Niehoff School of Nursing
Loyola University
Chicago

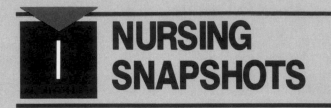

NURSING
SNAPSHOTS

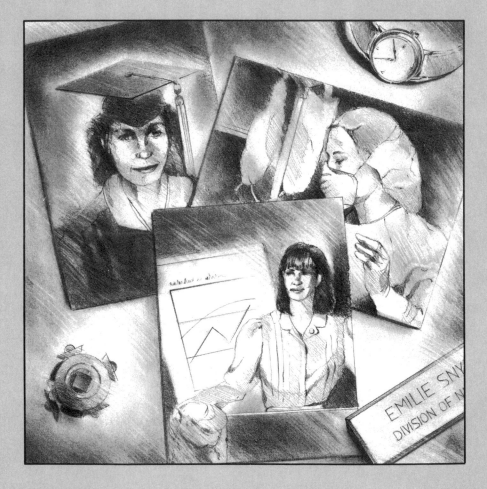

1 Yesterday, today, and tomorrow

A look at the past: Nursing's time line

1820
Florence Nightingale born. Thirty-one years later, she began her career as a caregiver, eventually building the foundations of modern nursing.

1833
The Institute of Deaconesses is established in Kaiserswerth, Germany, to train women to care for the sick and destitute.

1845
Elizabeth Blackwell becomes the first female doctor, opening the door for formal health sciences study by women.

1860
St. Thomas Hospital, in England, opens the first nursing school founded on Florence Nightingale's principles.

1861
The Union establishes the military nurse corps to care for the wounded during the Civil War.

1865
Harriet N. Philips, of the School of Nursing of the Women's Hospital of Philadelphia, becomes the first nurse diplomate in the United States.

1873
Bellevue Hospital, in New York City, opens the first U.S. nursing school founded on Florence Nightingale's principles.

1877
New York City Mission employs visiting nurses for the first time.

1879
Mary E.P. Mahoney, the first black woman to receive formal nursing training in the U.S., receives her diploma from the School of Nursing, New England Hospital for Women and Children in Boston.

1880
Nurses are allowed to use thermometers in patient care.

1881
Clara Barton organizes the American Red Cross.

1886
The Nightingale, the first nursing journal, is published in New York City.

1890
Uniforms are now established in nursing schools. To differentiate a "lady nurse" from a household servant, the uniform usually had such Victorian characteristics as frills, lace, long skirts and aprons, high collars, and black sateen sleeve protectors. (Rolled cuffs weren't considered ladylike.)

1891
First use of rubber gloves in surgery (to protect the nurse's hands).

1893
Lillian Wald establishes the Henry Street Settlement in New York City to provide nursing care for the poor. This marks the first time that nursing is associated with a municipal body instead of a religious order.

The first national nursing organization—the American Society of Superintendants of Training Schools for Nurses—comes into existence. In 1912, the organization was renamed the National League for Nursing Education.

1896
Ada Stewart employed as the first American industrial nurse by the Vermont Marble Company, Proctor, Vermont.

The American Nurses Alumnae comes into existence. In 1911, the organization was renamed American Nurses' Association (ANA).

1898
The National Association for the Daughters of the American Revolution recruits nurses to serve in Panama and Cuba in the Spanish-American War.

Nurses are permitted to administer ether for operations.

1899
Teachers College of Columbia University establishes a course in hospital economics to prepare nurses for administrative responsibilities. Practitioners receive a certificate upon completion.

Los Angeles beomes the first city to employ a public health nurse.

1901
Army Nurse Corps established, open only to women.

1902
Inception of public school nursing.

1903
North Carolina requires registration of nurses and establishes a board of nursing examiners.

1908
Naval Nurse Corps established.

First university-based (but non-degree) nursing program begins at University of Minnesota.

1909
Census Bureau survey indicates that 20% of U.S. wage-earners are women. Nursing employs one-half of these women.

1910
Helen Hartley starts the first endowment for nursing education with a $150,000 gift.

1911
California passes legislation reducing the number of hours a woman

can work from 14 to 8 per day. Nurses oppose the bill, feeling that it undercuts the profession's altruistic foundation.

1913
A study finds that nurses walk an average of 5.5 miles each day on the job, carry food trays weighing up to 15 pounds, and routinely move 31-pound bedscreens. The study recommends use of energy-saving devices, such as wheeled carts.

The U.S. extends protection of the 8-hour day to student nurses, whose health was found to decline during their nursing education.

1916
Margaret Sanger opens the first birth control clinic, in Boston.

1917
National League for Nursing calls for a standard curriculum in nursing schools.

1918
Army School of Nursing established.

Goldmark Report emphasizes the benefits of establishing autonomous schools of nursing within the university system.

1920
Hollywood films, "Nurse Marjorie" and "Goodnight, Nurse" begin to create an image problem for nurses.

1924
Yale University opens the first autonomous nursing school in a university.

1930
Estelle N. Massey and Mable Stauper become the first black nurses to join the National Organization of Public Health Nursing and to serve on committees.

"White Parade," a film starring Loretta Young, features idealism and self-sacrifice as essential characteristics of a good nurse.

1931
Nurses are hired by United Airlines as stewardesses to enhance the image of safe air travel.

1933
Federal aid programs hire more than 10,000 nurses to provide care for needy families.

1935
Social Security Act provides scholarship stipend for nurses to receive formal public health training.

1937
National League of Nursing Curriculum Guide states that the primary function of nursing schools is educating nurses rather than providing service to hospitals.

1938
New York City opens its first school for licensed practical nurses.

1940
Department of Commerce figures reveal 7,509 male nurses and students seeking employment.

1943
Bolton Act subsidizes entire education of nursing students in the U.S. Cadet Nurse Corps program.

1948
"Nursing for the Future," a report by Lucille Brown, PhD, emphasizes the need for university education of nurses and for nursing research.

1950
ANA establishes a program for nursing research.

1952
Almost 400,000 nurses work in U.S. hospitals.

Louise McManus initiates associate's degree program in nursing.

1955
2nd Lieutenant Edward L.T. Lyons is commissioned as the first male nurse in the U.S. Army.

1956
Health Amendment Act provides financial aid to RNs for full-time study of administration, supervision, and teaching in nursing.

1959
Nurses are reported to have the lowest income of all professional women: $3,200 per year.

1960
A Yale University study shows that a nurse in a college health service can safely replace a doctor in taking medical histories.

1964
First coronary care unit established at Presbyterian Hospital in Philadelphia.

1965
ANA recommends that BA be considered as entrance requirement for nursing. University of Colorado starts a nurse practitioner program.

1971
Idaho becomes the first state to authorize the expanded role of nurse practitioners.

1973
North American Nursing Diagnosis Association (NANDA) begins meeting biennially in an effort to define a conceptual framework for nursing practice.

1974
4,400 nurses of the California Nurses Association illegally strike San Francisco hospitals and clinics. Six weeks later, President Nixon amends the Taft-Hartley Act, allowing nurses to engage in collective bargaining.

1979
Growing numbers of nurses practice in nursing homes as geriatric care requirements expand.

1982
Nursing education programs continue to expand. In all, 1,432 programs are operation. About one-half are associate's degree programs; nearly one-third, bachelor's degree programs.

1983
Oregon and Washington allow nurses to write prescriptions.

1984
About 20,000 nurse practitioners are employed.

1986
Nursing shortage persists as issues of professionalism, educational preparation, and compensation continue to cause controversy.

1989
For the first time in 5 years, nursing school enrollments rise. They increase by almost 15%.

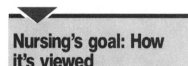

Nursing's goal: How it's viewed

Although nursing theorists have agreed that the nurse should work with—not for—the patient, they've historically differed on nursing's ultimate goal. Below, a look at some of the major nursing theorists and their perspectives on nursing's goal.

Florence Nightingale (1860s)
To put patients in the best possible condition so that nature can preserve or restore their health.

Hildegarde Peplau (1950s)
To help move the patient's personality and other human processes toward creative, productive, personal, and community living.

Virginia Henderson (1960s)
To substitute for what patients lack in physical strength, knowledge, or will to help them become whole or independent.

Dorothy Johnson (1960s)
To restore, preserve, or attain a patient's behavioral system balance and dynamic stability at the highest possible level.

Dorothea Orem (1970s)
To teach and manage continuous self-care to help patients sustain life and health, to recover from injury or disease, and to cope with their effects; also to move the patient toward responsible self-care and family members toward competent decision-making about the patient's daily care.

Martha Rogers (1970s)
To promote harmonious interaction between an individual and the environment, to strengthen an individual's integrity and coherence, and to direct the patterning of the individual and the environment to realize full human potential.

Sister Callista Roy (1970s)
To promote adaptation in each adaptive mode (psychological needs, self-concept, role function, and interdependence) to contribute to the patient's quality of life, health, and death with dignity.

Rosemary Parse (1980s)
To guide the patient, family and society in choosing among the possibilities in the changing health process.

Jean Watson (1980s)
To protect, enhance, and preserve humanity by helping a patient find meaning in illness, suffering, pain, and existence; to help a patient gain self-knowledge, control, and self-healing and restore a sense of harmony regardless of external circumstances.

Nursing's pioneers: Leading the way to better health care

Yesterday

Mary Breckinridge (1881-1965). Organized the first child hygiene and visiting nursing service in France, 1919. She also organized the Frontier Nursing Service in rural Kentucky in 1925.

Namahyoke S. Curtis (d. 1935). Active as a contract nurse during the Spanish-American War. She helped establish Provident Hospital in Chicago to care for black patients and train black nurses and doctors.

Dorothea Lynde Dix (1802-1887). Revolutionized care of the mentally ill by promoting legislation for government funding and care standards. She also was superintendant of Army nurses during the Civil War.

Clara Maas (1876-1901). Served as an Army nurse during the Spanish-American War. Died in 1901 from yellow fever while serving as a volunteer in experiments to isolate the mosquito vector of the disease.

Linda Richards (1841-1930). Pioneered industrial and psychiatric nursing in the United States.

Margaret Sanger (1883-1966). Established the first U.S. birth control clinic in New York City in 1916.

Lillian Wald (1867-1940). A leader of the public health nursing movement in the United States. She founded the Visiting Nurse Service in New York City.

Today

Ann Burgess. Co-founded one of the first rape victim counseling programs, at Boston City Hospital. She was also appointed to federal Rape Prevention and Control Advisory Committee.

Elaine D. Dyer. Invented positive pressure breathing therapy.

Eunice Ernst. A leader and consultant in nurse-midwifery. She developed alternative birthing centers and hospital nurse-midwifery centers in several states.

Where nurses practice: Ten settings significant

In the United States and Canada, about 1.2 million RNs and LPNs work in hospitals. Their typical workplace: a hospital with about 350 beds. Five times as many nurses, though, work in small hospitals (fewer than 100 beds) than in large ones (more than 1,000 beds).

Outside the hospital, more nurses work in nursing homes than anywhere else—200,000 in all. The chart below shows the percentage of nurses who work in hospitals, nursing homes, and eight other settings.

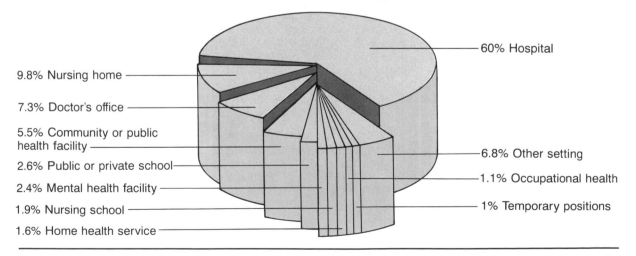

- 9.8% Nursing home
- 7.3% Doctor's office
- 5.5% Community or public health facility
- 2.6% Public or private school
- 2.4% Mental health facility
- 1.9% Nursing school
- 1.6% Home health service
- 60% Hospital
- 6.8% Other setting
- 1.1% Occupational health
- 1% Temporary positions

Where nurses work: A state-by-state roster

According to a recent study, California led the nation in employed RNs with 159,000. Wyoming, in turn, had the fewest, with 2,697. RN employment tended to be highest in the Northeast and lowest in the South.

For LPN/VNs, employment statistics are sketchier. Of 23 states responding to a recent survey, Texas led with 71,425 LPN/VNs. Once again, Wyoming trailed with just 787 LPN/VNs.

Pattern of RN employment

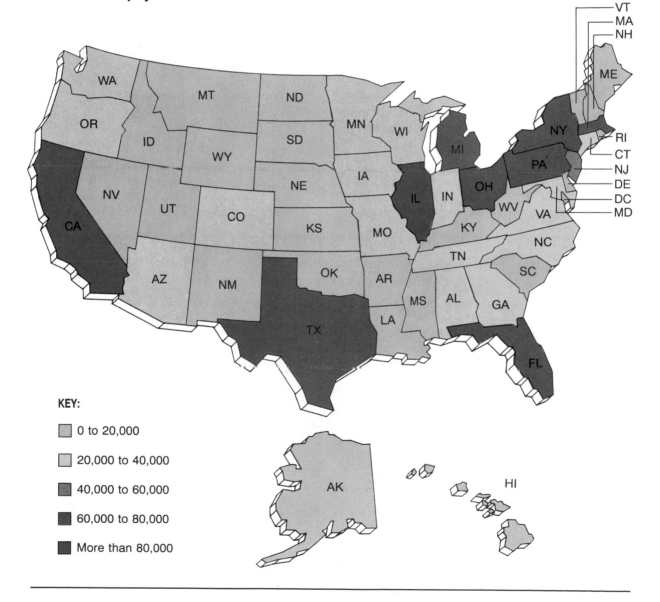

KEY:

- 0 to 20,000
- 20,000 to 40,000
- 40,000 to 60,000
- 60,000 to 80,000
- More than 80,000

Men and minorities in nursing: Slowly rising numbers

Nursing, of course, continues to be a profession chosen primarily by women. But during the 1980s, men made modest inroads. In 1980, men accounted for 2.7% of all nurses. Near the end of the decade, their share had risen to 3.6%.

Minority groups also posted slight gains in nursing during the 1980s. In 1980, minority groups made up 7.2% of all nurses. Near the end of the decade, they accounted for 7.6%, or almost 150,000 nurses. Minority group representation appears in the diagram at right.

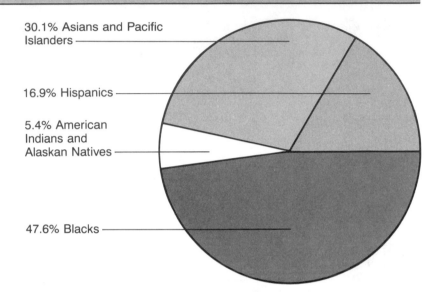

30.1% Asians and Pacific Islanders

16.9% Hispanics

5.4% American Indians and Alaskan Natives

47.6% Blacks

What nurses earn

A 1990 compensation survey conducted by the University of Texas found that nurses' salaries rose by an average of 14.7% over the previous year. The largest salary increase was realized by the nurse anesthetist, who averaged a 33% increase over the previous year.

Job title	National average	Salary range
Director of patient care services	$63,000	$54,800-79,100
Director of nursing	$55,900	$48,600-66,400
Nurse anesthetist	$53,800	$35,084-65,438
Clinical division head	$46,000	$40,800-53,700
Head nurse	$41,833	$26,655-55,568
Nurse practitioner	$40,327	$26,396-49,263
Clinical nurse specialist	$39,936	$27,119-49,921
Nursing supervisor	$39,200	$36,100-46,600
General duty/staff nurse	$32,257	$21,248-38,836
LPN	$20,900	$18,100-24,700

$65,000

$21,000

What staff RNs earn in major cities

What do RNs earn when they begin their careers? What salaries do experienced RNs command?
    You'll find the answers below for RNs in major U.S. cities. Salaries are based on a 40-hour week, and are reported as hourly and yearly figures. The consumer price index (CPI) represents Bureau of Labor Statistics estimates of price increases in each area for a recent 12-month period.

City	New RNs, $/hr	New RNs, $/yr	Top ranges RNs, $/hr	Top ranges RNs, $/yr	Increase in CPI
Atlanta	$11.00-13.93	$22,880-28,974	$15.40-20.89	$32,032-43,451	4.7%
Boston	$13.00-17.66	$27,040-36,733	$19.04-30.26	$39,603-62,941	6.6%
Chicago	$11.84-14.78	$24,627-30,742	$15.06-23.69	$31,325-49,275	5.3%
Dallas	$10.53-12.50	$21,902-26,000	$16.68-19.00	$34,694-39,520	3.5%
Denver	$10.16-12.87	$21,133-26,770	$16.23-26.94	$33,758-56,035	3.8%
Detroit	$10.76-15.05	$22,381-31,304	$13.73-21.76	$28,558-45,261	5.9%
Los Angeles	$12.27-17.22	$25,563-35,818	$16.73-27.40	$34,798-56,992	6.3%
Manhattan	$16.35-18.03	$34,000-37,500	$19.04-30.26	$39,603-62,941	5.3%
Bronx, Bklyn	$15.14-20.03	$31,491-41,662	$17.55-32.81	$36,500-68,250	N.A.
Suburban, LI	$16.11-18.27	$33,500-38,000	$18.03-25.12	$37,500-52,250	N.A.
Miami	$11.25-13.52	$23,400-28,122	$15.00-23.77	$31,200-49,422	5.6%
Milwaukee	$9.67-13.96	$20,114-29,037	$14.73-18.85	$30,638-39,208	3.0%
Minneapolis/ St. Paul	$12.94-13.35	$26,915-27,768	$19.65-20.06	$40,872-41,725	4.3%
Philadelphia	$13.50-15.81	$28,080-32,885	$17.37-22.74	$36,130-47,299	6.5%
Seattle	$12.82-13.50	$26,666-28,080	$19.53-22.48	$40,622-46,758	6.4%

Nursing shortage brings benefits boom

A survey of the National Association for Healthcare Recruitment shows that many nursing benefits have improved in response to the continuing nursing shortage. Of the nearly 400 nurse recruiters polled, 87% offered flexible staffing, up from 79% in 1988 and 63% in 1987.

Modest increases of 1% to 3% occurred in tuition reimbursement (98% of respondents reported offering this), paid time off for seminars or continuing education (85%), critical care internships (52%), clinical laddering (49%), and work-study programs for students (27%).

Evening and night differentials are almost universally offered (97%), with little regional variation. Weekend differential payment is relatively common nationwide (59%), but more common in the South (67%) than in the West (49%).

About one-third of the nurse recruiters reported that their institutions offered scholarships to student nurses. Scholarships, however, were most commonly awarded in the North Central states (46%) and least commonly awarded in the West (27%).

Nurse recruiters report little change in the percentage offering sign-on bonuses (22%) and retention bonuses (11%).

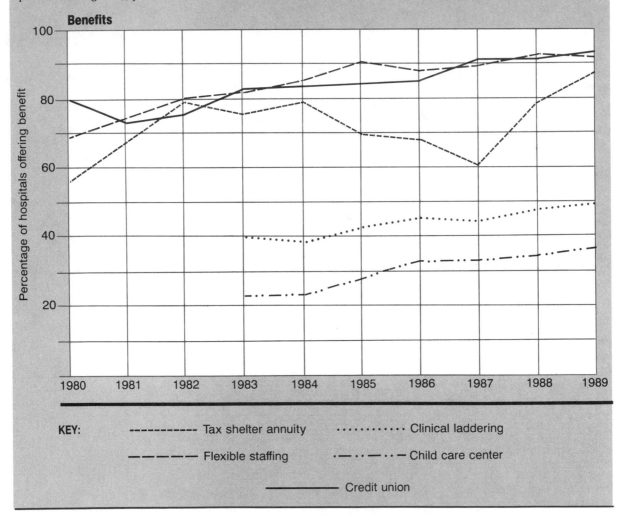

What nurses like most about their jobs

A survey conducted recently by *Nursing* magazine asked nurses if they would choose their profession if they had it to do all over again. Thirty-one percent of the 8,000 respondents said "Yes, definitely." Here are some reasons they gave.
• *The rewards of patient care.* You get satisfaction from knowing you can make a difference in a patient's life.
• *The belief that changes are possible.* You can make your job what you want it to be and can make constructive changes.
• *Job flexibility.* You can not only have a career but be a good wife and mother, too.
• *Personal enjoyment and fulfillment.* You can get paid for doing what you've always wanted to do.
• *A sense of mission.* You can be a voice for people who need help.
• *A belief in nursing's expanding opportunities.* A nursing career allows you to grow into other areas, such as a clinical specialist or management position.
• *Pride in the nursing profession.* No matter how frustrating your day is, you still feel proud of the work you do.

What nurses dislike most about their jobs

When asked about job dissatisfactions, nurses cited a lack of child care facilities as their chief complaint. Next, they cited:
• Insufficient support from nursing and hospital administration.
• Excessive paperwork.
• Low salaries.
• Lack of help when a patient needs extra care.

• Unfavorable nurse-patient ratio.
• Insufficient continuing education opportunities.
• Poor or absent in-service education.
• Inadequate fringe benefits.

What nurses read: The top five nursing journals

The first professional journal for nurses was a four-page monthly sheet, "The Nightingale," published from 1886 to 1891 in New York City. A year's subscription cost $2.

Today, the world's largest nursing journal is *Nursing91*. Roughly 500,000 nurses subscribe to it.

In second and third place are *RN* and *American Journal of Nursing*. Each of these nursing journals has about 270,000 subscribers.

Two other journals, *Heart & Lung* with about 65,000 subscribers and *Nursing Management* with about 17,000 subscribers, rank fourth and fifth.

Looking ahead: The nursing employment outlook

The Bureau of Labor Statistics projects that the health care industry will need more than 230,000 new LPNs, 430,000 nursing and psychiatric assistants, and 600,000 RNs over the next 15 years. This reflects the growth and aging of the population as well as emerging medical technologies. Unless nursing attracts more people at all levels, shortages will persist into the 21st century.

Projected new positions

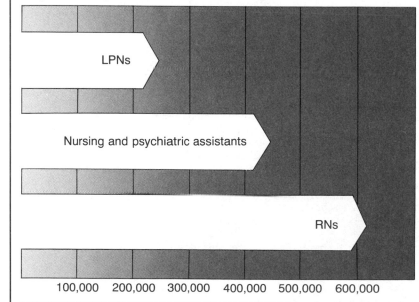

CLINICAL SKILLS

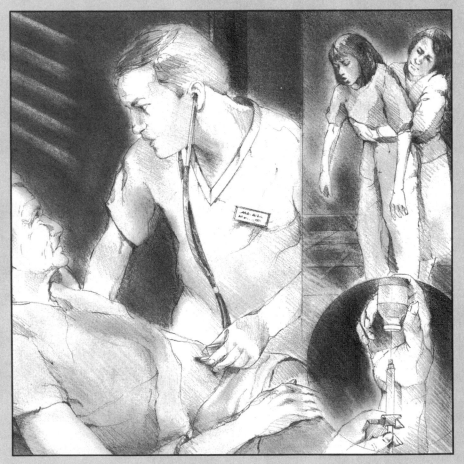

2 | Assessment: Tips and techniques

Properly conducted, the health history serves as the major subjective source of information about your patient's health status, and provides insights into actual or potential health problems. A useful guide to subsequent physical assessment, the health history organizes pertinent physiologic, psychological, psychosocial, and cultural information. It relates to the patient's current health status, and takes into account such factors as life-style, family relationships, and cultural influences.

In practice, the nursing health history differs from the medical history by its holistic focus on the patient's response to illness. Whereas the doctor takes a medical history to guide diagnosis and treatment of illness, you obtain a health history not only to provide health care, but also to assess the impact of illness on your patient and his family, to evaluate his health education needs, and to start discharge planning.

The health history includes biographical data, chief complaint, present illness, and other pertinent information.

Biographical data
Ask the patient's full name, address, telephone number, age, sex, date of birth, race, marital status, nationality, religion, occupation, and source of referral.

Chief complaint
Ask the patient to briefly describe his reasons for seeking health care.

Present illness
Have the patient describe the progression of his chief complaint or concern, with relevant symptoms. This clarifies clinical ramifications and provides a framework for nursing diagnosis.

Past illnesses
Elicit information about the patient's previous major health problems, experiences with health care system, and attitude toward it. This will give you important clues to the patient's present condition, help determine treatment plan, and may suggest prognosis. Be sure to ask about childhood and infectious diseases, immunizations, accidents, surgeries, hospitalizations, allergies, and medication use. You should note negative findings as well as positive ones.

Family history
Ask the patient to briefly describe his family's medical history. This helps identify familial patterns of some diseases, such as diabetes mellitus, cancer, migraine headaches, heart disease, and hypercholesterolemia.

Psychosocial history
Explore with the patient his place in society, relationships with others, and self-satisfaction. As appropriate, cover such topics as place of residence, economic situation, job situation, social life, coping mechanisms, and sex life.

Activities of daily living
Have the patient describe his daily activities to help determine how his personal habits affect his health. Probe the patient's diet and elimination habits, exercise and sleep patterns, recreation, and use of alcohol, tobacco, and drugs. Answers to these questions help you plan appropriate interventions and patient teaching.

Review of body systems
Questioning the patient about body systems, such as respiratory and GI, elicits subjective data about signs or symptoms of systemic disease.

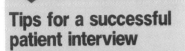

Tips for a successful patient interview

You'll get the most from a health history interview if you make the patient feel comfortable, gain his trust, and earn his respect. Effective interviewing helps the patient identify resources and improve problem-solving abilities.

Effective interviewing techniques

Offering general leads. Start with some general questions to encourage the patient to speak freely. Such questions as "What brought you here today?" or "Are you concerned about any other things?" help him talk about his most significant concerns. Give the patient a chance to do most of the talking, by allowing plenty of time for him to reflect and respond.

Restating. To help clarify what the patient means, restate the essence of his comments. If he confirms that he understood you correctly, you can confidently move on to the next question.

Reflecting (echoing). Repeating the patient's words back to him in an inquiring way gives him a chance to reconsider a response, and helps you avoid adding your personal viewpoint to what he's said.

Verbalizing the implied meaning. Stating what is implied or unspoken sometimes helps interpret a patient's statement accurately or yields additional insight into his symptoms or concerns.

Focusing the discussion. To help the patient identify significant health concerns, focus on certain discussion points. For example:
Nurse: "What do you do for a living?"
Patient: "I'm a coal miner."

Nurse: "Are you aware of any of the health hazards of your job?"

Placing a problem (or an event) in proper sequence. To identify a problem, determine its course and draw a conclusion. Define the time limits and other factors associated with the problem by asking, "What events led to this?" or "Did this happen before or after (another event)?"

Encouraging patient participation. This technique affirms the patient's individual value by encouraging him to express opinions, concerns or doubts. Ask questions like "What do you think about the stress-reduction plan we've discussed?" or "You said you couldn't get your breath; what happened after that?"

Encouraging patient evaluation. The patient will cooperate in developing a health care action plan if you encourage him to comment on implementation strategies. This technique ensures greater patient compliance, leading to a desired outcome.

Clarifying. Because many variables affect the interview and because interpretations of health behaviors or symptoms vary, you may have to clarify meanings. You can prevent misunderstandings by admitting "I'm not sure what you mean," or by clarifying a particular symptom or concern; for instance, "Was the mole as big as a dime?"

Presenting reality. When a patient makes unrealistic statements or exaggerates, presenting reality usually encourages the patient to reevaluate and modify statements. For example:
Patient: "I never get anything to eat."
Nurse: "But Mr. Johnson, when we discussed your eating patterns, you told me you had three meals a day."

Patient: "I meant I never get anything to eat that I like."

Making observations. Observing the patient helps you interpret and validate nonverbal behavior. Observations may increase the patient's situational awareness and suggest possible alternatives, or open new areas for discussion.

Giving information. Share facts and information with a patient to encourage direct involvement in health care decisions. For example, telling a mother about a vaccine for *Haemophilus influenzae* in young children can help her make informed health care choices.

Using silence. Periods of silence can help the patient reorganize thoughts and consider what to say next, while allowing you to observe. Although long silences can be awkward, avoid saying something just to reduce anxiety. Using silence effectively is a crucial skill; you can even use it to convey empathy.

Summarizing. To help clarify the information you've gathered and ease the transition from one part of the health history to the next, summarize what you've learned after you've covered each major health history component.

Techniques to avoid
Some interviewing techniques may hinder rather than help communication.

Asking why or how questions. Such questions may be perceived by the patient as a threat or challenge.

Using probing, persistent questioning. This may make the patient uncomfortable, arouse defensive feelings, and lead to a feeling of manipulation.

Employing inappropriate language. Avoid technical jargon or abstract terms not suited to the patient's developmental level, education, or background.

Giving advice. Doing so implies that you know what's best for the patient—the opposite of collaborating with him and encouraging his participation in health care decisions.

Giving false reassurance. This devalues the patient's feelings and conveys a lack of sensitivity.

Changing the subject or interrupting. By doing so, you prevent the patient from completing a thought and shift the conversation's focus.

Using clichés or stereotyped responses. Hackneyed responses make the patient feel uncomfortable or disappointed and may discourage him from expressing genuine feelings in return.

Giving excessive approval or agreement. This may make the patient feel that modifying his statements is wrong, or encourage him to tell the nurse only what he thinks she'll want to hear.

Jumping to conclusions. This invites inadequate or inaccurate information.

Using defensive responses. This implies to the patient that he has no right to his feelings and opinions concerning his treatment.

Responding too literally to the patient's statements. You run the risk of misunderstanding if a patient has difficulty stating his feelings directly. Avoid this by basing your responses on the patient's affect and the conversational context. For example, a patient might remark that he's "a real go-getter."

This could mean that the patient sees himself as ambitious and competitive, or, if stated ironically, as unsuccessful and a failure.

Asking leading questions. Doing so may force the patient to supply a socially acceptable response rather than an honest one.

Surveying activities of daily living

Recording daily activities can give you a comprehensive look at your patient's health and health history. To learn as much as possible, ask the patient questions in the following areas.

Diet and elimination
• How would you describe your appetite?
• What do you normally eat in a 24-hour period?
• What do you like and dislike eating? Is your diet restricted in any way?
• How much fluid do you drink during an average day?
• Are you allergic to any foods?
• When do you usually go to the bathroom? Has this pattern changed in any way recently?
• Do you take any foods, fluids, or drugs to help you maintain your normal bowel and urination patterns?

Exercise and sleep
• Do you have any special exercise program? What is it? How long have you been following it? How do you feel after exercising?
• How many hours do you sleep each day? When? Do you feel rested afterward?
• Do you fall asleep easily?
• Do you take any drugs or do anything special to help you fall asleep?

• What do you do when you can't sleep?
• Do you wake up during the night?
• Do you have sleepy spells during the day? When?
• Do you take naps routinely?

Recreation
• What do you do when you're not working?
• What kind of nonpaid work do you do for enjoyment?
• How much leisure time do you have?
• Are you satisfied with what you can do in your leisure time?
• Do you and your family share leisure time?
• How do your weekends differ from your weekdays?

Tobacco, alcohol, and drugs
• Do you use tobacco? What kind do you use? How much do you use each day? Each week? For how long have you used it? Have you ever tried to stop?
• Do you drink any alcoholic beverages?
• How much alcohol do you drink each day? Each week? What time of day do you drink, usually?
• What kind (beer, wine, whiskey) do you drink?
• Do you usually drink alone or with others?
• Do you drink more when you're under stress?
• Has drinking ever hampered your job performance?
• Do you or your family worry about your drinking?
• Do you feel dependent on alcohol, coffee, tea, or soft drinks? How much of these other beverages do you drink in an average day?
• Do you take any drugs not prescribed by a doctor (marijuana, sleeping pills, tranquilizers)?

Assessing body systems: What to ask your patient

When assessing your patient, ask about the function of each body system. Use the lists below as guidelines for your questions.

Overall health
• Unusual symptoms or problems
• Excessive fatigue
• Exercise intolerance
• Number of colds or other minor illnesses per year
• Unexplained episodes of fever, weakness, or night sweats
• Impaired ability to carry out daily activities

Skin, hair, and nails
• Known skin disease, such as psoriasis
• Itching
• Skin reaction to hot or cold weather
• Presence and location of scars, sores, and ulcers
• Presence and location of skin growths, such as warts, moles, masses, or tumors
• Color changes noted in any of the above lesions
• Changes in amount, texture, or character of hair
• Presence or development of baldness
• Hair care, including frequency of shampooing, permanents, or hair coloring
• Changes in nail color or texture
• Excessive nail splitting, cracking, or breaking

Head and neck
• Lumps, bumps, or scars from old injuries
• Headaches (explore symptoms)
• Recent head trauma, injury, or surgery
• Concussion or unconsciousness from head injury

• Dizzy spells or fainting
• Interference with normal range of motion
• Pain or stiffness (explore symptoms)
• Swelling or masses
• Enlarged lymph nodes or glands

Nose and sinuses
• History of frequent nosebleeds
• History of allergies
• Postnasal drip
• Frequent sneezing
• Frequent nasal drainage (note color, frequency, and amount)
• Impaired ability to smell
• Pain over the sinuses
• History of nasal trauma or fracture
• Difficulty breathing through the nostrils
• History of sinus infection and treatment received

Mouth and throat
• History of frequent sore throats—especially streptococcal (explore symptoms)
• Current or past mouth lesions, such as abscesses, ulcers, or sores
• History of oral herpes infections
• Date and results of last dental examination
• Overall description of dental health
• Use of proper dental hygiene, including fluoride toothpaste, where applicable
• Use of dentures or bridges
• Bleeding gums
• History of hoarseness
• Changes in voice quality
• Difficulty chewing or swallowing
• Changes in ability to taste

Eyes
• Date and results of last vision examination
• Date and results of last check for glaucoma (for patients over age 50 or those with a family history of glaucoma)
• History of eye infections or trauma
• Use of corrective lenses
• Itching, tearing, or discharge

(note color, amount, and time of occurrence as well as treatment received)
• Eye pain
• Spots or floaters in visual field
• History of glaucoma or cataracts
• Blurred or double vision
• Unusual sensations, such as twitching
• Light sensitivity
• Swelling around eyes or eyelids
• Visual disturbances, such as rainbows around lights, blind spots, or flashing lights
• History of retinal detachment
• History of strabismus or amblyopia

Ears
• Date and results of last hearing test
• Abnormal sensitivity to noise
• Ear pain
• Ringing or crackling in the ears
• Recent changes in hearing
• Use of hearing aids
• History of ear infection
• History of vertigo
• Feeling of fullness in the ear
• Ear care habits, including use of cotton-tipped swabs for ear wax removal
• Ear wax characteristics
• Number of ear infections per year (for pediatric patients)

Respiratory system
• History of asthma or other breathing problem (explore symptoms)
• Chronic cough (explore symptoms)
• History of hemoptysis
• Breathing problems after physical exertion
• Sputum production (note color, odor, and amount)
• Wheezing or noisy respirations
• History of pneumonia or bronchitis

Cardiovascular system
• History of chest pain, palpitations, heart murmur, or irregular pulse
• Hypertension
• Need to sit up to breathe, especially at night

- Coldness or numbness in extremities
- Color changes in fingers or toes
- Dependent edema
- Leg pain when walking, relieved by rest
- Hair loss on legs

Breasts
- Date and results of last breast examination (including mammography for women over age 40)
- Pattern of breast self-examination
- Breast pain, tenderness, or swelling (explore symptoms)
- History of nipple changes or nipple discharge (note color, odor, amount, and frequency)
- History of breast-feeding

GI system
- Indigestion or pain associated with eating (explore symptoms)
- History of ulcers or hematemesis
- Burning sensation in esophagus
- Frequent nausea and vomiting (explore symptoms)
- History of liver disease or jaundice
- History of gallbladder disease
- Abdominal swelling or ascites
- Changes in defecation pattern
- Stool characteristics
- History of diarrhea or constipation
- History of hemorrhoids
- Use of digestive aids or laxatives
- Date and results of last Hemoccult exam (for patients over age 50)

Urinary system
- Painful urination
- Urine characteristics
- Pattern of urination
- Hesitancy in starting urine stream
- Changes in urine stream
- History of renal calculi or flank pain
- Hematuria
- History of decreased or excessive urine output
- Dribbling, incontinence, or stress incontinence
- Frequent urination at night
- Toilet training problems or bed-wetting (for children)

- History of bladder or kidney infections
- History of urinary tract infections

Female reproductive system
- Menstrual history, including age of onset, duration, and amount of flow
- Date of last menstrual period
- Painful menstruation
- History of menorrhagia, metrorrhagia, or amenorrhea
- Date and results of last Pap smear
- Obstetrical history (for women of childbearing age), including number of pregnancies, miscarriages, abortions, live births, and stillbirths
- Sexual satisfaction
- History of painful intercourse
- Contraceptive practices
- History of sexually transmitted disease
- Knowledge of how to prevent sexually transmitted disease, including acquired immunodeficiency syndrome (AIDS)
- Problems with infertility

Male reproductive system
- Penile or scrotal lesions
- Prostate problems
- Pattern of testicular self-examination
- Sexual satisfaction
- History of venereal disease
- Contraceptive practices
- Knowledge of how to prevent sexually transmitted disease, including AIDS
- Concerns about impotence or sterility

Nervous system
- History of fainting or loss of consciousness
- History of seizures or use of anticonvulsant medication
- History of cognitive disturbances, including recent or remote memory loss, hallucinations, disorientation, speech and language dysfunction, or inability to concentrate
- History of sensory disturbances, including tingling, numbness, and sensory loss

- History of motor problems, including problems with gait, balance, coordination, tremor, spasm, or paralysis
- Interference by cognitive, sensory, or motor symptoms with activies of daily living (ADLs)

Musculoskeletal system
- History of fractures
- Muscle cramping, twitching, pain, or weakness (explore symptoms)
- Limitations on walking, running, or participation in sports
- Joint swelling, redness, or pain
- Joint deformity
- Joint stiffness, including time and duration
- Noise with joint movement
- Spinal deformity
- Chronic back pain (explore symptoms)
- Interference with ADLs

Immune and hematologic systems
- History of anemia, bleeding tendencies, easy bruising or fatigue, or low platelet count
- History of blood transfusion
- History of allergies, including eczema, hives, and itching
- Chronic clear nasal discharge
- Frequent sneezing
- Conjunctivitis
- Interference of allergies with ADLs
- Usual method for treating allergic symptoms
- History of frequent unexplained systemic infections
- Unexplained gland swelling

Endocrine system
- History of endocrine disease, such as thyroid problems, adrenal problems, or diabetes
- Unexplained changes in height or weight
- Increased appetite, thirst, or urinary output
- Heat or cold intolerance
- History of goiter
- Unexplained weakness
- Previous hormone therapy
- Changes in hair distribution or skin pigmentation

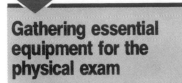

Gathering essential equipment for the physical exam

Here's a list of equipment you'll need to perform a basic physical examination. To help the examination run smoothly, gather all the equipment beforehand.
• Thermometer
• Scale for measuring height and weight

• Wristwatch (with sweep second-hand)
• Stethoscope (with diaphragm and bell)
• Sphygmomanometer and blood pressure cuff
• Ophthalmoscope
• Otoscope (with assorted specula)
• Nasoscope, nasal speculum, or nasal tip for otoscope
• Eye chart (Snellen) and newspaper clipping for close reading assessment
• Opaque card or eye cover
• Penlight or flashlight

• 2″ x 2″ and 4″ x 4″ sterile gauze pads and cotton swabs
• Tuning forks (512 to 1,024 cycles/second to test hearing acuity)
• Tongue depressors
• Laryngeal mirror
• Examination gloves and water-soluble lubricant
• Vaginal specula and slides
• Reflex or percussion hammer
• Safety pin
• Cloth tape measure (indicating centimeter measurements)
• Blood culture test slides
• Urine specimen container

Preparing for the physical exam: Positioning and draping the patient

Requirements for patient positioning and draping vary according to which body systems or regions you plan to examine. These illustrations show the primary positions and draping you'll use.

To examine the patient's head, neck, and anterior and posterior thorax and lungs, have him sit on the edge of the examining table.

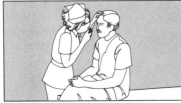

To examine the cardiovascular system and the abdomen, place the patient in the supine position.

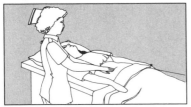

Ensure privacy for a female patient by placing a towel over her breasts and upper thorax. Pull down the sheet only as far as, but not exposing, her symphysis pubis.

To examine the female patient's breasts, have her sit down.

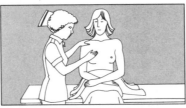

For the second part of the exam, ask her to lie down. Place a small pillow beneath her shoulder on the side being examined, to spread her breast evenly.

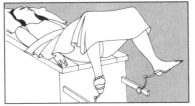

To examine the reproductive system, place her in the lithotomy position. Drape a sheet over her chest, knees, and legs. Her buttocks should border the table's edge and her feet should be in stirrups.

To perform a rectal examination, position the male patient so that he's leaning across the table.

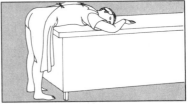

If he can't stand upright, have him lie on his left side, with his right hip and knee slightly flexed and his buttocks close to the table's edge.

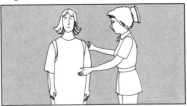

To perform some parts of the neurologic and musculoskeletal examinations, have the patient stand, when feasible, or sit.

Assessing body systems: What to examine

Physical examination findings help you identify and explore the patient's chief complaint, arrive at a nursing diagnosis, and develop a sound nursing care plan. Read over this list to outline what you need to cover during the physical examination.

General
• Identify the patient's sex and race.

Observe overall appearance
• Apparent state of health, mental status, and signs of distress
• Appearance in relation to chronologic age
• Facial expression, mood, and speech
• Skin color
• Body development and apparent nutritional state
• Dress and personal hygiene
• Stature, posture, motor activity, and gait

Monitor vital signs
• Temperature (oral, rectal, or axillary)
• Pulse rate
• Respiratory rate
• Blood pressure

Measure height and weight

Identify accessory equipment
• I.V. line
• Nasogastric or chest tubes
• Oxygen, ventilator, or cardiac monitor

Skin
• Examine facial skin for abnormal color, lesions, periorbital edema, masses, or abnormal hair growth (in females).
• Assess quantity, distribution, texture, and color of hair.

• Inspect scalp for scaliness, lumps, lesions, or parasites.
• Check color, texture, turgor.

Eyes
• Observe conjugate gaze.
• Inspect for redness, jaundice, or discharge.
• Test for blurring, diplopia, field cuts, photophobia, or decreased vision (R/L blindness, R/L glasses, R/L contact lens).

Test pupillary reaction
• Pupil size
• Reaction to light
• Consensual movement

Ears
• Inspect for size, shape, and any deformities, lumps, or skin lesions.
• Assess for drainage, pain on manipulation, and tinnitus.
• Test for hearing loss.

Respiratory system
• Assess rate, rhythm, and depth of respirations, and identify abnormal breathing patterns.

Look for signs of respiratory distress
• Lips and nail beds, noting color
• Fingers, noting any clubbing

Inspect nasal airway
• Deformity, asymmetry, or inflammation
• Drainage or nosebleed
• Sneezing or obstruction

Palpate neck, checking for asymmetry and enlargement
• Lymph nodes (preauricular, posterior auricular, occipital, tonsillar, submaxillary, submental, anterior cervical, supraclavicular, and infraclavicular)
• Trachea
• Thyroid gland

Inspect thorax
• Check posterior and anterior thorax for configuration and skin integrity

Palpate, percuss, and auscultate lung fields
• Note tenderness, thoracic expansion, tactile fremitus, crepitus, and diaphragmatic excursion

Cardiovascular system

Inspect, palpate, and auscultate thorax
• Precordium, noting any heave or lift
• Jugular vein, noting distention
• Apical impulse, noting any sternal lift or thrills
• Heart sounds, noting rate, rhythm, and any abnormalities
Auscultate at apical impulse and at mitral, tricuspid, aortic, and pulmonic areas.

Examine peripheral vessels
• *Carotid vessels:* Palpate each carotid artery, noting rate, quality, and equality of pulses, as well as presence of thrills. Auscultate over carotid arteries for bruits or referred cardiac murmurs.
• *Arms and hands:* Inspect skin color, noting any lesions or swelling. Also inspect nail color and condition, noting any clubbing. Check skin temperature, texture, and turgor. Take radial and brachial pulses, noting rate, quality, and equality.
• *Legs and feet:* Inspect skin color, noting lesions, edema, or varicosities. Note pattern of hair distribution and inspect nail color and condition. Check skin temperature, texture, and turgor. Also check the femoral, popliteal, posterior tibial, and dorsalis pedis pulses, noting rate, quality, and equality. Next, test for Homans' sign, a possible indication of phlebitis.

GI system
• Examine lips for color and moisture, noting lumps, ulcers, and cracking.

Examine oral cavity
• Tongue and papillae for color and smoothness

• Buccal mucosa for color and pigmentation, noting any ulcers or nodules
• Gums for condition and color, noting any retraction, bleeding, or inflammation
• Teeth for position, shape, and sturdiness, noting any caries
• Hard and soft palates for color and shape
• U-shaped area under tongue for color and condition, noting any white areas, nodules, or ulcerations
• Salivation, noting excessiveness

Inspect, auscultate, percuss, and palpate abdomen
• Skin for color, color symmetry, hair distribution, and presence of lesions, surgical scars, rashes, striae, and dilated vessels
• Umbilicus for color and contour, noting any herniation and drainage
• Abdominal contour, noting whether it's flat, scaphoid, rounded, or distended (protuberant)
• Abdominal movements caused by respiration, peristalsis, or arterial pulsation
• Bowel sounds in each quadrant (beginning in lower left quadrant and working clockwise)
• Presence of vascular bruits
• Presence of solid, fluid, or gas (auscultate from thorax down, following right and left midclavicular lines)
• Abdomen, noting firmness or tenderness and the presence of any large masses
• Stool for color and consistency; test for occult blood
• Aspirate, if nasogastric tube is in place, for color, odor, consistency, and volume

Urinary system
• Check for urinary drainage tubes (Foley, cystostomy, or urethral catheter).
• Examine urine color, concentration, odor, and quantity.

Reproductive system

Inspect and palpate male genitalia
• Penis, urethral opening, and scrotum, noting size, as well as any lesions, edema, or swelling
• Scrotal contents for any masses or tumors
• External inguinal ring for any hernias or enlarged nodes

Examine female genitalia
• Urethral, vaginal, and rectal openings, noting any lesions, varicosities, hernias, tumor masses, edema, or swelling; examine with vaginal speculum; note color, consistency, and odor of discharge; take smears and cultures
• Inguinal nodes, noting enlargement

Inspect and palpate breasts
• Breasts for size, shape, symmetry, and position, noting any localized redness, inflammation, skin retraction, and dimpling
• Nipples, noting any pigment change, erosions, crusting, scaling, discharge, edema, or inversion
• Nipple secretion
• Axillary and supraclavicular regions, noting any retractions, bulging, discoloration, rashes, and edema
• Breasts and lymph nodes in axillary and supraclavicular regions; palpate systematically, in clockwise fashion, from nipple to periphery

Nervous system

Assess level of consciousness
• Use the Glasgow coma scale or other appropriate tests
• Eye response
• Verbal response
• Motor response

Test reflexes
• Gag reflex
• Swallowing reflex
• Corneal reflex
• Neural reflexes
• Sensory reflexes

Musculoskeletal system

Examine head and neck
• Skull for symmetry, size, and contour
• Head and neck for involuntary movements
• Neck for range of motion

Examine spine
• Contour, position, motion, and tenderness

Assess upper extremity function and strength
• Note contractures, cast, or traction
• Inspect arms and hands for muscle mass and skeletal configuration
• Palpate joints for any swelling, stiffness, tenderness, or bony enlargement
• Assess motor strength of both small and large muscle groups
• Test joint range of motion by passively flexing and extending elbow, wrist, and metacarpal joints

Assess lower extremity function and strength
• Note contractures, cast, or traction
• Inspect legs and feet for muscle mass and skeletal configuration
• Palpate joints for any swelling, stiffness, sponginess, tenderness, or bony enlargement
• Assess motor strength of both small and large muscle groups
• Test joint range of motion by passively flexing and extending knee, ankle, and metatarsal joints

Performing the physical exam: Four basic techniques

To perform the physical exam, you'll use four basic techniques: inspection, palpation, percussion, and auscultation. Here's a brief review of each.

Inspection

Critical observation or inspection is the most commonly used assessment technique. Unlike palpation, percussion, and auscultation, inspection isn't a single, self-contained assessment step. Instead, it begins on first contact with the patient and continues throughout the health history interview, general survey, vital sign measurement, and detailed body systems assessment. Through each of these phases, your inspection findings enhance and refine the knowledge base.

Inspection can be direct or indirect. During direct inspection, rely totally on sight, hearing, and smell. During indirect inspection, you'll use equipment, such as a nasal or vaginal speculum or an ophthalmoscope, to expose internal tissues or to enhance the view of a specific body area.

To inspect a specific body area, first make sure the area is sufficiently exposed and adequately lit. Then, survey the entire area, noting key landmarks and checking the overall condition. Next, focus on specifics—color, shape, texture, size, and movement.

While inspecting the patient, always maintain objectivity: Don't be misled by preconceived ideas and expectations. Stay alert for unusual and unexpected findings as well as for predictable ones.

Palpation

During palpation, you'll touch the patient's body to feel pulsations and vibrations, to locate body structures (particularly in the ab-

---

Using the hands in palpation

To enhance palpation technique, you can take advantage of the tactile sensitivity specific to each hand region. The tips and pads of the fingers can best distinguish texture and shape. The back, or dorsal surface, of the hand can best feel for warmth. The ulnar surface, or ball, of the hand (at the base of the fingers on the palmar side) can best feel thrills (fine vibrations over the precordium) and fremitus (tremulous vibrations over the chest wall) as well as vocal vibrations through the chest wall. The thumb and index finger can best assess hair texture, grasp tissues, and feel for lymph node enlargement. The flattened finger pads can best palpate tender tissues, feel for crepitus (crackling) at joints, and lightly probe the abdomen. A single finger or nail tip can best stroke the skin when attempting to elicit the cremasteric (testicular retraction) or abdominal reflexes in the neurologic examination. The whole hand can best test handgrip strength.

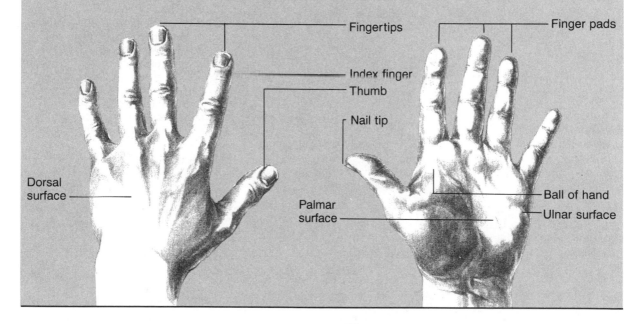

Palpation techniques

Light palpation involves using the tips and pads of the fingers to apply light pressure to the skin surface. *Ballottement,* a light palpation variation, involves gentle, repetitive bouncing of tissues against the hand (think of bouncing a small ball gently). *Deep palpation* requires use of both hands and heavier pressure.

Light palpation
To perform light palpation, press gently on the skin, indenting it to ½" to ¾" (1 to 2 cm). Use the lightest touch possible; too much pressure blunts your sensitivity. Close your eyes to concentrate on what your fingers are feeling.

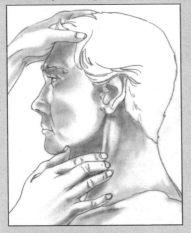

Deep palpation (bimanual palpation)
To perform deep palpation, increase your fingertip pressure, indenting the skin about 1½" (4 cm). Place your other hand on top of the palpating hand to control and guide your movements. To perform a variation of deep palpation that allows pinpointing an inflamed area, press firmly with one hand, then lift your hand away quickly. If the patient reports increased pain as you release pressure, you've identified rebound tenderness. (Suspect peritonitis if you elicit rebound tenderness when examining the abdomen.)

Use both hands (bimanual palpation) to trap a deep, underlying, hard-to-palpate organ (such as the kidney or spleen) or to fix or stabilize an organ (such as the uterus) with one hand and palpate it with the other.

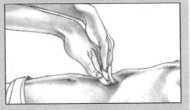

Light ballottement
To perform light ballottement, apply light, rapid pressure from quadrant to quadrant of the patient's abdomen. Keep your hand on the skin surface to detect any tissue rebound.

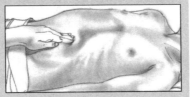

Deep ballottement
To perform deep ballottement, apply abrupt, deep pressure; then release the pressure, but maintain fingertip contact with the skin.

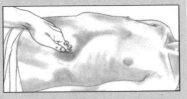

domen), and to assess such characteristics as size, texture, warmth, mobility, and tenderness. Palpation allows detection of a pulse, muscle rigidity, enlarged lymph nodes, dry skin or hair, organ tenderness or breast lumps, and measurement of the chest rising and falling with each respiration.

Usually, palpation follows inspection as the second technique in physical assessment. For example, if a rash is present on inspection, you can determine through palpation if the rash has a raised surface or feels tender or warm. However, during an abdominal or urinary system assessment, palpation should come at the end of the examination to avoid causing patient discomfort and stimulating peristalsis.

Correct palpation requires a highly developed sense of touch. Learn to use the various parts of the fingers and hands for different purposes; also expect to learn several palpation techniques. (For more information, see *Using the hands in palpation,* page 19, and *Palpation techniques.*)

A patient may react to palpation with anxiety, embarrassment, or discomfort. This, in turn, can lead to muscle tension or guarding, possibly interfering with palpation and causing misleading results. To put the patient at ease and thus enhance the accuracy of palpation findings, follow these simple guidelines:
• Warm your hands before beginning.
• Explain what you will do and why, and describe what the patient can expect, especially in sensitive areas.
• Encourage the patient to relax by taking several deep breaths, concentrating on inhaling and exhaling.
• Stop palpating immediately if the patient complains of pain.

Percussion
During percussion, you'll use

quick, sharp tapping of your fingers or hands against body surfaces (usually the chest and abdomen) to produce sounds, detect tenderness, or assess reflexes. Percussing for sound – the most common percussion goal – helps locate organ borders, identify organ shape and position, and determine if an organ is solid or filled with fluid or gas.

Three basic percussion methods include indirect (mediate), direct (immediate), and blunt (fist) percussion. In indirect percussion, the most common method, the examiner taps one finger against an object – usually the middle finger of the other hand – held against the skin surface. Although indirect percussion commonly produces clearer, crisper sounds than direct and blunt percussion, this technique requires practice to achieve good sound quality. (For more information, see *Percussion techniques*.)

Percussing for sound – perhaps the hardest assessment method to master – requires a skilled touch and an ear trained to detect slight sound variations. Organs and tissues produce sounds of varying loudness, pitch, and duration, depending upon their density. For instance, air-filled cavities, such as the lungs, produce markedly different sounds from those produced by the liver and other dense tissues.

When percussing for sound, use quick, light blows to create vibrations that penetrate about 1½″ to 2″ (4 to 5 cm) under the skin surface. The returning sounds reflect the contents of the percussed body cavity.

Normal percussion sounds over the chest and abdomen include:
• *resonance* – the long, low, hollow sound heard over an intercostal space lying above healthy lung tissue
• *tympany* – the loud, high-pitched, drumlike sound heard over a gastric air bubble or gas-filled bowel

Percussion techniques

To assess patients completely, you need to be able to perform these three percussion techniques: indirect, direct, and blunt.

Indirect percussion
To perform indirect percussion, use the second finger of your nondominant hand as the pleximeter (the mediating device used to receive the taps) and the middle finger of your dominant hand as the plexor (the device used to tap the pleximeter). Place the pleximeter finger firmly against a body surface, such as the upper back. With your wrist flexed loosely, use the tip of your plexor finger to deliver a crisp blow just beneath the distal joint of the pleximeter. Be sure to hold the plexor perpendicular to the pleximeter. Tap lightly and quickly, removing the plexor as soon as you have delivered each blow.

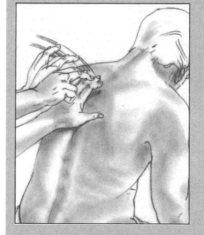

Direct percussion
To perform direct percussion, tap your hand or fingertip directly against the body surface. This method helps assess an

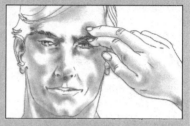

adult's sinuses for tenderness or elicit sounds in a child's thorax.

Blunt percussion
To perform blunt percussion, strike the ulnar surface of your fist against the body surface. Alternatively, use both hands by placing the palm of one hand over the area to be percussed, then making a fist with the other hand and using it to strike the back of the first hand.

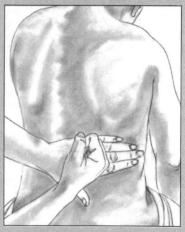

Both techniques aim to elicit tenderness – *not* to create a sound – over such organs as the kidneys, gallbladder or liver. (Another blunt percussion method, used in the neurologic exam, involves tapping a rubber-tipped reflex hammer against a tendon to create a reflexive muscle contraction.)

Using stethoscope heads effectively

To properly assess high-frequency sounds, such as breath sounds and first and second heart sounds, use the diaphragm side of the stethoscope's chest piece. Make sure the entire surface of the diaphragm is positioned firmly on your patient's skin. If there is much hair on the chest, reduce extraneous noise and improve diaphragm contact by applying water or water-soluble jelly to your patient's chest before auscultating.

To assess low-frequency sounds, such as heart murmurs and third and fourth heart sounds, lightly place the stethoscope's bell on the appropriate skin area. Don't exert pressure. If you do, your patient's chest will act as a diaphragm, and you'll miss low-frequency sounds. If your patient is extremely thin or emaciated, use a stethoscope with a pediatric chestpiece.

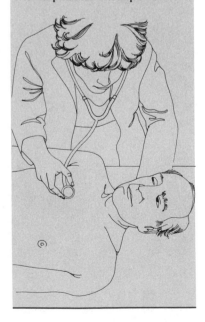

• *dullness* — the soft, high-pitched, thudding sound normally heard over more solid organs, such as the liver and heart. (*Note:* Dullness heard in a normally resonant or tympanic area warrants further investigation.)

Abnormal percussion sounds may be heard over body organs. Hyperresonance — a long, loud, low-pitched sound — is a classic sign of lung hyperinflation, as in emphysema. Flatness — similar to dullness but shorter in duration and softer in intensity — may also be heard over pleural fluid accumulation or pleural thickening.

When percussing, move from resonant areas to dull areas to accentuate any sound differences, as in these examples: to identify the lower border of liver dullness, begin percussing over the tympanic abdominal regions, then move up toward the dull liver area. To identify the upper border of liver dullness, begin over the lungs and percuss downward. Compare from side to side, tapping a few times in each area. Except for areas over such organs as the liver, gallbladder, and spleen, percussion findings should be symmetrical.

To enhance percussion technique and improve results, follow these guidelines:
• Keep your fingernails short, and warm your hands before starting.
• Have the patient void before you begin; otherwise, you could mistake a full bladder for a mass or could cause him discomfort.
• Make sure the examination room or area is quiet and distraction-free.
• Remove any jewelry or other items that could clatter and interfere with the ability to hear returning sounds.
• Before performing blunt percussion, briefly explain to the patient what you will do and why. This technique may startle and upset an unprepared client.
• In an obese patient, expect percussion sounds to be muffled by a thick subcutaneous fat layer. To help overcome this problem, use the lateral aspect of the thumb as the pleximeter and tap sharply on the last thumb joint with your plexor finger.

Auscultation
During auscultation, you'll listen for sounds produced by the heart, lungs, vessels, stomach, and intestines. Most sounds result from air or fluid movement, such as the rush of air through respiratory pathways, the turbulent flow of blood through vessels, or the movement of gas (agitated by peristalsis) through the bowels.

Usually, you perform auscultation after the other assessment techniques. When examining the abdomen, however, always auscultate second — *after* inspecting but *before* percussing and palpating. That way, bowel sounds are heard before palpation disrupts them.

You can hear body sounds, such as the voice, loud wheezing, or stomach growls, fairly easily, but you'll need a stethoscope to hear softer ones. An appropriate procedure is this one: use a high-quality, properly fitting stethoscope, provide a quiet environment, and make sure that the body area to be auscultated is sufficiently exposed. Remember that a gown or bed linens can interfere with sound transmission. Instruct the patient to remain quiet and still. Before starting, warm the stethoscope head (diaphragm and bell) in your hand; otherwise, the cold metal may make the patient shiver, possibly producing unwanted sounds. Position the diaphragm or bell over the appropriate area. Focusing your attention, listen intently to individual sounds and try to identify their characteristics. Determine the intensity, pitch, and duration of each sound and check the frequency of recurring sounds. (See *Using stethoscope heads effectively*.)

Normal body temperature fluctuations: What causes them?

When you check your patient's body temperature, keep in mind the factors listed below that can affect the reading.

Factor	Temperature rise	Temperature fall
Time of day	99.5° F (37.5° C) between 4 and 8 p.m., with increased activity	97.7° F (36.5° C) between 4 and 6 a.m., with decreased activity
Age	100° F (37.8° C) in infants and 98.9° F (37.2° C) in children because of increased growth, metabolic rate, and activity	95° F (35° C) in the elderly because of slower metabolic rate and decreased muscular activity
Exercise	100° F (37.8° C) with exertion; temperature returns to normal within 30 minutes	97.7° F (36.5° C) during sleep because of decreased metabolic rate and muscular activity, and increased heat loss
Menstrual cycle	99.6° F (37.6° C) during ovulation because of increased progesterone level	97.7° F (36.5° C.) in early morning just before onset of menstruation
Pregnancy	100.4° F (38° C) during first 4 months	97° F (36° C) during last 5 months

How to identify pulse patterns

Type of pulse rate and rhythm	Causes and incidence
Normal pulse rate 60 to 80 beats/minute; in newborns, 120 to 140 beats/minute	• Varies with such factors as age, physical activity, and sex (men usually have lower pulse rates than women)
Tachycardia Pulse rate above 100 beats/minute	• Accompanies stimulation of the sympathetic nervous system by emotional stress — anger, fear, anxiety — or certain drugs, such as caffeine • May result from exercise and conditions, such as congestive heart failure, anemia, and fever (which increases oxygen requirements and therefore pulse rate)
Bradycardia Pulse rate below 60 beats/minute	• Accompanies stimulation of the parasympathetic nervous system by drugs — especially digitalis — and such conditions as cerebral hemorrhage and heart block • May also be present in fit athletes
Irregular pulse Uneven time intervals between beats (for example, periods of regular rhythm interrupted by pauses or premature beats)	• *Premature beats:* occasional — may occur normally; frequent — may indicate cardiac irritability, hypoxia, digitalis overdose, potassium imbalance, or sometimes more serious dysrhythmias

How to identify respiratory patterns

Respiratory pattern		Possible causes
Eupnea Normal rate and rhythm. Rate varies with age: adult, usually 15 to 17 breaths/min; teenagers, usually 12 to 20 breaths/min; ages 2 to 12, usually 20 to 30 breaths/min; infants, usually 30 to 50 breaths/min. Two or three deep breaths normally occur each minute.		• Normal respiration
Tachypnea Rapid respirations. Rate rises with body temperature—about 4 breaths/min for every degree Fahrenheit above normal.		• Fever, as the body tries to rid itself of excess heat • Pneumonia, compensatory respiratory alkalosis, respiratory insufficiency, lesions of the lateral medulla oblongata, and salicylate poisoning
Bradypnea Slow, regular respirations		• Conditions affecting the respiratory center in the lateral medulla oblongata: tumors, metabolic disorders, respiratory decompensation; use of opiates and alcohol • Normal pattern during sleep
Hyperpnea Deep respirations, normal rate		• Strenuous exercise
Kussmaul's Fast (over 20 breaths/min), deep (resembling sighs), labored respirations without pause		• Renal failure or metabolic acidosis, particularly diabetic ketoacidosis
Apneustic Prolonged, gasping inspiration, followed by extremely short, inefficient expiration		• Lesions of the lateral medulla oblongata
Biot's Fast, deep respirations marked by abrupt pauses. Each breath has the same depth.		• Spinal meningitis or other central nervous system condition
Cheyne-Stokes Fast, deep respirations, punctuated by a period of apnea. Respirations increase and decrease for 30 to 170 seconds and stop for 20 to 60 seconds.		• Increased intracranial pressure, severe congestive heart failure, renal failure, meningitis, drug overdose, cerebral anoxia
Apnea Absence of breathing may be periodic		• Mechanical airway obstruction • Conditions affecting the brain's respiratory center

How age affects vital signs

Normal vital sign ranges vary with age, as this chart shows.

Age	Temperature Fahrenheit	Temperature Centigrade	Pulse rate	Respiratory rate	Blood pressure
Newborn	98.6 to 99.8	37 to 37.7	70 to 190	30 to 80	Systolic: 50 to 52 Diastolic: 25 to 30
3 years	98.5 to 99.5	36.9 to 37.5	80 to 125	20 to 30	Systolic: 78 to 114 Diastolic: 46 to 78
10 years	97.5 to 98.6	36.3 to 37	70 to 110	16 to 22	Systolic: 90 to 132 Diastolic: 56 to 86
16 years	97.6 to 98.8	36.4 to 37.1	55 to 100	15 to 20	Systolic: 104 to 108 Diastolic: 60 to 92
Adult	96.8 to 99.5	36 to 37.5	60 to 100	12 to 20	Systolic: 95 to 140 Diastolic: 60 to 90
Older adult	96.5 to 97.5	35.9 to 36.3	60 to 100	15 to 25	Systolic: 140 to 160 Diastolic: 70 to 90

Auscultating breath sounds

Breath sounds are produced by air moving through the tracheobronchoalveolar system. Normal breath sounds are labeled *bronchial*, *bronchovesicular*, and *vesicular*. They're described according to location, ratio of inspiration to expiration, intensity, and pitch.

Abnormal (adventitious) breath sounds occur when air passes either through narrowed airways or through moisture, or when the membranes lining the chest cavity and the lungs become inflamed. These sounds include *crackles, rhonchi, wheezes,* and *pleural friction rub.* You may hear them superimposed over normal breath sounds.

Use this chart as a guide to assess both normal and abnormal breath sounds. Document your findings.

Type	Location	Description
Normal sounds		
Bronchial	Over trachea	Loud, high-pitched, and hollow, harsh, or coarse
Bronchovesicular	Anteriorly, near the mainstem bronchi in the first and second intercostal spaces; posteriorly, between the scapulae	Soft, breezy, and pitched about two notes lower than bronchial sounds
Vesicular	In most of the lungs' peripheral parts (can't be heard over the presternum or the scapulae)	Soft, swishy, breezy, and about two notes lower than bronchovesicular sounds

(continued)

Auscultating breath sounds (continued)

Type	Location	Description
Abnormal sounds		
Crackles	Anywhere. Heard in lung bases first with pulmonary edema, usually during inspiratory phase	Air passing through moisture, especially in the small airways and alveoli Light crackling, popping, nonmusical; can be further classified by pitch: high, medium, or low
Rhonchi	In larger airways, usually during expiratory phase	Fluid or secretions in the large airways or narrowing of large airways Coarse rattling, usually louder and lower pitched than rales; can be described as sonorous, bubbling, moaning, musical, sibilant, and rumbly
Wheezes	May occur during inspiration or expiration	Narrowed airways Creaking, groaning; always high-pitched, musical squeaks
Pleural friction rub	Anterolateral lung field, on both inspiration and expiration (with the patient in an upright position)	Inflamed parietal and visceral pleural linings rubbing together Superficial squeaking or grating

▼

Auscultating bowel sounds

Auscultate bowel sounds as part of a baseline assessment and whenever the patient develops acute abdominal pain, distention, or rigidity.

Switch in sequence
Normally, you'd percuss and palpate before auscultating, but in this case, percussing and palpating can stimulate intestinal activity and produce misleading sounds on auscultation.

Stethoscope diaphragm first
After inspecting your patient's ab-

domen, auscultate it (see *Locating abdominal sounds*). Use the diaphragm of the stethoscope first. Exerting only light pressure, listen for bowel sounds in all quadrants. Normally, air and fluid movement through the bowel create irregular bubbling or soft, gurgling noises about every 5 to 15 seconds. If you don't hear bowel sounds immediately, listen for at least 5 minutes to confirm the absence of bowel sounds, which may indicate paralytic ileus or peritonitis. Report this finding. Conversely, rapid, high-pitched, tinkling bowel sounds or loud, gurgling noises with visible peristaltic waves commonly accompany diarrhea or gastroenteritis and indicate a hyperactive bowel. These findings may also serve as an early signal of intestinal obstruction.

Stethoscope bell next
Use the bell of the stethoscope to listen to vascular sounds. Place the bell lightly over the midline to check for *bruits,* blowing sounds that seem to elongate the pulsation normally heard over a vessel.

Check also for bruits over the renal vessels, the result of dilatation or constriction. If you note any bruits in the abdominal aorta, assess arterial perfusion in the patient's legs. Absence of pulses indicates decreased blood flow to the legs; notify the doctor promptly. Meanwhile, keep your patient quiet and *don't* palpate his abdomen, because these symptoms may reflect a dissecting aneurysm, which is a surgical emergency. The same symptoms may indicate arteriosclerosis obliterans, a chronic condition.

You can also use the bell of the stethoscope to detect other abnormal abdominal sounds. If you hear a *venous hum* — a hum of medium tone created by blood flow in a large, engorged, vascular organ such as the liver or spleen — check for other signs of fluid overload. A *friction rub,* which sounds like two pieces of sandpaper being rubbed together, may originate in an inflamed spleen or a neoplastic liver.

Edema's telltale sign

While auscultating the patient's abdomen, assess the abdominal surface for edema by watching the imprint left by the bell of the stethoscope. If the circular imprint of a *lightly* placed stethoscope remains visible on the skin, fluid has probably accumulated within the abdominal wall. This often results from a nutritional deficiency, such as low circulating protein levels.

Locating abdominal sounds

In abdominal auscultation, you'll find you can hear some sounds better in certain areas than in others. This illustration shows the best place to listen for each sound.

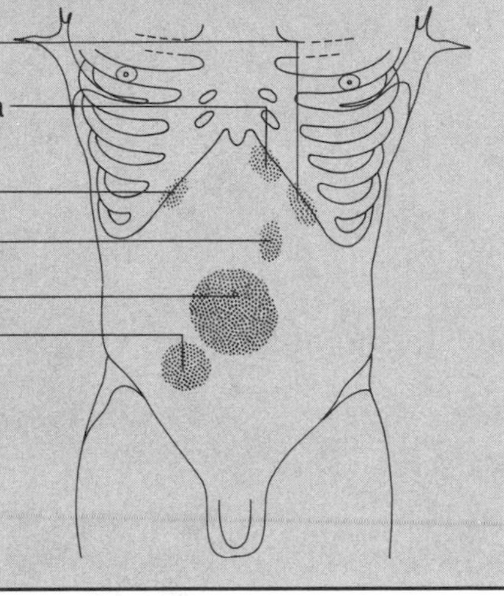

Splenic friction rub

Bruit of pancreatic carcinoma

Hepatic rubs or hum

Abdominal aorta bruits

Renal artery bruit

Peristaltic sounds

What abnormal heart sounds signify

Auscultating and interpreting heart murmurs, clicks, and rubs may sound like a formidable challenge. But it's one you can meet as along as you're familiar with the two normal heart sounds and the basic dynamics of systole and diastole.

Condition	Cause	Findings on auscultation	Other assessment findings	Signs and symptoms
Aortic stenosis	• Congenital bicuspid valve • Rheumatic heart disease • Calcification	*Moderate cases* — • Aortic ejection sound • Systolic ejection murmur • Normal split S_1 • Normal split S_2 *Severe cases* — • M_1 (mitral component of S_1) closure muffled • Ejection sound absent • A_2 (aortic component of S_2) absent, delayed, or paradoxically split • Systolic ejection murmur • S_4	• Narrow pulse pressure • Weak, slow-rising arterial pulses • Pulsus alternans • Forceful, sustained apical impulse • Systolic thrill (at right heart base, supraclavicular notch, or carotids)	• Dyspnea, orthopnea, paroxysmal nocturnal dyspnea (PND) • Nonproductive cough (with congestive heart failure [CHF]) • Pressing substernal pain • Syncope on exertion

(continued)

What abnormal heart sounds signify (continued)

Condition	Cause	Findings on auscultation	Other assessment findings	Signs and symptoms
Pulmonic stenosis	• Congenital (10% of patients) • Calcification	• Pulmonic ejection sound • Systolic ejection murmur • P_2 (pulmonic component of S_2) delayed and soft, producing wide, split S_2	*Moderate cases—* • Normal arterial pulse • Normal blood pressure or narrow pulse pressure • Sustained impulse at left sternal border (LSB) *Severe cases—* • Moon face • Cyanosis • Increased A wave in jugular venous pulse (JVP)	• Exertional dyspnea • Fatigue • Orthopnea and PND absent
Mitral regurgitation	• Rheumatic heart disease • Congenital malformation of mitral valve, mitral ring, or chordae tendineae • Mitral valve prolapse • Ruptured chordae tendineae	• Late systolic murmur (less severe cases) • Pansystolic murmur • Wide, split S_2 • S_3 • Intense P_2	• Vigorous apical impulse (may be sustained) • Palpitations (usually from atrial fibrillation)	• Asymptomatic (mild cases) • Fatigue, cough, palpitations (moderate cases) • Dyspnea, orthopnea, or PND from CHF (severe cases)
Mitral valve prolapse	• Myxomatous degeneration, possibly from autosomal dominant gene or form of Marfan's syndrome (valvular theory) • Dysfunction of papillary muscles, causing papillary muscles and chordae tendineae to rise and valve to billow during systole (myocardial theory)	• Midsystolic or late systolic clicks • Late systolic murmur	• Thin, pectus excavatum, pectus carinatum, scoliosis, or kyphosis • Abnormal apical impulse	• Asymptomatic (common) • Atypical or nonanginal chest pain • Fatigue and dyspnea • Palpitations • Transient ischemic attacks • Anxiety and lassitude
Tricuspid regurgitation	• Rheumatic heart disease • Commonly seen in pulmonary hypertension	• Pansystolic murmur (increases with inspiration) • S_2 • Intense P_2 (with pulmonary hypertension)	• Palpable right ventricular hypertrophy (at LSB) • Dominant systolic wave in JVP • Hepatomegaly • Peripheral edema	• Exertional dyspnea • Anorexia, nausea, vomiting, and abdominal pain

What abnormal heart sounds signify (continued)

Condition	Cause	Findings on auscultation	Other assessment findings	Signs and symptoms
Aortic regurgitation	• Congenital bicuspid valve • Rheumatic heart disease • Trauma • Infective endocarditis • Cystic aortic medial necrosis (as in Marfan's syndrome), hypertension, atherosclerosis	• Aortic ejection sound (not always present) • Systolic ejection murmur (not always present) • Early diastolic murmur	• Wide pulse pressure • Corrigan's or water-hammer pulse (rapidly rising and collapsing) • Visible carotid pulse • Pulsating nail bed (Quincke's pulse) • Systolic head nodding (Mussel's sign)	• Commonly asymptomatic (unless lesion is severe) • Exertional dyspnea • Dyspnea at rest • Angina • CHF
Pulmonic regurgitation	*With normal pulmonary artery pressure (PAP)—* • Congenitally absent pulmonary valves • Postoperative effect of surgery for pulmonary stenosis • Dilated pulmonary artery from atrial septal defect or ventricular septal defect • Idiopathic dilation of pulmonary artery *with high PAP—* • Mitral stenosis causing increased PA pressure (Graham Steell's murmur) • Pulmonary hypertension • Patent ductus arteriosus	*With normal PAP—* • Slight delay after P_2 before murmur is heard • Murmur tends to be short (increases with inspiration) *with high PAP—* • Loud P_2 (also heard at apex and right heart base) • Pulmonic ejection sound • S_4 gallop (increases with inspiration) • Tricuspid regurgitation murmur • Ejection murmur (increases with expiration)	• Occasional pulsation at second or third left intercostal space • Cyanosis	• Exertional dyspnea • Cough • Hemoptysis
Mitral stenosis	• Usually rheumatic heart disease	• Loud S_1 • Opening snap • Middiastolic rumble • Presystolic accentuation murmur • Loud P_2 (with pulmonary hypertension)	• Mitral facies • Abnormal A wave in JVP • Right ventricular hypertrophy • Bilateral moist crackles on inspiration • Wheezes (from associated bronchitis)	• Exertional dyspnea • Atrial fibrillation • Orthopnea and PND (with severe stenosis) • Hemoptysis (15% of patients) • Embolization • Fatigue from decreased cardiac output

(continued)

What abnormal heart sounds signify (continued)

Condition	Cause	Findings on auscultation	Other assessment findings	Signs and symptoms
Pericardial friction rub	• Myocardial infarction • Pericarditis • Uremia	• One systolic sound (any time during systole) • Two diastolic sounds (when ventricles are stretched)	• Sharp, stabbing pain, aggravated by deep inspiration • Fever	
Pleural friction rub	• Pneumonia • Viral infections • Tuberculosis • Pulmonary emboli	• Coarse, grating, or creaking sound on inspiration • Similar sound on expiration (sometimes absent) • Increased tactile fremitus • Dull percussion note over affected area • Abnormal breath sounds	• Atrial dysrhythmia • Tachycardia	• Precordial pain • Dyspnea • Fever, sweating, chills • Fatigue and weakness

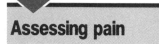

Assessing pain

Assessing your patient's pain is no simple matter. How much pain medication is enough? What other measures can be used to alleviate the patient's pain? And when should you use them?

You'll have to work to uncover the answers to these questions, using a focused approach to pain assessment. Presented here is a specific "pain model," developed by Loeser, that will help you assess your patient's pain systematically. It's an excellent tool for organizing and analyzing pain assessment data.

The Loeser model suggests that you consider four factors when assessing pain: *nociception, pain, suffering,* and *pain behaviors.* These factors, which build on one another, can all contribute to the experience of pain.

Nociception: Nervous system activation

In nociception, the free nerve endings found throughout body tissues detect a pain stimulus and send pain signals to the central nervous system. When assessing for nociception, think in terms of tissue damage that has activated the nervous system. Ask yourself, "What is happening in this patient's body tissues? What is initiating pain signals?"

Specifically, you're looking for actual or potential tissue damage from thermal, mechanical, or chemical causes, such as infection, inflammation, bowel or bladder distention, and physical trauma from a nasogastric tube or an I.V. catheter.

Pain: How do you know it's present?

As a result of nociception, noxious stimuli are transmitted to the central nervous system. And your patient feels *pain.*

But how do you *know* she's in pain? What tells you she's in pain? Ask yourself these key questions when considering this second factor in the pain assessment model.

You'll know your patient feels pain by subjective and objective evidence. First, the patient tells you she's in pain. She describes what she's feeling and she calls it pain. Objective evidence, for example, includes signs of sympathetic nervous system activation, such as changes in blood pressure, heart rate, or respiratory status.

Suffering: Emotional impact

Although *suffering* isn't synonymous with pain, people often talk in terms of pain when they discuss suffering. They have trouble talking about suffering itself, perhaps because they don't have the vocabulary for it; they find it hard to put their emotions into words. It's easier for them to talk in terms of pain.

But people *show* suffering in many different ways. Anxiety, fear, anger, depression, stoic endurance—these are all ways in which people express suffering. Often their feelings are related to a sense of loss—the loss of a job, for example, or an alteration in body image.

So the key question you want to ask yourself when assessing for suffering is: "How is the pain affecting this patient emotionally?"

Pain behaviors: Measurable and changeable
A patient's *pain behaviors* are her way of telling you she's in pain.

These highly individualized behaviors are shaped by the patient's personality and background. Cultural and social factors also come into play.

Pain behaviors are measurable—for example, an increase or decrease in range of motion. And they can be affected, for better or worse, by pain management interventions. As a nurse, you can track and record pain behaviors to monitor the effectiveness of such interventions.

These behaviors can also change with time, with the course of a disease, and with reinforcement from family members and

health care providers. The key question to ask yourself: "What is this patient doing that tells me she is in pain?"

The chart will give you more information on the four parts of the pain model.

Uncovering important information
By spending extra time with the patient and using the pain model to assess her pain systematically, you can uncover both physical and psychosocial factors affecting the patient's recovery.

The Loeser model: What to consider

Nociception	Pain	Suffering	Pain behaviors
What is happening in the tissues to initiate pain signals? •intraoperative factors (such as positioning or towel clips) •infection •incision •pressure (from dressing, swelling, positioning, or immobility, for example) •drugs (such as infiltration into tissues) •anoxia •vasoconstriction •irritation (physical trauma from nasogastric tube or I.V. catheter, for example) •distention (bowel or bladder) •viral causes (such as neuralgias) •pulled, tightened muscles (from positioning, tension, or fear, for example) •withdrawal (such as low glucose, caffeine, or nicotine level)	How do you know the patient is in pain? *Subjective factors:* •patient's description of the pain (such as what it feels like, when it occurs) *Objective factors:* •blood pressure changes •heart rate changes •respiratory changes •vasoconstriction •pallor •sweating •restlessness •reflexive withdrawal from nociception	How is the pain affecting the patient emotionally? •sadness •fear •anxiety •anger •depression •disorientation •anguish •actual or potential losses (such as loss of job, financial security, independence, important relationship, or body part) •altered perceptions (related to drugs, for example, or hospital environment) •meaning of pain (may be seen as punishment, for example)	What is the patient doing that tells you he's in pain? *Specific behaviors:* •taking pain medication •limping, groaning, grimacing, guarding •refusing to participate in activities *Characteristics of all behaviors:* •measurable (such as decreased range of motion) •changeable (through education or reinforcement) •culturally and socially influenced •individual •not always related to severity of pain •verbal or nonverbal

Assessing the substance abuser

Substance abusers regularly use alcohol or drugs that affect the central nervous system and cause behavioral changes. Such abuse may lead to dependency, in which the patient can't control his use of the substance and develops withdrawal symptoms if he attempts to stop or reduce intake.

Your assessment approach will depend on the patient's condition. If he suffers from such complications as alcohol withdrawal syndrome (commonly known as delerium tremens), hepatic coma, esophageal varices, respiratory depression, gastric bleeding, or dysrhythmias, treat these problems first. Afterward, you can address the chemical dependency.

If the patient is obviously intoxicated or high, keep your questions simple and to the point. Ask when he last took a drink or a drug. If he has taken one or more drugs, find out which ones. Then ask about symptoms. Try to establish rapport quickly. If friends or relatives have accompanied the patient to the hospital, ask them for relevant information. Also study any previous medical records. The patient may have to be examined for an accompanying condition, such as hypertension or diabetes. If the patient appears coherent, seek more detail on his pattern of abuse.

Physical examination

Substance abuse affects every organ and body system. While many symptoms are specific to particular substances, common indicators of abuse do exist. When assessing for substance abuse, form an impression of the patient's appearance. Note if he seems unkempt, nervous, or agitated. Does he pace around the room? Does he show signs of tremors? Ask the patient if he's had difficulty sleeping. Also take his vital signs, being alert for increased blood pressure (common in alcohol intoxication and withdrawal).

Central nervous system. Assess for alertness, coherence, and orientation to time, person, and place. Does the patient walk with an unsteady or awkward gait? You may perform the Romberg test to assess for cerebellar dysfunction. To perform the test, have the patient stand erect with his feet together and his arms at his sides. Ask him to hold this position with his eyes open, then closed. In cerebellar dysfunction, the patient will have difficulty keeping his balance.

Head and neck. Check for lesions or injuries, head lice (common in some juveniles and in homeless or indigent patients), distended neck veins, petechiae on the nose and cheeks, and ruddy complexion. Observe the sclera of his eyes for redness or yellowing. Test pupillary response.

Chest. Assess for irregular heart rate and rhythm, wheezing, abnormal breath sounds (such as crackles or rhonchi), and symptoms of obstructive pulmonary disease. Patients who smoke marijuana regularly or freebase cocaine commonly have difficulty breathing. Cocaine freebasers may feel as if their hearts are racing.

Abdomen. Observe for ascites, distended or tender abdomen, and enlarged liver or spleen. If the liver appears large, assess for ecchymoses or other signs of bleeding. The patient may spit up blood or have dark, foul, tarry stools.

Skin. Observe for spider hemangiomas, yellowed skin (a sign of liver damage), bruised or edematous legs, poor skin turgor in the legs, weak pedal pulses, and loss of muscle mass.

Nutritional status. The chemically dependent patient usually doesn't eat regularly and may become severely malnourished. Ask the patient what he usually eats, if he's experienced recent weight changes, what he considers a balanced diet, whether he cooks for himself, and whether he takes vitamin supplements. Alcoholics need more vitamin B complex because alcohol interferes with vitamin B metabolism. If the patient is homeless, ask if he can obtain regular meals at a shelter.

Emotional assessment

Note any signs of depression, excitation, suicidal ideation, suspiciousness, anger, or anxiety. Observe for signs of instability, mood swings, unreasonable resentments, remorse, grandiosity, self-pity, and pathologic jealousy. Ask the patient if he's experienced hallucinations, memory loss, or problems with communication, following directions, finishing work, or controlling violent impulses. Also ask if he's ever received treatment for emotional problems. If so, determine the type and effectiveness.

Motivation. Ask why the patient decided to seek treatment. Did his family or employer insist? Did the courts require it? Or did he enter treatment seeking relief from symptoms caused by abuse? If he entered the hospital on his own, verify who he wants informed about his admission. Because of social stigma, many patients don't want others to know they're being treated.

Social support. Find out about social and family support to help plan the patient's treatment and discharge. If the patient identifies certain people as especially supportive, involve them in his treatment and ask them to help in his recovery after discharge.

Understanding body systems and structures

SKIN

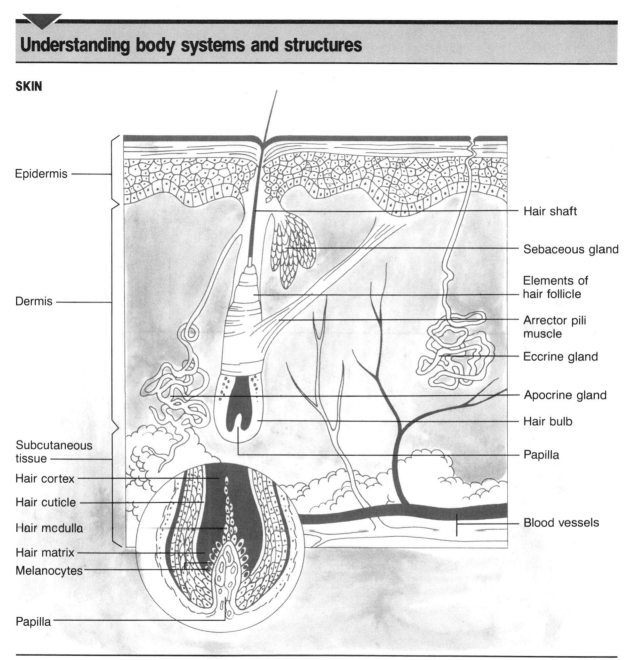

Epidermis

Dermis

Subcutaneous tissue

Hair cortex

Hair cuticle

Hair medulla

Hair matrix

Melanocytes

Papilla

Hair shaft

Sebaceous gland

Elements of hair follicle

Arrector pili muscle

Eccrine gland

Apocrine gland

Hair bulb

Papilla

Blood vessels

(continued)

Understanding body systems and structures (continued)

EYE

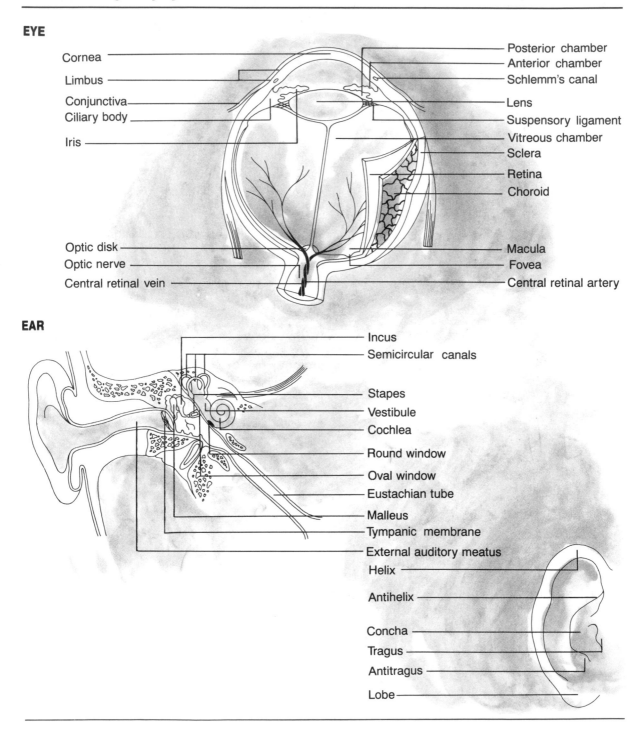

Cornea
Limbus
Conjunctiva
Ciliary body
Iris

Posterior chamber
Anterior chamber
Schlemm's canal
Lens
Suspensory ligament
Vitreous chamber
Sclera
Retina
Choroid

Optic disk
Optic nerve
Central retinal vein

Macula
Fovea
Central retinal artery

EAR

Incus
Semicircular canals

Stapes
Vestibule
Cochlea

Round window

Oval window
Eustachian tube

Malleus
Tympanic membrane
External auditory meatus
Helix

Antihelix

Concha
Tragus
Antitragus

Lobe

Understanding body systems and structures *(continued)*

UPPER AND LOWER AIRWAYS

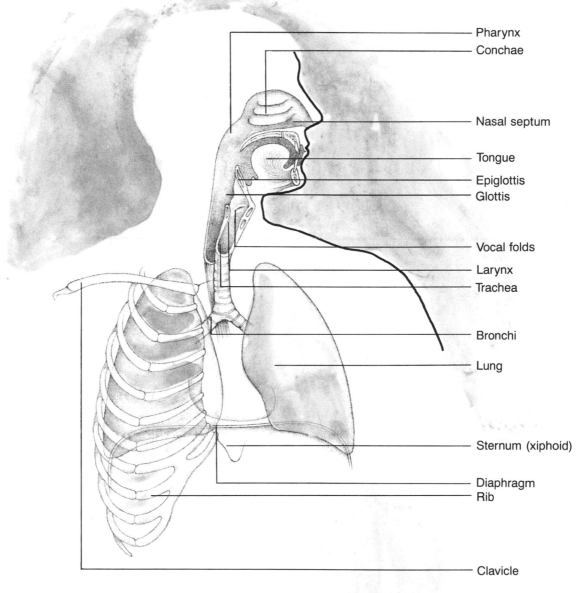

Pharynx
Conchae
Nasal septum
Tongue
Epiglottis
Glottis
Vocal folds
Larynx
Trachea
Bronchi
Lung
Sternum (xiphoid)
Diaphragm
Rib
Clavicle

(continued)

Understanding body systems and structures *(continued)*

CARDIOVASCULAR SYSTEM

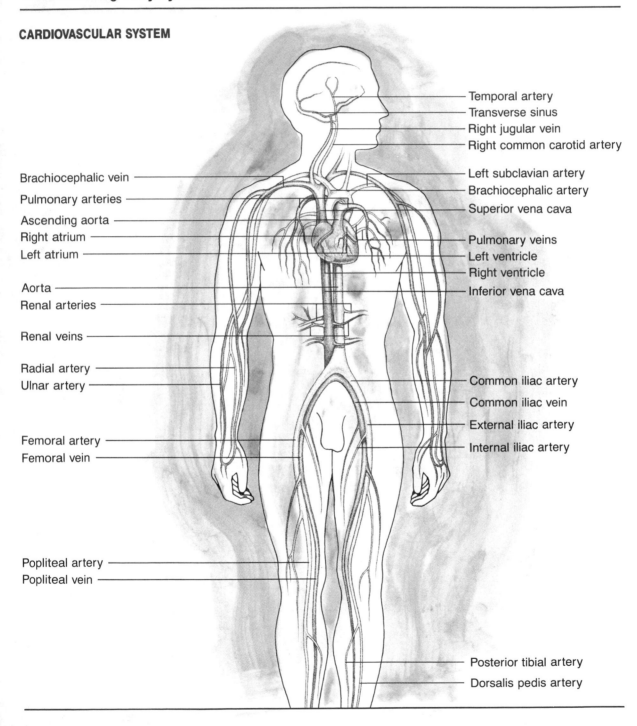

- Temporal artery
- Transverse sinus
- Right jugular vein
- Right common carotid artery
- Left subclavian artery
- Brachiocephalic artery
- Superior vena cava
- Pulmonary veins
- Left ventricle
- Right ventricle
- Inferior vena cava
- Common iliac artery
- Common iliac vein
- External iliac artery
- Internal iliac artery
- Posterior tibial artery
- Dorsalis pedis artery

- Brachiocephalic vein
- Pulmonary arteries
- Ascending aorta
- Right atrium
- Left atrium
- Aorta
- Renal arteries
- Renal veins
- Radial artery
- Ulnar artery
- Femoral artery
- Femoral vein
- Popliteal artery
- Popliteal vein

Understanding body systems and structures *(continued)*

NERVOUS SYSTEM

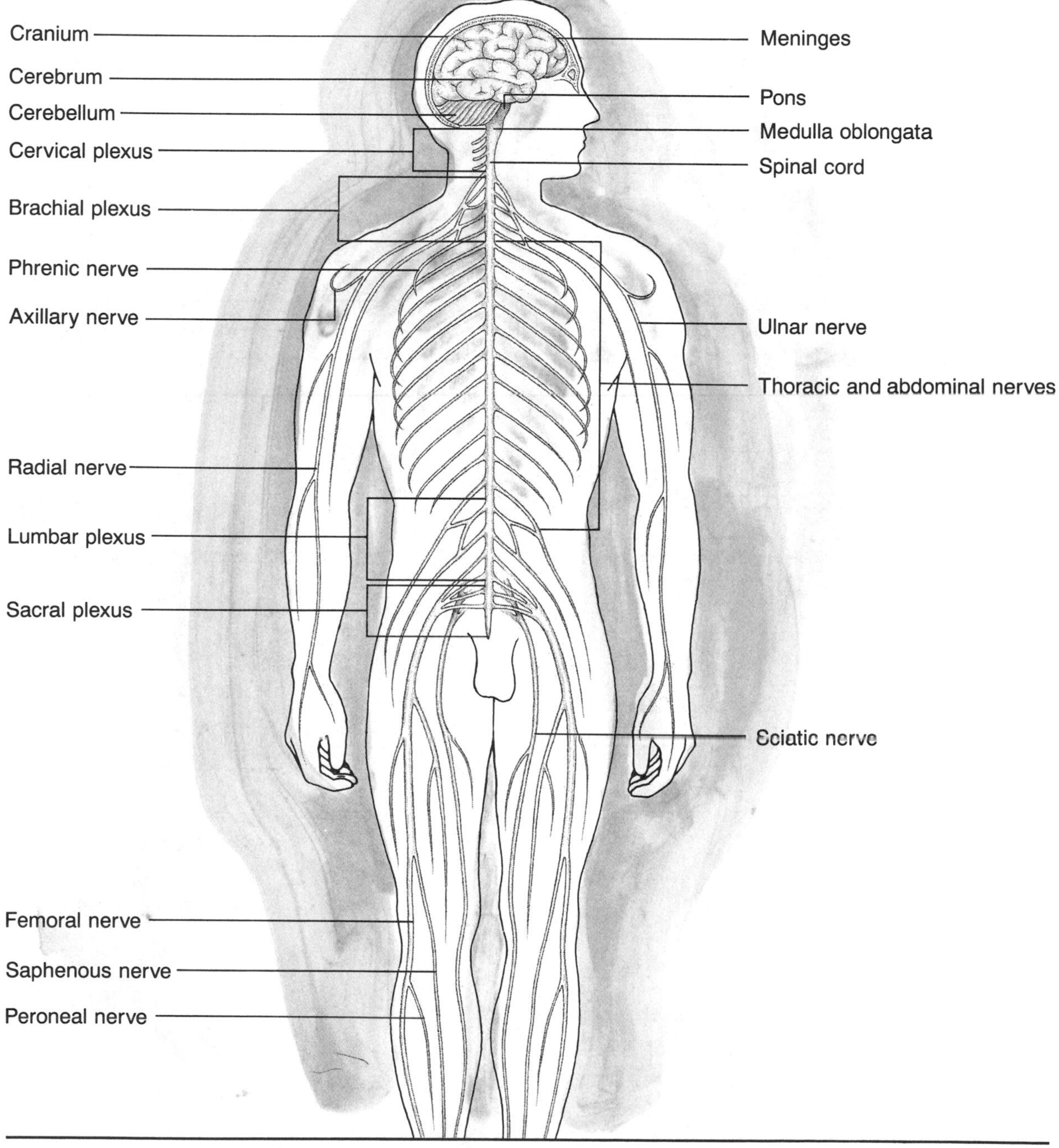

Cranium

Cerebrum

Cerebellum

Cervical plexus

Brachial plexus

Phrenic nerve

Axillary nerve

Radial nerve

Lumbar plexus

Sacral plexus

Femoral nerve

Saphenous nerve

Peroneal nerve

Meninges

Pons

Medulla oblongata

Spinal cord

Ulnar nerve

Thoracic and abdominal nerves

Sciatic nerve

(continued)

Understanding body systems and structures *(continued)*

MUSCULOSKELETAL SYSTEM

Anterior view

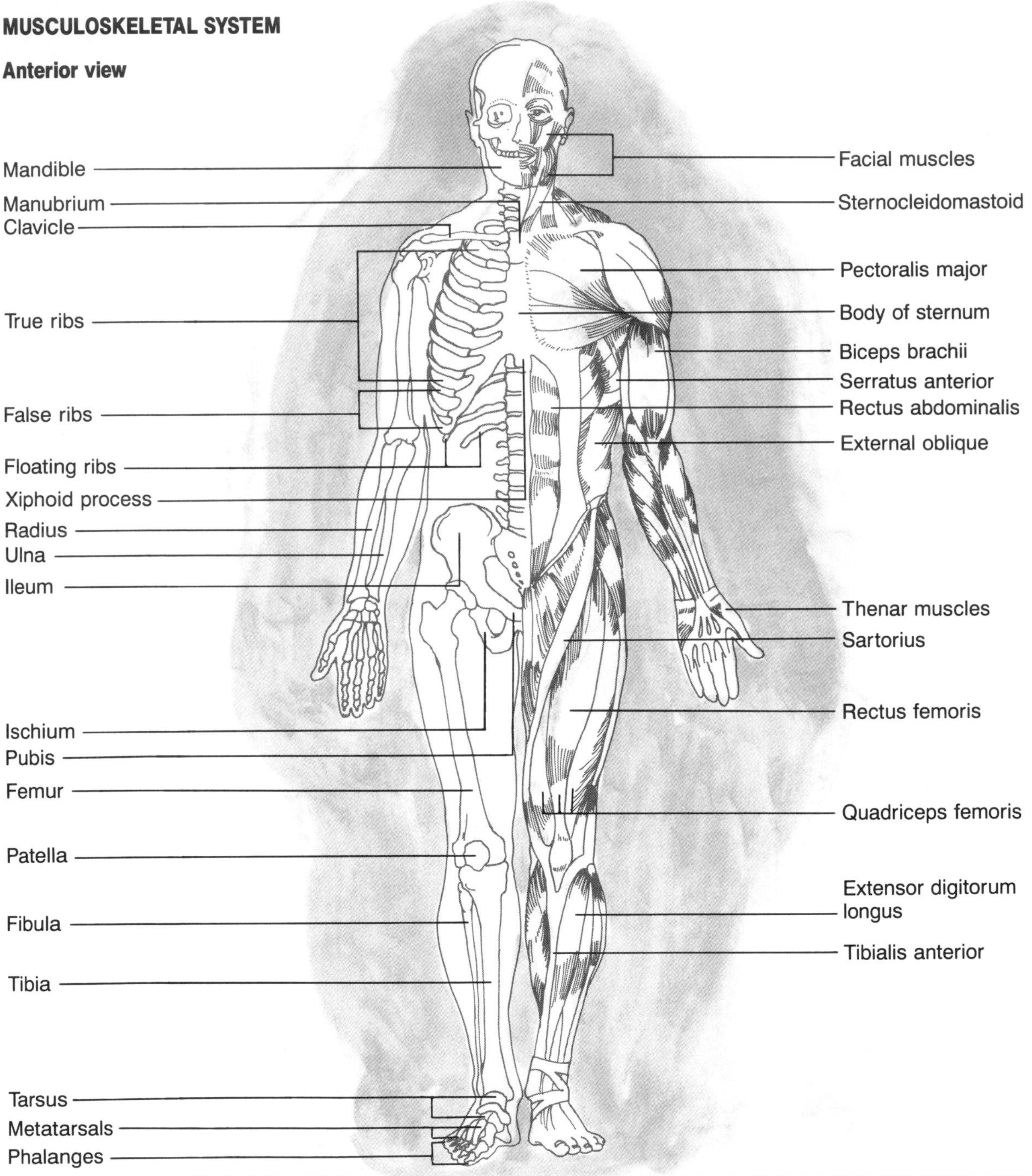

Mandible

Manubrium
Clavicle

True ribs

False ribs

Floating ribs
Xiphoid process
Radius
Ulna
Ileum

Ischium
Pubis
Femur

Patella

Fibula

Tibia

Tarsus
Metatarsals
Phalanges

Facial muscles
Sternocleidomastoid

Pectoralis major
Body of sternum
Biceps brachii
Serratus anterior
Rectus abdominalis
External oblique

Thenar muscles
Sartorius

Rectus femoris

Quadriceps femoris

Extensor digitorum longus
Tibialis anterior

Understanding body systems and structures *(continued)*

Posterior view

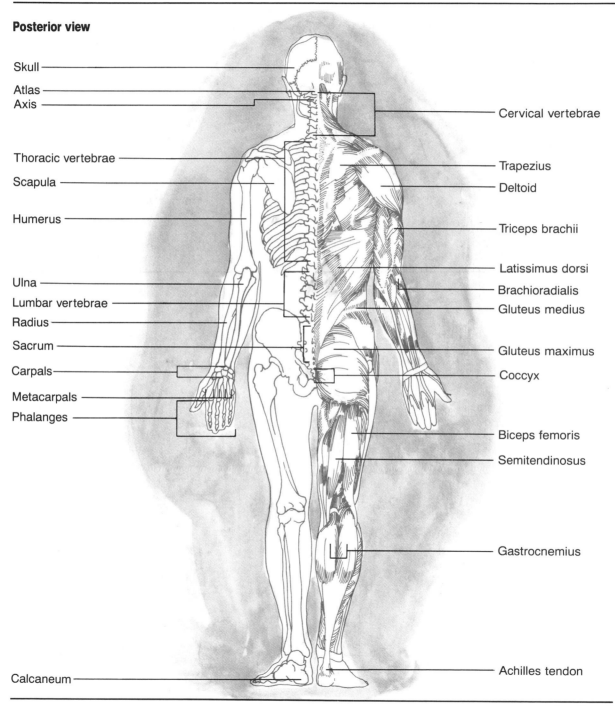

Skull

Atlas

Axis

Cervical vertebrae

Thoracic vertebrae

Scapula

Trapezius

Deltoid

Humerus

Triceps brachii

Latissimus dorsi

Ulna

Brachioradialis

Lumbar vertebrae

Gluteus medius

Radius

Sacrum

Gluteus maximus

Carpals

Coccyx

Metacarpals

Phalanges

Biceps femoris

Semitendinosus

Gastrocnemius

Calcaneum

Achilles tendon

(continued)

Understanding body systems and structures *(continued)*

GASTROINTESTINAL SYSTEM

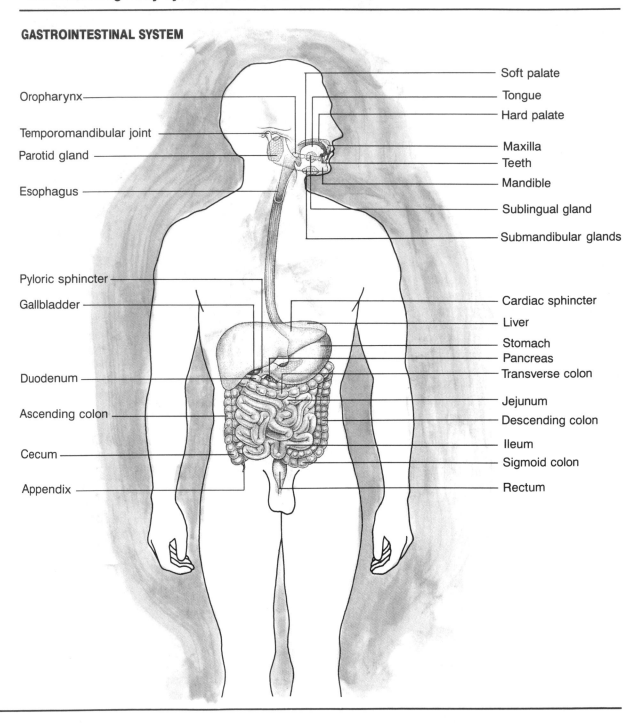

Oropharynx

Temporomandibular joint

Parotid gland

Esophagus

Pyloric sphincter

Gallbladder

Duodenum

Ascending colon

Cecum

Appendix

Soft palate

Tongue

Hard palate

Maxilla

Teeth

Mandible

Sublingual gland

Submandibular glands

Cardiac sphincter

Liver

Stomach

Pancreas

Transverse colon

Jejunum

Descending colon

Ileum

Sigmoid colon

Rectum

Understanding body systems and structures (continued)

URINARY SYSTEM

ENDOCRINE SYSTEM

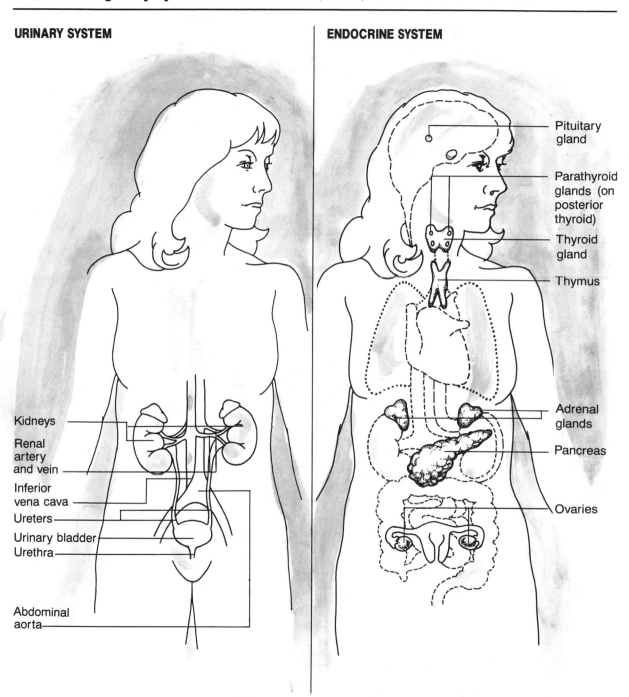

Pituitary gland

Parathyroid glands (on posterior thyroid)

Thyroid gland

Thymus

Adrenal glands

Pancreas

Ovaries

Kidneys

Renal artery and vein

Inferior vena cava

Ureters

Urinary bladder

Urethra

Abdominal aorta

(continued)

Understanding body systems and structures (continued)

FEMALE REPRODUCTIVE SYSTEM

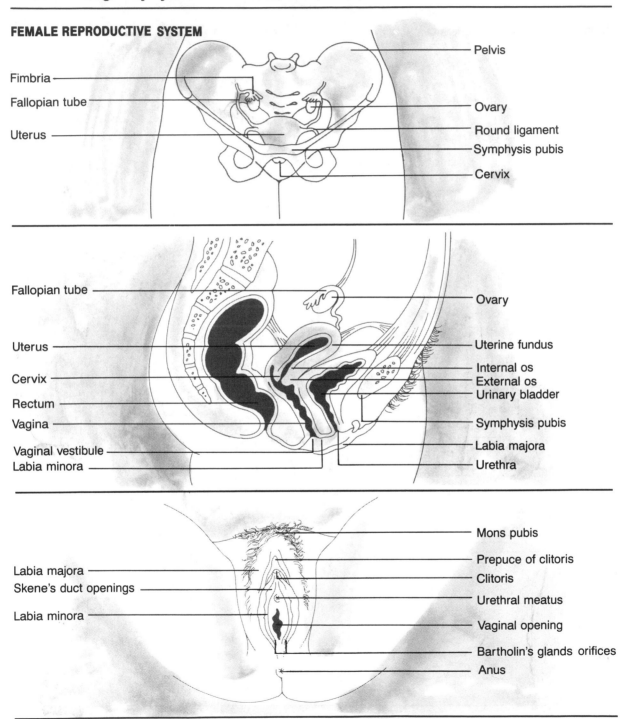

Fimbria

Fallopian tube

Uterus

Pelvis

Ovary

Round ligament

Symphysis pubis

Cervix

Fallopian tube

Uterus

Cervix

Rectum

Vagina

Vaginal vestibule

Labia minora

Ovary

Uterine fundus

Internal os

External os

Urinary bladder

Symphysis pubis

Labia majora

Urethra

Labia majora

Skene's duct openings

Labia minora

Mons pubis

Prepuce of clitoris

Clitoris

Urethral meatus

Vaginal opening

Bartholin's glands orifices

Anus

Understanding body systems and structures *(continued)*

MALE REPRODUCTIVE SYSTEM

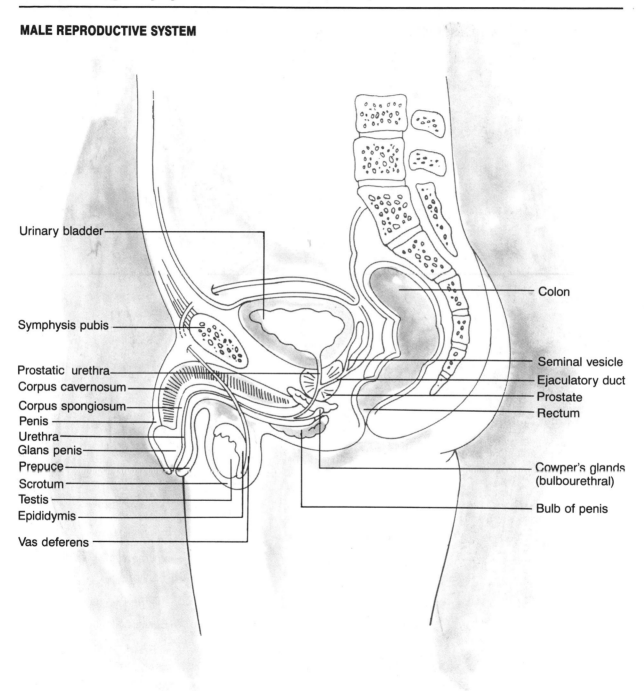

Urinary bladder

Symphysis pubis

Prostatic urethra
Corpus cavernosum
Corpus spongiosum
Penis
Urethra
Glans penis
Prepuce
Scrotum
Testis
Epididymis

Vas deferens

Colon

Seminal vesicle
Ejaculatory duct
Prostate
Rectum

Cowper's glands
(bulbourethral)

Bulb of penis

(continued)

Understanding body systems and structures (continued)

HEMATOLOGIC AND IMMUNE SYSTEMS

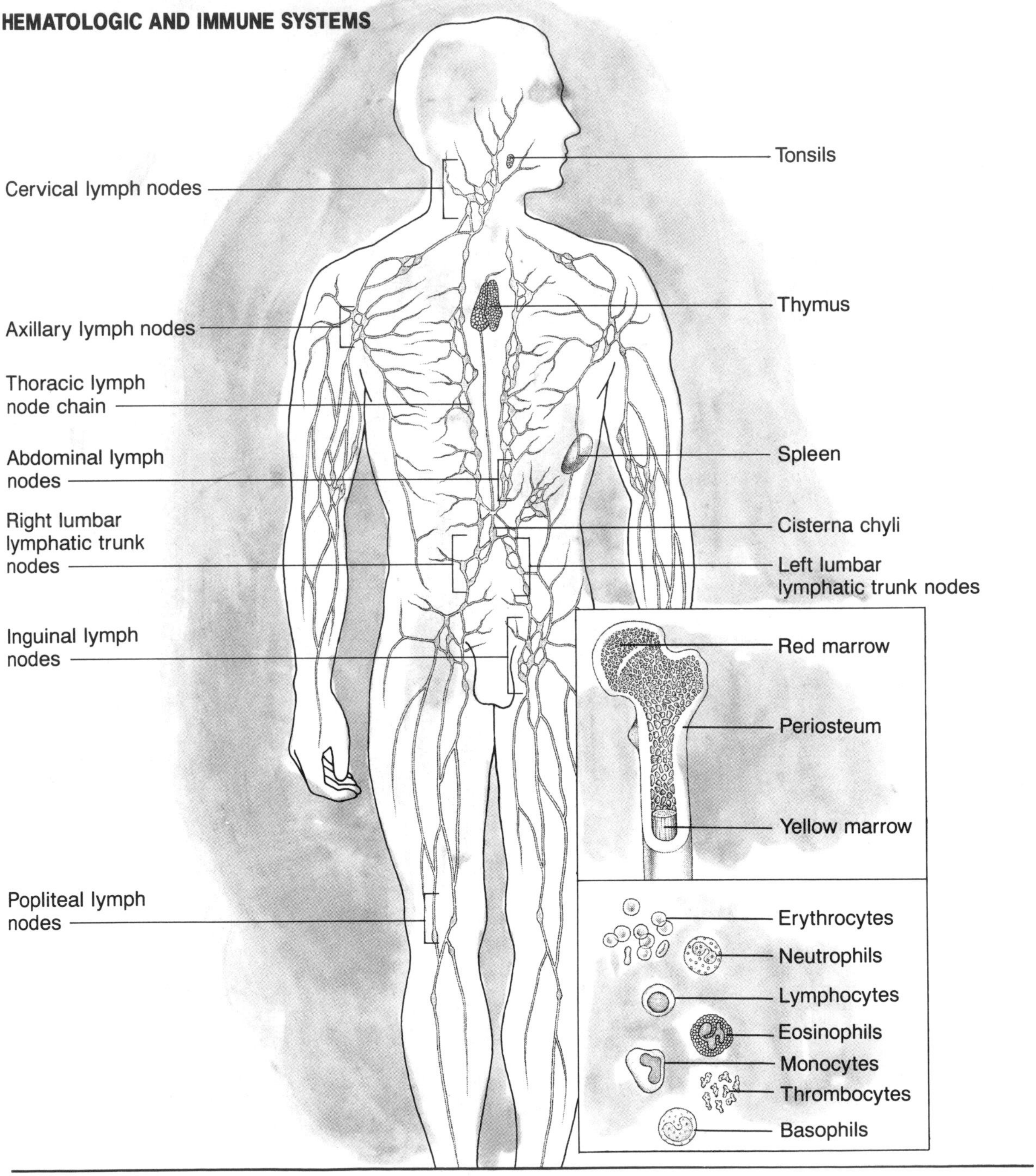

Cervical lymph nodes

Axillary lymph nodes

Thoracic lymph node chain

Abdominal lymph nodes

Right lumbar lymphatic trunk nodes

Inguinal lymph nodes

Popliteal lymph nodes

Tonsils

Thymus

Spleen

Cisterna chyli

Left lumbar lymphatic trunk nodes

Red marrow

Periosteum

Yellow marrow

Erythrocytes

Neutrophils

Lymphocytes

Eosinophils

Monocytes

Thrombocytes

Basophils

3 | Nursing diagnoses: An evolving framework

Approved nursing diagnoses

Your nursing diagnosis is a "problem statement" that describes the cluster of symptoms and signs indicating an actual or potential health problem you can identify and resolve. The chart below lists the latest diagnoses approved by the North American Nursing Diagnosis Association (NANDA).

Nursing diagnosis	Definition
Activity intolerance, related to imbalance between supply and demand	Extreme fatigue or other physical symptoms caused by simple activity
Activity intolerance, related to immobility	Extreme fatigue or other physical symptoms caused by simple activity
Adjustment impairment, related to disability	Inability to modify life-style or behavior consistent with changed health status
Airway clearance, ineffective, related to decreased energy or fatigue	Anatomic or physiologic obstruction of the airway that interferes with normal ventilation
Airway clearance, ineffective, related to presence of tracheobronchial obstruction or secretions	Anatomic or physiologic obstruction of the airway that interferes with normal ventilation
Anxiety, related to environmental conflict (phobia)	Feeling of threat or danger to self arising from an unidentifiable source
Anxiety, related to situational crisis	Feeling of threat or danger to self arising from an unidentifiable source
Anxiety, related to threat of death	Feeling of threat or danger to self arising from an unidentifiable source
Aspiration, potential, related to absence of protective mechanisms	State of being at risk for aspiration of gastrointestinal or oropharyngeal secretions, food, or fluids into tracheobronchial passages
Body temperature alteration, potential, related to aging	State of being at risk for failure to maintain body temperature within normal range

(continued)

Approved nursing diagnoses (continued)

Nursing diagnosis	Definition
Breastfeeding, effective	State in which mother, infant, or family experiences satisfaction with breastfeeding process.
Breastfeeding, ineffective, related to dissatisfaction with breastfeeding process	State in which mother, infant, or family experiences dissatisfaction or difficulty with breastfeeding process
Breathing pattern, ineffective, related to decreased energy or fatigue	Change in rate, depth, or pattern of breathing that alters normal gas exchange
Breathing pattern, ineffective, related to pain	Change in the rate, depth, or pattern of breathing that alters normal gas exchange
Cardiac output, decreased, related to reduced stroke volume	Cardiovascular or respiratory symptoms resulting from insufficient blood being pumped by the heart
Constipation, related to gastrointestinal obstruction	Interruption of normal bowel movements resulting in infrequent or absent stools
Constipation, related to inadequate intake of fluid and bulk	Interruption of normal bowel movements resulting in infrequent or absent stools
Constipation, related to personal habits	Interruption of normal bowel movements resulting in infrequent or absent stools
Constipation, colonic	Elimination pattern characterized by hard, dry stool resulting from delayed passage of food residue
Constipation, perceived	State in which an individual makes a self-diagnosis of constipation and ensures daily bowel movements through use of laxatives, enemas, or suppositories
Coping, defensive, related to perceived threat to positive self-regard	Falsely positive self-evaluation based on a self-protective pattern that defends against underlying perceived threats to positive self-regard
Coping, family: Potential for growth, related to self-actualization needs	Inability to use adaptive behaviors in response to difficult life situations
Coping, ineffective family, related to inadequate or incorrect information held by primary caregiver	Inability to use adaptive behaviors in response to difficult life situations
Coping, ineffective individual, related to situational crisis	Inability to use adaptive behaviors in response to such difficult life situations as loss of health, a loved one, or job
Decisional conflict (specify), related to perceived threat to value system	State of uncertainty about health-related course of action when choice involves risk, loss, or challenge to personal life values
Denial, related to fear or anxiety	Conscious or unconscious attempt to disavow the knowledge or meaning of an event to reduce anxiety or fear to the detriment of health
Diarrhea, related to malabsorption, inflammation, or irritation of bowel	Interruption of normal elimination pattern characterized by frequent, loose stools

Approved nursing diagnoses (continued)

Nursing diagnosis	Definition
Diarrhea, related to stress and anxiety	Interruption of normal bowel movements resulting in frequent, loose stools
Diversional activity deficit, related to lack of environmental stimulation	Restriction or decline in ability to use unoccupied time to patient's advantage or satisfaction
Diversional activity deficit, related to long-term hospitalization or frequent, lengthy treatments	Restriction or decrease in ability to use unoccupied time to patient's advantage or satisfaction
Dysreflexia, related to spinal cord trauma	State in which a patient with spinal cord injury at T6 or above experiences or risks life-threatening, uninhibited sympathetic response to a noxious stimulus
Family process alteration, related to situational crisis	Disruption in expected role functions within the family structure because of such situational crises as protracted physical or emotional illness
Fatigue	Overwhelming sense of exhaustion and decreased capacity for physical and mental work, regardless of adequate sleep
Fear, related to separation from support system	Feeling of physiologic or emotional disruption related to an identifiable source
Fear, related to unfamiliarity	Feelings of threat or danger to self arising from an identifiable source
Fluid volume deficit, related to actual loss	Excessive loss of body fluid and electrolytes
Fluid volume deficit, potential, related to excessive loss through artificial routes (such as indwelling tubes)	Presence of risk factors that can lead to excessive fluid and electrolyte loss
Fluid volume deficit, potential, related to excessive loss through physiologic routes	Presence of risk factors that could lead to excessive fluid and electrolyte loss
Fluid volume excess, related to compromised regulatory mechanisms	Excess fluid resulting from compromised regulatory mechanisms (internal physiologic controls that help the body adjust to changing needs, such as renin-angiotensin, antidiuretic hormone, aldosterone, hydrogen-bicarbonate ion exchange)
Fluid volume excess, related to excess fluid intake or retention or excess sodium intake or retention	Imbalance of water or sodium causing increased total body fluid or fluid volume shift from one compartment to another
Gas exchange impairment, related to altered oxygen-carrying capacity of the blood	Interference in cellular respiration resulting from inadequate exchange or transport of oxygen or carbon dioxide
Gas exchange impairment, related to altered oxygen supply	Interference in cellular respiration resulting from inadequate exchange or transport of oxygen or carbon dioxide
Grieving, anticipatory, related to perceived potential loss of significant object (person, job, possessions, etc.)	Grief response in anticipation of perceived personal loss

(continued)

Approved nursing diagnoses *(continued)*

Nursing diagnosis	Definition
Grieving, dysfunctional, related to actual object loss	Prolongation of the normal grief response beyond the time one would expect resolution to have occurred
Growth and development alteration, related to effects of physical disability	State in which an individual deviates from norms for age
Health maintenance alteration, related to lack of motor skills	Inability to maintain a healthy state
Health maintenance alteration, related to perceptual or cognitive impairment	Inability to maintain a healthy state
Health-seeking behaviors, related to absence of aerobic exercise as a risk factor for coronary artery disease	State in which a patient in stable health actively seeks ways to alter personal health habits or the environment in order to move toward optimal health
Health-seeking behaviors, related to elevated serum cholesterol level as a risk factor for coronary disease	State in which a patient in stable health actively seeks ways to alter personal health habits or the environment in order to move toward optimal health
Health-seeking behaviors, related to hypertension as a risk factor for coronary artery disease	State in which a patient in stable health actively seeks ways to alter personal health habits or the environment in order to move toward optimal health
Health-seeking behaviors, related to smoking as a risk factor for coronary artery disease	State in which a patient in stable health actively seeks ways to alter personal health habits or the environment in order to move toward optimal health
Health-seeking behaviors, related to stress as a risk factor for coronary artery disease	State in which a patient in stable health actively seeks ways to alter personal health habits or the environment in order to move toward optimal health
Home maintenance management impairment, related to inadequate support system	Insufficient resources available to meet self-care needs adequately and safely in the patient's home
Hopelessness, related to failing or deteriorating physiologic condition	Subjective state in which an individual sees few or no available alternatives or personal choices and cannot mobilize energy on own behalf
Hopelessness, related to prolonged activity restriction, creating isolation	Subjective state in which an individual sees few or no available alternatives or personal choices and cannot mobilize energy on own behalf
Hyperthermia, related to dehydration	Elevation of body temperature above normal range
Hypothermia, related to exposure to cold or cold environment	State in which body temperature is reduced below normal range
Incontinence, bowel, related to neuromuscular involvement	Involuntary passage of stool
Incontinence, bowel, related to perceptual or cognitive impairment	Involuntary passage of stool
Incontinence, functional, related to sensory or mobility deficits	Involuntary and unpredictable passage of urine in socially unacceptable situations, where patient usually does not recognize warning signs of bladder fullness

Approved nursing diagnoses *(continued)*

Nursing diagnosis	Definition
Incontinence, functional, related to cognitive deficits	Involuntary and unpredictable passage of urine in socially unacceptable situations, where patient usually does not recognize warning signs of bladder fullness
Incontinence, reflex, related to sensory or neuromuscular impairment	Involuntary loss of urine, controlled by spinal cord reflex, occurring at somewhat predictable intervals when a specific bladder volume is reached
Incontinence, stress, related to weak pelvic musculature	Loss of urine (less than 50 ml) resulting from increased abdominal pressure
Incontinence, total, related to neurologic dysfunction	Continuous and unpredictable passage of urine
Incontinence, urge, related to decreased bladder capacity	Involuntary passage of urine occurring shortly after a strong sense of urgency to void
Infection, potential, related to external factors	Presence of internal or external hazards that threaten physical well-being
Knowledge deficit, related to cognitive impairment	Inadequate understanding of information or inability to perform skills needed to practice health-related behaviors
Knowledge deficit, related to lack of exposure	Inadequate understanding of information or inability to perform skills needed to practice health-related behaviors
Knowledge deficit, related to lack of motivation	Inadequate understanding of information or inability to perform skills needed to practice health-related behaviors
Mobility impairment, related to neuromuscular impairment	Limitation of physical movement
Mobility impairment, related to pain or discomfort	Limitation of physical movement
Mobility impairment, related to perceptual or cognitive impairment	Limitation of physical movement
Neglect, unilateral, related to neurologic illness or trauma	Lack of awareness of a body part
Noncompliance, related to patient's value system	Unwillingness to practice prescribed health-related behaviors
Nutrition alteration: Less than body requirements, related to inability to digest or absorb nutrients resulting from biological factors	Change in normal eating pattern that results in changed body weight
Nutrition alteration: Less than body requirements, related to inability to digest foods	Change in normal eating pattern that results in changed body weight
Nutrition alteration: Less than body requirements, related to psychological factors	Change in normal eating pattern that results in changed body weight
Nutrition alteration: More than body requirements, related to excessive intake	Change in normal eating pattern that results in changed body weight

(continued)

Approved nursing diagnoses (continued)

Nursing diagnosis	Definition
Oral mucous membrane alteration, related to dehydration	Altered mouth integrity
Oral mucous membrane alteration, related to mechanical trauma	Altered mouth integrity
Oral mucous membrane alteration, related to pathologic condition	Altered mouth integrity
Pain, related to physical, biological, or chemical agents	Subjective sensation of discomfort derived from multiple sensory nerve interactions generated by physical, chemical, biological or psychological stimuli
Pain, related to psychological agents	Subjective sensation of discomfort derived from multiple sensory nerve interactions generated by physical, chemical, biological or psychological stimuli
Pain, chronic, related to physical disability	Pain complaints that last longer than the expected healing process, which is usually 6 to 12 weeks
Parental role conflict, related to crisis (child's hospitalization)	State in which one or both parents experience role confusion and conflict in response to crisis
Parenting alteration: Actual or potential, related to lack of knowledge	Inability of a nurturing figure to promote optimum growth and development in an infant or child
Personal identity disturbance, related to change in body image	Negative perception of self that makes healthful functioning more difficult
Personal identity disturbance, related to lowered self-esteem	Uncertainty about components of self regarding choices of vocation, intimacy and life-style
Poisoning, potential, related to external factors	Accentuated risk of accidental exposure to or ingestion of drugs or dangerous products in doses sufficient to cause poisoning
Poisoning, potential, related to internal factors (biological, psychological, developmental)	Accentuated risk of accidental exposure to or ingestion of drugs or dangerous products in doses sufficient to cause poisoning
Posttrauma response, related to accidental injury	Sustained painful response to an unexpected life event
Posttrauma response, related to assault	Sustained painful response to an unexpected life event
Potential for disuse syndrome, related to prolonged inactivity	State of being at risk for deterioration of body systems as a result of prescribed or unavoidable inactivity
Powerlessness, related to the health care environment	Perceived loss of control over what happens to oneself and one's environment
Protection, altered	Decreased ability to guard against internal or external threats
Rape-trauma syndrome	Physical and emotional trauma that occurs as a result of sexual assault

Approved nursing diagnoses *(continued)*

Nursing diagnosis	Definition
Self-care deficit: Feeding, related to musculoskeletal impairment	Inability to carry out the self-care activity: feeding
Self-care deficit: Feeding, bathing and hygiene, dressing and grooming, toileting, related to musculoskeletal impairment	Inability to carry out some aspects of self-care, such as bathing, dressing, feeding
Self-care deficit: Feeding, bathing and hygiene, dressing and grooming, toileting, related to perceptual or cognitive impairment	Inability to carry out some aspects of self-care, such as bathing, dressing, feeding
Self-esteem, chronic low	Long-standing negative self-evaluation or feelings about self or capabilities
Self-esteem disturbance	Negative self-evaluation or feelings about self or capabilities that may be directly or indirectly expressed
Self-esteem, situational low	Negative self-evaluation or feelings about self that develop in response to a loss or change in an individual who previously had a positive self-evaluation
Sensory or perceptual alteration (auditory), related to altered sensory reception, transmission, or integration	Change in the characteristics of auditory stimuli
Sensory or perceptual alteration (specify), related to sensory deprivation	Change in the characteristics of incoming stimuli
Sensory or perceptual alteration (specify), related to sensory overload	Change in the characteristics of incoming stimuli
Sensory or perceptual alteration (visual), related to altered sensory reception, transmission, or integration	Change in the characteristics of visual stimuli
Sexual dysfunction, related to altered body structure or function	Presence of physical or emotional factors that alter one's usual pattern of sexual function
Sexual pattern alteration, related to illness or medical treatment	State in which an individual expresses concern about personal sexuality
Sexual pattern alteration, related to separation from significant other	State in which an individual expresses concern about personal sexuality
Skin integrity impairment, related to external (environmental) factors	Interruption in skin integrity
Skin integrity impairment, related to internal (somatic) factors	Interruption in skin integrity
Skin integrity impairment, potential	Presence of risk factors for interruption or destruction of skin surface
Sleep pattern disturbance, related to external factors, such as environmental changes	Inability to meet individual need for sleep or rest arising from internal or external factors

(continued)

Approved nursing diagnoses (continued)

Nursing diagnosis	Definition
Sleep pattern disturbance, related to internal factors, such as illness, psychological stress, drug therapy, biorhythm disturbance	Inability to meet individual need for sleep or rest arising from internal or external factors
Social interaction impairment, related to altered thought processes	Insufficient quantity or ineffective quality of social exchange
Social interaction impairment, related to sociocultural dissonance	Insufficient quantity or ineffective quality of social exchange
Social isolation, related to altered state of wellness	Self-imposed or environmentally imposed lack of contact with support systems
Social isolation, related to inadequate personal resources	Self-imposed or environmentally imposed lack of contact with support systems
Spiritual distress, related to separation from religious and cultural ties	Separation or alienation from religious traditions or values
Spiritual distress, related to situational crisis	Separation or alienation from religious tradition or values
Suffocation, potential, related to external factors	Accentuated risk of accidental suffocation (inadequate air available for inhalation)
Suffocation, potential, related to internal factors	Accentuated risk of accidental suffocation (inadequate air available for inhalation)
Swallowing impairment, related to neuromuscular impairment	Inability to move food, fluid, or saliva from the mouth through the esophagus
Thermoregulation, ineffective, related to trauma or illness	Fluctuations in body temperature caused by thermoregulatory disturbances
Thought process alteration, related to loss of memory	Inability to process thoughts accurately and correctly
Thought process alteration, related to physiologic causes	Inability to process thoughts accurately and correctly
Tissue integrity impairment, related to peripheral vascular changes	Damage to mucous membranes or to corneal, integumentary or subcutaneous tissue
Tissue integrity impairment, related to radiation	Damage to mucous membranes or to corneal, integumentary or subcutaneous tissue
Tissue perfusion alteration (peripheral), related to reduced arterial blood flow	Decrease in cellular nutrition and respiration because of decreased capillary blood flow
Tissue perfusion alteration (specify), related to hypovolemia	Decrease in cellular nutrition and respiration because of decreased capillary blood flow
Tissue perfusion alteration (venous), related to reduced venous blood flow	Decrease in cellular nutrition and respiration because of decreased capillary blood flow
Trauma, potential, related to external factors (environmental, physical, chemical agents)	Accentuated risk of accidental tissue injury such as burns or fractures
Trauma, potential, related to internal factors	Accentuated risk of accidental tissue injury such as burns or fractures

Approved nursing diagnoses (continued)

Nursing diagnosis	Definition
Urinary elimination pattern alteration, related to obstruction	Alteration or impairment of urinary function
Urinary elimination pattern alteration, related to sensory or neuromuscular impairment	Alteration or impairment of urinary function
Urinary retention, related to obstruction, sensory or neuromuscular impairment	Incomplete emptying of bladder
Verbal communication impairment, related to decreased circulation to the brain	Decreased ability to speak, understand, or use words appropriately
Verbal communication impairment, related to physical barriers	Decreased ability to speak, understand or use words appropriately
Verbal communication impairment, related to psychological barriers	Decreased ability to speak, understand, or use words appropriately
Violence, potential, related to panic state	Presence of risk factors for self-directed or other-directed violence
Violence, potential: Self-directed, related to suicide attempt	Presence of risk factors for self-directed violence
Violence, potential: Self-directed or directed at others, related to organic brain dysfunction	Presence of risk factors for self-directed violence

Home health care: What it costs

The Visiting Nurses Association of Eastern Montgomery County, Pennsylvania, monitored the cost of care by nursing diagnosis for fiscal years 1986 through 1989. The average charge per diagnosis was $606.08, with an average of 9 visits during a 34-day length of stay on service. The table below provide breakdowns of the most frequently identified nursing diagnoses, the most expensive nursing diagnoses, and the least expensive nursing diagnoses, based on 5,937 cases over 4 years.

Ten most common nursing diagnoses

	Charge per case, $	Average number of visits	Number of cases
Health maintenance alteration	431	9	2,334
Self-care deficit	165	11	1,546
Knowledge deficit	371	8	1,274
Skin integrity impairment, actual	559	13	1,269
Breathing pattern, ineffective	408	9	1,019
Urinary elimination pattern alteration	309	11	500

(continued)

Home health care: What it costs *(continued)*

	Charge per case, $	Average number of visits	Number of cases
Ten most common nursing diagnoses *(continued)*			
Pain	304	9	383
Nutrition alteration: less than body requirements	292	10	348
Constipation	200	7	346
Mobility impairment	271	9	275
Ten most expensive nursing diagnoses			
Tissue integrity impairment	1,001	11	1
Sexual dysfunction	854	29	2
Verbal communication impairment	724	22	3
Parenting alteration	635	14	2
Skin integrity impairment: potential	586	12	52
Family process alteration	579	26	4
Skin integrity impairment: actual	559	13	1,269
Cardiac output, decreased	531	14	11
Airway clearance, ineffective	519	12	8
Noncompliance	455	10	1
Ten least expensive nursing diagnoses			
Coping, ineffective family: compromised	129	13	11
Self-esteem disturbance	103	8	8
Grieving, anticipatory	101	9	3
Coping, ineffective family: disabling	92	5	6
Spiritual distress	62	22	6
Fear	50	2	1
Thermoregulation, ineffective	50	2	1
Incontinence, total	25	1	1
Coping, family: potential for growth	23	1	1
Nutrition alteration: potential, more than body requirements	23	1	1

4 Diagnostic tests: What you need to know

Changing the outlook for diagnosis and treatment

New diagnostic tests are helping specialists in dozens of ways: to detect the acquired immunodeficiency syndrome (AIDS) virus sooner, to characterize biologic markers of depression, to apply imaging technology in new ways, and to evaluate the integrity of nerve pathways in comatose patients.

Detecting AIDS earlier
This 24-hour enzyme immunoassay, developed by Abbott Laboratories, can detect the p24 viral core protein of human immunodeficiency virus (HIV) in serum before any HIV antibodies develop. The antigen can be detected within 2 weeks of exposure to the virus.

The FDA has approved the new test for diagnostic and prognostic use, but not for screening blood donors, because little evidence exists that earlier detection of HIV antigens will reduce the already small risk of infection from plasma products.

Distinguishing depression
Researchers at Duke University have devised a blood test that can distinguish depression from Alzheimer's disease, and perhaps from other disorders. They found that platelets in patients with major depression have significantly fewer binding sites for imipramine, a tricyclic antidepressant, than those in patients who are healthy or who have Alzheimer's disease.

This parallels the finding that depressed patients have fewer binding sites in the hippocampus and cortex compared to healthy or Alzheimer controls. Platelets are physiologically similar to serotonergic neurons in the brain. Both platelets and neurons take up serotonin. When serotonin reaches high levels, a feedback mechanism inhibits further serotonin release. Imipramine prolongs serotonin's effect.

The number of imipramine binding sites on platelets may be a biochemical index of depression. If that's the case, blood samples, rather than brain biopsy specimens, could be used for diagnosis.

"Strokeless" digital subtraction angiography (DSA)
DSA uses video equipment and computer-assisted image enhancement to examine the cerebral vasculature. It takes fluoroscopic images before and after injection of a contrast medium. The information is digitized by a computer, which then "subtracts" the first image from the second, emphasizing the vascular picture at the expense of bone and soft tissue.

Besides providing superior image quality, the technique allows intravenous rather than arterial injection of the contrast medium, thus eliminating one of the major risks of conventional angiography—stroke. The test is most useful in diagnosing cerebrovascular disorders such as carotid stenosis and occlusion, arteriovenous malformation, aneurysms, and vascular tumors.

Diagnosing head trauma with MRI
Magnetic resonance imaging (MRI) uses a magnetic field and radiofrequency energy to produce cross-sectional scans of body tissues, which are processed by a computer into high-resolution images. The test, used primarily to aid diagnosis of intracranial and spinal lesions and soft-tissue abnormalities, proves more accurate than computed tomography (CT) scans for evaluating head trauma in an emergency department setting. In a study at the University of New Mexico, 100 head trauma patients were scanned with both

MRI and CT within 48 hours of admission. Of the 191 lesions found, CT detected 46%, while MRI detected 83%.

Magnetoencephalography (MEG): A window to the brain

Used to study epilepsy, the test employs a neuromagnetometer, a kind of supersensitive antenna, to record magnetic fields generated during neuronal transmission. A computer collects the information and generates a map of electrical activity in selected areas of the brain. The technique is more accurate than electroencephalography (EEG) because it provides readings that are more easily converted into three-dimensional information to localize areas of abnormal neuronal activity. Identifying an abnormal electrical source within the brain can guide the choice of medical or surgical treatment.

Monitoring cancer treatment with PET scans

Positron emission tomography (PET) monitors brain function by measuring emissions of injected radioisotopes. It's being used experimentally to study various disorders, such as amyotrophic lateral sclerosis, Parkinson's disease, and multiple sclerosis. Some researchers have found that PET scanning also shows promise in tracking the progress of hormonal treatment of breast cancer. The technique allows investigators to view the concentration of estrogen receptors in breast tumors and to monitor the uptake of estrogen. PET scans reduce by up to three-fourths the time needed to determine effectiveness of hormonal treatments.

Evoked potential studies

Evoked potentials refer to the brain's electrical response to stimulation of sense organs or peripheral nerves. They're recorded as electronic impulses by surface electrodes attached to the scalp and skin over various peripheral sensory nerves. A computer enhances the resulting impulses and averages the signals from repeated stimuli to supply EEG tracings that can be analyzed for abnormal conduction patterns along the nerve pathways under study.

Three types of responses are measured:

Visual evoked potentials, produced by exposing the eye to a rapidly reversing checkerboard pattern, help evaluate demyelinating disease, traumatic injury, and puzzling visual complaints.

Somatosensory evoked potentials, which are produced by electrically stimulating a peripheral sensory nerve, help diagnose peripheral nerve disease and locate brain and spinal cord lesions.

Auditory brain stem evoked potentials, produced by delivering clicks to the ear, help locate auditory lesions and evaluate brain stem integrity.

Evoked potential studies are also useful for monitoring comatose patients and patients under anesthesia, for monitoring spinal cord function during surgery, and for evaluating neurologic function in infants whose sensory systems can't be assessed.

Hematologic tests: What they measure and mean

Erythrocyte sedimentation rate

The erythrocyte sedimentation rate (ESR) measures the time required for erythrocytes in a whole blood sample to settle to the bottom of a vertical tube. Plasma proteins (notably fibrinogen and globulin) encourage aggregation, thereby increasing ESR. This test is sensitive and nonspecific, and frequently indicates disease when other physical or chemical signs are normal. It often rises significantly in widespread inflammatory disorders due to infection or autoimmune mechanisms; such elevations may be prolonged in localized inflammation and malignancy. The test is used to monitor inflammatory or malignant disease, and to aid detection and diagnosis of occult disease, such as tuberculosis, tissue necrosis, or connective tissue disease.

Normal values. Normal ESRs range from 0 to 20 mm/hour. Rates gradually rise with age.

Abnormal results. *Increased ESR* may indicate pregnancy, acute or chronic inflammation, tuberculosis, paraproteinemias (especially multiple myeloma and Waldenström's macroglobulinemia), rheumatic fever, rheumatoid arthritis, some malignancies, or anemia.

Decreased ESR may indicate polycythemia, sickle cell anemia, hyperviscosity, or low plasma protein levels.

Hematocrit

This common, reliable test measures the percentage by volume of packed red blood cells (RBCs) in a whole blood sample. For instance, a hematocrit (HCT) of 40% means that a 100-ml sample contains 40 ml of packed RBCs. This packing is achieved by centrifuging anticoagulated whole blood in a capillary tube, so that RBCs are tightly packed without hemolysis. Test results may be used to calculate mean corpuscular volume (MCV) and mean corpuscular hemoglobin (MCH) concentration, and to aid diagnosis of abnormal states of hydration, polycythemia, and anemia.

Normal values. Hematocrit values vary, depending on the patient's sex and age, type of sample and the laboratory performing the test. (See *Normal hematocrit levels.*)

Normal hematocrit levels

Age	Hematocrit level
Newborn	55% to 68%
1 week	47% to 65%
1 month	37% to 49%
3 months	30% to 36%
1 year	29% to 41%
10 years	36% to 40%
Adult male	42% to 54%
Adult female	38% to 46%

Abnormal results. *Reduced levels* may indicate anemia or hemodilution, whereas *elevated levels* may indicate polycythemia or hemoconcentration due to blood loss.

Hemoglobin

This test measures the grams of hemoglobin (Hgb) found in a deciliter (100 ml) of whole blood. Hgb concentration correlates closely with the RBC count and is affected by the Hgb-RBC ratio (MCH) and free plasma Hgb. The test is usualy performed as part of a complete blood count; it helps measure the severity of anemia or polycythemia and monitors response to therapy.

Normal values. Hgb concentration varies, depending on the patient's age and sex, and on the type of blood sample drawn. Except for infants, values for age groups listed in the accompanying chart are based on venous blood samples. (See *Normal hemoglobin levels,* page 57.)

Abnormal results. *Elevated Hgb levels* suggest hemoconcentration from polycythemia or dehydration. *Decreased Hgb levels* may indicate anemia, recent hemorrhage, or fluid retention causing hemodilution.

Red blood cell count

This test reports the number of RBCs found in a microliter (cubic millimeter) of whole blood and is included in the complete blood count. By itself, the RBC count may be used to calculate MCV and MCH. The test is also used to support other hematologic tests in diagnosis of anemia and polycythemia.

Normal values. Normal RBC values vary with age, sex, sample, and geographic location. In adult males, red cell counts range from 4.5 to 6.2 million/μl of venous blood; in adult females, 4.2 to 5.4 million/μl; and in children, 4.6 to 4.8 million/μl. In full-term infants, values range from 4.4. to 5.8 million/μl of capillary blood at birth, fall to 3.8 million/μl at age 2 months, and rise slowly thereafter. Values are typically higher in persons living at high altitudes.

Abnormal results. An *elevated RBC count* may indicate primary or secondary polycythemia. A *diminished RBC count* may indicate anemia, fluid overload, or recent hemorrhage.

Reticulocyte count

Reticulocytes are nonnucleated, immature RBCs that remain in the peripheral blood for 24 to 48 hours while maturing. In this test, reticulocytes in a whole blood sample are counted and expressed as a percentage of the total red cell count. The reticulocyte count is useful in evaluating anemia and is an index of effective erythropoiesis and bone marrow response to anemia. The test is also used to help assess blood loss, bone marrow response to anemia, and therapy for anemia. Since the error rate for a single test is very high, patients with abnormal values should be tested repeatedly.

Normal values. Reticulocytes account for 0.5% to 2% of the total

Normal hemoglobin levels

Age	Hemoglobin level
Newborn	17 to 22 g/dl
1 Week	15 to 20 g/dl
1 Month	11 to 15 g/dl
Children	11 to 13 g/dl
Men	14 to 18 g/dl
Men after middle age	12.4 to 14.9 g/dl
Women	12 to 16 g/dl
Women after middle age	11.7 to 13.8 g/dl

RBC count. In infants, the percentage is normally higher, ranging from 3.2% at birth to 0.7% at age 12 weeks.

Abnormal results. An *above-normal reticulocyte count* indicates a bone marrow response to anemia caused by hemolysis or blood loss, and may also occur after therapy for iron deficiency anemia or pernicious anemia. A *below-normal count* occurs in hypoplastic and pernicious anemias.

Iron and total iron-binding capacity

Iron is essential to the formation and function of hemoglobin, as well as many other heme and nonheme compounds. It appears in the plasma, bound to a glycoprotein called transferrin.

The test measures the amount of iron bound to transferrin; total iron-binding capacity (TIBC) measures the amount of iron that would apear in plasma if all the transferrin were saturated with iron. The saturation percentage is obtained by dividing the serum iron result by the TIBC, which reveals the actual amount of satu-

WBC differential: Reference values

| Cells | For adults | | For children (age 6 to 18) | |
| | Relative value | Absolute value | Relative value | |
			Boys	Girls
Neutrophils	47.6% to 76.8%	1,950 to 8,400/μl	38.5% to 71.5%	41.9% to 76.5%
Lymphocytes	16.2% to 43%	660 to 4,600/μl	19.4% to 51.4%	16.3% to 46.7%
Monocytes	0.6% to 9.6%	24 to 960/μl	1.1% to 11.6%	0.9% to 9.9%
Eosinophils	0.3% to 7%	12 to 760/μl	1% to 8.1%	0.8% to 8.3%
Basophils	0.3% to 2%	12 to 200/μl	0.25% to 1.3%	0.3% to 1.4%

rated transferrin. Normally, transferrin is about 30% saturated. This test is used to estimate total iron storage; aid diagnosis of hemochromatosis; help distinguish between iron deficiency anemia and anemia of chronic disease; and help evaluate nutritional status.

Normal values. Normal serum iron ranges from 70 to 150 μg/dl in men and 80 to 150 μg/dl in women. TIBC ranges from 300 to 400 μg/dl in men and 300 to 450 μg/dl in women. The solution percentage varies from 20 to 50%.

Abnormal results. *Decreased serum iron level and increased TIBC* suggest iron deficiency. *Reduced serum iron level (in presence of adequate body stores) and normal or slight drop in TIBC* suggest chronic inflammation, such as in rheumatoid arthritis.

Increased serum iron level and normal TIBC suggest iron overload (may not alter serum levels until relatively late).

White blood cell count
Part of the complete blood count, the white blood cell (WBC) count reports the number of white cells found in a microliter (mm³) of whole blood. On any given day, WBC counts may vary by as much as 2,000/μl. Such variation can result from strenuous exercise, stress, or digestion. The WBC count may rise or fall significantly in certain diseases, but is diagnostically useful only when interpreted in light of the white cell differential and of the patient's current clinical status. The test is used to determine infection or inflammation, to determine the need for further tests (such as WBC differential or bone marrow biopsy), and to monitor response to chemotherapy or radiation therapy.

Normal values. The WBC count ranges from 4,100 to 10,900/μl.

Abnormal results. An *elevated WBC count (leukocytosis)* may suggest infection or inflammation, such as an abscess, meningitis,

appendicitis, or tonsilitis. It may also suggest leukemia or tissue necrosis due to burns, MI, or gangrene.

A *diminished WBC count (leukopenia)* may suggest bone marrow depression, possibly due to a viral infection or to toxic reactions, such as those following treatment with antineoplastics, ingestion of mercury or other heavy metals, or exposure to benzene or arsenicals. It may also suggest influenza, typhoid, measles, infectious hepatitis, mononucleosis, or rubella.

White blood cell differential
Because the WBC differential evaluates the distribution and morphology of white cells, it provides more specific information about a patient's immune system than the WBC count. In this test, the laboratory classifies 100 or more white cells in a stained film of peripheral blood according to two major types of leukocytes — granulocytes (neutrophils, eosinophils, and basophils) and nongranulocytes (lymphocytes and basophils) — and determines the percentage of each type. The differential count is the relative number of each type of white cell in the blood. The test is used to evaluate the body's capacity to resist and overcome infection; to detect and identify various types of leukemia; to determine the stage and severity of an infection; and to detect and stage allergic reactions and parasitic infections.

Normal values. Normal values for the five types of WBCs classified in the differential are given for adults and children in the accompanying chart. (See *WBC differential: Reference values.*)

Abnormal results. A wide range of diseases and other conditions produces abnormal differential patterns. (See *How disorders affect WBC values.*)

How disorders affect WBC values

WBC type	How affected
Neutrophils	**Increased by:** • Infections: osteomyelitis, otitis media, salpingitis, septicemia, gonorrhea, endocarditis, smallpox, chickenpox, herpes, Rocky Mountain spotted fever • Ischemic necrosis due to myocardial infarction, burns, carcinoma • Metabolic disorders: diabetic acidosis, eclampsia, uremia, thyrotoxicosis • Stress response due to acute hemorrhage, surgery, excessive exercise, emotional distress, third trimester of pregnancy, childbirth • Inflammatory disease: rheumatic fever, rheumatoid arthritis, acute gout, vasculitis and myositis **Decreased by:** • Bone marrow depression due to radiation or cytotoxic drugs • Infections: typhoid, tularemia, brucellosis, hepatitis, influenza, measles, mumps, rubella, infectious mononucleosis • Hypersplenism: hepatic disease amd storage diseases • Collagen vascular disease, such as systemic lupus erythematosus (SLE) • Deficiency of folic acid or vitamin B_{12}
Eosinophils	**Increased by:** • Allergic disorders: asthma, hay fever, food or drug sensitivity, serum sickness, angioneurotic edema • Parasitic infections: trichinosis, hookworm, roundworm, amebiasis • Skin diseases: eczema, pemphigus, psoriasis, dermatitis, herpes • Neoplastic diseases: chronic myelocytic leukemia, Hodgkin's disease, metastases and necrosis of solid tumors • Collagen vascular disease, adrenocortical hypofunction, ulcerative colitis, polyarteritis nodosa, postsplenectomy, pernicious anemia, scarlet fever, excessive exercise **Decreased by:** • Stress response due to trauma, shock, burns, surgery, mental distress • Cushing's syndrome
Basophils	**Increased by:** • Chronic myelocytic leukemia, polycythemia vera, some chronic hemolytic anemias, Hodgkin's disease, systemic mastocytosis, myxedema, ulcerative colitis, chronic hypersensitivity states, nephrosis **Decreased by:** • Hyperthyroidism, ovulation, pregnancy, stress
Lymphocytes	**Increased by:** • Infections: pertussis, brucellosis, syphilis, tuberculosis, hepatitis, infectious mononucleosis, mumps, German measles, cytomegalovirus • Thyrotoxicosis, hypoadrenalism, ulcerative colitis, immune diseases, lymphocytic leukemia **Decreased by:** • Severe debilitating illness, such as congestive heart failure, renal failure, advanced tuberculosis • Defective lymphatic circulation, high levels of adrenal corticosteroids, immunodeficiency
Monocytes	**Increased by:** • Infections: subacute bacterial endocarditis, tuberculosis, hepatitis, malaria, Rocky Mountain spotted fever • Collagen vascular disease: SLE, rheumatoid arthritis, polyarteritis nodosa • Carcinomas, monocytic leukemia, lymphomas

Coagulation tests: What they measure and mean

Activated partial thromboplastin time (APTT)

The APTT test evaluates all the clotting factors of the intrinsic pathway—except Factors VII and XIII—by measuring the time required to form a fibrin clot. Since most congenital coagulation deficiencies occur in the intrinsic pathway, APTT is valuable in preoperative screening for bleeding tendencies. It is also the test of choice for monitoring heparin therapy.

Normal values. A fibrin clot forms 25 to 36 seconds after reagent is added.

Abnormal results. Prolonged APTT may indicate deficiency of certain plasma clotting factors; presence of heparin; presence of fibrin split products, fibrinolysins, or circulating anticoagulants that are antibodies to specific clotting factors.

Bleeding time

This test measures the duration of bleeding after a standardized skin incision. It's used to assess overall hemostatic function and to detect congenital and acquired platelet function disorders. Although this test is usually performed on patients with personal or family histories of bleeding disorders, it's also performed for preoperative screening, along with a platelet count. Bleeding time may be measured by one of four methods: Duke, Ivy, template, or modified template. The template methods are the most frequently used and the most accurate, since they standardize the incision size, making test results reproducible.

Normal values. Normal range of bleeding time is from 2 to 8 minutes in template method; from 2 to 10 minutes in modified template method; from 1 to 7 minutes in Ivy method; and from 1 to 3 minutes in Duke method.

Abnormal results. Prolonged bleeding time with a low platelet count occurs in Hodgkin's disease, acute leukemia, disseminated intravascular coagulation (DIC), Schönlein-Henoch purpura, severe hepatic disease, and severe deficiency of Factors I, II, V, VII, VIII, IX, and XI.
Prolonged bleeding time with normal platelet count occurs in platelet function disorders, such as thrombasthenia and thrombocytopathia.

Platelet count

One of the most important screening tests of platelet function, the platelet count proves vital for monitoring chemotherapy, radiation therapy, and severe thrombocytosis and throbocytopenia. A platelet count that falls below 50,000 can cause spontaneous bleeding; when it drops below 5,000, fatal central nervous system bleeding or massive gastrointestinal hemorrhage is possible.

This test is used to evaluate platelet production, to assess effects of chemotherapy or radiation therapy on platelet production, to aid diagnosis of thrombocytopenia and thrombocytosis, and to confirm a visual estimate of platelet number and morphology from a stained blood film.

Normal values. Normal platelet counts range from 130,000 to 370,000/mm³.

Abnormal results. Increased platelet count (thrombocytosis) may indicate hemorrhage, infectious disorders, malignancies, iron deficiency anemia, and recent surgery or pregnancy. It may also suggest inflammatory disorders, such as collagen vascular disease; primary thrombocytosis; polycythemia vera; and chronic myelogenous leukemia.
Decreased platelet count (thrombocytopenia) may indicate aplastic or hypoplastic bone marrow; infiltrative bone marrow disease, such as carcinoma, leukemia or disseminated infection; megakaryocytic hypoplasia; ineffective thrombopoiesis due to folic acid or vitamin B_{12} deficiency; pooling of platelets in an enlarged spleen; increased platelet destruction due to drugs or immune disorders; disseminated intravascular coagulation; Bernard-Soulier syndrome; or mechanical injury to platelets.

Prothrombin time

Also known as pro time or PT, this test indirectly measures prothrombin and is an excellent screening procedure for overall evaluation of extrinsic coagulation Factors V, VII, and X, and of prothrombin and fibrinogen. PT is the test of choice for monitoring oral anticoagulant therapy. In a patient receiving oral anticoagulants, PT is usually kept one and a half to two times the normal control value. Prolonged PT that exceeds two and a half times the control value is commonly associated with abnormal bleeding.

Normal values. Normal PT values range from 9.6 to 11.8 seconds in males and from 9.5 to 11.3 seconds in females. Values may vary depending on source of tissue thromboplastin and type of devices used to measure clot formation.

Abnormal results. Increased PT may indicate deficiencies in fibrinogen, prothrombin, or Factors V, VII, or X (specific assays can pinpoint such deficiencies); vitamin K deficiency; hepatic disease; or ongoing anticoagulant therapy.

Whole blood clotting time

This test measures the interval required for fresh whole blood to clot in vitro at 98.6° F (37° C) and grossly evaluates the intrinsic clotting mechanism. Unfortunately, the test is lengthy, nonspecific for any coagulation factor, and unreliable as a screening test. Abnormal clotting time requires further tests, such as prothrombin time, APTT, and specific factor assays.

Normal values. Normal blood clotting time is 5 to 15 minutes.

Abnormal results. Increased whole blood clotting time may indicate severe deficiency of coagulation factors (except Factors VII and XIII), or presence of anticoagulants.

ABGs and electrolytes: What they measure and mean

Arterial blood gas analysis

This test helps evaluate the efficiency of pulmonary gas exchange, assess ventilatory control, determine the acid-base level of the blood, and monitor respiratory therapy. Five values are commonly measured:
• partial pressure of oxygen dissolved in arterial blood (PaO_2), which indicates how much oxygen the lungs are delivering to the blood
• partial pressure of carbon dioxide ($PaCO_2$) dissolved in arterial blood, which indicates how efficiently the lungs eliminate carbon dioxide
• hydrogen ion concentration (pH), which indicates the acid-base level of the blood
• oxygen saturation (O_2 Sat), which is the percentage of hemoglobin carrying oxygen

• bicarbonate levels (HCO_3-), which indicates the amount of alkaline substance dissolved in the blood.

Another value, oxygen content (O_2Ct) measures the volume of oxygen combined with hemoglobin in arterial blood. This value isn't commonly measured.

Normal values.
PaO_2: 75 to 100 mm Hg
$PaCO_2$: 35 to 45 mm Hg
pH: 7.35 to 7.42
O_2 Sat: 94% to 100%
HCO_3- : 22 to 26 mEq/liter
O_2Ct: 15% to 23%

Abnormal results. (See *Abnormal ABG values,* and *Acid-base disorders,* page 62.)

Serum calcium

This test measures levels of calcium, a predominantly extracellular cation that helps regulate and promote neuromuscular and enzyme activity, skeletal development, and blood coagulation. Over 98% of the body's calcium is found in the bones and teeth. However, calcium can shift in and out of these structures. For example, when calcium concentrations in the blood fall below normal, calcium ions move out of the bones and teeth to help restore blood levels. This test is used to aid diagnosis of neuromuscular, skeletal, and endocrine disorders; dysrhythmias; blood-clotting deficiencies; and acid-base imbalance.

Normal values. Serum levels range from 8.9 to 10.1 mg/dl (atomic absorption), or from 4.5 to 5.5 mEq/liter. In children, serum calcium levels are higher than in adults. Calcium levels can rise as high as 12 mg/dl or 6 mEq/liter during phases of rapid bone growth.

Abnormal results. Increased levels (hypercalcemia) may indicate hyperparathyroidism, parathyroid tumors, Paget's disease of bone, multiple myeloma, metastatic car-

Abnormal ABG values

PaO_2

Value less than 50 mm Hg indicates hypoxia. PaO_2 between 0 and 80 mm Hg may or may not indicate hypoxia, depending on age of patient and oxygen concentration being given. A newborn has a PaO_2 between 40 and 60 mm Hg. After age 60, PaO_2 may fall below 80 mm Hg without hypoxia.

$PaCO_2$

Value above 45 mm Hg indicates hypoventilation (hypercapnia). Value below 35 mm Hg indicates hyperventilation (hypocapnia). $PaCO_2$ level may also indicate respiratory (lung-regulated) acid-base imbalance. If patient's pH shows an imbalance, $PaCO_2$ above 45 mm Hg indicates respiratory acidosis; $PaCO_2$ below 35 mm Hg indicates respiratory alkalosis.

pH

Value greater than 7.45 indicates alkalosis. Value less than 7.35 indicates acidosis.

O_2 Sat

If PaO_2 is between 60 and 95 mm Hg, O_2 Sat should remain above 85%. Sharply decreased values usually indicate drop in PaO_2 below 50 mm Hg.

HCO_3-

Value greater than 26 mEq/liter indicates metabolic (kidney-regulated) alkalosis. Value less than 22 mEq/liter indicates metabolic acidosis.

Acid-base disorders

Disorders and ABG findings	Possible causes
Respiratory acidosis (excess CO_2 retention) pH < 7.35 HCO_3^- > 26 mEq/liter (if compensating) $PaCO_2$ > 45 mm Hg	• Central nervous system depression from drugs, injury, or disease • Asphyxia • Hypoventilation due to pulmonary, cardiac, musculoskeletal, or neuromuscular disease
Respiratory alkalosis (excess CO_2 excretion) pH > 7.42 HCO_3^- < 22 mEq/liter (if compensating) $PaCO_2$ < 35 mm Hg	• Hyperventilation due to anxiety, pain, or improper ventilator settings • Respiratory stimulation by drugs, disease, hypoxia, fever, or high room temperature • Gram-negative bacteremia
Metabolic acidosis (HCO_3^- loss, acid retention) pH < 7.35 HCO_3^- < 22 mEq/liter $PaCO_2$ < 35 mm Hg (if compensating)	• HCO_3^- depletion due to renal disease, diarrhea, or small-bowel fistulas • Excessive production of organic acids due to hepatic disease; endocrine disorders, including diabetes mellitus; hypoxia; shock; or drug intoxication • Inadequate excretion of acids due to renal disease
Metabolic alkalosis (HCO_3^- retention, acid loss) pH > 7.42 HCO_3^- > 26 mEq/liter $PaCO_2$ > 45 mm Hg (if compensating)	• Loss of hydrochloric acid from prolonged vomiting, gastric suctioning • Loss of potassium from increased renal excretion (as in diuretic therapy), steroid overdose • Excessive alkali ingestion

cinoma, multiple fractures, prolonged immobilization, inadequate calcium secretion (as in adrenal insufficiency and renal disease), excessive calcium ingestion, or overuse of antacids such as calcium carbonate.

Diminished levels (hypocalcemia) may indicate hypoparathyroidism, total parathyroidectomy, malabsorption, Cushing's syndrome, renal failure, acute pancreatitis, or peritonitis.

Serum chloride
This test measures serum levels of chloride, the major extracellular fluid anion. Interacting with sodium, chloride helps maintain the osmotic pressure of blood and so helps regulate blood volume and arterial pressure. Chloride levels relate inversely to those of bicarbonate and thus reflect acid-base balance. They're regulated by aldosterone, secondarily to regulation of sodium.

The test is used to detect acid-base imbalance (acidosis and alkalosis) and to aid in evaluating fluid status and extracellular cation-anion balance.

Normal values. Serum chloride levels range from 100 to 108 mEq/liter.

Abnormal results. *Elevated levels (hyperchloremia)* can indicate severe dehydration, complete renal shutdown, head injury producing neurogenic hyperventilation, or primary aldosteronism.

Depressed levels (hypochloremia) can indicate prolonged vomiting, gastric suctioning, intestinal fistula, chronic renal failure, Addison's disease, congestive heart failure (dilutional hypochloremia), or edema (dilutional hypochloremia).

Serum magnesium
This test measures serum levels of magnesium, the most abundant intracellular cation after potassium. Vital to neuromuscular function, this often overlooked electrolyte helps regulate intracellular metabolism, activates many essential enzymes, and affects the metabolism of nucleic acids and proteins. Magnesium also helps transport sodium and potassium across cell membranes and, through its effect on parathyroid hormone secretion, influences intracellular calcium levels. The test helps to evaluate electrolyte status and neuromuscular or renal function.

Normal values. Serum magnesium levels range from 1.7 to 2.1 mg/dl (atomic absorption) or from 1.5 to 2.5 mEq/liter.

Abnormal results. *Increased levels* can result from renal failure and Addison's disease.

Lowered levels can result from chronic alcoholism, malabsorption syndrome, diarrhea, faulty absorption following bowel resection, prolonged bowel or gastric aspiration, acute pancreatitis, primary aldosteronism, or severe burns. They can also result from hypercalcemic conditions (including hyperparathyroidism) or certain diuretic therapies.

Serum phosphates

This test measures serum levels of phosphates, the dominant cellular anions. Phosphates help store and utilize body energy and help regulate calcium levels, carbohydrate and lipid metabolism, and acid-base balance. Phosphates are essential to bone formation; about 85% of the body's phosphates are found in bone. Calcium and phosphate interact reciprocally, so that urinary excretion of phosphates increases or decreases in inverse proportion to serum calcium levels. Since serum phosphate values alone have limited diagnostic value, they should be interpreted in light of serum calcium results. The test is used to aid diagnosis of renal disorders and acid-base balance, and to detect endrocrine, skeletal, and calcium disorders.

Normal values. Serum levels range from 2.5 to 4.5 mg/dl (atomic absorption), or from 1.8 to 2.6 mEq/liter. Children have higher serum phosphate levels than adults. Phosphate levels can rise as high as 7 mg/dl or 4.1 mEq/liter during periods of increased bone growth.

Abnormal results. Elevated levels (hyperphosphatemia) can stem from skeletal disease, healing fractures, hypoparathyroidism, acromegaly, diabetic acidosis, high intestinal obstruction, or renal failure.

Diminished levels (hypophosphatemia) can stem from malnutrition, malabsorption syndrome, hyperparathyroidism, renal tubular acidosis, or treatment of diabetic acidosis.

Serum potassium

This test measures serum levels of potassium, the major intracellular cation. Vital to homeostasis, potassium maintains cellular osmotic equilibrium and helps regulate muscle activity (it is essential in maintaining electrical conduction within the cardiac and skeletal muscles). Potassium also helps regulate enzyme activity and acid-base balance, and influences kidney function.

Although serum values and clinical symptoms can indicate a potassium imbalance, an ECG provides the definitive diagnosis. The test is used to evaluate clinical signs of potassium excess (hyperkalemia) or potassium depletion (hypokalemia); to monitor renal function, acid-base balance, and glucose metabolism; and to detect the origin of dysrhythmias.

Normal values. Serum levels range from 3.8 to 5.5 mEq/liter.

Abnormal results. Heightened levels (hyperkalemia) can result from burns, crush injuries, diabetic ketoacidosis, MI, renal failure, and Addison's disease.

Diminished levels (hypokalemia) can result from aldosteronism, Cushing's syndrome, loss of body fluids, and excessive licorice ingestion.

Serum sodium

This test measures serum levels of sodium, the major extracellular cation. Sodium affects body water distribution, maintains osmotic pressure of extracellular fluid, and helps promote neuromuscular function; it also helps maintain acid-base balance and influences chloride and potassium levels. Because extracellular sodium concentration helps the kidneys regulate body water, serum sodium levels are evaluated in relation to the amount of water in the body. Urine sodium determinations are commonly more sensitive to early changes in sodium balance and should always be evaluated simultaneously with serum sodium findings. The test is used to evaluate fluid-electrolyte and acid-base balance, and related neuromuscular, renal, and adrenal functions.

Normal values. Serum sodium levels range from 135 to 145 mEq/liter.

Abnormal results. Sodium imbalance can result from loss or gain of sodium, or from a change in water volume. Remember, serum sodium results must be interpreted in light of the patient's state of hydration. (See *Fluid imbalances,* page 64.)

Increased sodium levels (hypernatremia) can indicate inadequate water intake, excessive sodium intake, diabetes insipidus, impaired renal function, prolonged hyperventilation, severe vomiting (occasionally), severe diarrhea (occasionally), and sodium retention (as in aldosteronism).

Reduced sodium levels (hyponatremia) can indicate inadequate sodium intake, excessive sodium loss due to profuse sweating, GI suctioning, diuretic therapy, diarrhea, vomiting, adrenal insufficiency, burns, and chronic renal insufficiency with acidosis.

Total carbon dioxide content

This test measures the total concentration of all forms of dissolved CO_2 (H_2CO_3, $H+$, and HCO_3-) in serum, plasma, or whole blood samples. Because about 90% of CO_2 in serum is in the form of bicarbonate, the test closely assesses bicarbonate levels. Total CO_2 content reflects the adequacy of gas exchange in the lungs and the efficiency of the carbonic acid-bicarbonate buffer system, which maintains acid-base balance and normal pH. Consequently, this test is commonly ordered for patients with respiratory insufficiency and is usually included in any assessment of electrolyte balance. For maximum clinical significance, test results must be considered with both pH and arterial blood gas values.

Normal values. Total CO_2 levels range from 22 to 34 mEq/liter.

Abnormal results. *Increased CO₂ content* may occur in:
- metabolic alkalosis, such as in severe vomiting or continuous gastric drainage.
- respiratory acidosis, as in hypoventilation from emphysema or pneumonia.

- primary aldosteronism and Cushing's syndrome.
  Decreased CO₂ content may occur in:
- metabolic acidosis, such as in diabetic acidosis, renal tubular acidosis, severe diarrhea, and intestinal drainage.

- respiratory alkalosis, such as in hyperventilation.

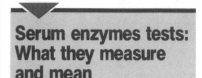

Serum enzymes tests: What they measure and mean

Acid phosphatase
A group of phosphatase enzymes most active at a pH of about 5.0, acid phosphatase appears primarily in the prostate gland and semen, and to a lesser extent in the liver, spleen, red blood cells, bone marrow, and platelets. Prostatic and erythrocytic enzymes are this group's two major isoenzymes that can be separated in the laboratory; the prostatic isoenzyme is more specific for prostatic cancer. The more widespread the tumor, the more likely it is to produce high serum acid phosphatase levels. This test is used to detect prostatic cancer and to monitor response to therapy.

Normal values. Serum values for total acid phosphatase depend on the test method, and range from 0 to 1.1 Bodansky units/ml; 1 to 4 King-Armstrong units/ml; 0.13 to 0.63 Bessey-Lowery-Brock (BLB) units/ml.

Abnormal results. *Markedly increased levels* indicate a tumor that has spread beyond the prostatic capsule. *Moderately increased levels* can indicate prostatic infarction, Paget's disease, Gaucher's disease, and other conditions, such as multiple myeloma.
  Declining high acid phosphatase levels point toward successful treatment of prostatic cancer.

Alanine aminotransferase (ALT)
Also known as serum glutamic-pyruvic transaminase (SGPT), this test

Fluid imbalances

Causes	Signs and symptoms	Laboratory findings
Hypervolemia		
• Increased water intake • Decreased water output due to renal disease • Congestive heart failure • Excessive ingestion or infusion of sodium chloride • Long-term administration of adrenocortical hormones • Excessive infusion of isotonic solutions	• Increased — blood pressure — pulse rate — body weight — respiratory rate • Bounding peripheral pulses • Moist pulmonary crackles • Moist mucous membranes • Moist respiratory secretions • Edema • Weakness • Convulsions and coma due to swelling of brain cells	• Decreased — red cell count — hemoglobin concentration — packed cell volume — serum sodium concentration (dilutional decrease) — urine specific gravity
Hypovolemia		
• Diminished water intake • Fluid loss due to diarrhea, fever, vomiting • Systemic infection • Impaired renal concentrating ability • Fistulous drainage • Severe burns • Hidden fluid in body cavities	• Elevated — pulse rate — respiratory rate • Decreased — blood pressure — body weight • Weak and thready peripheral pulses • Thick, slurred speech • Thirst • Oliguria (diminished urine output compared with fluid intake) • Anuria • Dry skin	• Elevated — red cell count — hemoglobin concentration — packed cell volume — serum sodium concentration — urine specific gravity

measures serum ALT levels. An enzyme necessary for tissue energy production, ALT primarily appears in hepatocellular cytoplasm, with lesser amounts in the kidneys, heart, and skeletal muscles. The enzyme is a relatively specific indicator of acute hepatocellular damage. When such damage occurs, ALT is released from the cytoplasm into the bloodstream, often before jaundice appears, resulting in abnormally high serum levels that may not return to normal for days or weeks.

The test is used to help detect acute hepatic disease—especially hepatitis, and cirrhosis without jaundice—and to evaluate treatment. It's also used to help distinguish between myocardial and hepatic tissue damage, and to assess hepatoxicity of some drugs.

Normal values. Serum ALT levels in men range from 10 to 32 units/liter; in women, from 9 to 24 units/liter. The normal range for infants is twice that of adults.

Abnormal results. Extremely high ALT levels (up to 50 times normal) can indicate viral or severe drug-induced hepatitis and other hepatic disease with extensive necrosis.

Moderately high to high ALT levels can stem from infectious mononucleosis, intrahepatic cholestasis, cholecystitis, early or improving viral hepatitis, and severe hepatic congestion due to heart failure.

Slightly to moderately high ALT levels can result from active cirrhosis, drug-induced alcoholic hepatitis, and other conditions that cause acute hepatocellular injury.

Marginal ALT elevations occasionally occur in acute MI.

Alkaline phosphatase
This test measures serum levels of alkaline phosphatase, an enzyme that influences bone calcification and lipid and metabolite transport.

Total serum levels reflect the combined activity of several alkaline phosphatase isoenzymes. The test is especially sensitive to mild biliary obstruction and is a primary indicator of space-occupying hepatic lesions. However, because both skeletal and hepatic diseases can raise alkaline phosphatase levels, the test's most specific application is in diagnosing metabolic bone disease. Additional liver function studies are usually needed to identify hepatobiliary disorders. The test may also be used to assess response to vitamin D in treatment of rickets.

Normal values. Normal values vary with test method used. Total alkaline phosphatase levels, when measured by chemical inhibition, range from 90 to 239 units/liter for males; for females under age 45, the range is 76 to 196 units/liter; for women over age 45, the range widens from 87 to 250 units/liter, for unknown reasons. Because alkaline phosphatase concentrations rise during active bone formation in growth, infants, children, and adolescents normally have levels that may be 3 times as high as those of adults. Pregnancy also elevates alkaline phosphatase levels. When the Bodansky method is used, normal range is from 1.5 to 4 units/dl; for the King-Armstrong method, normal adult values range from 4 to 13.5 units/dl.

Abnormal results. Markedly elevated levels can stem from severe biliary obstruction by gallstones, malignant or infectious infiltrations or fibrosis, Paget's disease, bone metastasis, and hyperparathyroidism.

Moderately elevated levels suggest cirrhosis, mononucleosis, viral hepatitis, osteomalacia, and deficiency-induced rickets.

Reduced levels can indicate hypophosphatasia or protein or magnesium deficiency.

Amylase
Synthesized primarily in the pancreas and salivary glands, amylase is secreted into the GI tract. This enzyme helps digest starch and glycogen in the mouth, stomach, and intestine. In suspected acute pancreatic disease, measurement of serum or urine amylase is the most important laboratory test. Highest serum levels occur 4 to 8 hours after onset of acute pancreatitis, then drop to normal in 48 to 72 hours. Determination of urine levels should follow normal serum amylase results, to rule out pancreatitis.

More than 20 methods of measuring serum amylase exist, with different ranges of normal values that cannot always be converted to a standard measurement. The classic saccharogenic method described here reports serum amylase in Somogyi units/dl.

Normal values. Serum levels range from 60 to 180 Somogyi units/dl.

Abnormal results. Markedly increased levels occur 4 to 12 hours after the onset of acute pancreatitis. *Moderately increased levels* can signal obstruction of the common bile duct, pancreatic duct, or ampulla of Vater; pancreatic injury from perforated peptic ulcer; pancreatic cancer; or acute salivary gland disease.

Decreased levels can indicate chronic pancreatitis, pancreatic cancer, cirrhosis, hepatitis, or toxemia of pregnancy.

Aspartate aminotransferase (AST)
Also known as serum glutamic-oxaloacetic transaminase (SGOT), this enzyme occurs primarily in cells of the liver, heart, heart, skeletal muscles, kidneys, pancreas, and, to a lesser extent, in red blood cells. It's released into serum in proportion to the extent of cellular damage. Depending on when during the course of the disease the initial sample was drawn,

AST levels can rise—indicating increasing disease severity and tissue damage—or fall—indicating disease resolution and tissue repair. Thus, the relative change in AST values serves as a reliable monitoring mechanism. The test is commonly used to detect recent MI, to help detect and diagnose acute hepatic disease, and to monitor patient progress and prognosis in cardiac and hepatic diseases.

Normal values. AST levels range from 8 to 20 units/liter. Normal

AST elevations in MI and hepatic disease

In acute myocardial infarction (MI), aspartate aminotransferase (serum glutamic-oxaloacetic transaminase [SGOT]) levels rise 6 to 10 hours after onset of chest pain, peak in 24 to 48 hours, and—if the infarct doesn't extend or another MI doesn't occur—drop to normal in 4 or 5 days. The degree of elevation is roughly proportional to the number of damaged cells, and to the interval between the beginning of the infarction and the time the sample is drawn. Values 15 to 20 times normal indicate extensive myocardial damage and a guarded prognosis. Variable increases occur in congestive heart failure and shock, due to hypoxia and hepatic congestion.

In hepatic disease, AST (SGOT) levels usually rise within 4 to 8 hours of onset of acute disease, peak in 24 to 48 hours, and drop to normal in 4 to 8 days or longer, depending on the disease. Subsequent elevations generally indicate a relapse. Serum levels commonly rise before symptoms (such as jaundice) appear.

values for infants may be four times higher than those for adults.

Abnormal results. *Extremely high levels (more than 20 times normal)* occur in acute viral hepatitis, severe skeletal muscle trauma, extensive surgery, drug-induced hepatic injury, and severe passive liver congestion.

High levels (10 to 20 times normal) occur in severe MI, severe infectious mononucleosis, and alcoholic cirrhosis. They also occur in the prodromal or resolving stages of conditions that cause extremely high levels.

Moderately high to high levels (5 to 10 times normal) can signal Duchenne muscular dystrophy, dermatomyositis, chronic hepatitis, prodromal or resolving stages of above conditions causing high levels.

Slightly to moderately high levels (2 to 5 times normal) can indicate hemolytic anemia, metastatic hepatic tumors, acute pancreatitis, pulmonary emboli, alcohol withdrawal syndrome, fatty liver, or biliary obstruction. (See *AST elevations in MI and hepatic disease.*)

Creatine phosphokinase
This enzyme catalyzes the creatine-creatinine metabolic pathway in muscle cells and brain tissue. Because of its intimate role in energy production, CPK relects normal tissue catabolism; an increase above normal serum levels indicates trauma to cells with high CPK content. CPK may be separated into three isoenzymes: CPK-BB, which occurs primarily in brain tissue; CPK-MB, which occurs in cardiac muscle (some also occurs in skeletal muscle); and CPK-MM, which occurs in skeletal muscle. CPK-MM constitutes over 99% of total CPK normally present in serum.

This test is used to detect and diagnose acute MI and reinfarction

(CPK-MB primarily used); to evaluate possible causes of chest pain and to monitor severity of myocardial ischemia after cardiac surgery, cardiac catheterization, or cardioversion (CPK-MB primarily used); and to detect non-neurogenic skeletal muscle disorders, such as Duchenne muscular dystrophy (total CPK primarily used), and early dermatomyositis.

Normal values. Total CPK values determined by ultraviolet or kinetic measurement range from 23 to 99 units/liter for men, and from 15 to 57 units/liter for women. CPK levels may be significantly higher in extremely muscular people. Infants up to age 1 have levels 2 to 4 times higher than adult levels, possibly reflecting birth trauma and striated muscle development. Normal ranges for isoenzyme levels are as follows: CPK-BB, undetectable; CPK-MB, undetectable to 7 IU/liter; CPK-MM, 5 to 70 IU/liter.

Abnormal results. *Detectable CPK-BB isoenzyme* can indicate brain tissue injury, certain widespread malignant tumors, severe shock, or renal failure.

CPK-MB isoenzyme greater than 5% of total CPK (or more than 10 IU/liter) can result from MI or cardiac surgery. In acute MI and after cardiac surgery, CPK-MB begins to rise in 2 to 4 hours, peaks in 12 to 24 hours, and usually returns to normal in 24 to 48 hours. Persistent elevations or increasing levels indicate ongoing myocardial damage.

A *slight rise in CPK-MB isoenzyme* occurs in muscular dystrophies, polymyositis, and severe myoglobinuria.

Increased CPK-MM isoenzyme may reflect trauma to skeletal muscle, such as surgery and I.M. injections; dermatomyositis and muscular dystrophy; hypothyroidism; or muscular activity due to agitation as in acute psychotic episode.

Elevated total CPK levels may indicate severe hypokalemia, carbon monoxide poisoning, malignant hyperthermia, postconvulsions, or alcoholic cardiomyopathy. They occur occasionally in pulmonary or cerebral infarction.

Lactic dehydrogenase

Because lactic dehydrogenase (LDH) occurs in almost all body tissues, cellular damage causes an elevation of total serum LDH, thus limiting the diagnostic usefulness of the test. However, five tissue-specific isoenzymes can be identified and measured. Two of these, LDH_1 and LDH_2, appear primarily in the heart, red blood cells (RBCs) and kidneys; LDH_3, primarily in the lungs; and LDH_4 and LDH_5, in the liver and the skeletal muscles.

The specificity of these isoenzymes proves useful in diagnosing hepatic, pulmonary, and erythrocytic damage. But their widest clinical application (with other cardiac enzyme tests) is in diagnosing acute MI. LDH isoenzyme assay is also useful when CPK hasn't been measured within 24 hours of an acute MI. The myocardial LDH level rises later than CPK (12 to 48 hours after infarction begins), peaks in 2 to 5 days, and drops to normal in 7 to 10 days, if tissue necrosis does not persist.

Normal values. Total LDH levels range from 48 to 115 IU/liter. Distribution is as follows:
LDH_1: 18.1% to 29% of total
LDH_2: 29.4% to 37.5% of total
LDH_3: 18.8% to 26% of total
LDH_4: 9.2% to 16.5% of total
LDH_5: 5.3% to 13.4% of total

Abnormal results. See *Diagnostic LDH isoenzyme variations in disease.*

Diagnostic LDH isoenzyme variations in disease

Diseases	LDH_1	LDH_2	LDH_3	LDH_4	LDH_5
Cardiovascular					
Myocardial infarction					
Myocardial infarction with hepatic congestion					
Rheumatic carditis					
Myocarditis					
Congestive heart failure (decompensated)					
Shock					
Angina pectoris	Normal				
Pulmonary					
Pulmonary embolism	Normal				
Pulmonary infarction			Not diagnostic		
Hematologic					
Pernicious anemia					
Hemolytic anemia					
Sickle cell anemia					
Hepatobiliary					
Hepatitis					
Active cirrhosis					
Hepatic congestion					

Normal ■   Diagnostic □   Not diagnostic ▢

Hormone tests: What they measure and mean

Free thyroxine

This test measures serum levels of free thyroxine (FT_4), the minute portion of T_4 not bound to thyroxine-binding globulin (TBG) and other serum proteins. As the active component of T_4, this un-bound hormone enters target cells and is responsible (along with free T_3) for the thyroid's effects on cellular metabolism. The test may be useful in the 5% of patients in whom the standard T_3 or T_4 tests fail to produce diagnostic results.

Normal values. Values vary, depending on the laboratory. The range for FT_4 is 0.8 to 3.3 ng/dl.

Abnormal results. *Increased levels* occur in hyperthyroidism.

Diminished levels occur in hypothyroidism (except in patients receiving T_3 replacement therapy).

Thyroxine
Thyroxine (T_4) is secreted by the thyroid gland in response to thyroid-stimulating hormone (TSH) from the pituitary gland, and, indirectly, to thyrotropin-releasing hormone (TRH) from the hypothalamus. The rate of secretion is normally regulated by a complex system of negative and positive feedback involving the thyroid, anterior pituitary, and hypothalamus. Only a fraction of T_4 (about 0.3%) circulates freely in the blood; the rest binds strongly to plasma proteins, primarily to thyroxine-binding globulin (TBG). This radioimmunoassay is one of the most common diagnostic indicators of thyroid function and measures the total circulating T_4 level when TBG is normal.

Normal values. Total T_4 levels range from 5 to 13.5 mcg/dl.

Abnormal results. Heightened levels occur in primary hyperthyroidism as well as in secondary hyperthyroidism, including excessive T_4 (L-thyroxine) replacement therapy.
Depressed levels occur in primary hypothyroidism; secondary hypothyroidism; T_4 suppression by normal, elevated, or replacement levels of triiodothyronine (T_3).

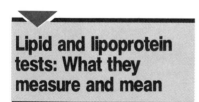

Lipid and lipoprotein tests: What they measure and mean

Lipoprotein-cholesterol fractionation
Cholesterol fractionation tests isolate and measure the cholesterol in serum—low-density lipoprotein (LDL) and high-density lipoprotein (HDL)—by ultracentrifugation or electrophoresis. They are used to assess the risk of coronary artery disease (CAD). The cholesterol in LDL and HDL fractions is significant, since the Framingham Heart Study has shown that cholesterol in HDL is inversely related to the incidence of CAD—the higher the HDL level, the lower the incidence of CAD; conversely, the higher the LDL level, the higher the incidence of CAD.

Normal values. Because normal cholesterol levels vary according to age, sex, geographic region, and ethnic group, check the laboratory for the normal values in your hospital. An alternate method—measuring cholesterol and trigylceride levels, separating out HDL and using these values to calculate LDL—provides HDL-cholesterol levels that range from 29 to 77 mg/100 ml and LDL-cholesterol levels that range from 62 to 185 mg/100 ml.

Abnormal results. Increased LDL levels indicate a heightened risk of CAD. *Elevated HDL levels* usually reflect a healthy state, but can indicate chronic hepatitis, early primary biliary cirrhosis, or alcohol consumption.
Sharp increases in alpha-2-HDL levels may indicate CAD.

Total cholesterol
This quantitative analysis of serum cholesterol measures the circulating levels of free cholesterol and cholesterol esters. Total cholesterol is the only cholesterol routinely measured. High serum cholesterol levels may be associated with an increased risk of CAD. Besides assessing the risk of CAD, the test is used to evaluate fat metabolism, and to aid in diagnosing nephrotic syndrome, pancreatitis, hepatic disease, and hypothyroidism and hyperthyroidism.

Normal values. Total cholesterol concentrations vary with age and sex. The ideal level is < 200 mg/dl;

borderline high levels are 200 to 239 mg/dl; high levels are > 240 mg/dl.

Abnormal results. Increased levels (hypercholesterolemia) can indicate a risk of CAD, incipient hepatitis, lipid disorders, bile duct blockage, nephrotic syndrome, obstructive jaundice, pancreatitis, or hypothyroidism.
Decreased levels (hypocholesterolemia) can stem from malnutrition, cellular necrosis of the liver, or hyperthyroidism.

Triglycerides
This test provides quantitative analysis of triglycerides—the main storage form of lipids—which constitute about 95% of fatty tissue. Increased or decreased serum triglyceride levels merely suggest a clinical abnormality, and additional tests are required for definitive diagnosis. However, serum triglyceride analysis permits early identification of hyperlipemia (characteristic in nephrotic syndrome and other conditions) and risk of CAD.

Normal values. Triglyceride values are age-related. Some controversy exists over the most appropriate normal ranges, but the following are fairly widely accepted:

Age	Triglycerides (mg/dl)
0 to 29	10 to 140
30 to 39	10 to 150
40 to 49	10 to 160
50 to 59	10 to 190

Abnormal results. Increased triglycerides and cholesterol levels indicate an exaggerated risk of CAD. *Mildly to moderately increased triglycerides* can idicate biliary obstruction, diabetes, nephrotic syndrome, endocrinopathies, and overconsumption of alcohol. *Markedly increased levels* without an identifiable cause suggest congenital hyperlipoproteinemia.

Decreased levels occur in malnutrition and abetalipoproteinemia.

▼
Protein and pigment tests: What they measure and mean

Bilirubin
This test measures serum levels of bilirubin, the most abundant bile pigment and the major product of hemoglobin catabolism. Effective conjugation and excretion of bilirubin depends on a properly functioning hepatobiliary system and a normal red blood cell turnover rate. As a result, measurement of unconjugated (indirect), or prehepatic, bilirubin and conjugated (direct), or posthepatic, bilirubin, can help evaluate hepatobiliary and erythropoietic functions. Serum bilirubin measurements are especially important in the newborn, because elevated unconjugated bilirubin can accumulate in the brain and cause irreparable tissue damage.

The test is used to evaluate liver function; to aid differential diagnosis of jaundice and monitor its progression; to aid diagnosis of biliary obstruction and hemolytic anemia; and to determine whether a newborn requires an exchange transfusion or phototherapy because of dangerously high unconjugated bilirubin levels.

Normal values. In an adult, indirect serum bilirubin measures 1.1 mg/dl or less; direct serum bilirubin, less than 0.5 mg/dl. Total serum bilirubin in the newborn measures 1 to 12 mg/dl.

Abnormal results. Increased indirect serum bilirubin levels can idicate hepatic damage, hemolytic anemia; congenital enzyme deficiencies, such as Gilbert's disease. *Elevated direct serum bilirubin levels* can stem from biliary obstruction. *Heightened direct and indirect serum bilirubin levels* can result from continued hemolysis, continued biliary obstruction with resulting hepatic damage.

Blood urea nitrogen (BUN)
This test measures the nitrogen fraction of urea, the chief end product of protein metabolism. Urea constitutes 40% to 50% of the blood's nonprotein nitrogen. The BUN level reflects protein intake and renal excretory capacity, but is a less reliable indicator of uremia than the serum creatinine level. The test is used to evaluate renal function and aid in diagnosing renal disease, and to help assess hydration.

Normal values. BUN values normally range from 8 to 20 mg/dl.

Abnormal results. Elevated BUN levels can signal renal disease; reduced renal blood flow, as in dehydration; urinary tract obstruction; increased protein catabolism, as in burns.

Diminished levels can result from severe hepatic damage, malnutrition, overhydration.

Creatinine
This test provides a more sensitive measure of renal damage than blood urea nitrogen (BUN) levels, because renal impairment is virtually the only cause of creatinine elevation. Creatinine is a nonprotein end product of creatine metabolism. Like creatine, creatinine appears in serum in amounts proportional to the body's muscle mass; unlike creatine, it is easily excreted by the kidneys, with minimal or no tubular reabsorption. Creatinine levels, therefore, are di-

rectly related to the glomerular filtration rate. Since creatinine levels normally remain constant, elevated levels usually indicate diminished renal function. The test is used to assess renal glomerular function and to screen for renal damage.

Normal values. Serum creatinine concentrations in males normally range from 0.8 to 1.2 mg/dl; in females, from 0.6 to 0.9 mg/dl.

Abnormal results. Increased creatinine levels indicate renal disease that has seriously damaged 50% or more of the nephrons, gigantism, or acromegaly.

Proteins
This test measures serum albumin and globulins, the major blood proteins, by fractionating them in an electric field at pH 8.6. Albumin maintains oncotic pressure (preventing leakage of capillary plasma) and transports substances that are insoluble in water alone, such as bilirubin, fatty acids, hormones, and drugs.

Four types of globulins exist—alpha$_1$, alpha$_2$, beta, and gamma. The first three types act primarily as carrier proteins that transport lipids, hormones and metals through the blood. The fourth type, gamma globulin, is an important immune system component. When the relative percentage of each component protein fraction is multiplied by the total protein concentration, the proportions can be converted into absolute values.

The test helps detect hepatic disease, protein deficiency, blood dyscrasias, renal disorders, and GI and neoplastic diseases.

Normal values. Total serum protein ranges from 6.6 to 7.9 g/dl. Values for the protein fractions are:
• Albumin: 3.3 to 4.5 g/dl (53%)
• Alpha$_1$ globulin: 0.1 to 0.4 g/dl (14%)

- Alpha$_2$ globulin: 0.5 to 1 g/dl (14%)
- Beta globulin: 0.7 to 1.2 g/dl (12%)
- Gamma globulin: 0.5 to 1.6 g/dl (20%)

Abnormal results. See *What abnormal protein levels mean.*

Uric acid
Used primarily to detect gout and help detect kidney dysfunction,

---

What abnormal protein levels mean

Abnormal levels of albumin or globulin are characteristic in many pathologic states, such as those listed below.

Total proteins	Albumin	Globulins
Elevated levels		
• Dehydration • Vomiting, diarrhea • Diabetic acidosis • Fulminating and chronic infections • Multiple myeloma • Monocytic leukemia • Chronic inflammatory disease (such as rheumatoid arthritis or early stage Laennec's cirrhosis)	• Multiple myeloma only	• Chronic syphilis • Tuberculosis • Subacute bacterial endocarditis • Multiple myeloma • Collagen diseases • Systemic lupus erythematosus • Rheumatoid arthritis • Diabetes mellitus • Hodgkin's disease
Diminished levels		
• Malnutrition • Gastrointestinal disease • Blood dyscrasias • Essential hypertension • Hodgkin's disease • Uncontrolled diabetes mellitus • Malabsorption • Hepatic dysfunction • Toxemia of pregnancy • Nephroses • Surgical and traumatic shock • Severe burns • Hemorrhage • Hyperthyroidism • Benzene and carbon tetrachloride poisoning • Congestive heart failure	• Malnutrition • Nephritis or nephrosis • Diarrhea • Plasma loss from burns • Hepatic disease • Hodgkin's disease • Hypogamma-globulinemia • Peptic ulcer • Acute cholecystitis • Sarcoidosis • Collagen diseases • Systemic lupus erythematosus • Rheumatoid arthritis • Essential hypertension • Metastatic carcinoma • Hyperthyroidism	• Levels are variable in neoplastic and renal diseases, hepatic dysfunction, and blood dyscrasias

---

this test measures serum levels of uric acid, the major end metabolite of purine. Large amounts of purines are present in nucleic acids and derive from dietary and endogenous sources. Uric acid clears the body by glomerular filtration and tubular secretion. However, uric acid is not very soluble at pH 7.4 or lower. Disorders of purine metabolism, rapid destruction of nucleic acids, and conditions marked by impaired renal excretion characteristically raise serum uric acid levels.

Normal values. Uric acid concentrations in men commonly range from 4.3 to 8 mg/dl; in women, from 2.3 to 6 mg/dl.

Abnormal results. Elevated levels occur in gout, impaired renal function, and congestive heart failure. They also occur in von Gierke's disease, infections, hemolytic anemia, sickle cell anemia, polycythemia, neoplasms, and psoriasis.
  Depressed levels occur in Fanconi's syndrome, Wilson's disease, and acute hepatic atrophy.

Carbohydrate tests: What they measure and mean

Fasting plasma glucose
This test is commonly used to screen for diabetes mellitus and to monitor drug or dietary therapy in patients with diabetes mellitus. The test measures plasma glucose levels following a 12- to 14-hour fast; however, borderline or transient elevated levels require the 2-hour postprandial plasma glucose test or the oral glucose tolerance test to confirm the diagnosis. In the fasting state, falling plasma glucose levels stimulate release of

the hormone glucagon. Glucagon then acts to raise plasma glucose by accelerating glycogenolysis, stimulating glyconeogenesis, and inhibiting glycogen synthesis. Normally, secretion of insulin checks this rise in glucose levels. But in diabetes, absence or deficiency of insulin allows persistently high glucose levels.

Normal values. The range varies with the laboratory procedure. Generally, normal values after a 12- to 14-hour fast are 70 to 100 mg of "true glucose"/100 ml of blood when measured by the glucose oxidase and hexokinase methods.

Abnormal results. *Increased fasting plasma glucose levels:*
• confirm diabetes mellitus with levels of 140 mg/dl on two or more occasions
• may also occur with pancreatitis; recent acute illness, such as MI; Cushing's syndrome; acromegaly; pheochromocytoma; hyperlipoproteinemia (especially Type III, IV or V); chronic hepatic disease; nephrotic syndrome; brain tumor; sepsis; dumping syndrome; eclampsia; anoxia; and convulsive disorders.
Decreased fasting plasma glucose levels can indicate hyperinsulinism, insulinoma, von Gierke's disease, functional or reactive hypoglycemia, myxedema, adrenal insufficiency, congenital adrenal hyperplasia, hypopituitarism, malabsorption syndrome, or possible hepatic insufficiency.

Lactic acid
Lactic acid, present in blood as lactate ion, is the reduction product of pyruvate, a byproduct of carbohydrate metabolism. Together these compounds form a reversible reaction that is regulated by oxygen supply. When oxygen levels are low, pyruvate converts to lactate; when they are adequate, lactate converts to py-

ruvate. When the hepatic system fails to metabolize lactate sufficiently, or when excess pyruvate converts to lactate due to tissue hypoxia and circulatory collapse, lactic acidosis may result.

Comparison of pyruvate and lactate levels reliably mirrors tissue oxidation, but measurement of pyruvate is technically difficult and infrequently performed. Blood lactic acid is tested to assess tissue oxidation and to help determine the cause of lactic acidosis.

Normal values. Blood lactate values range from 0.93 to 1.65 mEq/liter; pyruvate levels, from 0.08 to 0.16 mEq/liter. The lactate-pyruvate ratio is less than 10:1.

Abnormal results. *Increased blood lactate levels* can reflect strenuous muscle exercise; shock; hemorrhage; septicemia; MI; pulmonary embolism; cardiac arrest; diabetes mellitus; leukemias; lymphomas; hepatic disease; renal failure; enzymatic defects, such as glycogen storage disease; ingestion of large doses of acetaminophen and ethanol; and IV infusion of epinephrine, glucagon, fructose, and sorbitol.

Oral glucose tolerance test (OGTT)
The OGTT, the most sensitive method of evaluating borderline cases of diabetes mellitus in selected patients, measures carbohydrate metabolism after ingestion of a challenge dose of glucose. The body absorbs this dose rapidly, causing plasma glucose levels to rise and peak within 30 minutes to 1 hour. The pancreas responds by secreting more insulin, causing glucose levels to return to normal after 2 to 3 hours. During this period, plasma and urine glucose levels are monitored to assess insulin secretion and the body's ability to metabolize glucose. In a patient with mild or diet-controlled diabetes, fasting

plasma glucose levels may be within normal range; however, insufficient secretion of insulin after ingestion of carbohydrates causes plasma glucose to rise sharply and return to normal slowly. This decreased glucose tolerance helps confirm mild diabetes.

Normal values. Plasma glucose levels peak at 160 to 180 mg/dl within 30 minutes to 1 hour after administration of an oral glucose test dose and return to fasting levels or lower within 2 or 3 hours. Urine glucose tests remain negative throughout.

Abnormal results. *Sustained elevated plasma glucose levels during at least two OGTTs* help confirm diabetes mellitus. Many other diseases may cause abnormal glucose tolerance curves; these include myasthenia gravis, brain injury, Cushing's syndrome, acromegaly (early), hemochromatosis, alimentary glycosuria, pituitary deficiency, myxedema, anorexia nervosa, panhypopituitarism, hyperinsulinism, and Addison's disease.

Two-hour postprandial plasma glucose
This test is a valuable screen for diabetes mellitus, and is also used to monitor drug or diet therapy in patients with the disease. It is performed when the patient demonstrates symptoms of diabetes (polydipsia and polyuria) or when results of the fasting plasma glucose test suggest diabetes. The greatest difference between normal and diabetic insulin responses, and thus in plasma glucose concentration, occurs about 2 hours after a glucose challenge. Values of this test, however, can fluctuate according to the patient's age. After age 50, for example, normal levels rise markedly and steadily, sometimes reaching 160 mg/dl or higher. In younger patients, glucose concentration over 145 mg/dl

suggests incipient diabetes and requires further evaluation. When postprandial results are borderline, the OGTT may confirm diagnosis.

Normal values. In a person without diabetes, postprandial glucose values are < 145 mg/dl by the glucose oxidase or hexokinase method; levels are slightly elevated in persons over age 50.

Abnormal results. *Increased 2-hour postprandial blood glucose:*
• indicates diabetes mellitus when values exceed 200 mg/dl or above on two occasions.
• may also occur with pancreatitis, Cushing's syndrome, acromegaly, pheochromocytoma, hyperlipoproteinemia, chronic hepatic disease, nephrotic syndrome, brain tumor, sepsis, gastrectomy with dumping syndrome, eclampsia, anoxia, or convulsive disorders.
Decreased glucose levels can indicate hyperinsulinism, insulinoma, von Gierke's disease, hypoglycemia, myxedema, adrenal insufficiency, congenital adrenal hyperplasia, hypopituitarism, malabsorption syndrome, or hepatic insufficiency.

Immunologic tests: What they measure and mean

Antinuclear antibodies
In conditions such as systemic lupus erythematosus (SLE), systemic sclerosis, and certain infections, the body's immune system may perceive portions of its own cell nuclei as foreign, and may produce antinuclear antibodies (ANA). Specific ANA include antibodies to DNA, nucleoprotein, histones, nuclear ribonucleoprotein, and other nuclear constitu-

ents. Although ANA are harmless in themselves, because they do not penetrate living cells, they sometimes form antigen-antibody complexes that cause tissue damage (as in SLE).

Because of multiorgan involvement, test results aren't diagnostic, and can only partly validate clinical evidence. Although the ANA test can't confirm SLE, the higher the titer, the more specific the test is for SLE. This test is commonly used to screen for the disease, and to monitor effectiveness of immunosuppressive therapy. The test is gradually replacing the less reliable LE cell preparation test for these purposes.

Normal values. Negative for ANA at a titer of 1:32 or below.

Abnormal results. *High ANA titers* can indicate SLE. *Lower but still elevated titers* may occur in patients with viral diseases, chronic hepatic diseases, collagen vascular diseases, and autoimmune diseases. They also may occur in some healthy adults; incidence increases with age.

Complement assays
Complement refers to a group of at least 20 serum proteins designed to destroy foreign cells and to help remove foreign materials. The complement system may be triggered by contact with antigen-antibody complexes or by clotting factor XIIa. A cascade of events follows, which results in formation of a complex that ruptures cell membranes. Complement components are numerically designated as C1 through C9, with C1 having three subcomponents: C1q, C1r, and C1s. Complement comprises 3% to 4% of total serum globulins, and plays a key role in antibody-mediated immune reactions. Complement assays are indicated in patients with known or sus-

pected immunomediated disease or repeatedly abnormal response to infection.

Normal values. Total complement ranges from 41 to 90 hemolytic units. Values for components are:
• C1 esterase inhibitor: 16 to 33 mg/dl
• C3: in males, 88 to 252 mg/dl; in females, 88 to 206 mg/dl
• C4: in males, 12 to 72 mg/dl; in females, 13 to 75 mg/dl.

Abnormal results. *Increased total complement levels* can signal obstructive jaundice, thyroiditis, acute rheumatic fever, rheumatoid arthritis (RA), acute MI, ulcerative colitis, or diabetes. *Reduced levels* characteristically occur in SLE, acute poststreptococcal glomerulonephritis, and acute serum sickness. They may occur in advanced cirrhosis of the liver, multiple myeloma, and hypogammaglobulinemia.
Decreased C1 esterase inhibitor can indicate hereditary angioedema. *Diminished C3* can result from recurrent pyrogenic infection, whereas *decreased C4* can result from SLE.

Heterophil agglutination
Heterophil agglutination tests detect and identify two IgM antibodies in human serum that react against foreign red blood cells (RBCs). In the Paul-Bunnell or "presumptive" test, Epstein-Barr virus (EBV) antibodies found in the sera of patients with infectious mononucleosis (IM) agglutinate with sheep RBCs in a test tube. However, Forssman antibodies, present in some normal serum as well as in conditions such as serum sickness, also agglutinate with sheep RBCs, thus rendering test results inconclusive for IM. If the Paul-Bunnell test establishes a presumptive titer, the Davidsohn differential absorption test can then distinguish between EBV antibodies and Forssman antibodies.

Although heterophil antibodies occur in the sera of approximately 80% of patients with IM 1 month after onset, a positive finding—a titer higher than 1:56—does not confirm this disorder. Confirmation depends on heterophil agglutination tests that show absolute lymphocytosis, with 10% to 30% or more atypical lymphocytes.

Normal values. Negative, no reaction; titer < 1:56 (may be higher in the elderly).

Abnormal results. *Positive, or a titer greater than 1:56* can indicate infectious mononucleosis, SLE, cryoglobulinemia, or presence of antibodies to nonsyphilitic treponema (yaws, pinta, bejel).

Rheumatoid factor (RF)

In rheumatoid arthritis, "renegade" IgG antibodies, produced by lymphocytes in the synovial joints, react with other IgG or IgM to produce immune complexes, complement activation, and tissue destruction. How IgG molecules become autogenic is still unknown, but they may be altered by aggregating with viruses or other antigens. These immune complexes can migrate from the synovial fluid to other areas of the body, causing vasculitis, subcutaneous nodules, or lymphadenopathy. The IgG or IgM molecules that react with altered IgG are called rheumatoid factors.

Agglutination and flocculation tests—the sheep cell agglutination test (SCAT) and the latex fixation text—are used to detect RF, especially when clinical diagnosis is doubtful. SCAT is the better test for confirming RA, while latex fixation is the better screen.

Normal values. The normal RF titer is less than 1:20. The normal rheumatoid screening test is nonreactve or negative.

Normal findings in routine urinalysis

Element	Findings
Macroscopic	
Color	Straw
Odor	Slightly aromatic
Appearance	Clear
Specific gravity	1.005 to 1.020
pH	4.5 to 8.0
Protein	None
Glucose	None
Ketones	None
Other sugars	None
Microscopic	
Red blood cells	0 to 3/high-power field
White blood cells	0 to 4/high-power field
Epithelial cells	Few
Casts	None, except occasional hyaline casts
Crystals	Present
Yeast cells	None
Parasites	None
Bacteria	None

Abnormal results. *Titers above 1:80* can indicate RA (usually considered confirming if patient also meets criteria for clinical diagnosis).

Titers between 1:20 and 1:80 can indicate SLE, systemic sclerosis, polymyositis, tuberculosis, infectious mononucleosis, leprosy, syphilis, sarcoidosis, chronic hepatic disease, subacute bacterial endocarditis, and chronic interstitial fibrosis.

Urine tests: What they measure and mean

Urinalysis

Routine urinalysis is an important, commonly used screening test for renal, urinary tract disease, and for helping to detect metabolic or systemic disease un-

related to renal disorders. Normal urine findings suggest the absence of major disease, while abnormal findings suggest its presence and require further urine or blood tests to pinpoint a disease. The elements of routine urinalysis include evaluation of physical characteristics (color, odor, opacity); determination of specific gravity and pH; detection and rough measurement of protein, glucose, and ketone bodies; and examination of sediment for red and white blood cells, casts, and crystals.

Normal values. See *Normal findings in routine urinalysis.*

Abnormal results. *Color:* Changes in color can result from diet, drugs, and many metabolic, inflammatory, or infectious diseases. (See *How drugs influence urinalysis results,* pages 74 and 75.)

How drugs influence urinalysis results

Drugs that change urine color
Alcohol (light, due to diuresis)
Chlorpromazine hydrochloride
   (dark)
Chlorzoxazone (orange to
   purple-red)
Deferoxamine mesylate (red)
Fluorescein sodium I.V. (yellow-
   orange)
Furazolidone (brown)
Iron salts (black)
Levodopa (dark)
Metronidazole (dark)
Methylene blue (blue-green)
Nitrofurantoin (brown)
Oral anticoagulants, indanedione
   derivatives (orange)
Phenazopyridine (orange-red,
   orange-brown, or red)
Quinacrine (deep yellow)
Riboflavin (yellow)
Rifampin (red-orange)
Sulfasalazine (orange-yellow)

Drugs that cause urine odor
Antibiotics
Paraldehyde
Vitamins

**Drugs that raise specific
gravity**
Albumin
Dextran
Glucose
Radiopaque contrast media

Drugs that lower pH
Ammonium chloride
Ascorbic acid
Diazoxide
Methenamine
Metolazone

Drugs that raise pH
Acetazolamide
Amphotericin B
Mafenide
Sodium bicarbonate
Potassium citrate

**Drugs that cause false-positive
result for proteinuria**
Acetazolamide (Combistix or
   Labstix)
Aminosalicylic acid (sulfosali-
   cylic acid or Extons method)
Cephalothin in large doses (sul-
   fosalicylic acid method)
Nafcillin (sulfosalicylic acid
   method)
Sodium bicarbonate (all methods)
Tolbutamide (sulfosalicylic acid
   method)
Tolmetin (sulfosalicylic acid
   method)

**Drugs that cause true
proteinuria**
Amikacin
Amphotericin B
Bacitracin
Gentamicin
Gold preparations
Kanamycin
Neomycin
Netilmicin
Phenylbutazone
Polymyxin B
Streptomycin
Tobramycin
Trimethadione

**Drugs that can cause true
proteinuria or false-positive
results**
Penicillin in large doses (except
   with Ames reagent strips);
   however, some penicillins
   cause true proteinuria
Sulfonamides (sulfosalicylic acid
   method)

**Drugs that cause false-positive
glycosuria**
Aminosalicylic acid (Benedict's
   test)
Ascorbic acid (Clinistix, Diastix,
   or Tes-Tape)
Ascorbic acid in large doses
   (Clinitest tablets)

Cephalosporins (Clinitest tablets)
Chloral hydrate (Benedict's test)
Chloramphenicol (Benedict's test
   or Clinitest tablets)
Isoniazid (Benedict's test)
Levodopa (Clinistix, Diastix, or
   Tes-Tape)
Levodopa in large doses (Clini-
   test tablets)
Methyldopa (Tes-Tape)
Nalidixic acid (Benedict's test or
   Clinitest tablets)
Nitrofurantoin (Benedict's test)
Penicillin G in large doses (Ben-
   edict's test)
Phenazopyridine (Clinistix, Dias-
   tix, or Tes-Tape)
Probenecid (Benedict's test or
   Clinitest tablets)
Salicylates in large doses (Clini-
   test tablets, Clinistix, Diastix,
   or Tes-Tape)
Streptomycin (Benedict's test)
Tetracycline (Clinistix, Diastix,
   Tes-Tape)
Tetracyclines, due to ascorbic
   acid buffer (Benedict's test or
   Clinitest tablets)

**Drugs that cause true
glycosuria**
Ammonium chloride
Asparaginase
Carbamazepine
Corticosteroids
Dextrothyroxine
Lithium carbonate
Nicotinic acid (large doses)
Phenothiazines (long-term)
Thiazide diuretics

**Drugs that cause false-positive
results for ketonuria**
Levodopa (Ketostix or Labstix)
Phenazopyridine (Ketostix or
   Gerhardt's reagent strip shows
   atypical color)
Phenothiazines (Gerhardt's reagent
   strip shows atypical color)
Salicylates (Gerhardt's reagent
   strip shows reddish color)

Sulfobromophthalein (Bili-
Labstix)

Drugs that cause true ketonuria
Ether (anesthesia)
Isoniazid (intoxication)
Isopropyl alcohol (intoxication)
Insulin (excessive doses)

Drugs that increase white blood cells
Allopurinol
Ampicillin
Aspirin toxicity
Kanamycin
Methicillin

Drugs that cause hematuria
Amphotericin B
Coumarin derivatives
Methenamine in large doses
Methicillin
Para-aminosalicylic acid
Phenylbutazone
Sulfonamides

Drugs that cause casts
Amphotericin B
Aspirin toxicity
Bacitracin
Ethacrynic acid
Furosemide
Gentamicin
Griseofulvin
Isoniazid
Kanamycin
Neomycin
Penicillin
Radiographic agents
Streptomycin
Sulfonamides

Drugs that cause crystals (if urine is acidic)
Acetazolamide
Aminosalicylic acid
Ascorbic acid
Nitrofurantoin
Theophylline
Thiazide diuretics

• *Odor:* In diabetes mellitus, starvation, and dehydration, a fruity odor accompanies formation of ketone bodies. In urinary tract infection, a fetid odor is common, especially if *Escherichia coli* is present. Maple syrup urine disease and phenylketonuria also cause distinctive odors.

• *Turbidity:* Turbid urine may contain red or white cells, bacteria, fat, or chyle and may reflect renal infection.

• *Specific gravity:* Low specific gravity (< 1.005) is characteristic of diabetes inspidus, nephrogenic diabetes insipidus, acute tubular necrosis, and pyelonephritis. Fixed specific gravity (value remains 1.010 regardless of fluid intake) occurs in chronic glomerulonephritis with severe renal damage. High specific gravity (> 1.020) occurs in nephrotic syndrome, dehydration, acute glomerulonephritis, congestive heart failure, liver failure, and shock.

• *pH:* Alkaline urine pH may result from Fanconi's syndrome, urinary tract infection, and metabolic or respiratory alkalosis. Acid pH is associated with renal tuberculosis, pyrexia, phenylketonuria and alkaptonuria, and all forms of acidosis.

• *Protein:* Proteinuria suggests renal disease, such as nephrosis, glomerulosclerosis, polycystic kidney disease, or renal failure. Proteinuria can also result from multiple myeloma.

• *Sugars:* Glycosuria usually indicates diabetes mellitus but may also result from pheochromocytoma, Cushing's syndrome, and increased intracranial pressure. Fructosuria, galactosuria, and pentosuria suggest rare metabolic disorders.

• *Ketones:* Ketonuria occurs in diabetes mellitus when cellular energy needs exceed available cellular glucose. It may also occur in starvation, and in conditions of acutely increased metabolic demand associated with decreased food intake, such as diarrhea or vomiting.

• *Cells:* Hematuria indicates bleeding within the genitourinary tract and may result from infection, obstruction, inflammation, trauma, tumors, glomerulonephritis, renal hypertension, lupus nephritis, renal tuberculosis, renal vein thrombosis, hydronephrosis, pyelonephritis, scurvy, malaria, parasitic infection of the bladder, subacute bacterial endocarditis, polyarteritis nodosa, and hemorrhagic disorders. Numerous white cells in urine usually imply urinary tract inflammation, especially cystitis or pyelonephritis. White cells and white cell casts in urine suggest renal infection. An excessive number of epithelial cells suggests renal tubular degradation.

• *Casts:* Excessive numbers of casts indicate renal disease. Hyaline casts are associated with renal parenchymal disease, inflammation, and trauma to the glomerular capillary membrane; epithelial casts, with renal tubular damage, nephrosis, eclampsia, amyloidosis, and heavy metal poisoning; coarse and fine granular casts, with acute or chronic renal failure, pyelonephritis, and chronic lead intoxication; fatty and waxy casts, with nephrotic syndrome, chronic renal disease, and diabetes mellitus; red blood cell casts, with renal parenchymal disease (especially glomerulonephritis), renal infarction, subacute bacterial endocarditis, vascular disorders, sickle cell anemia, scurvy, blood dyscrasias, malignant hypertension, collagen disease, and acute inflammation; and white blood cell casts, with acute pyelonephritis and glomerulonephritis, nephrotic syndrome, pyogenic infection, and lupus nephritis.

• *Crystals:* Some crystals normally appear in urine, but numerous calcium oxalate crystals suggest hypercalcemia. Cystine crystals

Dehydration test for diabetes insipidus

The dehydration test measures urine osmolality, which reflects renal concentrating capacity after a period of dehydration and after subcutaneous injection of the pituitary hormone vasopressin. Comparison of the two osmolalities permits reliable diagnosis of diabetes insipidus, a metabolic disorder characterized by vasopressin (antidiuretic hormone) deficiency. Simply measuring urine osmolality after a period of water deprivation doesn't itself confirm vasopressin deficiency; however, subsequent injection of vasopressin raises urine osmolality beyond normal limits only in patients with diabetes insipidus.

To achieve dehydration, withhold fluids the evening before and the morning of the test. Collect a urine sample at hourly intervals in the morning for osmolality measurement. At noon, or after osmolality increases less than 30 mOsm/kg each hour for 3 consecutive hours, draw a blood sample for osmolality measurement. If serum osmolality exceeds 288 mOsm/kg, the level of adequate dehydration, inject 5 units of vasopressin subcutaneously. Within an hour, collect a urine specimen for osmolality measurement.

Clinical alert: During dehydration, weigh the patient and monitor vital signs every 2 hours; a 1-kg weight loss normally accompanies adequate dehydration. In a patient with polyuria exceeding 10 liters/day, withhold fluids only during the morning of the test; if his weight loss exceeds 2 kg, discontinue the test.

In a patient with normal neurohypophyseal function, urine osmolality after vasopressin injection doesn't rise more than 9% of the maximum dehydration osmolality. A larger increase indicates diabetes insipidus. In a patient with polyuria caused by renal disease, potassium depletion, or nephrogenic diabetes insipidus, urine osmolality increases slightly during dehydration but not at all after vasopressin injection.

(cystinuria) reflect an inborn error of metabolism.

• *Other components:* Bacteria, yeast cells, and parasites in urinary sediment reflect genitourinary tract infection, as well as contamination of external genitalia. Yeast cells, which may be mistaken for red cells, can be identified by their ovoid shape, lack of color, variable size, and frequently, signs of budding. The most common parasite in sediment is *Trichomonas vaginalis,* a flagellated protozoan that commonly causes vaginitis, urethritis, and prostatovesiculitis.

Urine concentration and dilution tests

The kidneys normally concentrate or dilute urine according to fluid intake. When this intake is excessive, the kidneys excrete more water in the urine; when intake is limited, they excrete less. This test measures specific gravity or osmolality; it evaluates renal capacity to concentrate urine in response to fluid deprivation, or to dilute it in response to fluid overload. Specific gravity, the ratio of urine mass to an equal volume of water, is usually high in small volumes of output (concentrated urine) and low in large volumes (dilute urine). Osmolality, a more sensitive index of renal function, measures the number of osmotically active ions or particles present per kilogram of water. Osmolality is high in concentrated urine and low in dilute urine.

Normal values. In the *concentration test,* specific gravity ranges from 1.025 to 1.032, and osmolality rises above 800 mOsm/kg water, in patients with normal renal function.

In the *dilution test,* specific gravity falls below 1.003 and osmolality below 100 mOsm/kg for at least one specimen; 80% or more of the ingested water is eliminated in 4 hours. In elderly persons, depressed values can be associated with normal renal function.

Abnormal results. Impaired renal capacity to concentrate urine in response to fluid deprivation, or to dilute urine in response to fluid overload, may indicate tubular epithelial damage, decreased renal blood flow, loss of functional nephrons, or pituitary or cardiac dysfunction.

Amylase

A starch-splitting enzyme primarily produced in the pancreas and salivary glands, amylase is usually secreted into the alimentary tract and absorbed into the blood. Small amounts of amylase are also absorbed into the blood directly from these organs. Following glomerular filtration, amylase is excreted in the urine.

With adequate renal function, serum and urine levels usually rise in tandem. However, within 2 or 3 days of onset of acute pancreatitis, serum amylase levels fall to normal, but elevated urine amylase persists for 7 to 10 days. The test is used to diagnose acute pancreatitis when serum amylase levels are normal or borderline; and to aid diagnosis of chronic

17-ketosteroid fractionation: Normal test values (mg/24 hours)

Steroid	Adult male	Adult female	Male (age 10 to 15)	Female (age 10 to 15)	Both sexes (age 0 to 9)
Androsterone	2.2 to 5	0.5 to 2.4	0.2 to 2	0.2 to 2.5	≤ 1
Dehydroepiandrosterone	0 to 2.3	0 to 1.2	< 0.4	< 0.4	< 0.2
Etiocholanolone	1.9 to 4.7	1.1 to 3	0.1 to 1.6	0.7 to 3	≤ 1
11-hydroxyandrosterone	0.5 to 1.3	0.2 to 0.6	0.1 to 1.1	0.2 to 1	≤ 1
11-hydroxyetiocholanolone	0.3 to 0.7	0.2 to 0.6	< 0.3	0.1 to 0.5	≤ 0.5
11-ketoandrosterone	0 to 0.1	0 to 0.2	< 0.1	< 0.1	< 0.1
11-ketoetiocholanolone	0.2 to 0.7	0.2 to 0.6	0.2 to 0.6	0.1 to 0.6	≤ 0.7
Pregnanediol	0.6 to 1.6	0.2 to 2.4	0.1 to 0.7	0.1 to 1.2	< 0.5
Pregnanetriol	0.6 to 1.3	0.1 to 1	0.2 to 0.6	0.1 to 0.6	< 0.3
5-pregnanetriol	0 to 0.3	0 to 0.3	< 0.3	< 0.3	< 0.2
11-ketopregnanetriol	0 to 0.2	0 to 0.4	< 0.3	< 0.2	< 0.2

Through gas-liquid chromatography, this fractionation test shows which specific steroids in the 17-ketosteroid (KS) group are elevated or suppressed, and thus aids differential diagnosis of conditions suggested by abnormal 17-KS levels.

pancreatitis and salivary gland disorders.

Normal values. Urine amylase is reported in various units of measure, so values differ from laboratory to laboratory. The Mayo Clinic reports urinary excretion of 10 to 80 amylase units/hour as normal.

Abnormal results. *Increased levels* can signal acute pancreatitis, destruction of pancreatic duct, intestinal obstruction, obstruction of salivary duct, carcinoma of head of pancreas, mumps, acute spleen injury, renal disease with impaired absorption, perforated peptic or duodenal ulcers, or gallbladder disease.

Reduced levels can stem from chronic pancreatitis, cachexia, alcoholism, cancer of the liver, cirrhosis, hepatitis, or hepatic abscess.

17-ketosteroids (17-KS)
This test measures urine levels of 17-KS, which are steroids and steroid metabolites characterized by a ketone group on carbon 17 in the steroid nucleus. They originate primarily in the adrenal glands and also in the testes, which produce one-third of 17-KS in males, and in the ovaries, which produce a small amount of 17-KS in females. Although not all 17-KS are adrenogens, they cause androgenic effects. Because 17-KS do not include all of the androgens (testosterone, for instance, the most potent androgen, isn't a 17-KS), these levels provide only a rough estimate of androgenic activity.

The test aids diagnosis of adrenal and gonadal dysfunction and adrenogenital syndrome (congenital adrenal hyperplasia). It also helps monitor cortisol therapy in adrenogenital syndrome.

Normal values. Urine 17-KS values range from 6 to 21 mg/24 hours in men, and from 4 to 17 mg/24 hours in women. Children between the ages of 11 and 14 excrete 2 to 7 mg/24 hours; younger children and infants excrete 0.1 to 3 mg/24 hours. (See *17-ketosteroid fractionation: Normal test values.*)

Abnormal results. *Elevated urine 17-KS levels* may result from adrenal hyperplasia, carcinoma, or adenoma or from adrenogenital syndrome. They may also result from Stein-Leventhal syndrome, lutein cell tumor of the ovary, adrenogenic arrhenoblastoma, or interstitial cell tumor of the testes.

Reduced urine 17-KS levels may result from Addison's disease, panhypopituitarism, eunuchoidism, or castration. They may also occur in cretinism, myxedema, or nephrosis.

Creatinine clearance

An anhydride of creatine, creatinine is formed and excreted in constant amounts by an irreversible reaction, and functions solely as the main end product of creatine. Creatine production is proportional to total muscle mass and is relatively unaffected by normal physical activity, diet, or urine volume.

An excellent diagnostic indicator of renal function, the creatinine clearance test determines how efficiently the kidneys remove creatinine from the blood. The clearance rate is expressed as the volume of blood (in ml) that can be cleared of creatinine in 1 minute. Creatinine levels become abnormal when more than 50% of the total nephron units have been damaged. High creatinine clearance rates have little diagnostic significance. The test is used to assess renal function (primarily glomerular filtration) and to monitor progression of renal insufficiency.

Normal values. For young men (age 20), creatinine clearance is 90 ml/minute/1.73 m² of body surface; for young women (age 20), 84 ml/minute/1.73 m². For older patients, concentrations normally decline by 6 ml/minute/decade.

Abnormal results. *Diminished creatinine clearance levels* stem from conditions causing reduced renal blood flow. These include shock, congestive heart failure, and severe dehydration. Local conditions include renal artery obstruction; acute tubular necrosis, acute or chronic glomerulonephritis, advanced bilateral chronic pyelonephritis; advanced bilateral renal lesions, as in polycystic kidney disease, renal tuberculosis, and malignancy; or nephrosclerosis.

Protein

This is a quantitative test for proteinuria. Normally, the glomerular membrane allows only proteins of low molecular weight to enter the filtrate. The renal tubules then reabsorb most of these proteins, normally excreting a small amount that's undetectable by a screening test.

Proteinuria can result from glomerular leakage of plasma proteins (a major cause of protein excretion), from overflow of filtered proteins of low molecular weight (when these are present in excessive concentrations), from impaired tubular reabsorption of filtered proteins, and from the presence of renal proteins derived from the breakdown of kidney tissue. Some forms of proteinuria are transient and nonpathologic (such as changes in body position, or emotional or physiologic stress). Many drugs, such as amphotericin B, gold preparations, aminoglycosides, polymyxins, and trimethadione, cause true proteinuria, making routine evaluation of urine proteins essential when these are in use.

Normal values. Up to 150 mg of protein is excreted in 24 hours.

Abnormal results. *Persistent proteinuria* indicates renal disease resulting from increased glomerular permeability.

Minimal proteinuria (< 0.5 g/24 hours) commonly signals a renal disease in which glomerular involvement isn't a major factor, such as chronic pyelonephritis.

Moderate proteinuria (0.5 to 4 g/24 hours) commonly indicates acute or chronic glomerulonephritis, amyloidosis, or toxic nephropathies. It also can indicate diseases in which renal failure develops as a late complication, such as diabetes or heart failure.

Heavy proteinuria (> 4 g/24 hours) commonly indicates nephrotic syndrome.

When accompanied by an elevated WBC count, proteinuria indicates urinary tract infection.

When accompanied by hematuria, it indicates local or diffuse urinary tract disorders. Other pathologic states (for example, infections and central nervous system (CNS) lesions) can also cause proteinuria.

Uric acid

A quantitative analysis of urine uric acid levels, this test supplements serum uric acid testing for identifying disorders that alter production or excretion of uric acid (such as leukemia, gout, and renal dysfunction). It helps detect enzyme deficiencies and metabolic disturbances that affect uric acid production. What's more, it helps measure the efficiency of renal clearance.

Normal values. Urine uric acid values vary with diet, but characteristically range from 250 to 750 mg/24 hours.

Abnormal results. *Heightened uric acid levels* may result from chronic myeloid leukemia, polycythemia vera, multiple myeloma, early remission in pernicious anemia, Fanconi's syndrome, or Wilson's disease. They also may occur in lymphosarcoma and lymphatic leukemia during radiotherapy.

Glucose oxidase

This test—involving the use of commercial, plastic-coated reagent strips (Clinistix, Diastix) or Tes-Tape—is a specific, qualitative test for glycosuria. Although indicated in routine urinalysis, the test is used primarily to monitor urine glucose in patients with diabetes. Because of this test's simplicity and convenience, patients can perform it at home. However, no standardized test values exist, so it's necessary to note the type of test used along with the results.

Normal values. No glucose is present in urine.

Abnormal results. *Glycosuria* usually indicates diabetes mellitus. It also occurs in adrenal disorders, thyroid disorders, hepatic disease, CNS disease, Fanconi's syndrome, conditions involving low renal threshold, toxic renal tubular disease, heavy metal poisoning, glomerulonephritis, nephrosis, and pregnancy.

Glycosuria occurs with administration of hyperalimentation, large amounts of glucose or nicotinic acid, asparaginase, corticosteroids, carbamazepine, ammonium chloride, thiazide diuretics, dextrothyroxine, lithium carbonate, or phenothiazines (long term).

Ketones
In this routine, semiquantitative screening test, the action of urine on a commercially prepared product (Acetest tablet, Chemstrip K, Ketostix, or Keto-Diastix) measures the urine level of ketone bodies. Each product measures a specific ketone body. For example, Acetest measures acetone, while Ketostix measures acetoacetic acid. Urine determinations reflect serum concentration.

The tests are used to screen for ketonuria; to identify diabetic ketoacidosis and carbohydrate deprivation; to distinguish between a diabetic and a nondiabetic coma; and to monitor control of diabetes mellitus, ketogenic weight reduction, and treatment of diabetic ketoacidosis.

Normal values. No ketones are present in urine.

Abnormal results. *Ketonuria* is present in uncontrolled diabetes mellitus, starvation, and as a metabolic complication of hyperalimentation.

Calcium and phosphates
This test measures urine levels of calcium and phosphates, elements essential in bone formation and

Disorders affecting urine calcium and phosphate levels

Disorder	Urine calcium level	Urine phosphate level
Hyperparathyroidism	Elevated	Elevated
Vitamin D intoxication	Elevated	Suppressed
Metastatic carcinoma	Elevated	Normal
Sarcoidosis	Elevated	Suppressed
Renal tubular acidosis	Elevated	Elevated
Multiple myeloma	Elevated or normal	Elevated or normal
Paget's disease	Normal	Normal
Milk-alkali syndrome	Suppressed or normal	Suppressed or normal
Hypoparathyroidism	Suppressed	Suppressed
Acute nephrosis	Suppressed	Suppressed or normal
Chronic nephrosis	Suppressed	Suppressed
Acute nephritis	Suppressed	Suppressed
Renal insufficiency	Suppressed	Suppressed
Osteomalacia	Suppressed	Suppressed
Steatorrhea	Suppressed	Suppressed

resorption. It's used to evaluate calcium and phosphate metabolism and excretion, and to monitor treatment of calcium or phosphate deficiency. Urine calcium and phosphate levels generally parallel serum levels. These minerals help maintain tissue and fluid pH, electrolyte balance in cells and extracellular fluids, and permeability of cell membranes. Calcium promotes enzymatic processes, aids blood coagulation, and lowers neuromuscular irritability; phosphates aid carbohydrate metabolism.

Normal values. Values depend on dietary intake. Males excrete < 275 mg of calcium/24 hours; females, < 250 mg/24 hours. Normal excretion of phosphate is < 1,000 mg/24 hours.

Abnormal results. See *Disorders affecting urine calcium and phosphate levels.*

Sodium and chloride
This test determines urine levels of sodium, the major extracellular cation, and of chloride, the major extracellular anion. Less significant than serum levels (and thus performed less frequently), measurement of urine sodium and chloride concentrations is used to evaluate renal conservation of these two electrolytes and to confirm serum sodium and chloride values. The test is also used to monitor the effects of a low-salt diet, and to help evaluate renal and adrenal disorders.

Sodium and chloride help maintain osmotic pressure and water and acid-base balance. After these ions are absorbed by the alimentary tract, they are regulated by the kidneys and rise and fall in tandem. The kidneys conserve constant serum levels of sodium and chloride — even at the risk of dehydration or edema — or excrete excessive amounts.

Normal values. Normal ranges of urine sodium and chloride vary greatly with dietary salt intake and perspiration. Urine sodium excretion is 30 to 280 mEq/24 hours; normal urine chloride excretion, 110 to 250 mEq/24 hours; and normal urine sodium-chloride excretion, 5 to 20 g/24 hours.

Abnormal results. *Elevated sodium levels* may reflect increased salt intake, adrenal failure, salicylate toxicity, diabetic acidosis, salt-losing nephritis, or water-deficient dehydration. *Lowered levels* suggest decreased salt intake, primary aldosteronism, acute renal failure, or congestive heart failure. *Increased chloride levels* may result from water-deficient dehydration, salicylate toxicity, diabetic acidosis, Addison's disease, or salt-losing renal disease. *Elevated chloride levels* may result from excessive diaphoresis, congestive heart failure, or hypochloremic metabolic acidosis.

Stool tests: What they measure and mean

Fecal occult blood
Fecal occult blood, invisible because of its minute quantity, can be detected by microscopic analysis or by chemical tests for hemoglobin, such as the guaiac or orthotolidine test. Because small amounts of blood (2 to 2.5 ml/day) normally appear in

the feces, tests for occult blood are designed to detect quantities larger than this. These tests are indicated in patients whose clinical symptoms and preliminary blood studies suggest GI bleeding. However, further tests are required to pinpoint the origin of the bleeding.

This test is particularly important for early diagnosis of colorectal cancer, since 80% of persons with this type of cancer demonstrate positive results.

Normal values. Less than 2.5 ml of blood is present, resulting in a green reaction.

Abnormal results. A positive test indicates GI bleeding.

Fecal urobilinogen
Urobilinogen, the end product of bilirubin metabolism, is a brown pigment formed by bacterial enzymes in the small intestine. It is excreted in feces or reabsorbed into portal blood, where it is returned to the liver and reexcreted in bile; a small amount of urobilinogen is also excreted in urine. Because bilirubin metabolism depends on a properly functioning hepatobiliary system and a normal erythrocyte life span, measurement of fecal urobilinogen is a useful indicator of hepatobiliary and hemolytic disorders.

Normal values. Fecal urobilinogen values range from 50 to 300 mg/24 hours.

Abnormal results. *Decreased levels* may indicate obstructed bile flow, as in cirrhosis; hepatitis; tumor of the head of the pancreas, the ampulla of Vater, or the bile duct; choledocholithiasis. Reduced levels may also reflect depressed erythropoiesis in aplastic anemia. *Increased levels* may indicate hemolytic jaundice, thalassemia; hemolytic, sickle-cell, or pernicious anemia.

What other commonly done tests reveal

Cerebrospinal fluid analysis
Cerebrospinal fluid (CSF), a clear substance that circulates in the subarachnoid space, has many vital functions. It protects the brain and spinal cord from injury and transports products of neurosecretion, cellular biosynthesis, and cellular metabolism through the central nervous system. Samples are commonly obtained by lumbar puncture (usually between the third and fourth vertebrae) and, occasionally, by cisternal or ventricular puncture. The test is used to measure CSF pressure to help detect obstruction of CSF circulation; to help diagnose viral or bacterial meningitis, subarachnoid or intracranial hemorrhage, tumors, and brain abscesses; and to help diagnose neurosyphilis and chronic CNS infections.

Normal and abnormal results. See *CSF findings* for a summary of findings in CSF analyses.

Papanicolaou test
This cytologic test is widely used for early detection of cervical cancer. However, although cervical scrapings are the most common test specimen, this test also permits cytologic examination of the vaginal pool, prostatic secretions, urine, gastric secretions, cavity fluids, bronchial aspirations, sputum, and solid tumor cells obtained by fine-needle aspiration. It also shows cell maturity, metabolic activity, and morphologic variations.

The American Cancer Society recommends a Pap test every 3 years for women between ages 20 and 40 who aren't in a high-risk category and who have had negative results from two previous Pap tests. Yearly tests (or at intervals dictated by the patient's doctor) are advisable for women over age 40, for those in a high-risk category, and for those who have had a positive test.

Normal values. No malignant, abnormal, or atypical cells are present.

Abnormal results. A Pap test may be graded in different ways. The following system is the traditional classification method:
• *Class I:* normal pattern; absence of atypical or abnormal cells.

CSF findings

Test	Normal	Abnormal	Implications
Pressure	50 to 180 mm H_2O	Increase	Increased intracranial pressure due to hemorrhage, tumor, or edema caused by trauma
		Decrease	Spinal subarachnoid obstruction above puncture site
Appearance	Clear, colorless	Cloudy	Infection (elevated white blood cell count and protein, or many microorganisms)
		Xanthochromic or bloody	Subarachnoid, intracerebral, or intraventricular hemorrhage; spinal cord obstruction; traumatic tap (usually noted only in initial specimen)
		Brown, orange, or yellow	Elevated protein, red blood cell (RBC) breakdown (blood present for at least 3 days)
Protein	15 to 45 mg/ 100 ml	Marked increase	Tumors, trauma, hemorrhage, diabetes mellitus, polyneuritis, blood in cerebrospinal fluid (CSF)
		Marked decrease	Rapid CSF production
Gamma globulin	3% to 12% of total protein	Increase	Demyelinating disease (such as multiple sclerosis), neurosyphilis, Guillain-Barré syndrome
Glucose	50 to 80 mg/ 100 ml (2/3 of blood glucose)	Increase	Systemic hyperglycemia
		Decrease	Systemic hypoglycemia, bacterial or fungal infection, meningitis, mumps, postsubarachnoid hemorrhage
Cell count	0 to 5 WBCs	Increase	Active disease: meningitis, acute infection, onset of chronic illness, tumor, abscess, infarction, demyelinating disease (such as multiple sclerosis)
	No RBCs	RBCs	Hemorrhage or traumatic tap
VDRL and other serologic tests	Nonreactive	Positive	Neurosyphilis
Chloride	118 to 130 mEq/liter	Decrease	Infected meninges (as in tuberculosis or meningitis)
Gram's stain	No organisms	Gram-positive or gram-negative organisms	Bacterial meningitis

•*Class II:* benign abnormality; atypical, but nonmalignant, cells present.
•*Class III:* atypical cells consistent with dysplasia.
•*Class IV:* suggestive of, but inconclusive for, malignancy.
•*Class V:* conclusive for malignancy.

Normal laboratory test values

Hematologic tests

Erythrocyte sedimentation rate
0 to 20 mm/hour; rates gradually increase with age.

Hematocrit
Adult males: 42% to 52%
Adult females: 38% to 46%

Hemoglobin
Adult males: 14 to 18 g/dl
Adult females: 12 to 16 g/dl

Iron and total iron-binding capacity (TIBC)

	Men	Women
Serum Iron	70 to 150 µg/dl	80 to 150 µg/dl
TIBC	300 to 400 µg/dl	300 to 450 µg/dl
Saturation	20% to 50%	20% to 50%

Red blood cell count
•Adult males: 4.5 to 6.2 million/µl of venous blood
•Adult females: 4.2 to 5.4 million/µl of venous blood

Reticulocyte count
0.5% to 2% of total RBC count

White blood cell count
4,100 to 10,900 /µl.

White blood cell differential
Adult values—
•Neutrophils: 47.6% to 76.8%
•Lymphocytes: 16.2% to 43%
•Monocytes: 0.6% to 9.6%
•Eosinophils: 0.3% to 7%
•Basophils: 0.3% to 2%

Coagulation tests

Activated partial thromboplastin time (APTT)
25 to 36 seconds

Bleeding time
•Template: 2 to 8 minutes
•Ivy: 1 to 7 minutes
•Duke: 1 to 3 minutes

Platelet count
130,000 to 370,000/mm³

Prothrombin time
•Males: 9.6 to 11.8 seconds
•Females: 9.5 to 11.3 seconds

Whole blood clotting time
5 to 15 minutes

Arterial blood gases

PaO₂
75 to 100 mm Hg

PaCO₂
35 to 45 mm Hg

pH
7.35 to 7.42

O₂ Sat
94% to 100%

HCO₃ –
22 to 26 mEq/liter

O₂Ct
15% to 23%

Total carbon dioxide content
22 to 34 mEq/liter

Serum electrolytes

Calcium
4.5 to 5.5 mEq/liter (Atomic absorption: 8.9 to 10.1 mg/dl)

Chloride
100 to 108 mEq/liter

Magnesium
1.5 to 2.5 mEq/liter (atomic absorption: 1.7 to 2.1 mg/dl)

Phosphates
1.8 to 2.6 mEq/liter (atomic absorption: 2.5 to 4.5 mg/dl)

Potassium
3.8 to 5.5 mEq/liter

Sodium
135 to 145 mEq/liter

Serum enzymes

Acid phosphatase
•0 to 1.1 Bodansky units/ml
•1 to 4 King-Armstrong units/ml
•0.13 to 0.63 BLB units/ml

Alanine aminotransferase (ALT)
•Adult males: 10 to 32 units/liter
•Adult females: 9 to 24 units/liter

Alkaline phosphatase
•1.5 to 4 Bodansky units/dl
•4 to 13.5 King-Armstrong units/dl
•Chemical inhibition method: Men, 90 to 239 units/dl; Women < age 45, 76 to 196 units/liter; women > age 45, 87 to 250 units/liter

Amylase
60 to 180 Somogyi units/dl

Angiotensin converting enzyme
18 to 67 U/liter (adults)

Aspartate aminotransferase (AST)
8 to 20 units/liter

Creatine phosphokinase
•Total: Men, 23 to 99 units/liter; women, 15 to 57 units/liter
•CPK-BB: none
•CPK-MB: 0 to 7 IU/liter
•CPK-MM: 5 to 70 IU/liter

Hydroxybutyric dehydrogenase (HBD)
•Serum HBD: 114 to 290 units/ml
•LDH/HBD ratio: 1.2 to 1.6:1

Lactic dehydrogenase
- Total: 48 to 115 IU/liter
- LDH_1: 18.1% to 29% of total
- LDH_2: 29.4% to 37.5% of total
- LDH_3: 18.8% to 26% of total
- LDH_4: 9.2% to 16.5% of total
- LDH_5: 5.3% to 13.4% of total

Serum hormones

Aldosterone
1 to 21 ng/dl

Antidiuretic hormone
1 to 5 pg/ml

Chorionic gonadotropin
< 3 mIU/ml

Cortisol (plasma)
7 to 28 μg/dl in the morning to 2 to 18 μg/dl in the afternoon

Estrogens
- Premenopausal women: 24 to 68 pg/ml on days 1 to 10, 50 to 186 pg/ml on days 11 to 20, and 73 to 149 pg/ml on days 21 to 28
- Men: 12 to 34 pg/ml

Free thyroxine (FT₄)
0.8 to 3.3 ng/dl

Free triiodothyronine
0.2 to 0.6 ng/dl

Growth hormone
- Men: 1 to 5 ng/ml
- Women: 0 to 10 ng/ml

Insulin
0 to 25 μU/ml

Parathyroid hormone
210 to 310 pg/ml

Prolactin
0 to 23 ng/dl in nonlactating females

Thyroxine (T₄)
5 to 13.5 μg/dl

Triiodothyronine
90 to 239 ng/dl

Serum lipids and lipoproteins

Lipoprotein-cholesterol fractionation
- HDL: 29 to 77 mg/dl
- LDL: 62 to 185 mg/dl

Total cholesterol
- Ideal: < 200 mg/dl
- Borderline high: 200 to 239 mg/dl
- High: > 240 mg/dl

Triglycerides
- Ages 0 to 29: 10 to 140 mg/dl
- Ages 30 to 39: 10 to 150 mg/dl
- Ages 40 to 49: 10 to 160 mg/dl
- Ages 50 to 59: 10 to 190 mg/dl

Serum proteins and pigments

Bilirubin, serum
Adult: direct, < 0.5 mg/dl; indirect, ≤ 1.1 mg/dl

Blood urea nitrogen (BUN)
8 to 20 mg/dl

Creatinine
Males: 0.8 to 1.2 mg/dl
Females: 0.6 to 0.9 mg/dl

Proteins
- Total serum protein: 6.6 to 7.9 g/dl (100%)
- Albumin: 3.3 to 4.5 g/dl (53%)
- Alpha₁ globulin: 0.1 to 0.4 g/dl (14%)
- Alpha₂ globulin: 0.5 to 1 g/dl (14%)
- Beta globulin: 0.7 to 1.2 g/dl (12%)
- Gamma globulin: 0.5 to 1.6 g/dl (20%)

Uric acid
- Men: 4.3 to 8 mg/dl
- Women: 2.3 to 6 mg/dl

Serum carbohydrates

Fasting plasma glucose
70 to 100 mg/dl

Lactic acid
0.93 to 1.65 mEq/liter

Oral glucose tolerance test (OGTT)
Peak at 160 to 180 mg/dl, 30 to 60 minutes after challenge dose

Two-hour postprandial plasma glucose
< 145 mg/dl

Urinalysis

Routine urinalysis
- *Appearance:* clear
- *Casts:* none, except ocasional hyaline casts
- *Color:* straw
- *Crystals:* present
- *Epithelial cells:* none
- *Odor:* slightly aromatic
- *pH:* 4.5 to 8.0
- *Specific gravity:* 1.025 to 1.030
- *Sugars:* none
- *Red blood cells:* 0 to 3 per high-power field
- *White blood cell count:* 0 to 4 per high-power field
- *Yeast cells:* none

Urine concentration test
- Specific gravity: 1.025 to 1.032
- Osmolality: > 800 mOsm/kg water

Urine dilution test
- Specific gravity: < 1.003
- Osmolality: < 100 mOsm/kg; 80% of water excreted in 4 hours

Urine chemistry tests

Amylase
10 to 80 amylase units/hour

17-ketosteroids (17-KS)
Men: 6 to 21 mg/24 hours
Women: 4 to 17 mg/24 hours

Creatinine clearance
- Men (age 20): 90 ml/minute/1.73 m²
- Women (age 20): 84 ml/minute/1.73 m²

Protein
< 150 mg/24 hours

Uric acid
250 to 750 mg/24 hours

Glucose oxidase
Negative

Ketones
Negative

Calcium
Males: < 275 mg/24 hours
Females: < 250 mg/24 hours

Phosphate
< 1,000 mg/24 hours

Sodium
30 to 280 mEq/24 hours

Chloride
110 to 250 mEq/24 hours

Cerebrospinal fluid

Glucose
50 to 80 mg/100 ml (two-thirds of blood glucose)

Pressure
50 to 180 mm H_2O

Protein
15 to 45 mg/dl

Stool tests

Lipids
Less than 20% of excreted solids, with excretion of less than 7 g/24 hours

Occult blood
2.5 mg/24 hours

Urobilinogen
50 to 300 mg/24 hours

Crisis values of laboratory tests

The abnormal laboratory test values listed below have immediate life-and-death significance to the patient. Report each value to the patient's doctor immediately.

Test	Low value	Common causes and effects	High value	Common causes and effects
Calcium, serum	< 7 mg/dl	*Vitamin D or parathyroid hormone deficiency:* tetany, convulsions	> 12 mg/dl	*Hyperparathyroidism:* coma
Carbon dioxide/bicarbonate, blood	< 10 mEq/liter	Complex pattern of metabolic and respiratory factors	> 40 mEq/liter	Complex pattern of metabolic and respiratory factors
Creatinine, blood			> 4 mg/dl	*Renal failure:* coma
Glucose, blood	< 40 mg/dl	*Excess insulin administration:* brain damage	> 400 mg/dl (with ketonemia and electrolyte imbalance)	*Diabetes:* diabetic coma
Hemoglobin	< 8 g/dl	*Hemorrhage, vitamin B_{12} or iron deficiency:* heart failure	> 18 g/dl	*Chronic obstructive pulmonary disease:* thrombosis, polycythemia vera
Partial thromboplastin time			> 60 sec	*Hemorrhage:* anticoagulation factor deficiency
$PaCO_2$, arterial	< 20 mm Hg	Complex pattern of metabolic and respiratory factors	> 70 mmHg	Complex pattern of metabolic and respiratory factors

Crisis values of laboratory tests *(continued)*

Test	Low value	Common causes and effects	High value	Common causes and effects
pH, blood	< 7.2	Complex pattern of metabolic and respiratory factors	> 7.6	Complex pattern of metabolic and respiratory factors
Platelet count	< 50,000/μl	*Bone marrow suppression:* hemorrhage	> 1,000,000/μl	*Leukemia, reaction to acute bleeding:* hemorrhage
PO₂, blood	< 50 mmHg	Complex pattern of metabolic and respiratory factors		
Potassium, serum	< 3 mEq/liter	*Vomiting and diarrhea, diuretic therapy:* cardiotoxicity, dysrhythmia, cardiac arrest	> 6 mEq/liter	*Renal disease, diuretic therapy:* cardiotoxicity, dysrhythmia
Prothrombin time			> 32 sec	*Anticoagulant therapy, anticoagulation factor deficiency:* hemorrhage
Sodium, serum	< 120 mEq/liter	*Diuretic therapy:* cardiac failure	> 160 mEq/liter	*Dehydration:* vascular collapse
White blood cell count	< 2,000/μl	*Bone marrow suppression:* infection	> 50,000/μl	*Leukemia:* infection
White blood cell count, CSF			> 10/μl	*Meningitis, encephalitis:* infection

Blood tests requiring immediate specimen transport

Each test is listed together with its appropriate color-top specimen collection tube. To review these briefly:
• *Red-top* tubes contain no additives, and are used to test serum samples.
• *Lavender-top* tubes contain EDTA, and are used to test whole blood samples.

• *Green-top* tubes contain heparin and are used to test plasma samples.
• *Blue top* tubes contain sodium citrate and citric acid, and are used for coagulation studies of plasma samples.
• *Black-top tubes* contain sodium oxalate, and are used for coagulation studies of plasma samples.
• *Gray-top* tubes contain a glycolytic inhibitor, and are used most often for glucose determinations in serum or plasma samples.

ABO blood typing (Red)
Acetylcholine receptor antibodies (Red)

Acid phosphatase (Red)
ACTH, plasma (Green)
Activated partial thromboplastin time (Blue)
Alkaline phosphatase (Red)
Ammonia, plasma (Green)
Angiotensin converting enzyme (Red for serum; Green for plasma)
Antibodies to extractable nuclear antigen (Red)
Antibody screening test (Red)
Antiglobulin, direct (Red)
Arginine test (Red)
Arterial blood gas analysis (Heparinized syringe)
Aspartate aminotransferase (Red)
Bilirubin, serum (Red)

Calcitonin, plasma (Green)
Carcinoembryonic antigen (Red)
Catecholamines, plasma (Special
  tube usually supplied)
Ceruloplasmin, serum (Red)
Cholinesterase (Red)
Coagulation, extrinsic system
  (Blue)
Coagulation, intrinsic system
  (Blue)
Cold agglutinins (Red)
Complement assays (Red)
Creatine phosphokinase (Red)
Creatine, serum (Red)
Creatinine, serum (Red)
Crossmatching (Red)
Cryoglobulins (Red)
Erythrocyte sedimentation
  (Lavender)
Estrogen, serum (Red)
Euglobulin lysis time (Blue)
Febrile agglutination tests (Red)
Fibrinogen, plasma (Blue)
Folic acid, serum (Red)
Fungal serology (Red)
Gastrin, serum (Red)
Glucose, fasting plasma (Gray)
Glucose, plasma, 2-hour postpran-
  dial (Gray)

Glucose tolerance, oral (Gray)
Growth hormone, serum (Red)
Growth hormone suppression
  (Red)
Hematocrit (Lavender)
Human chorionic gonadotropin,
  serum (Red)
Human placental lactogen, serum
  (Red)
Hydroxybutyric dehydrogenase
  (Red)
Immune complex assays, serum
  (Red)
Immunoglobulins G, A, and M
  (Red)
Insulin, serum (Red)
Insulin tolerance test (Gray)
Iron, serum (Red)
Isocitrate dehydrogenase (Red)
Lactic acid and pyruvic acid
  (Gray)
Lactic dehydrogenase (Red)
Lipoprotein-cholesterol fractiona-
  tion (Red)
Lymphocyte transformation
  (Green)
Manganese, serum (Metal-free
  tube)
Parathyroid hormone, serum (Red)

Phospholipids (Red)
Plasma thrombin time (Blue)
Progesterone, plasma (Green)
Prothrombin consumption time
  (Red)
Prothrombin time (Blue)
Renin, plasma (Lavender for pe-
  ripheral vein sample)
Rh typing (Red for serum; Laven-
  der for whole blood)
T- and B-lymphocyte counts
  (Green)
Tolbutamide tolerance test (Gray)
Total CO_2 (Red with electrolytes;
  Green alone)
Total cholesterol (Red)
Total iron-binding capacity (Red)
Transferrin, serum (Red)
Triglycerides (Red)
Vitamin A and carotene, serum
  (Red)
Vitamin B_{12}, serum (Red)
Vitamin C, plasma (Black)
Zinc, serum (Metal-free tube)

How an ECG reflects cardiac conduction

An ECG is a graphic display of the heart's electrical activity. The electrical currents produced by the heart are transmitted to the skin's surface and recorded by electrodes attached to the chest wall and extremities. The resulting electrical ebb and flow are amplified before being printed on moving graph paper or displayed on an oscilloscope. The deflections in each ECG waveform reflect the electrical status (depolarized and repolarized) of cardiac muscle. In the illustration, colors on the ECG pattern correspond to the colored areas of the heart's conduction system.

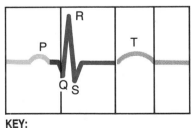

KEY:

P wave: atrial depolarization

QRS complex: ventricular depolarization

T wave: ventricular repolarization

Conduction system

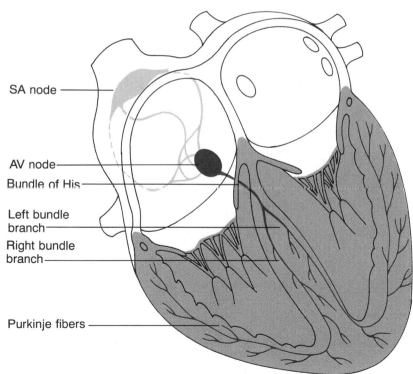

SA node

AV node

Bundle of His

Left bundle branch

Right bundle branch

Purkinje fibers

Understanding the 12-lead ECG

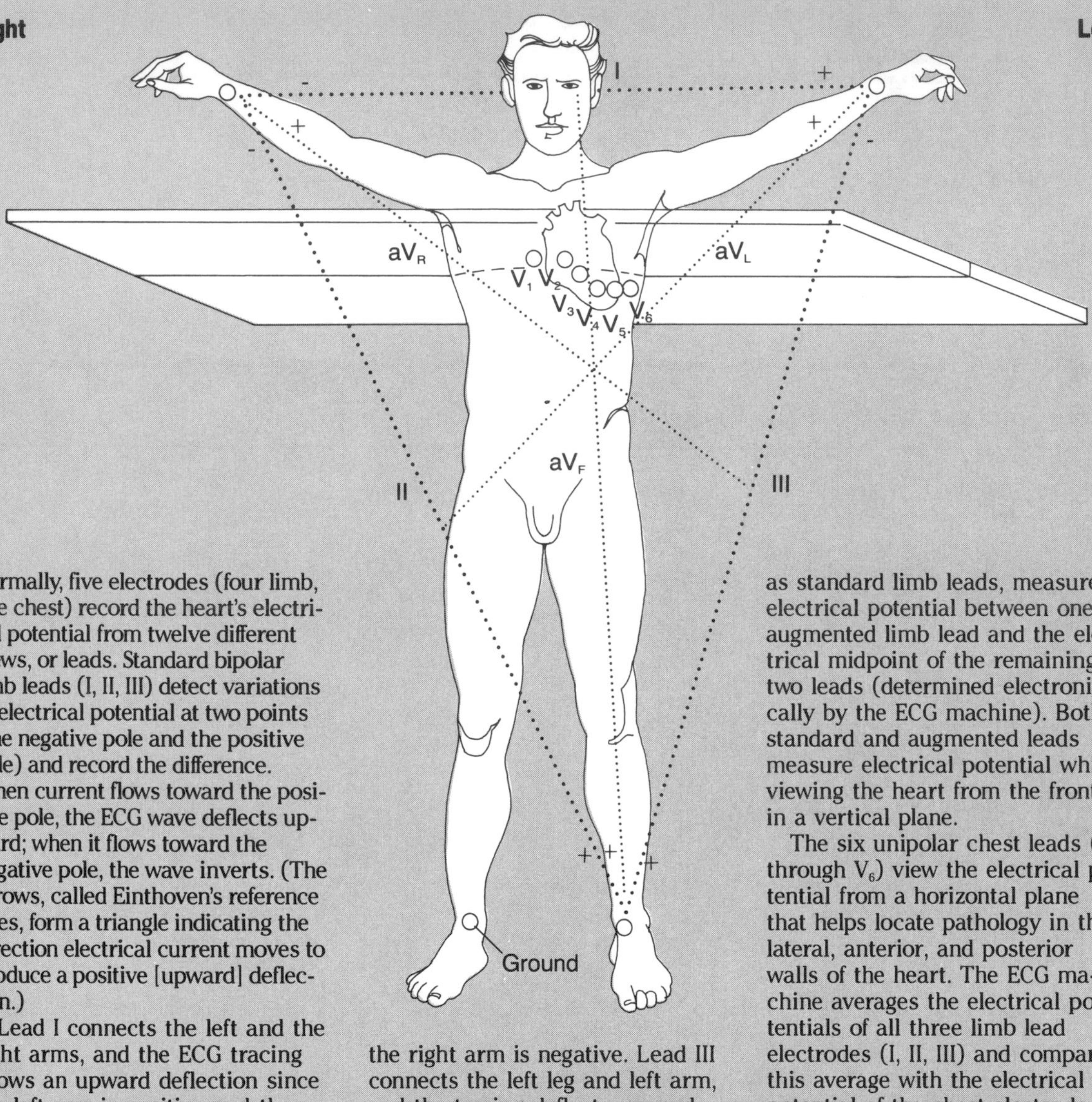

Right   **Left**

I

aV$_R$ aV$_L$

V$_1$ V$_2$
V$_3$ V$_4$ V$_5$ V$_6$

aV$_F$

II   III

Ground

Normally, five electrodes (four limb, one chest) record the heart's electrical potential from twelve different views, or leads. Standard bipolar limb leads (I, II, III) detect variations in electrical potential at two points (the negative pole and the positive pole) and record the difference. When current flows toward the positive pole, the ECG wave deflects upward; when it flows toward the negative pole, the wave inverts. (The arrows, called Einthoven's reference lines, form a triangle indicating the direction electrical current moves to produce a positive [upward] deflection.)

Lead I connects the left and the right arms, and the ECG tracing shows an upward deflection since the left arm is positive and the right arm is negative. Lead II connects the left leg and right arm, and the tracing deflects upward since the left leg is positive and

the right arm is negative. Lead III connects the left leg and left arm, and the tracing deflects upward since the left leg is positive and the left arm negative.

The unipolar augmented limb leads (aV$_R$, aV$_L$, and aV$_F$), which use the same electrode placement

as standard limb leads, measure electrical potential between one augmented limb lead and the electrical midpoint of the remaining two leads (determined electronically by the ECG machine). Both standard and augmented leads measure electrical potential while viewing the heart from the front, in a vertical plane.

The six unipolar chest leads (V$_1$ through V$_6$) view the electrical potential from a horizontal plane that helps locate pathology in the lateral, anterior, and posterior walls of the heart. The ECG machine averages the electrical potentials of all three limb lead electrodes (I, II, III) and compares this average with the electrical potential of the chest electrode. Recordings made with the V connection show electrical potential variations that occur under the chest electrode as its position is changed.

How to read any ECG: An 8-step guide

An ECG waveform has three basic elements: a *P wave,* a *QRS complex,* and a *T wave.* These are joined by five other useful diagnostic elements: the *PR interval,* the *U wave,* the *ST segment,* the *J-point,* and the *QT interval.* The diagram below shows how they're related.

The following 8-step guide will enable you to read any ECG.

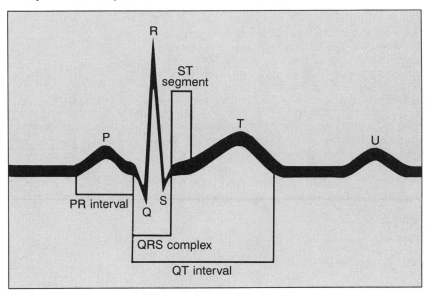

Step 1: Evaluate the P wave
Observe the P wave's size, shape and location in the waveform. If the P wave consistently precedes the QRS complex, the electrical impulse is being initiated by the sinoatrial (SA) node, as it should be.

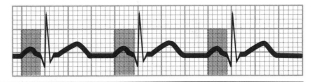

Step 2: Evaluate the atrial rhythm
The P wave should occur at regular intervals, with only small variations associated with respiration. Using calipers, you can easily measure the interval betwen P waves (the *P-P interval*). Compare the P-P intervals in several ECG cycles. Make sure the calipers are set at the same point—at the beginning of the wave or on its peak. Instead of lifting the calipers, rotate one of its legs to the next P wave, to ensure accurate measurements.

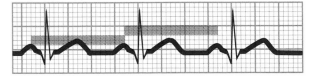

(continued)

How to read any ECG: An 8-step guide *(continued)*

Step 3: Determine the atrial rate

To determine the atrial rate quickly, count the number of P waves in two 3-second segments. Multiply this number by 10.

For a more accurate determination, count the number of small squares between two P waves using either the apex of the wave or the initial upstroke of the wave. Each small square equals 0.04 second; 1,500 squares equal 1 minute (0.04 x 1,500 = 60 seconds). So, divide 1,500 by the number of squares you counted between the P waves. This gives you the atrial rate—the number of contractions per minute.

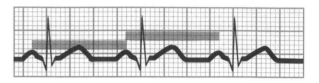

Step 4: Calculate duration of the P-R interval

Count the number of small squares between the beginning of the P wave and the beginning of the QRS complex. Multiply the number of squares by 0.04 second. The normal interval is between 0.12 and 0.20 second, or between 3 and 5 small squares wide. A wider interval indicates delayed conduction of the impulse to the ventricles.

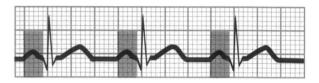

Step 5: Evaluate the ventricular rhythm

Use the calipers to measure the R-R intervals. Remember to place the calipers on the same point of the QRS complex. If the R-R intervals remain consistent, the ventricular rhythm is regular.

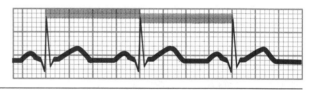

Step 6: Determine the ventricular rate

To determine the ventricular rate, use the same formula as in Step 3. In this case, however, count the number of small squares between two R waves to do the calculation. Also check that the QRS complex is shaped appropriately for the lead you're monitoring.

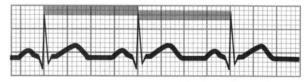

Step 7: Calculate the duration of the QRS complex

Count the number of squares between the beginning and the end of the QRS complex and multiply by 0.04 second. A normal QRS complex is less than 0.12 second, or less than 3 small squares wide. Some references specify 0.06 to 0.10 second as the normal duration for the QRS complex.

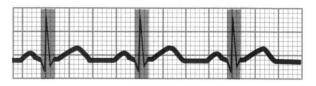

Step 8: Calculate the duration of the QT interval

Count the number of squares from the beginning of the QRS complex to the end of the T wave. Multiply this number by 0.04 second. The normal range is 0.36 to 0.44 second, or 9 to 11 small squares wide.

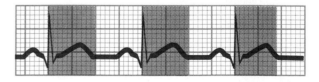

Marking an ECG strip

Use the marking button on the ECG machine to identify chest leads and limb leads. Depress the button to print a code of long and short dashes (shown below) directly on the ECG strip. (*Note:* Since code varies, check manufacturer's instructions.)

Limb leads

I: -   aV$_R$: - —
II: - -   aV$_L$: - - —
III: - - -   aV$_F$: - - - —

Chest leads

V$_1$: — -   V$_4$: — - - - -
V$_2$: — - -   V$_5$: — - - - - -
V$_3$: — - - -   V$_6$: — - - - - - -

Positioning chest leads

To prevent spurious test results, position chest electrodes as follows:
V$_1$: fourth intercostal space at right border of sternum
V$_2$: fourth intercostal space at left border of sternum
V$_3$: halfway between V$_2$ and V$_4$
V$_4$: fifth intercostal space at midclavicular line
V$_5$: anterior axillary line (halfway between V$_4$ and V$_6$)
V$_6$: midaxillary line, level with V$_4$

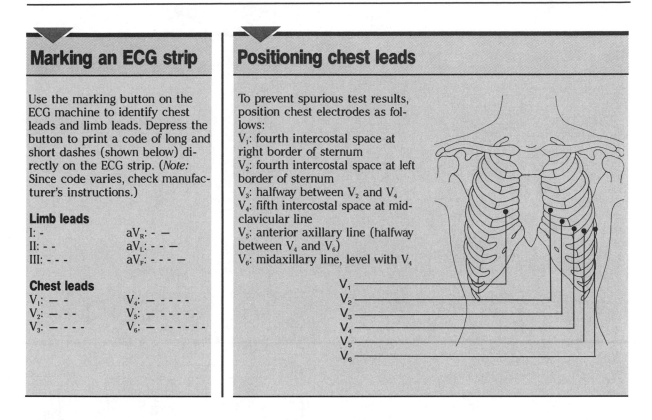

Normal 12-lead ECG waveforms: What they look like

Because each lead takes a different view of heart activity, it generates its own characteristic tracing. The traces shown here are representative of each of the 12 leads. Leads aV$_R$, V$_1$, V$_2$, and V$_3$ normally show strong negative deflections below the baseline. Negative deflections indicate that the current is flowing away from the positive electrode; positive deflections, that the current's flowing toward the positive electrode.

Lead I

Lead V$_1$

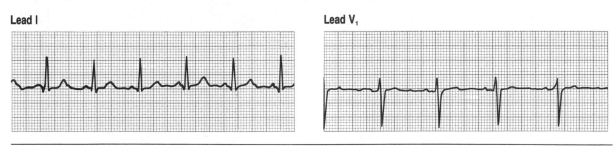

(continued)

Normal ECG waveforms: What they look like (continued)

Lead II

Lead V₂

Lead III

Lead V₃

Lead aV_R

Lead V₄

Lead aV_L

Lead V₅

Lead aV_F

Lead V₆

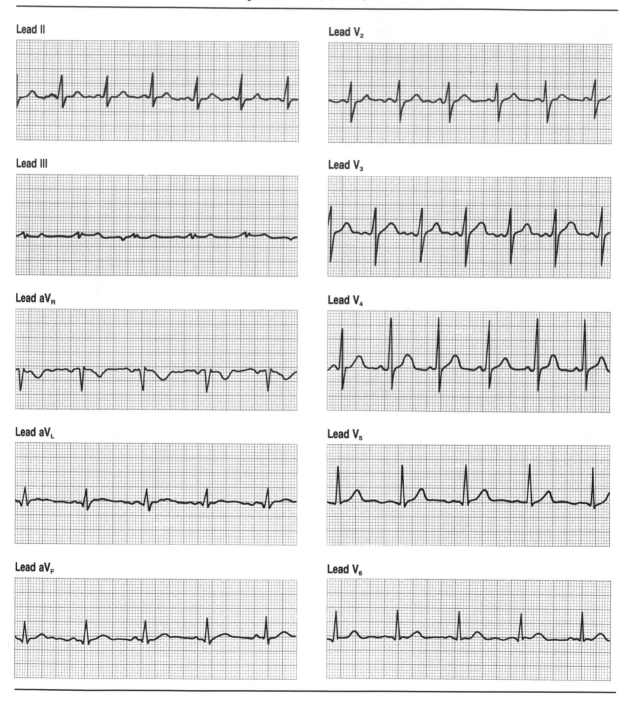

Where to place electrodes for an exercise ECG

If you're working with a three-electrode monitor, you can establish the three standard leads (I, II, III) and the three augmented limb leads (aV_R, aV_L, aV_F). However, if you want to obtain readings similar to the V_1 and V_6 chest leads, you can use modified chest leads (MCL_1, MCL_6). If you're using a five-electrode monitor, the most sensitive of these recording devices, you can record standard and augmented leads as well as six chest leads.

Type	Lead	Electrode placement	
Three-electrode monitor	Lead II	Positive (+): left side of chest, lowest palpable rib, midclavicular Negative (−): right shoulder, below clavicular hollow Ground (G): left shoulder, below clavicular hollow	
	MCL_1	Positive (+): right sternal border, lowest palpable rib Negative (−): left shoulder, below clavicular hollow Ground (G): right shoulder, below clavicular hollow	
	MCL_6	Positive (+): left side of chest, lowest palpable rib, midclavicular line Negative (−): left shoulder, below clavicular hollow Ground (G): right shoulder, below clavicular hollow	
Five-electrode monitor	V_1 through V_6	Positive (+): left side of chest, just below lowest palpable rib Negative (−): right shoulder, midclavicular Ground (G): right side of chest, just below lowest palpable rib Inactive (I): left shoulder, midclavicular Chest V_1: fourth intercostal space to right of sternum Chest V_2: fourth intercostal space to left of sternum Chest V_3: halfway between V_2 and V_4 Chest V_4: fifth intercostal space, midclavicular, left side Chest V_5: halfway between V_4 and V_6 Chest V_6: same line as V_5 at midaxillary line	

Identifying abnormal exercise ECG tracings

These tracings are from an abnormal exercise ECG obtained during a treadmill test performed on a patient who had just undergone a triple coronary artery bypass graft. The first tracing shows the heart at rest, blood pressure 124/80. In the second tracing, the patient worked up to a 10% grade at 1.7 mph before experiencing angina at 2 minutes 25 seconds. The tracing shows a depressed ST segment; heart rate was 85, blood pressure 140/70. The third tracing shows the heart at rest 6 minutes after the test; blood pressure was 140/90.

(Tracings courtesy of Arlene Strong, RN, MN)

Resting

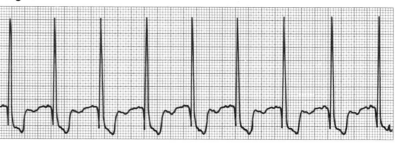

Angina

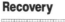
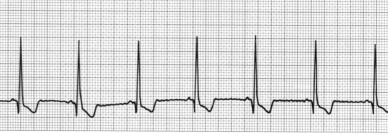

Recovery

Detecting common cardiac dysrhythmias

In cardiac dysrhythmias, abnormal electrical conduction or automaticity changes heart rate and rhythm. Dysrhythmias are generally classified according to their origin (ventricular or supraventricular). Their effect on cardiac output and blood pressure, partially influenced by the site of origin, determines their clinical significance. Depicted here are several of the more common dysrhythmias to look out for.

Sinus arrhythmia

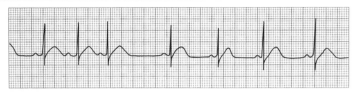

Causes
• Usually a normal variation of normal sinus rhythm (NSR); associated with sinus bradycardia

Description
• Slight irregularity of heartbeat, usually corresponding to respiratory cycle
• Rate increases with inspiration and decreases with expiration

Treatment
• None

Sinus tachycardia

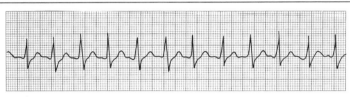

Causes
• Normal physiologic response to fever, exercise, anxiety, pain, dehydration; may also accompany shock, left ventricular failure, cardiac tamponade, anemia, hyperthyroidism, hypovolemia, pulmonary embolus
• May result from treatment with vagolytic and sympathetic stimulating drugs

Description
• Rate > 100 beats/minute; rarely, > 160 beats/minute
• Every QRS complex follows a P wave

Treatment
• Correct underlying cause

Sinus bradycardia

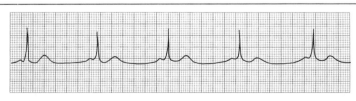

Causes
• Increased intracranial pressure; increased vagal tone due to bowel straining, vomiting, intubation, mechanical ventilation; sick sinus syndrome or hypothyroidism
• Treatment with beta-blockers and sympatholytic drugs
• May be normal in athletes

Description
• Rate < 60 beats/minute
• A QRS complex follows each P wave

Treatment
• For low cardiac output, dizziness, weakness, altered level of consciousness, or low blood pressure, 0.5 mg atropine every 5 minutes to total of 2.0 mg
• Temporary pacemaker or isoproterenol, if atropine fails

(continued)

Detecting common cardiac dysrhythmias (continued)

Sinus arrest

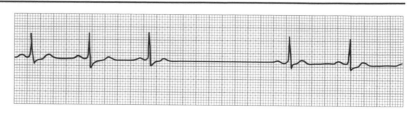

Causes
• Vagal stimulation, digitalis or quinidine toxicity
• Often a sign of sick sinus syndrome

Description
• NSR interrupted by unexpectedly prolonged P-P interval, often terminated by a junctional escape beat, or return to NSR
• QRS complexes uniform but irregular

Treatment
• A pacemaker for repeated episodes

Wandering pacemaker

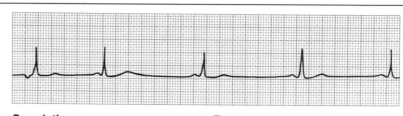

Causes
• Seen in rheumatic pericarditis as a result of inflammation involving the SA node, digitalis toxicity, and sick sinus syndrome

Description
• Rate varies
• QRS complexes uniform in shape but irregular in rhythm
• P waves irregular with changing configuration, indicating they're not all from sinus node or single atrial focus
• PR interval varies from short to normal

Treatment
• Patient should use digitalis cautiously
• No other treatment

First-degree AV block

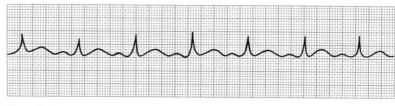

Causes
• Inferior myocardial ischemia or infarction, hypothyroidism, digitalis toxicity, potassium imbalance

Description
• PR interval prolonged > 0.20 seconds
• QRS complex normal

Treatment
• Patient should use digitalis cautiously
• Correct underlying cause; otherwise, be alert for increasing block

Detecting common cardiac dysrhythmias (continued)

Type I second-degree AV block (Wenckebach or Mobitz I)

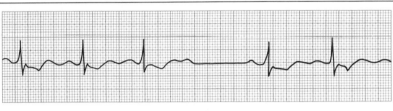

Causes
• *Mobitz Type I:* Inferior wall myocardial infarction, digitalis toxicity, vagal stimulation

Description
• *Mobitz Type I:* PR interval becomes progessively longer with each cycle until QRS disappears (dropped beat). After a dropped beat, PR interval is shorter.
• Ventricular rate is irregular; atrial rhythm, regular.

Treatment
• *Mobitz Type I:* Atropine, if patient is symptomatic
• Discontinue digitalis

Type II second-degree AV block (Mobitz Type II)

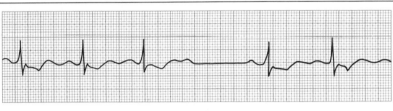

Causes
• *Mobitz Type II:* Degenerative disease of conduction system, ischemia of AV node in anterior myocardial infarction, digitalis toxicity, anteroseptal infarction

Description
• *Mobitz Type II:* PR interval is constant, with QRS complexes dropped
• Ventricular rhythm may be irregular, with varying degree of block
• Atrial rate regular

Treatment
• *Mobitz Type II:* Temporary pacemaker, sometimes followed by permanent pacemaker
• Atropine, for slow rate
• If patient is taking digitalis, it is discontinued

Junctional tachycardia

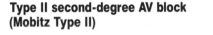
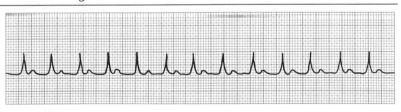

Causes
• Digitalis toxicity, myocarditis, cardiomyopathy, myocardial ischemia or infarct

Description
• Onset of rhythm often sudden, occurring in bursts
• Ventricular rate > 100 beats/ minute
• Other characteristics same as junctional rhythm

Treatment
• Vagal stimulation
• Propranolol, quinidine, digitalis (if cause is not digitalis toxicity)
• Elective cardioversion

How drugs affect ECGs

Digitalis

This potent cardiac glycoside increases the force of myocardial contraction, decreases conduction velocity through the AV node to slow heart rate, and prolongs the effective refractory period of the AV node by direct and sympatholytic effects on the SA node. Excess amounts of digitalis can slow conduction through the AV node and cause irritable ectopic foci in the ventricles.

ECG characteristics

P wave: decreased voltage, may be notched
Atrial rhythm: regular
Atrial rate: usually within normal limits, but may be bradycardic
PR interval: May be within normal limits or prolonged
Ventricular rhythm: regular
Ventricular rate: usually within normal limits, but may be bradycardic
QRS complex: within normal limits
QT interval duration: often shortened

Signs and symptoms

• None unless digitalis toxicity is present.
• Severity depends on degree of toxicity.
• Common toxic effects·may include abdominal pain, almost any type of rhythm disturbance, anorexia, change in mental status, diarrhea, nausea and vomiting, visual disturbances such as altered color perception and blurred vision, weakness, and fatigue.

Interventions

• None unless digitialis toxicity occurs.
• If toxicity occurs, stop the drug and treat the cause and any dysrhythmia

Special considerations

• Gradual sloping occurs in ST segment, causing ST depression in a direction opposite to the QRS deflection.
• T wave may be flattened and inverted in a direction opposite to the QRS deflection.
• ST depression and T-wave inversion in leads with negatively deflected QRS complexes may indicate a need to reduce the digitalis dose.
• Virtually any dysrhythmia may be caused by digitalis excess. The most common dysrhythmias that occur include premature ventricular contractions (PVCs), especially bigeminy, paroxysmal supraventricular tachycardias with or without block, second-degree heart block, and sinus arrest.

Digitalis effects

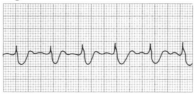

Quinidine

Quinidine is an antiarrhythmic drug that decreases sodium transport through cardiac tissues, slowing conduction through the AV node. It also prolongs the effective refractory period and decreases automaticity. At toxic levels, quinidine can cause SA and AV block and ventricular dysrhythmias.

ECG characteristics

P wave: May be widened and notched, especially evident in leads I and II
Atrial rhythm: regular
Atrial rate: within normal limits
PR interval: within normal limits
Ventricular rhythm: regular
Ventricular rate: within normal limits
QRS complex: widens slightly
QT interval duration: may be prolonged

Signs and symptoms

• None unless toxicity is present.
• Severity depends on degree of toxicity.
• Common toxic effects may include diarrhea, dizziness, fever, headache, hypotension, nausea and vomiting, tinnitus, SA and AV block, rash, syncope, ventricular tachycardia.

Interventions

• None unless toxicity occurs. Check patient's ECG before dose. If QRS complex shows 50% increase or greater, or if bundle branch block is present and QRS complex has increased 25% or greater, hold dose and notify doctor.
• If toxicity occurs, stop drug and treat dysrhythmia, if present.

Special considerations

• U waves are apparent.
• If quinidine levels climb to toxic levels, a "roller coaster" pattern of toxicity can occur. The QRS complex continues to widen as serum quinidine levels increase.
• Dysrhythmias caused by quinidine toxicity include SA and AV block, torsades de pointes, ventricular tachycardia, and ventricular fibrillation.

Quinidine effects

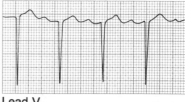

Lead V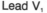

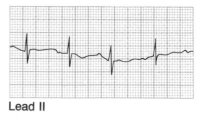

Lead II

How electrolyte imbalances affect ECGs

Potassium or calcium imbalance—either an excess or a deficiency—will have a marked effect on your patient's cardiac conduction system, as shown on his ECG strip. Learn to recognize these ECG abnormalities—they may help you prevent serious and possibly life-threatening problems.

KEY:
◻ **Abnormal** ◼ **Normal**

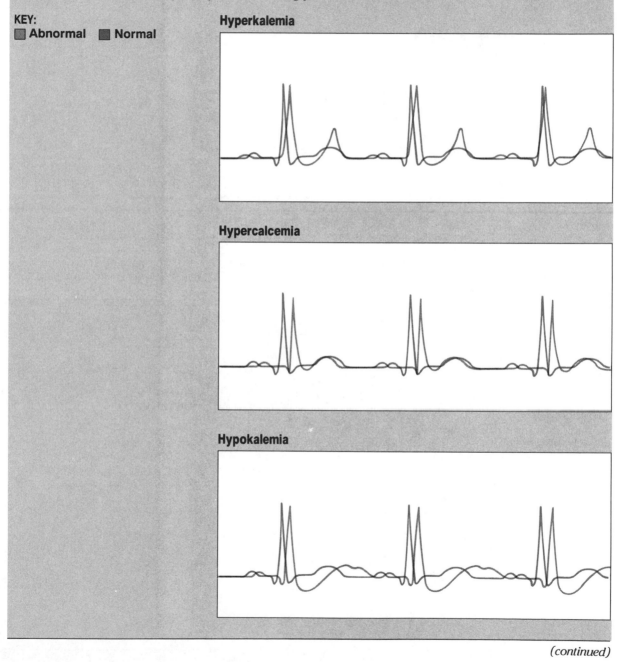

Hyperkalemia

Hypercalcemia

Hypokalemia

(continued)

How electrolyte imbalances affect ECGs *(continued)*

KEY:
🔲 **Abnormal**   🔲 **Normal**

Hypocalcemia

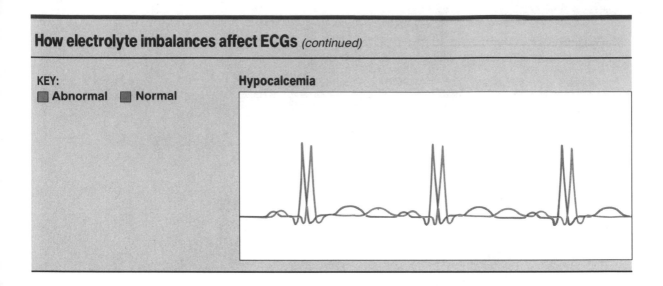

Identifying life-threatening ECG waveforms

As you monitor your patient on a cardiac monitor or 12-lead ECG, watch for any of the waveforms shown here. They indicate that your patient faces an immediate life-threatening situation. Notify the doctor; then prepare to perform the nursing interventions described.

**Ventricular asystole
(Cardiac standstill)**

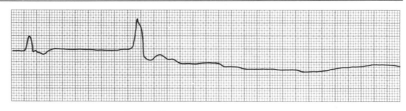

Characteristics
• Totally absent ventricular electrical activity
• Possible P waves
• Possibly the main event in cardiac arrest (may also occur after ventricular fibrillation)
• May occur in a patient with complete heart block and no pacemaker
• Possible severe metabolic deficit or extensive myocardial damage

Interventions
• Begin CPR.
• Assist with endotracheal intubation.
• Start an I.V.
• Prepare to give epinephrine, sodium bicarbonate, atropine, calcium chloride, and isoproterenol, as ordered.
• Prepare to assist with temporary pacemaker insertion and defibrillation.

Identifying life-threatening ECG waveforms (continued)

Ventricular fibrillation

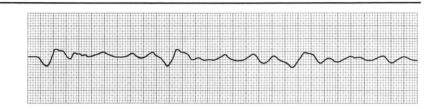

Characteristics
- Possible ventricular fibrillation arising spontaneously or triggered by premature ventricular contractions or ventricular tachycardia
- Ventricular rhythm rapid and chaotic, indicating varying degrees of depolarization and repolarization; QRS complexes not identifiable
- Patient unconscious at onset
- Absent pulses, heart sounds, and blood pressure
- Dilated pupils, rapid development of cyanosis
- Possible convulsions
- Possible death of patient within minutes, depending on his age (ventricular fibrillation is the most common cause of sudden death in patients with coronary heart disease)

Interventions
- Give precordial thump if ventricular fibrillation appears on the monitor.
- Defibrillate the patient.
- Begin CPR.
- Administer bretylium, epinephrine, and sodium bicarbonate, as ordered. (Sodium bicarbonate is given according to the patient's arterial blood gas levels, after dysrhythmia terminates, to treat lactic acidosis.)
- Prepare to give lidocaine to treat myocardial irritability and to prevent recurring dysrhythmias.

Ventricular tachycardia

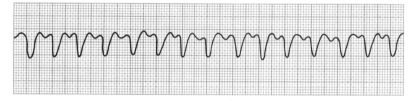

Characteristics
- Dangerously low cardiac output that may produce hypotension, chest pain, palpitations, dyspnea, anxiety, shock, coma, and sudden death resulting from ventricular fibrillation
- Wide, bizarrely shaped QRS complexes
- Regular rhythm, rapid rate
- Absent P waves
- T waves pointing in direction opposite that of QRS complexes

Interventions
- Perform precordial thump if the patient's pulseless and on a monitor.
- Prepare to give lidocaine to treat the dysrhythmia.
- Prepare to give defibrillation immediately if lidocaine's ineffective.
- Administer lidocaine drip, procainamide, and bretylium, as ordered.
- Suspect hypokalemia if the patient's tachycardia returns despite antiarrhythmic drugs.
- Prepare to give potassium chloride for hypokalemia.
- Suspect lactic acidosis if the patient's tachycardia persists for more than 5 minutes, and prepare to give sodium bicarbonate.
- Prepare to assist with temporary pacemaker insertion for recurrent tachycardia.

(continued)

Identifying life-threatening ECG waveforms (continued)

Premature ventricular contractions (PVCs)

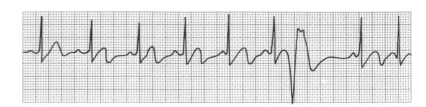

Characteristics
• Common form of dysrhythmia
• Longer-than-normal pause occurring immediately after premature beats (compensatory pause)
• Indicator of myocardial irritability
• May initiate ventricular tachycardia, then ventricular fibrillation when they occur *frequently* (six or more times/minute), strike on the T wave of preceding complex (R on T pattern), have more than one configuration (multiple form PVCs), occur sequentially for two or three beats (coupling or short runs of PVCs), or when every second beat is a PVC (bigeminy)
• Trigeminy: pattern of two normal beats followed by a PVC
• Increased risk of sudden death if occurring with angina

Interventions
• Prepare to give lidocaine (sometimes procainamide or later potassium) as ordered to suppress the irritable ventricular focus.
• Be aware that digitalis or diuretic therapy can cause PVCs, and anticipate continuing the drug or giving the patient potassium to restore electrolyte balance and to correct drug-induced ectopic beats.
• Watch the patient for signs and symptoms of lidocaine overdose—such as seizures.
• With procainamide, watch the patient for hypotension.

Sinus bradycardia

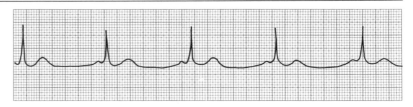

Characteristics
• Normal rhythm but with rate less than 60 beats/minute.
• Bradydysrhythmias, possibly including sinus bradycardia, junctional rhythm, idioventricular rhythm, heart block
• Reentry facilitated, possible ectopic rhythms when ventricular rate is low
• Reduced threshold for ventricular fibrillation, possible decreased cardiac output

Interventions
• Start an I.V. and prepare to give atropine, then isoproterenol, as ordered.
• Assist with temporary pacemaker insertion, as ordered, if the patient's heartbeat doesn't respond to drugs.
• Restore volume status if the patient's hypotensive. (If hypotension persists, you may be ordered to start an infusion of dopamine or norepinephrine.)

Identifying life-threatening ECG waveforms *(continued)*

Third-degree AV block
(Complete heart block)

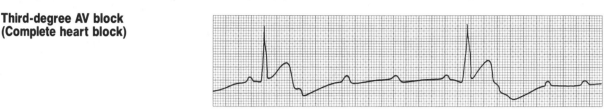

Characteristics
• Atria beating independently of the ventricles
• Possible episodes of syncope and convulsions, left ventricular failure
• Cardiac output insufficient to meet circulatory demands
• Potential cessation of ventricular impulse or replacement by irritable ventricular foci

Interventions
• Prepare to assist with temporary pacemaker insertion.
• Prepare to give atropine, as ordered.
• Prepare to give an infusion of isoproterenol, as ordered.
• Bring a defibrillator to the patient's bedside, and be ready to use it.

Troubleshooting ECG artifacts

Even minor disturbances in the ECG monitoring system—electrical interference, loose electrodes, and patient movement, for example—can create major interference with the ECG tracing. Your first step whenever you notice an artifact should be to check the patient for medical causes. If his condition appears stable, check the monitor for mechanical causes. Some common mechanical artifacts are listed here.

False high-rate alarms
The rate alarm averages the number of heartbeats per minute by counting the QRS complexes. But if a tracing contains tall waves from sources other than the heart, the monitor may record them as QRS complexes and falsely sound the high-rate alarm.

One possible cause of false high-rate alarms is skeletal muscle activity, which causes tall waves in a tracing.

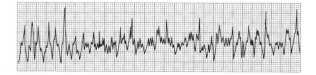

Avoid this by applying electrodes away from large muscle masses, such as the pectoral muscles.

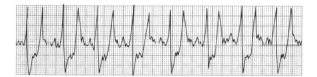

Another cause is T waves as tall as, or taller than, the QRS complexes.

Once you've ruled out hyperkalemia as the cause of abnormally high T waves, check for other problems with the monitor. Try repositioning the electrodes. If the T waves are still too tall, select a different lead—one where the QRS complexes have a higher amplitude than the T waves.

If the problem persists, check for loose electrodes, damaged or broken wires or cables, or improper cable connections. If you still have no luck, you may have set the alarm system too close to the patient's normal pulse rate. Reset the high-rate alarm slightly higher.

(continued)

Troubleshooting ECG artifacts (continued)

False low-rate alarms
Poor contact between the skin and electrodes may cause a false-low rate alarm to sound. The tracings may resemble idioventricular rhythm or asystole. Check the patient. If he's not distressed, check the electrodes. You may find at least one electrode making poor skin contact.

Patient movement may also cause a false low-rate alarm. For example, if a patient turns on his side, the axis of his heart shifts slightly, which reduces the QRS amplitude and triggers the low rate alarm. Instead of disturbing the patient, reset the gain control to enlarge the QRS complexes.

If you get a baseline but no tracing, check the gain knob and the lead selector control to make sure they're positioned properly. If they are, check the cable connections. Also check the low-rate setting on the pulse-rate meter. If the patient's heart rate is too close to the low-rate setting, increase the setting slightly, but be sure it's within a safe margin.

Electrical interference
Interference caused by external electrical voltage (60-cycle alternating current) appears on the oscilloscope and rhythm strip as a widened baseline that distorts the ECG and obscures parts of the cardiac cycle.

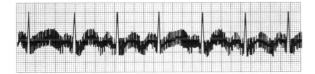

It may also create a hazard for the patient and staff. Check power plugs for third prongs (ground) and report the problem to the electrician. Also move nearby electrical devices away from the monitor, if at all possible. If the patient is on an electrically operated bed, disconnect the bed's cable from the wall socket. Sometimes you can eliminate interference just by replacing the electrodes.

Weak signals
Indistinct or defective patterns on a monitor (see figure) may result from an improper gain-dial setting, poor electrode-skin contact, improper small-electrode cable connection, or monitor malfunction. If turning up the gain doesn't remedy the problem, look for improperly attached electrodes, too little or too much electrode jelly, and moist skin from perspiration. Correct the problem and reapply electrodes.

Wandering baseline
Inadequate electrode connections or a patient's movements or respirations may cause a wandering baseline to appear.

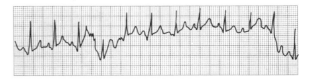

Replace the electrodes and check cable tension to ensure that it's not pulling the electrode away from the patient's body. If respiratory movement is the problem, try moving the electrode to another part of the patient's chest, away from his ribs. If the problem persists, it may be caused by external voltage variations. Inform the electrician.

6 Disorders: Signs, significance, trends

Danger signs and symptoms

Some signs and symptoms, like cyanosis and bulging fontanelles, clearly alert you to danger. Others, like headache, are less dramatic, but can prove to be subtle signals of an emergency.

Abdominal rigidity
This abnormal muscle tension or inflexibility of the abdomen can be detected by palpation.

Rigidity may be voluntary or involuntary. Involuntary rigidity reflects peritoneal irritation or inflammation. Although involuntary rigidity commonly results from GI disorders, it may indicate pneumonia or dissecting aortic aneurysm, or mesenteric artery ischemia or other vascular disorders. Insect toxins may also cause involuntary rigidity. Nausea, vomiting and abdominal tenderness, distention, and pain frequently accompany this sign.

Voluntary rigidity simply reflects the patient's fear or nervousness upon palpation.

Absent bowel sounds
When are bowel sounds considered absent? If you auscultate us-

ing a stethoscope for 5 minutes in each abdominal quadrant and don't hear any sounds, you've detected this sign.

Bowel sounds cease when mechanical or vascular obstruction or neurogenic inhibition halts peristalsis. When peristalsis halts, gas from bowel contents and fluid secreted from the intestinal walls accumulate and distend the lumen. This accumulation leads to life-threatening complications such as perforation, peritonitis and sepsis, or hypovolemic shock.

Abrupt cessation of bowel sounds accompanied by abdominal pain, rigidity, and distention signals a life-threatening crisis. Absent bowel sounds following a period of hyperactivity may indicate strangulation of a mechanically obstructed bowel.

Absent or weak pulse
Absent or weak pulse may indicate a number of potentially life-threatening conditions, including aortic aneurysm, aortic arch syndrome, aortic bifurcation occlusion, aortic stenosis, cardiac tamponade, dysrhythmias, peripheral vascular disease, pulmonary embolism, and shock. Localized loss or weakness of a pulse that's normally strong may indicate arterial occlusion, possibly calling for emergency surgery.

Altered level of consciousness
Consciousness is controlled by an intricate network of neurons whose axons extend from the brain stem, thalamus, and hypothalamus to the cerebral cortex. Disturbance in any part of this network alters consciousness. Level of consciousness may deteriorate suddenly or gradually and may remain altered temporarily or permanently.

Progression from lethargy to stupor to coma usually results from neurologic disorders and often signals life-threatening complications of hemorrhage, trauma, or cerebral edema. The sign can also result from metabolic, gastrointestinal, musculoskeletal, urologic, and cardiopulmonary disorders; severe nutritional deficiency; the effects of toxins; and drug use.

Apnea
The cessation of spontaneous respiration, apnea almost always represents a life-threatening emergency. Pathophysiologic mechanisms that can lead to this sign include airway obstruction, alveolar gas diffusion impairment, brain stem dysfunction, pleural pressure gradient disruption, pulmonary capillary perfusion decrease, and respiratory muscle failure. Common causes include

trauma, cardiac arrest, neurologic disease, aspiration of foreign objects, bronchospasm, and drug overdose.

Occasionally, apnea is temporary and self-limiting, as in Cheyne-Stokes and Biot's respirations.

Bradycardia
By itself, a heart rate of fewer than 60 beats/minute is a nonspecific sign. However, in conjunction with such symptoms as chest pain, dizziness, and shortness of breath, bradycardia can signal a life-threatening disorder. When bradycardia results from an illness, heart rate may slow to as little as 1 beat/minute. Possible causes include cardiomyopathy, cervical spine injury, hypothermia, hypothyroidism, increased intracranial pressure (ICP), and myocardial infarction (MI).

Bradycardia occurs normally in young adults, trained athletes, and the elderly. Bradycardia can also occur during sleep.

Chest pain
Chest pain may arise suddenly or gradually. It can radiate to the arms, neck, jaw, or back. It can be steady or intermittent, mild or acute. And it can range in character from a sharp, shooting sensation to a feeling of heaviness, fullness, or even indigestion.

This symptom most often results from disorders that affect thoracic or abdominal organs — the heart, pleurae, lungs, gallbladder, pancreas, or stomach. It's an important indicator of several acute cardiopulmonary and GI disorders and may also result from musculoskeletal and hematologic disorders, anxiety, or drug therapy.

Chest pain can stem from angina pectoris, aortic aneurysm, acute asthma, bronchitis, cardiomyopathy, cholecystitis, interstitial lung disease, lung abscess, lung cancer, mitral prolapse, MI, pan-

creatitis, peptic ulcer, pericarditis, pleurisy, pneumonia, pneumothorax, pulmonary embolism, and pulmonary hypertension.

Cheyne-Stokes respirations
A waxing and waning period of hyperpnea that alternates with a shorter period of apnea, Cheyne-Stokes respirations most commonly indicate increased ICP from a deep cerebral or brain stem lesion (usually bilateral) or a metabolic disturbance in the brain.

Usually, Cheyne-Stokes respirations indicate a change for the worse in the patient's condition. For example, in a patient who's had head trauma or brain surgery, Cheyne-Stokes respirations may signal increased ICP. However, this breathing pattern also occurs normally among people who live at high altitudes and among the elderly during sleep.

Cyanosis
When the patient develops bluish or bluish black discoloration of the skin and mucous membranes, the concentration of unoxygenated hemoglobin in his blood has become excessive.

Central cyanosis reflects inadequate oxygenation of arterial blood caused by right-to-left cardiac shunting or pulmonary disease, or by hematologic disorders. *Peripheral cyanosis* results from sluggish peripheral circulation caused by vasoconstriction, reduced cardiac output, or vascular occlusion.

Possible causes of cyanosis include chronic arteriosclerotic occlusive disease, bronchiectasis, Buerger's disease, chronic obstructive pulmonary disease (COPD), congestive heart failure (CHF), deep vein thrombosis, lung cancer, methemoglobinemia, acute peripheral arterial occlusion, pneumonia, pneumothorax, polycythemia, pulmonary edema, pulmonary embolism, Raynaud's disease, and shock.

Dyspnea
Patients with cardiopulmonary dysfunction frequently experience difficulty or discomfort with breathing. Usually, such patients report shortness of breath. The severity of this symptom varies greatly, but is often unrelated to the severity of the underlying cause. Dyspnea may arise suddenly or slowly and may subside rapidly or persist for years.

Pathologic causes of dyspnea include adult respiratory distress syndrome, amyotrophic lateral sclerosis, aspiration of a foreign body, asthma, CHF, cor pulmonale, emphysema, flail chest, inhalation injury, lung cancer, myasthenia gravis, MI, pleural effusion, pneumonia, pneumothorax, pulmonary edema, pulmonary embolism, and shock.

People normally experience dyspnea if they overexert themselves; in a healthy individual, rest quickly relieves this condition.

Fontanelle bulging
In a normal infant, the anterior fontanelle, or soft spot, is flat, soft yet firm, and well demarcated against surrounding skull bones. You may be able to see subtle pulsations that reflect the arterial pulse. A bulging fontanelle — widened, tense, and with marked pulsations — is a cardinal sign of increased ICP.

Generalized tonic-clonic seizure
Like other types of seizure, a generalized tonic-clonic seizure reflects the paroxysmal, uncontrolled discharge of central nervous system (CNS) neurons, leading to neurologic dysfunction. Unlike most other seizures, cerebral hyperactivity doesn't remain confined to the original focus or to a localized area but extends to the entire brain.

The patient on the verge of a tonic-clonic seizure usually experiences a prodrome and may feel an aura. As seizure activity spreads to the subcortical structures, he loses consciousness, falls to the ground, and may utter a loud cry that's precipitated by air rushing from the lungs through the vocal cords. His body stiffens (tonic phase), then undergoes rapid, synchronous muscle jerking and hyperventilation (clonic phase). Tongue biting, incontinence, diaphoresis, profuse salivation, and signs of respiratory distress may also occur. The seizure usually lasts 2 to 5 minutes, until neurons finish conducting the abnormal electrical charge.

Headache
About 90% of the time, this common neurologic symptom results from muscle contraction or vascular abnormalities. Occasionally, though, headaches indicate a severe underlying disorder. Such disorders include brain abscess or tumor, ruptured cerebral aneurysm, encephalitis, acute epidural hemorrhage, acute closed angle glaucoma, intracerebral hemorrhage, meningitis, psittacosis, subarachnoid hemorrhage, subdural hematoma, typhoid fever, acute sinusitis, or temporal arteritis.

At a cellular level, these disorders may cause intracranial inflammation, increased ICP or meningeal irritation leading to headache pain.

Hematemesis
Usually, this sign indicates GI bleeding above the ligament of Treitz, which suspends the duodenum at its junction with the jejunum. If the patient vomits a large quantity of blood (500 to 1,000 ml), his life may be in danger.

Possible causes of hematemesis include GI disorders, coagulation disorders, treatments that irritate the GI tract, and swallowing blood from epistaxis or oropharyngeal erosions.

If the patient emits bright red or blood-streaked vomit, it indicates fresh or recent bleeding. Dark red, brown, or black vomitus indicates that the patient has retained blood in his stomach and has partially digested it.

Hemoptysis
Hemoptysis refers to the expectoration of blood or bloody sputum from the lungs or tracheobronchial tree. Massive expectoration (400 ml of blood in 3 hours or more than 600 ml in 16 hours) may cause airway obstruction, asphyxiation and death.

Hemoptysis most commonly results from chronic bronchitis, bronchogenic carcinoma, or bronchiectasis. However, it may also result from inflammatory, infectious, cardiovascular, or coagulation disorders. In up to 15% of patients, doctors cannot determine the cause. Rarely, it stems from a ruptured aortic aneurysm. Massive hemoptysis most commonly results from lung cancer, bronchiectasis, active tuberculosis, and cavitary pulmonary disease from necrotic infections or tuberculosis.

When assessing the patient, be careful not to confuse hemoptysis with bleeding from the mouth, throat, nasopharynx, or GI tract.

Hypertension
An intermittent or sustained increase in blood pressure exceeding 140/86 mm Hg, this sign is especially dangerous because patients all too frequently ignore it. During a hypertensive crisis, blood pressure may exceed 200/120 mm Hg. A less dramatic rise may also herald life-threatening conditions, such as dissecting aortic aneurysm, increased ICP, preeclampsia or eclampsia, thyrotoxicosis, atherosclerosis, or MI. Hypertension may also result from anemia; renal disorders (polycystic kidney disease, chronic pyelonephritis, renovascular stenosis); endocrine disorders (aldosteronism,

Cushing's syndrome, pheochromocytoma); or drug side effects.

Hypotension
Typically, a reading below 90/60 mm Hg or a drop of 30 mm Hg from the baseline indicates that the patient's blood pressure is no longer adequate to perfuse or oxygenate the body's tissues. Physiologic mechanisms that contribute to low blood pressure include expanded intravascular space, reduced intravascular volume, and decreased cardiac output.

Hypotension can result from acute adrenal insufficiency, alcohol toxicity, anaphylactic shock, cardiac contusion, cardiac dysrhythmias, cardiac tamponade, cardiogenic shock, CHF, diabetic ketoacidosis, hypovolemic shock, hypoxemia, MI, neurogenic shock, pulmonary embolism, septic shock, or vasovagal syncope.

Narrowed pulse pressure
Normally, systolic pressure exceeds diastolic pressure by about 40 mm Hg. This difference may narrow down to less than 30 mm Hg, however, if peripheral vascular resistance increases, cardiac output declines, or intravascular volume decreases. Usually a late sign, narrowed pulse pressure alone doesn't signal an emergency. But it commonly occurs in shock, aortic stenosis, cardiac tamponade, and CHF.

Posture changes
Neurologic dysfunction may lead to characteristic changes in posture. Severe damage to the cerebral cortex, the subcortical cerebrum, and the upper brain stem may cause decerebrate posture, characterized by adduction and extension of the patient's arms, with wrists pronated and the fingers flexed. The patient's legs are stiffly extended, with plantar flexion of the feet. In severe cases, his back is acutely arched (opisthotonos). Damage

may result from primary lesions such as infarction, hemorrhage, or tumor; metabolic encephalopathy; or brain stem compression associated with increased ICP.

Severe damage to the cerebral cortex resulting from cerebrovascular accident or head injury may lead to decorticate posture. The patient's arms are adducted and flexed, with the wrists and fingers flexed on the chest. His legs are extended and internally rotated with plantar flexion of the feet.

Decorticate posture carries a more favorable prognosis than decerebrate posture. However, if the causative disorder extends lower in the brain stem, decorticate posture may progress to decerebrate posture. The two postures may alternate as the patient's neurologic status fluctuates. Generally, the duration of each posturing episode correlates with the severity of brain stem damage.

Pulsus paradoxus

Also called paradoxical pulse, this sign refers to a pulse that fades on inspiration and strengthens on expiration. During inspiration, systolic pressure falls more than the normal amount—10 mm Hg. If systolic pressure falls more than 20 mm Hg, the peripheral pulses may be barely palpable or may disappear. This pulse abnormality occurs when a condition such as cardiac tamponade or COPD impedes the blood flow from the left ventricle during inspiration. Its causes also include pericarditis, massive pulmonary embolism, and right ventricular infarction.

Tachycardia

A heart rate greater than 100 beats/minute, tachycardia represents the heart's effort to deliver more oxygen to body tissues by increasing the rate at which blood passes through the vessels. Usually, the patient complains of palpitations, or of his heart's racing.

It may be an early sign of a life-threatening disorder, such as cardiogenic shock, septic shock, or MI.

Tachycardia frequently occurs in patients with such respiratory disorders as adult respiratory distress syndrome (ARDS), COPD, pneumothorax, or pulmonary embolism. It also occurs in numerous cardiovascular disorders: aortic insufficiency, aortic stenosis, cardiac contusion, cardiac dysrhythmias, cardiac tamponade, CHF, hypertensive crisis, and hypovolemic shock. The list of medical causes of tachycardia also includes adrenocortical insufficiency, alcohol withdrawal syndrome, anaphylactic shock, anemia, diabetic ketoacidosis, hyperosmolar nonketotic syndrome, hypoglycemia, hyponatremia, hypovolemia, hypoxemia, neurogenic shock, pheochromocytoma, and thyrotoxicosis.

Tachycardia may represent a response to emotional or physical stress or use of stimulants, such as caffeine and tobacco.

Tachypnea

Tachypnea is an abnormally fast respiratory rate, where the patient takes 20 or more breaths/minute. CNS disorders that cause tachypnea include head trauma, neurogenic shock, and respiratory shock. Respiratory disorders associated with this sign include ARDS; aspiration of a foreign body; asthma; bronchiectasis; emphysema; flail chest; lung abscess; lung, pleural or mediastinal tumor; bacterial pneumonia; pneumothorax; pulmonary edema; acute pulmonary embolism; and primary pulmonary hypertension. Cardiovascular causes of tachypnea include cardiac dysrhythmias, cardiac tamponade, cardiogenic shock, and hypovolemic shock. Other causes include anemia, hyperosmolar nonketotic syndrome, anaphylactic shock, al-

cohol withdrawal syndrome, malignant mesothelioma, and septic shock.

Wheezes

Wheezes refer to adventitious breath sounds with a high-pitched, musical, squealing, creaking, or groaning quality. Coughing will not clear wheezes, as it will crackles and rhonchi.

Prolonged wheezing during expiration indicates shortening and narrowing of the bronchi. Causes may include bronchospasm; mucosal thickening or edema; partial obstruction from a tumor, foreign body, or secretions; and extrinsic pressure from tension pneumothorax, thyroid goiter, or other cause. If wheezing occurs during inspiration, it's a sign of airway obstruction.

Potentially life-threatening disorders associated with wheezing include acute chemical pneumonitis, anaphylaxis, aspiration pneumonitis, asthma, bronchiectasis, bronchogenic carcinoma, chronic bronchitis, emphysema, pulmonary edema, and tracheobronchitis.

▼
Disorders A-to-Z: What they are, why they occur

Disease, like health, is a dimension of every human life. Below you'll read about the most common ailments, the deadliest, the rarest, and those brought to the public spotlight by their peculiar or contemporary significance. Some strike children, others affect adults, and still others reach both groups.

Acquired immunodeficiency syndrome (AIDS)

An immunodeficiency of epidemic proportions, AIDS is one of the

Opportunistic infections in AIDS

Besides the HIV infection itself, most patients with AIDS develop ravaging opportunistic infections. Pathogens easily take advantage of the patient's suppressed immune system, specifically the weakened T cell-mediated response. The subsequent infections are often complicated and disseminated, and tend to resist treatment or recur in spite of conventional

therapy. The most common opportunistic infection in AIDS patients is *Pneumocystis carinii*.

The chart below discusses infections that commonly appear in AIDS patients. Keep in mind that the type, location, and severity relate directly to the degree of the patient's immunosuppression.

Infection	Affected areas	Treatment
Viruses		
Cytomegalovirus (CMV)	• Lungs: pneumonia • GI tract: diarrhea, colitis • Liver: elevated liver enzymes • Retina: large hemorrhages, white exudates, visual changes leading to blindness • Lymphocytes: positive antibody titers • Brain: encephalitis	• Acyclovir • Ganciclovir (also known as DHPG) for CMV retinitis
Herpes simplex	• Perineal, perianal, and scrotal areas; face; esophagus; colon: mucocutaneous ulcers lasting longer than 1 month	• Acyclovir, vidarabine, fluoroidoaracytosine (also known as FIAC)
Herpes zoster	• Disseminated: weeping, raised, coalesced, pruritic rash, usually on buttocks, back, and legs	• Acyclovir, vidarabine, FIAC
Fungi		
Candida albicans	• Mouth, esophagus: difficult, painful swallowing; white coating or plaque in oral mucosa • Anus: white coating or plaque in rectal mucosa • Axilla, groin, systemic: skin lesions	• Miconazole, nystatin, clotrimazole, mycelex, ketoconazole, I.V. amphotericin B, 5-flucytosine
Cryptococcus neoformans	• Brain: meningitis • Blood: fungicemia	• Amphotericin B, 5-flucytosine, ketoconazole
Protozoa		
Pneumocystis carinii	• Disseminated: initially, diarrhea, night sweats, fever, weight loss, unexplained lymphadenopathy; later, dyspnea, dry cough, tachypnea, cyanosis, diffuse crackles, severe hypoxemia • Retina: cotton-wool exudates	• Trimethoprim-sulfamethoxazole (also known as TMP-SMX) • Pentamidine • Trimetrexate with leucovorin • Experimental: dapsone-trimethoprim; sulfadoxine-pyrimethamine; dapsone; BW301; difluromethylornithane (also known as DFMO)

(continued)

Opportunistic infections in AIDS *(continued)*

Infection	Affected areas	Treatment
Protozoa *(continued)*		
Toxoplasma gondii	• Brain: abscess, diffuse encephalopathy, meningoencephalitis	• Sulfadiazine and pyrimethamine with leucovorin
Cryptosporidium	• GI tract: soft stools to severe diarrhea	• No effective treatment known • Possible spiramycin or combined quinine and clindamycin • Opiate-based antidiarrheal drugs • I.V. hyperalimentation, fluid replacements
Mycobacteria		
Mycobacterium avium and *M. tuberculosis*	• Lungs: chronic cough, hemoptysis • Liver, spleen, lymph nodes, bone marrow: fatigue, weakness, weight loss, fever	• Usually a combination of two or more of the following: rifampin, isoniazid, ethambutol, ethionamide, streptomycin, capreomycin, cycloserine, pyrazinamide • Experimental: ansamycin, clofazamine

most serious health challenges of our time. It results from infection with human immunodeficiency virus (HIV), leading to destruction of T4 (T-helper) cells and immunodeficiency. It's characterized by chronic wasting syndrome, dementia, opportunistic infection (such as *Pneumocystis carinii* pneumonia), or malignancy (such as Kaposi's sarcoma) — or from some combination of these conditions.

HIV infection can result from transfusion of contaminated blood or blood products, sharing of contaminated needles, accidental needlesticks, exposure through open wounds or mucous membranes. Sexual and perinatal transmission also occur. High-risk groups include sexually active homosexual and bisexual men; I.V. drug abusers; hemophiliacs, especially if they have received Factor VIII concentrate; heterosexual partners and children of patients with AIDS; and recipients of multiple blood transfusions. Until the late 1980s, patients rarely lived beyond 2 years after diagnosis; more effec-

tive treatments are now extending lives.

AIDS-related complex (ARC). Patients with ARC display some nonspecific symptoms of AIDS, but not the typical opportunistic infections. Most of them have a history of unexplained fever, lymphadenopathy, weight loss, diarrhea, sore throat, fatigue, and night sweats. Scientists don't know whether all patients with ARC will eventually develop AIDS.

Acute poststreptococcal glomerulonephritis

Fairly common, this bilateral inflammation of the glomeruli may follow a streptococcal infection of the respiratory tract or, less often, a skin infection, such as impetigo. The disorder results from entrapment and collection of antigen-antibody (produced as an immunologic mechanism in response to streptococcus) in the glomerular capillary membranes, inducing inflammatory damage and impeding glomerular filtration. Symptoms include mild to moderate edema, proteinuria, azotemia, hematuria,

oliguria, and fatigue.

Acute poststreptococcal glomerulonephritis occurs most commonly among boys aged 3 to 7, but may strike at any age. Up to 95% of children and up to 70% of adults will recover fully; the rest may progress to chronic renal failure within months.

Acute respiratory failure

This condition occurs when the lungs no longer efficiently exchange carbon dioxide for oxygen and can't keep pace with cellular metabolism. It has many causes. In many patients, such as those with respiratory failure caused by sedative overdose, the lungs appear completely normal.

Arterial blood gas levels provide important clues to acute respiratory failure. For most patients, a PaO_2 less than 50 mm Hg or a $PaCO_2$ more than 50 mm Hg indicates respiratory failure. Patients with COPD, however, have chronically low PaO_2 levels and high $PaCO_2$ levels. Therefore, any sudden or extreme shift in baseline values suggests acute respiratory failure.

Acute transverse myelitis

A form of spinal cord inflammation, acute transverse myelitis affects the entire thickness of the spinal cord. Onset is rapid; motor and sensory dysfunction below the level of spinal cord damage appears in 1 to 2 days. The patient develops flaccid paralysis of the legs with loss of sensory and sphincter function. Pain in the legs or trunk may precede sensory loss. Reflexes disappear in the early stages but may return later. The extent of damage depends on the level of the spinal cord affected. In severe cases, the patient may go into shock.

Possible causes of acute transverse myelitis include acute infectious diseases, such as measles or pneumonia; primary infections of the spinal cord such as syphilis or acute disseminated encephalomyelitis; demyelinating diseases such as acute multiple sclerosis; and inflammatory and necrotizing disorders of the spinal cord, such as hematomyelia.

Acute tubular necrosis

Accounting for about 75% of all cases of acute renal failure, acute tubular necrosis (ATN) injures the tubular segment of the nephron, causing renal failure and uremic syndrome. Mortality ranges from 40% to 70%, depending on complications from underlying diseases. Nonoliguric forms of ATN have a better prognosis.

In critically ill patients and individuals who have undergone extensive surgery, ATN may result from ischemic or nephrotoxic injury. In ischemic injury, disruption of blood flow to the kidneys may result from circulatory collapse, severe hypotension, trauma, hemorrhage, dehydration, cardiogenic or septic shock, surgery, anesthetics, or reaction to transfusions. Nephrotoxic injury may follow ingestion of certain chemical agents or result from a hypersensitive reaction of the kidneys.

Adrenal insufficiency

Also called Addison's disease, adrenal insufficiency occurs when more than 90% of the adrenal gland is destroyed. It usually results from an autoimmune process; circulating antibodies react specifically against the adrenal tissue. Other possible causes include tuberculosis, bilateral adrenalectomy, hemorrhage into the adrenal gland, neoplasms, and infections, such as histoplasmosis and cytomegalovirus.

The patient exhibits a conspicuous bronze discoloration of the skin—he appears to be deeply suntanned, especially over the metacarpophalangeal joints, the elbows, and the knees. Other signs and symptoms include weakness, fatigue, weight loss, nausea, vomiting, anorexia, and chronic diarrhea. Associated cardiovascular abnormalities include postural hypotension, decreased cardiac size and output, and a weak, irregular pulse. The patient may also experience decreased tolerance for even minor stress, poor coordination, fasting hypoglycemia, and a craving for salty food.

Adult respiratory distress syndrome

A form of pulmonary edema, adult respiratory distress syndrome (ARDS) results from increased permeability of the alveolar capillary membrane. Fluid accumulates in the lung interstitium, alveolar spaces, and small airways, causing the lung to stiffen. This impairs ventilation and prohibits adequate oxygenation of pulmonary capillary blood, thereby leading to acute respiratory failure.

ARDS may result from aspiration of gastric contents; sepsis; head trauma; oxygen toxicity; viral, bacterial, or fungal pneumonia; microemboli; drug overdose; blood transfusion; smoke or chemical inhalation; hydrocarbon or paraquat ingestion; pancreatitis; uremia; or near-drowning. If severe enough, ARDS can cause intractable and fatal hypoxemia; however, patients who recover may suffer little or no permanent lung damage.

Alzheimer's disease

This disease is characterized by reduced levels of choline acetyltransferase, the enzyme that synthesizes acetylcholine in the brain. This reduction causes a loss of neurons in the cortical area along with characteristic neurofibrillary tangles and senile plaques. Steady progressive intellectual deterioration occurs without remission.

Initially, the patient experiences less conspicuous changes such as forgetfulness, recent memory loss, difficulty learning and remembering new information, deterioration in personal hygiene and appearance and an inability to concentrate. As intellectual disability progresses, he may eventually forget how to write or speak, lose control of his emotions, experience delusions, and cease to recognize family members. Motor function remains unaffected until late stages.

Amebiasis

This acute or chronic protozoal infection results from *Entamoeba histolytica*. It produces varying degrees of illness, from no symptoms at all to mild diarrhea to fulminating dysentery. Extraintestinal amebiasis can induce hepatic abscess and infections of the lungs, pleural cavity, pericardium, peritoneum, and, rarely, the brain. Prognosis is usually good, although complications such as ameboma, abscess, intussusception, and intestinal stricture, hemorrhage, and perforation increase mortality.

Amebiasis occurs worldwide but appears most frequently in the tropics, subtropics, and other areas with poor sanitation and health practices. Incidence in the United States averages between 1% and 3% but may be higher among homosexuals and institutionalized populations where a high rate of fecal oral contamination is common.

Amyloidosis

In this rare chronic disease, abnormal fibrillar scleroprotein (amyloid) accumulates and infiltrates body organs and soft tissues. *Perireticular type* amyloidosis affects the inner coats of blood vessels. *Pericollagen type* amyloidosis affects the outer coat of blood vessels and also involves the parenchyma.

Effects of this disorder include proteinuria, CHF, stiffness and enlargement of the tongue, malabsorption, GI bleeding, infiltration of blood vessel walls, abdominal pain, constipation, diarrhea, peripheral neuropathy, and (less commonly) liver enlargement. Prognosis varies but the disorder can cause permanent and life-threatening organ damage.

Amyotrophic lateral sclerosis

Also called Lou Gehrig's disease, this neurologic disease causes progressive physical degeneration but leaves the patient's mental status intact, enabling him to perceive every change acutely.

During the course of illness, the patient develops fasciculations, accompanied by atrophy and weakness, especially in the muscles of the forearms and the hands. Other signs include impaired speech; difficulty chewing, swallowing, and breathing, particularly if the brain stem is affected; and, occasionally, choking and excessive drooling. Progressive bulbar palsy may cause crying spells or inappro-

priate laughter. Onset generally occurs between ages 40 and 70 and death usually occurs within 3 to 10 years, usually a result of aspiration pneumonia or respiratory failure.

Anxiety disorders

Typically, people experience anxiety as a feeling of worry, insecurity, apprehension, and foreboding. Such feelings may represent a transient emotional reaction, or may persist and strongly shape personality development. When anxiety and inner conflict become overwhelming, a psychiatric disorder develops.

Based on symptoms, the Diagnostic and Statistical Manual of Mental Disorders subdivides anxiety disorders into the following categories:
• generalized anxiety disorder
• panic disorder (repeated experience of panic attacks—a sudden, intense feeling of terror)
• phobic disorders (an irrational, persistent fear of specific activities, objects, or situations)
• obsessive-compulsive disorders (uncontrolled, recurrent thoughts, impulses or images or ritualized repetition of bizarre and irrational activities)
• post-traumatic stress disorder (the psychological consequences of a traumatic event).

Arthritis

Arthritis encompasses various diseases involving inflammation and, possibly, degeneration of joints or surrounding structures. Subsequent damage may cause anatomic changes that impair joint mobility and lead to deformity and disability.

Each arthritic disorder carries a distinctive pathogenesis. *Gouty arthritis* is a metabolic disease marked by urate deposits, which cause painfully arthritic joints. It most often strikes joints in the feet and legs. *Infectious arthritis*

constitutes a medical emergency. Bacterial invasion of a joint leads to inflammation of the synovial lining, and can lead to eventual destruction of bone and cartilage. A chronic, recurrent inflammatory disorder of connective tissue, *rheumatoid arthritis* attacks peripheral joints and surrounding, muscles, tendons, ligaments, and blood vessels. The cause isn't certain, but evidence suggests an immune or autoimmune process. *Juvenile rheumatoid arthritis* affects children under age 16. It causes joint swelling, pain, and tenderness, and may also involve the skin, heart, lungs, liver, spleen, and eyes, producing extra-articular signs and symptoms. *Psoriatic arthritis* has rheumatoid effects but is associated with skin and nail psoriasis.

Asthma

Patients with asthma experience episodic bronchospasm, increased mucous secretion, and mucosal edema leading to airway obstruction. In extrinsic asthma, external factors (allergens) trigger bronchospasm. In intrinsic asthma, internal causes such as stress or infection trigger an asthma attack. The cause of bronchospasm is not known. Although this common condition can strike at any age, half of all cases occur in children under age 10.

Atopic dermatitis

A patient with this chronic skin disorder experiences superficial skin inflammation and intense itching. Scratching the skin causes vasoconstriction and intensifies pruritus, resulting in erythematous, weeping lesions. Eventually, the lesions become scaly and lichenified. Atopic dermatitis may appear at any age, though it usually begins during infancy or early childhood. It may then subside spontaneously, followed by exacerbations in late childhood, adolescence, or early adulthood.

Exacerbating factors may include irritants, infections, and some allergens, particularly food allergens.

Bipolar affective disorder
This psychiatric disorder is characterized by severe pathologic mood swings from euphoria to sadness, by spontaneous recoveries, and by a tendency to recur. The cause of the disorder isn't clearly understood, but hereditary, biologic, and psychological factors may play a part. Bipolar affective disorder occurs more commonly among women than men. It's also more common in higher socioeconomic groups. The higher incidence in females suggests a socially learned or a sex-linked genetic cause. Twenty percent of patients who suffer from this disorder take their own lives, many just as the depression lifts.

Breast cancer
Initial symptoms of this disease, usually detected by self-examination, include a small, painless lump, thick or dimpled skin, or nipple retraction. Establishing a diagnosis requires careful physical examination, mammography, and cytologic examination of tumor cells obtained by biopsy. Depending on the assessment of the tumor, the patient may undergo a radical, modified radical, or simple mastectomy with dissection of the axillary nodes, or a lumpectomy. After surgery, the doctor will usually prescribe radiotherapy, chemotherapy, or both.

Bronchiectasis
An irreversible condition marked by chronic abnormal dilation of the bronchi and destruction of the bronchial walls, bronchiectasis can occur throughout the tracheobronchial tree or can be confined to one segment or lobe. However, it's usually bilateral and involves the basilar segments of the lower lobes. The classic symptom is a chronic cough that produces copious, foul-smelling, mucopurulent secretions, possibly totaling several cupfuls daily. The patient experiences repeated episodes of acute bronchial infection with heavy productive coughing, alternating with periods of chronic infection and mild coughing. The availability of antibiotics has dramatically decreased incidence of this disorder; Eskimos and the Maoris of New Zealand now have the highest rate of bronchiectasis.

Bronchitis
Chronic bronchitis results from repeated exposure to irritants such as cigarette smoke, environmental pollutants, or bacterial and viral infections that inflame the airways, causing them to swell and clog with mucus, leading to a chronic or recurrent productive cough. Other effects include airway edema, cilia loss, and hypertrophy and hyperplasia of the bronchial glands and goblet cells. Because the patient lacks effective mucociliary clearing mechanisms, mucus secretions stagnate in the airways, predisposing him to respiratory infections that exacerbate the condition.

Acute bronchitis is characterized by productive cough, fever, hypertrophy of mucus-secreting structures and back pain. Caused by the spread of upper respiratory viral infections, it often occurs with or follows childhood infections such as measles, pertussis, diphtheria, and typhoid fever.

Buerger's disease
An inflammatory, nonatheromatous occlusive condition, Buerger's disease causes segmental lesions and subsequent thrombus formation in the small and medium arteries (and sometimes the veins), resulting in decreased blood flow to the feet and legs. The disorder may produce ulceration and, eventually, gangrene. Probably linked to nicotine hypersensitivity, it occurs most commonly among Jewish men ages 20 to 40 who smoke heavily.

Chicken pox
Also called varicella, this common, acute, and highly contagious infection results from the herpesvirus varicella zoster, the same virus that in its later stages causes herpes zoster. Chicken pox may occur at any time, though the risk is greatest between ages 2 to 8. The infection occurs worldwide and presents a constant threat in large cities. Outbreaks occur sporadically in areas with large groups of susceptible children. Most children recover completely.

This infection may be transmitted through air droplets or through contact with respiratory secretions or skin lesions. The incubation period lasts from 13 to 17 days. Afterward, the patient develops distinctive signs and symptoms. During the prodromal phase, he experiences slight fever, malaise, and anorexia. Within 24 hours, the characteristic rash appears; usually it begins as crops of small, erythematous macules on the trunk or scalp. These spots progress to papules or clear vesicles on an erythematous base. The vesicles become cloudy and break easily, then scabs form. Severe pruritus with this rash may provoke persistent scratching, which can lead to infection, scarring, impetigo, furuncles, and cellulitis.

Chlamydia infections
This is a group of infections linked to one organism: *Chlamydia trachomatis*. It includes urethritis in men, cervicitis in women, and lymphogranuloma venereum (LGV) in both. The most common sexually transmitted diseases in the United States, chlamydial infections afflict an estimated 34 million Americans

each year. One such infection, trachoma inclusion conjunctivitis, is the leading cause of blindness in the Third World.

Transmission of *C. trachomatis* follows vaginal or rectal intercourse or oral-genital contact with infected persons. Because symptoms appear late in the course of illness, sexual transmission occurs unknowingly. Patients may be asymptomatic or show a variety of signs depending on the type of chlamydial infection. The primary lesion of LGV is a painless vesicle or nodular ulcer 2 to 3 mm in diameter.

Untreated chlamydial infections can lead to such complications as acute epididymitis, salpingitis, pelvic inflammatory disease, and eventually, sterility. In pregnant women, chlamydial infections may contribute to spontaneous abortion, premature delivery, and neonatal death.

Cholelithiasis
Cholelithiasis, stones or calculi in the gallbladder, results from changes in bile components that occur during periods of sluggishness in the gallbladder due to pregnancy, oral contraceptives, diabetes mellitus, celiac disease, cirrhosis of the liver, and pancreatitis. Gallstones may consist of cholesterol, calcium bilirubinate, or a mixture of cholesterol and bilirubin pigment.

Cholelithiasis is the fifth leading cause of hospitalization among adults and accounts for 90% of all gallbladder and duct diseases. Prognosis is usually good with treatment. Although the patient doesn't always experience symptoms, acute cholelithiasis produces acute abdominal pain in the right upper quadrant. Pain may radiate to the back, between the shoulders, or to the front of the chest. Pain from acute cholelithiasis may be severe enough to cause the patient to seek emergency care.

Chronic obstructive pulmonary disease
The most common forms of COPD are chronic bronchitis, emphysema, and asthma. All share one important characteristic: airway obstruction leading to dyspnea. In *chronic bronchitis*, repeated exposure to irritants inflames the airways, causing them to swell and clog with mucus. In *emphysema,* such inflammation eventually destroys the alveoli and bronchioles, creating air spaces known as blebs or bullae. *Asthma* causes episodic bronchospasm, leading to bronchial hypertrophy with thickened epithelium and edematous walls. Then, airways become obstructed and secretions trapped. COPD may also include cystic fibrosis and bronchiectasis. Because COPD cannot be cured, treatment seeks to relieve symptoms and prevent complications.

Chronic renal failure
Usually the result of a gradually progressive loss of renal function, chronic renal failure occasionally results from rapidly progressive disease of sudden onset. Few symptoms develop until the patient loses more than 75% of glomerular filtration; then the remaining normal parenchyma deteriorates progressively and symptoms worsen as renal function decreases.

If this condition continues unchecked, uremic toxins accumulate and produce potentially fatal physiologic changes in all major organ systems. If the patient can tolerate it, maintenance dialysis can sustain life. Kidney transplant, when possible, offers a cure.

Cirrhosis
In this chronic degenerative hepatic disease, fibrous tissue covers the lobes, the parenchyma degenerates, and fat infiltrates the lobules. The liver ceases to function properly; gluconeogenesis, detoxification of drugs and alcohol, and

bilirubin metabolism deteriorate. Blood flow through the liver becomes obstructed, leading to portal hypertension and esophageal varices.

Most commonly the consequence of alcohol abuse, cirrhosis can also result from nutritional deprivation or infection such as hepatitis. Symptoms include nausea, flatulence, anorexia, weight loss, ascites, light-colored stools, weakness, abdominal pain, varicosities, and spider angiomas. Unchecked, the disorder leads to hepatic coma, gastrointestinal hemorrhage, and kidney failure.

Coal worker's pneumoconiosis
Also called black lung disease, this progressive, nodular pulmonary disease occurs in two forms. The simple form is characterized by small lung opacities. In the complicated form, also known as progressive massive fibrosis, masses of fibrous tissue develop.

The disease most often strikes anthracite coal workers in the eastern United States. The risk of developing it depends upon the duration of exposure to coal dust (usually 15 years or longer), intensity of exposure (dust count, particle size), location of the mine, silica content of the coal, and the worker's susceptibility.

Prognosis varies. Simple asymptomatic disease is self-limiting, although it may progress, especially if the disease appears after a relatively short period of exposure. Effects of complicated coal worker's pneumoconiosis include severe ventilatory failure and right heart failure secondary to pulmonary hypertension.

Common cold
The most common infectious disease, the cold is an acute, usually afebrile viral infection that causes upper respiratory tract inflammation. It's more prevalent in children than in adults; in adolescent boys than in girls; and in women

than men. More than a hundred viruses cause the common cold, including rhinoviruses, myxoviruses, adenoviruses, coxsackieviruses, and echoviruses. Transmission occurs through airborne respiratory droplets, contact with contaminated objects, and hand-to-hand transmission.

Congestive heart failure
This circulatory congestion results from cardiac disorders, especially MI. Common symptoms of CHF include dyspnea, high venous pressure, prolonged circulation time, peripheral edema, and decreased vital capacity.

CHF usually develops chronically in association with renal retention of sodium and water. Humoral agents that significantly affect such retention include renin, angiotensin, aldosterone, vasopressin, estrogen, and norepinephrine.

Acute CHF may follow MI of the left ventricle. A significant shift of blood from the systemic to the pulmonary circulation may occur before the body begins retaining sodium and water. Pulmonary congestion may result from mechanical obstruction in the left mitral valve or from ventricular failure.

Cor pulmonale
Caused by pulmonary hypertension and accompanied by hypertrophy of the right ventricle, cor pulmonale follows a disorder of the lungs, pulmonary vessels, chest wall, or respiratory control center. For instance, COPD produces pulmonary hypertension, which leads to right ventricular hypertrophy and failure. Because cor pulmonale usually occurs late during the course of COPD and other irreversible disorders, prognosis is poor.

As long as the heart compensates for the increased pulmonary vascular resistance, clinical features reflect the underlying disorder and occur mostly in the respiratory system. As the disorder progresses, the patient experiences resting dyspnea that worsens with exertion, tachypnea, orthopnea, edema, weakness, and right upper quadrant discomfort. Signs of cor pulmonale with right ventricular failure include dependent edema; distended neck veins; enlarged, tender liver; prominent parasternal or epigastric cardiac impulse; hepatojugular reflux; and tachycardia. Decreased cardiac output may cause a weak pulse and hypotension.

Coronary artery disease
Coronary artery disease (CAD) remains the most common cause of cardiac disease in adults and the leading cause of death in the United States. Characterized by narrowed or obstructed arterial lumina, CAD interferes with blood flow to the heart. It can cause various ischemic diseases, including angina pectoris, MI, CHF, sudden cardiac death, and cardiac dysrhythmias.

CAD most commonly results from atherosclerosis, a form of hardening of the arteries. Such atherosclerosis occurs primarily in arteries on the heart's epicardial surface.

Atherosclerosis evolves slowly, beginning in childhood and progressing throughout life. Certain factors, such as a sedentary lifestyle and a high-fat diet, increase the risk of CAD. Signs and symptoms usually don't appear until middle age or later. The classic symptom, angina, results from inadequate myocardial perfusion. The patient often describes angina as a burning, squeezing, or crushing tightness in the substernal or precordial chest. Nausea, vomiting, fainting, sweating, and cool extremities may accompany angina. Anginal episodes may follow physical exertion, exposure to cold, or a large meal.

Cytomegalic inclusion disease
Also called cytomegalovirus infection, this disease results from a DNA, ether-sensitive virus belonging to the herpes family, transmitted by human contact. About four out of five people over age 35 have been infected with cytomegalovirus, usually during childhood or early adulthood.

Most people overlook the cytomegalovirus infection because it's so mild. However, cytomegalovirus infection during pregnancy can lead to stillbirth, brain damage and other birth defects, or severe neonatal illness. Immunodeficient patients and individuals receiving immunosuppressant drugs may develop pneumonia or other secondary infections from the cytomegalovirus. Although usually asymptomatic, infected infants may develop hepatic dysfunction, hepatosplenomegaly, spider angiomas, pneumonitis, and lymphadenopathy.

Diabetes insipidus
This disorder results from a deficiency of antidiuretic hormone (ADH). *Primary diabetes insipidus* is familial or idiopathic in origin. *Secondary diabetes insipidus* results from intracranial neoplastic metastatic lesions, hypophysectomy or other neurosurgery, head trauma, infection, granulomatous disease, and vascular lesions. Incidence has risen slightly because of the increased use of hypophysectomy.

Diabetes insipidus produces extreme polyuria. The patient becomes extremely thirsty and drinks great quantities of water to compensate for the body's water loss. The disorder may result in slight to moderate nocturia and, in severe cases, extreme fatigue from inadequate rest caused by frequent voiding and excess thirst.

Uncomplicated diabetes insipidus has a good prognosis; patients usually lead normal lives, with adequate water replacement. In cases complicated by an underlying disorder, prognosis varies.

Diabetes mellitus

When pancreatic beta cells fail to secrete sufficient insulin, this complex disorder of carbohydrate, protein, and fat metabolism results. Energy deficiency and a catabolic state lead to fatigue. Insulin deficiency causes hyperglycemia, which pulls fluid from body tissues, causing osmotic diuresis, polyuria, and dehydration.

As the disorder progresses, the patient may also experience polydipsia, weight loss, polyphagia, and glycosuria. Long-term effects may include retinopathy, nephropathy, atherosclerosis, or peripheral and autonomic neuropathy. The patient faces a high risk of infection. During advanced stages of the disease (when the pancreas excretes no endogenous insulin), he risks developing ketoacidosis. Children with diabetes also face a high risk of ketoacidosis.

Discoid lupus erythematosus

In this form of lupus erythematosus, the patient experiences chronic skin eruptions that, if untreated, can lead to scarring and permanent disfigurement. Raised red, scaling plaques with follicle plugging and central atrophy may appear on the face, scalp, neck, arms, or any part of the body exposed to sunlight. Facial plaques sometimes assume the butterfly pattern characteristic of systemic lupus erythematosus (SLE). Hair tends to become brittle and may fall out in patches.

About 1 out of 20 patients with DLE develops SLE. The exact cause of DLE remains unknown, but evidence suggests an autoimmune defect. An estimated 60% of patients with DLE are women age 20 or older.

Disseminated intravascular coagulation

This disorder accelerates clotting, causing small vessel occlusion, organ necrosis, depletion of circulating clotting factors and platelets, and activation of the fibrinolytic system. The possible result: severe hemorrhage.

DIC is caused by a primary disorder (such as septicemia, acute hypotension, or neoplasms) that initiates generalized intravascular clotting, which in turn overstimulates fibrinolytic mechanisms. Clotting in the microcirculation usually affects the kidneys and the extremities but may occur in the brain, lungs, pituitary and adrenal glands, and GI mucosa. Prognosis depends on early detection and

Distinguishing between Type I and Type II diabetes

The leading cause of new blindness, diabetes mellitus contributes to about 50% of MIs and about 75% of cerebrovascular accidents. This chronic condition occurs in two forms: insulin-dependent diabetes mellitus and the more prevalent non-insulin-dependent diabetes mellitus. Use this chart to distinguish the two types.

Type I (Insulin-dependent)	Type II (Non-insulin-dependent)
Onset usually before age 20	Onset usually after age 30
Abrupt onset	Gradual onset
Symptoms include polydipsia, polyuria, appetite increase, weight loss, endogenous insulin absent, lethargy	Symptoms may not occur; endogenous insulin present
Wide fluctuations of blood glucose, with marked sensitivity to diet, exercise, and insulin; disease control difficult	Disease usually easily controlled if patient adheres to a proper diet
Insulin needed by all	Insulin needed by only 20% to 30%; usually diet-controlled
Oral hypoglycemic not indicated	Oral hypoglycemic useful for about 40% of patients

treatment, the severity of the hemorrhage, and treatment of the underlying disease or condition.

Diverticular disease
In diverticular disease, bulging pouches (diverticula) in the GI wall push the mucosal lining through the surrounding muscle. The most common site for diverticula is in the sigmoid colon, but they may develop anywhere from proximal end of the pharynx to the anus. Typical sites include the duodenum, jejunum, and ileum (Meckel's diverticulum). Diverticula probably result from high intraluminal pressure on areas of weakness in the GI wall where blood vessels enter. Lack of roughage in the patient's diet may contribute to development of this disease.

Diverticular disease has two forms. In *diverticulosis*, diverticula do not cause symptoms except for possible lower left quadrant pain accompanied by alternating constipation and diarrhea. In *diverticulitis*, diverticula become inflamed and may cause potentially fatal obstruction, infection, or hemorrhage.

Down's syndrome
The physical signs of Down's syndrome (especially hypotonia) are readily apparent at birth; mental retardation becomes obvious as the patient grows older. Craniofacial anomalies include slanting, almond-shaped eyes; protruding tongue; small opened mouth; a single transverse palmar crease; small white spots on the iris; strabismus; small skull; flat bridge across the nose; slow dental development; flattened face; small external ears; short neck; and occasionally, cataracts. Such patients have an IQ between 30 and 50; however, social performance usually exceeds mental age.

Life expectancy for patients with Down's syndrome has increased significantly because of improved treatment for related complications (heart defects, tendency toward respiratory and other infections, acute leukemia). Nevertheless, up to 44% of patients with congenital heart defects die before they're 1 year old.

Endometriosis
In this disorder, endometrial tissue lies outside the uterine lining. Usually, ectopic tissue appears in the pelvic area, most commonly around the ovaries, uterovesical peritoneum, uterosacral ligaments, and the cul-de-sac, but it can appear anywhere in the body. The classic symptom of endometriosis is acquired dysmenorrhea; the patient may experience constant pain in the lower abdomen, vagina, posterior pelvis, or back. Symptoms may develop abruptly or over many years. Active endometriosis usually occurs between ages 30 and 40, especially in women who postpone childbearing. Typically, it becomes progressively severe during the menstrual years and subsides after menopause.

The primary complication of endometriosis is infertility. The disorder can also cause spontaneous abortion. Treatment varies, from conservative therapy with androgens, progestins, and oral contraceptives, to total abdominal hysterectomy.

Gastroenteritis
Gastroenteritis produces diarrhea, nausea, vomiting, and abdominal cramping. Its possible causes include bacteria (*Staphyloccus aureus, Salmonella, Shigella, Clostridium botulinum, Escherichia coli, Clostridium perfringens*); amebae (*Entamoeba histolytica*); parasites (*Ascaris, Enterobius, Trichinella spiralis*); virus (adreno-, echo-, or coxsackieviruses); ingestion of toxins; reaction to antibiotic drugs; enzyme deficiencies; and food allergies.

In adults, gastroenteritis is usually self-limiting and nonfatal. When it afflicts a young child or elderly or debilitated person, treatment may necessitate hospitalization. In developing nations, it's a major cause of death.

Glaucoma
This dangerous rise in intraocular pressure can lead to irreversible blindness. *Chronic open angle glaucoma* results from overproduction of aqueous humor or obstruction of its outflow through the trabecular meshwork or the canal of Schlemm. Ninety percent of glaucoma patients suffer from this form of the disorder, which may be detected during a routine eye examination before symptoms become severe.

Acute closed-angle glaucoma occurs when the iris adheres more tightly to the lens than usual, narrowing the angle between the surface of the iris and the trabecular meshwork. If this angle closes, the drainage of aqueous humor stops, causing a sudden rise in intraocular pressure. Acute angle closure glaucoma constitutes an ophthalmic emergency.

Secondary glaucoma can result from uveitis, trauma, or adverse effects of drugs such as corticosteroids.

Gonorrhea
Transmission of *Neisseria gonorrhoeae* follows sexual contact with an infected person. This common venereal disease infects the genitourinary tract (especially the urethra and cervix) and, occasionally, the rectum, pharynx, and eyes. Although many infected males may not experience symptoms, after a 3- to 6-day incubation period some develop urethritis with redness and swelling at the site of infection. Infected females may remain asymptomatic or may develop inflammation and a greenish yellow discharge from the cervix.
(continued on page 124)

Electrolyte imbalances

Body fluids contain two kinds of dissolved substances: those that dissociate in solution (electrolytes) and those that do not. For example, glucose, when dissolved in water, doesn't break down into smaller particles; however, sodium chloride dissociates in solution into sodium cations (+) and chloride anions (-). The composition of these electrolytes in body fluids is electrically balanced so that the positively charged ions (cations: sodium, potassium, calcium, and magnesium) equal the negatively charged ions (anions: chloride, bicarbonate, sulfate, phosphate, proteinate, and carbonic and other organic acids). Although these particles are present in relatively low concentrations, any deviation from their normal levels can have profound physiological effects. This table details the causes, signs and symptoms, and treatments of the more important electrolyte imbalances.

Causes	Signs and symptoms	Nursing considerations
Sodium		
Hyponatremia (serum sodium below 135 mEq/liter)		
Hyponatremia associated with excess fluid • Syndrome of inappropriate secretion of ADH • Excessive intake of hypotonic fluids *Hyponatremia associated with dehydration* • Administration of salt-removing diuretics • Salt-wasting nephritis • Excessive GI fluid losses from nasogastric suctioning, vomiting, or diarrhea • Severe diaphoresis • Potassium depletion • Trauma, such as burns • Aldosterone deficiency • Severe malnutrition	*Hyponatremia associated with excess fluid* • Headache, anxiety, lassitude, apathy, confusion • Anorexia, nausea, vomiting, diarrhea, cramping • Hyperreflexia, muscle spasms, weakness *Hyponatremia associated with dehydration* • Irritability, tremors, seizures, coma • Dry mucous membranes • Low-grade fever • Hypotension, tachycardia • Decreased urine output ranging from oliguria to anuria	• Correct sodium and water imbalance through diet and administration of I.V. solutions, as ordered. • During administration of saline solution, observe patient closely for signs of hypervolemia (such as dyspnea, crackles, and engorged neck or hand veins). • During treatments, monitor neurologic and GI symptoms to detect improvement or deterioration. • Monitor sodium and potassium levels closely.
Hypernatremia (serum sodium above 145 mEq/liter)		
Hypernatremia associated with excess fluid • Excessive administration of large amounts of sodium chloride solution I.V. • Excessive aldosterone secretion *Hypernatremia associated with dehydration* • Dehydration *without sodium loss* from decreased water intake, severe vomiting, or diarrhea • Excessive use of osmotic diuretics • Hypercalcemia with polyuria and dehydration • Neurohypophyseal dysfunction (as in diabetes insipidus) • Renal tubular disease • Dysfunctional thirst mechanism	*Hypernatremia associated with excess fluid* • Weight gain • Pitting edema in extremities • Hypertension • Shortness of breath (only in severe imbalance) *Hypernatremia associated with dehydration* • Lethargy, irritability, tremors, seizures, coma • Dry mucous membranes; rough, dry tongue; flushed skin • Low-grade fever • Oliguria • Intense thirst	• Monitor hourly urine output. • Replace water volume, as ordered, administering fluids with caution. • Check serum sodium levels every 6 hours. • Monitor vital signs closely. Watch for increasing pulse rate and hypertension. • Observe patient for signs of hypervolemia.

Electrolyte imbalances *(continued)*

Causes	Signs and symptoms	Nursing considerations

Potassium

Hypokalemia *(serum potassium level below 3.5 mEq/liter)*

Causes	Signs and symptoms	Nursing considerations
• Thiazide and osmotic diuretic therapy • Prolonged potassium-free I.V. therapy (for a patient receiving nothing by mouth) • Renal disease such as tubular acidosis and Fanconi's syndrome • Excessive aldosterone secretion • Acid-base imbalance • Excessive GI fluid losses from nasogastric suctioning, vomiting, diarrhea, or intestinal fistula • Malnutrition or malabsorption syndrome • Laxative abuse • Trauma with associated loss of potassium in urine	• Dysrhythmias, enhanced effectiveness of digitalis (to the point of toxicosis), presence of U wave and depressed ST segment on ECG waveform • Muscle weakness, fatigue, leg cramps • Drowsiness, irritability, coma • Anorexia, vomiting, paralytic ileus • Polyuria	• Place patient on cardiac monitor, as ordered. Observe him for changes in heart rate, rhythm, and ECG pattern. • Treat dysrhythmias by correcting potassium imbalance, as ordered; method depends on serum level and severity of symptoms. Doctor may order increased potassium intake in diet or oral potassium supplements (diluted to prevent irritation and facilitate absorption); or, in emergency, slow administration of diluted potassium chloride I.V. (with patient on cardiac monitor). Monitor patient for signs and symptoms of sudden hypokalemia onset. • Monitor serum potassium level to determine effects of replacement therapy. • Determine source of potassium loss; for example, wound or fistula drainage. Analysis of drainage sample electrolyte content will help indicate amount of daily loss. • Observe patient for digitalis toxicosis. • Observe patient for signs of alkalosis, such as irritability, confusion, diarrhea, and nausea. • Never give potassium when patient's urine output is below 600 ml/day.

Hyperkalemia *(serum potassium level above 5.5 mEq/liter)*

Causes	Signs and symptoms	Nursing considerations
• Excessive administration of potassium chloride • Renal disease • Use of potassium-sparing diuretics by renal disease patients • Destruction of cells by burns or trauma, with subsequent potassium release	• Cardiac symptoms, including bradycardia, lethal dysrhythmias, and cardiac arrest; ECG waveform shows tented T wave, prolonged PR interval, widened QRS complex, flat-to-absent P wave and asystole • Apathy, confusion, tingling	• Place patient on cardiac monitor, as ordered. Observe him for changes in heart rate, rhythm, and ECG pattern. • Restrict ingestion of potassium in diet. • In an emergency (when potassium excess causes ECG changes

(continued)

Electrolyte imbalances *(continued)*

Causes	Signs and symptoms	Nursing considerations
Hyperkalemia *(continued)*		
• Aldosterone insufficiency • Acidosis, as in diabetic keotacidosis	• Hyperreflexia progressing to numbness, tingling, and flaccid weakness, paralysis • Abdominal cramping, nausea, diarrhea • Oliguria, anuria • Metabolic acidosis	or the serum potassium level exceeds 6 mEq/liter), administer I.V. glucose, insulin, and sodium bicarbonate, as ordered. This treatment will help shift potassium into the cell. *Note:* Treatment's effects last about 4 hours. • Check serum potassium levels to monitor shift of potassium in and out of cells. When I.V. treatment is discontinued, potassium shifts back into blood. • Follow I.V. treatment with one or both of the following, as ordered: sodium polystyrene sulfonate (Kayexalate), an exchange resin, administered orally, through a nasogastric tube, or as an enema; or dialysis. If these treatments are prolonged, monitor patient for resulting hypokalemia.
Calcium		
Hypocalcemia (serum calcium level below 4.5 mEq/liter)		
• Hypoparathyroidism • Chronic renal failure • Inadequate vitamin D and calcium intake • Chronic malabsorption syndrome • Cancer • Hyperphosphatemia • Hypomagnesemia • Cushing's syndrome • Acute pancreatitis	• Muscle cramps, muscle tremors, tetany, tonic-clonic seizures, paresthesia • Alteration in normal blood clotting mechanisms, causing bleeding • Dysrhythmias, hypotension, lengthened QT interval with normal T wave on ECG waveform • Anxiety, irritability, twitching, Chvostek's sign, Trousseau's sign	• Place patient on cardiac monitor, as ordered. Observe him for changes in heart rate, rhythm, and ECG pattern. • Administer calcium gluconate or calcium chloride 10% I.V., as ordered. • Provide calcium in diet, as ordered. • Monitor serum calcium levels every 12 to 24 hours. Report a serum calcium level of less than 8 mEq/liter. • Monitor blood's prothrombin time and platelet levels. • Administer any ordered antacids with caution; some contain phosphorus.

Electrolyte imbalances (continued)

Causes	Signs and symptoms	Nursing considerations

Hypercalcemia (serum calcium level above 5.5 mEq/liter)

Causes	Signs and symptoms	Nursing considerations
• Long-term immobilization (causes calcium displacement from bone to blood) • Hyperparathyroidism • Hypophosphatemia • Metastatic carcinoma • Alkalosis • Thyrotoxicosis • Vitamin D toxicosis • Prolonged thiazide diuretic therapy • Addison's disease	• Drowsiness, lethargy, headaches, depression, apathy, irritability, confusion, personality change • Increased incidence of kidney stones, with associated flank pain • Muscular flaccidity • Nausea, vomiting, anorexia, or constipation • Polydipsia • Polyuria • Hypertension; enhanced effectiveness of digitalis, to the point of toxicity (administration of digitalis may cause dysrhythmias); shortening of QT interval of ECG waveform; decreased effectiveness of cardiac contractions, leading to cardiac arrest • Pathologic fractures	• Place patient on cardiac monitor. Observe him for changes in heart rate, rhythm, and ECG pattern. • Monitor serum calcium level frequently. Watch for cardiac dysrhythmias if serum calcium level exceeds 5.5 mEq/liter. • If patient's on digitalis, check his digitalis serum level before administering each daily dose. Assess him for signs of digitalis toxicosis, such as vomiting, headache, fatigue, and dysrhythmias. • Administer the following medication, as ordered: loop diuretics (never thiazide diuretics) and fluid therapy, to enhance renal calcium excretion; mithramycin (Mithracin); corticosteroids; phosphate binders. • Administer any ordered antacids with caution; some contain calcium. • Check urine for renal calculi and acidity.

Magnesium

Hypomagnesemia (serum magnesium level below 1.5 mEq/liter)

Causes	Signs and symptoms	Nursing considerations
• Starvation syndrome • Malabsorption syndrome • Postoperative complications after bowel resection • Prolonged total parenteral nutrition (TPN) therapy without adequate magnesium • Excessive administration of mercurial diuretics • Excessive GI fluid losses from nasogastric suctioning, vomiting, diarrhea, or fistula • Hyper- and hypoparathyroidism	• Dizziness, confusion, delusions, hallucinations, convulsions • Tremors, hyperirritability, tetany, leg and foot cramps, Chvostek's sign • Dysrhythmias and vasomotor changes • Anorexia and nausea	• If patient needs antacids, give Maalox or Mylanta (as ordered). • Take seizure precautions, such as keeping side rails up and initiating neurochecks. • Replace magnesium losses, as ordered. Infuse magnesium replacement slowly, observing patient for bradycardia and decreased respirations. • Monitor serum magnesium levels every 6 to 12 hours during replacement therapy. Report abnormal levels immediately.

(continued)

Electrolyte imbalances *(continued)*

Causes	Signs and symptoms	Nursing considerations
Hypermagnesemia (serum magnesium level above 2.5 mEq/liter)		
• Renal failure • Adrenal insufficiency • Excessive ingestion of magnesium (for example, in the form of antacid gels such as Maalox or Mylanta) • Excessive use of magnesium-containing laxatives such as Milk of Magnesia	• Drowsiness, lethargy, confusion, coma • Bradycardia, weak pulse; hypotension, prolonged QT interval on ECG waveform, heart block, cardiac arrest (with serum levels of 25 mEq/liter) • Vague neuromuscular changes (may include tremors and hyporeflexia) • Vague GI symptoms, such as nausea	• Discontinue Maalox and Mylanta if patient's receiving them. • Administer calcium gluconate I.V. as ordered. Note that calcium enhances digitalis action. • In renal failure, perform dialysis, as ordered, to remove excess magnesium. • Monitor serum magnesium levels to determine effectiveness of treatment. Watch for respiratory distress if serum magnesium levels exceed 10 mEq/liter.

Phosphorus

Hypophosphatemia (serum phosphate level below 1.8 mEq/liter)		
• Chronic alcoholism (usually entails decreased phosphate intake) • Prolonged phosphate-free or low-phosphate TPN therapy • Hyperparathyroidism, with resultant hypercalcemia • Excessive use of phosphate-binding gels such as aluminum hydroxide • Malabsorption syndrome • Chronic diarrhea	• Anorexia • Mental confusion • Muscle weakness, muscle wasting, tremors, paresthesia • Hemolytic anemia • Hypoxia with peripheral cyanosis	• Monitor calcium, magnesium, and phosphorus levels, and report any changes immediately. • Administer potassium phosphate I.V., as ordered. • Provide phosphate in diet, or give oral phosphate supplements, as ordered. Monitor patient for signs of hypocalcemia when giving supplements. • If patient's receiving phosphate-binding gels such as aluminum hydroxide (Amphojel), discontinue their use.
Hyperphosphatemia (serum phosphate level above 2.6 mEq/liter)		
• Excessive use of phosphate-containing laxatives or enemas • Acute and chronic renal failure • Excessive I.V. or oral phosphate therapy • Cytotoxic agents • Vitamin D toxicosis • Hypocalcemia • Hypoparathyroidism	• Usually asymptomatic • Possible metastatic calcifications • With hypocalcemia, neuromuscular changes including cramps, tetany, or seizures	• Administer phosphate-binding gels such as aluminum hydroxide (Amphojel), as ordered. • Monitor serum calcium, magnesium, and phosphorus levels. Report any changes immediately. • Observe patient for signs of hypocalcemia, such as muscle twitching and tetany. • Discontinue antacids, such as Maalox and Mylanta.

Electrolyte imbalances *(continued)*

Causes	Signs and symptoms	Nursing considerations

Chloride

Hypochloremia (serum chloride level below 98 mEq/liter)

• Decreased chloride intake or absorption—as in low dietary sodium intake, sodium deficiency, potassium deficiency, metabolic alkalosis; prolonged use of mercurial diuretics; or administration of dextrose I.V. without electrolytes • Excessive chloride loss, resulting from prolonged diarrhea or diaphoresis; loss of hydrochloric acid in gastric secretions, due to vomiting, gastric suctioning, or gastric surgery	• Usually associated with hyponatremia and its characteristic muscular weakness and twitching, since renal chloride loss always accompanies sodium loss, and sodium reabsorption is not possible without chloride • If chloride depletion results from metabolic alkalosis secondary to loss of gastric secretions, chloride is lost independently from sodium; typical symptoms are muscle hypertonicity, tetany, and shallow, depressed breathing	• Monitor serum chloride levels frequently, especially during I.V. therapy. • Watch for signs of hyperchloremia or hypochloremia. Be alert for respiratory difficulty. • To prevent hypochloremia, monitor laboratory results (serum electrolytes and blood gases) and fluid intake and output of patients who are vulnerable to chloride imbalance, especially those recovering from gastric surgery. Record and report excessive or continuous loss of gastric secretions. Also report prolonged infusion of dextrose in water without saline.

Hyperchloremia (serum chloride level above 108 mEq/liter)

• Excessive chloride intake or absorption—as in hyperingestion of ammonium chloride, or ureterointestinal anastomosis—allowing reabsorption of chloride by the bowel. • Hemoconcentration, caused by dehydration • Compensatory mechanisms for other metabolic abnormalities, as in metabolic acidosis, brain stem injury causing neurogenic hyperventilation, and hyperparathyroidism	• Because of the natural affinity of sodium and chloride ions, hyperchloremia usually produces clinical effects associated with hypernatremia and resulting extracellular fluid volume excess (agitation, tachycardia, hypertension, pitting edema, dyspnea) • Hyperchloremia associated with metabolic acidosis is due to excretion of base bicarbonate by the kidneys, and induces deep, rapid breathing; weakness; diminished cognitive ability; and ultimately, coma	• Check serum electrolyte levels every 3 to 6 hours. If the patient is receiving high doses of sodium bicarbonate, watch for signs of overcorrection (metabolic alkalosis, respiratory depression) or lingering signs of hyperchloremia, which indicate inadequate treatment. • To prevent hyperchloremia, check laboratory results for elevated serum chloride or potassium imbalance if the patient is receiving I.V. solutions containing sodium chloride, and monitor fluid intake and output. Also, watch for signs of metabolic acidosis. When administering I.V. fluids containing lactated Ringer's solution, monitor flow rate according to the patient's age, physical condition, and bicarbonate level. Report any irregularities promptly.

Untreated gonorrhea can spread through the blood to the joints, tendons, meninges, and endocardium; in females, it can also lead to chronic pelvic inflammatory disease and sterility. After adequate treatment, prognosis is excellent, although reinfection is common.

A child born to an infected mother can contract gonococcal ophthalmia neonatorum. A patient with gonorrhea can contract gonococcal conjunctivitis by touching his eyes with contaminated hands. The disease occurs most frequently among people ages 19 to 25; individuals with multiple sexual partners have the greatest risk.

Graves' disease

The most common cause of hyperthyroidism, a metabolic imbalance that results from thyroid hormone overproduction, Graves' disease strikes women 5 times as often as men and occurs most frequently between ages 20 and 40. It often arises following an infection or physical and emotional stress. While researchers haven't identified the cause of Graves' disease, studies implicate abnormal T-lymphocyte function.

Graves' disease profoundly affects every body system. It affects the eyes, skin, and bones as well as the thyroid, commonly causing such problems as exophthalmos, infiltrative dermopathy (myxedema), acropachy (finger clubbing), and goiter.

The patient may also develop nervousness, a fine tremor of the hands, weight loss, fatigue, breathlessness, palpitations, heat intolerance, and increased metabolic rate and gastrointestinal motility.

With treatment—which may include antithyroid drugs and iodine preparations, or subtotal thyroidectomy—most patients can lead normal lives. However, if a patient has inadequately controlled Graves' disease, stressful conditions (in-

cluding surgery, infection, toxemia of pregnancy, and diabetic ketoacidosis) may precipitate a thyroid storm. This acute exacerbation of hyperthyroidism may lead to life-threatening cardiac, hepatic, or renal failure.

Guillain-Barré syndrome

This acute, rapidly progressive form of polyneuritis causes segmental demyelination of the peripheral nerves, resulting in weakness and mild distal sensory loss. Its exact cause remains unknown, but it may follow a cell-mediated immunologic attack on the peripheral nerves in response to a virus. Weakness usually appears in the legs first (ascending type), then extends to the arms and facial nerves in 24 to 72 hours. The course of illness includes 3 phases; an initial phase (lasting 1 to 3 weeks following the first definitive symptoms); a plateau phase (lasting several days to 2 weeks); and a recovery phase marked by remyelination and axonal process regrowth (usually over a period of 4 to 6 months). About 95% of patients experience complete and spontaneous recovery, although mild motor or reflex deficits in the feet or legs may persist.

Herpes simplex

A recurrent viral infection caused by the widespread infectious agent *Herpesvirus hominis* (HVH). Herpes Type I, transmitted by oral and respiratory secretions, affects the skin and mucous membranes. Herpes Type II, transmitted by sexual contact, primarily affects the genital areas.

One to two weeks after contact with the infected person, the patient may experience burning, tingling or itching sensations around the edges of the lips or nose. Several hours later, he may develop small red papules in the irritated area, followed by the eruption of small vesicles or fever blisters

filled with fluid and usually causing itching and pain. After the first infection, the patient is a carrier subject to recurrent infection.

Herpes Type II can pass to the fetus transplacentally and may cause spontaneous abortion or stillbirth. Infants born with HVH infection may experience localized skin lesions or disseminated infection of the lungs, liver, brain, or other organs; disseminated infection usually leads to death.

Herpes zoster

Acute unilateral and segmental inflammation of the dorsal root ganglia caused by infection with herpesvirus varicella-zoster. Herpes zoster produces localized vascular skin lesions confined to a dermatome, and severe neuralgic pain in peripheral areas innervated by nerves arising in the inflamed root ganglia.

Unless infection spreads to the brain, prognosis is good. Eventually most patients recover completely, except for possible scarring and, in cases of corneal damage, visual impairment. Occasionally, neuralgia persists for months or years.

Hiatal hernia

This type of hernia occurs when a defect in the diaphragm permits a portion of the stomach to pass through the diaphragmatic opening into the chest. In *paraesophageal hernia,* a part of the greater curvature of the stomach rolls through the diaphragmatic defect. Usually, this produces no symptoms. In a *sliding hernia,* both the stomach and the gastroesophageal junction slip up into the chest, so that the gastroesophageal junction is above the diaphragmatic hiatus. This usually doesn't produce symptoms, but if the patient also has an incompetent sphincter he may experience heartburn and chest pain. Treatment of hiatal hernia seeks to prevent complications, such as strangulation of the herniated intrathoracic portion of the stomach.

Hirschsprung's disease

A congenital disorder of the large intestine, Hirschsprung's disease is characterized by absence or marked reduction of parasympathetic ganglion cells in the colorectal wall. The patient suffers from impaired intestinal motility which causes severe, intractable constipation. Clinical effects usually appear shortly after birth but mild symptoms may not be recognized until later in childhood, adolescence, or in rare cases, adulthood. Without prompt treatment, an infant with colonic obstruction may die within 24 hours from enterocolitis leading to severe diarrhea and hypovolemic shock. Prognosis improves greatly with prompt treatment.

Hodgkin's disease

This neoplastic disease begins as a painless lymph node enlargement, usually starting in one node, then spreading to the spleen and throughout the lymphatic system. Eventually, the disease travels through the bloodstream to organs close to lymph nodes, such as the uterus, bronchi, or vertebrae.

In Hodgkin's disease, abnormal, enlarged, multinucleated macrophages called Reed-Sternberg cells gradually replace normal lymph node structure. Lymphocytes, histiocytes, eosinophils, plasma cells, and neutrophils also proliferate. Characteristic symptoms include night sweats, unexplained weight loss and itching, and lymph nodes that enlarge rapidly during fever, then revert to normal size afterward.

Untreated, Hodgkin's disease follows a relentless and ultimately fatal course. Conventional treatments have a good success rate, and even in advanced stages, chances for successful treatment are good to excellent. Ninety percent of patients survive past 5 years and patients with localized disease often live 10 years or more without a recurrence.

Huntington's chorea

This hereditary disease causes degeneration in the cerebral cortex and basal ganglia. The patient experiences progressive chorea with rapid, often violent and purposeless movements, and mental deterioration. Personality changes include obstinacy, carelessness, untidiness, moodiness, apathy, inappropriate behavior, loss of memory, and sometimes paranoia. Eventually, the patient develops dementia. Death usually results 10 to 15 years after onset, from suicide, CHF, or pneumonia.

Hypertension

Hypertension refers to an intermittent or sustained elevation in diastolic or systolic blood pressure. Most patients develop essential (idiopathic) hypertension. Secondary hypertension results from renal or vascular disease; primary hypoaldosteronism; Cushing's syndrome; dysfunctions of the thyroid, pituitary or parathyroid glands; or other causes. Malignant hypertension is a severe fulminant form of hypertension common to both types.

Hypertension affects 15% to 20% of adults in the United States. Risk factors for essential hypertension include family history, race (most common in blacks), stress, obesity, a high dietary intake of saturated fats or sodium, use of tobacco or oral contraceptives, a sedentary life-style, and aging.

Hypertension represents a major cause of cerebrovascular accident, cardiac disease, and renal failure. If detected and treated before complications develop, however, the disorder carries a good prognosis.

Infectious mononucleosis

Infectious mononucleosis is an acute infectious disease caused by the Epstein-Barr virus (EBV), a member of the herpes group. It primarily affects young adults and children, although in children it's often so mild that it's overlooked. Characteristically, infectious mononucleosis produces fever, sore throat, cervical lymphadenopathy, hepatic dysfunction, increased lymphocytes and monocytes, and the development and persistence of heterophil antibodies. Most patients recover completely and major complications are rare.

Legg-Calve-Perthes disease

In this disease, vascular interruption causes ischemic necrosis and eventual flattening of the head of the femur. It most frequently affects boys age 4 to 10 and usually occurs unilaterally. The patient first experiences a persistent thigh pain or limp that becomes progressively severe. He may also experience mild pain in the hip, thigh or knee that is aggravated by activity and relieved by rest; muscle spasm; atrophy of muscles in the upper thigh; slight shortening of the leg; and severely restricted abduction and internal rotation of the hip. Although this disease usually runs its course in 3 to 4 years, misalignment of the acetabulum and flattening of the femoral head may lead to premature osteoarthritis. Legg-Calve-Perthes disease tends to recur in families.

Legionnaire's disease

This acute bronchopneumonia derives its name and notoriety from the peculiar, highly publicized outbreak among attendees at an American Legion Convention in July 1976. It results from infection by a fastidious gram-negative bacillus, *Legionella pneumophila,* that probably is transmitted by an airborne route. It doesn't spread from person to person. Severity of Legionnaire's disease ranges from a mild illness (with or without pneumonitis) to multilobar pneumonia, with a mortality rate as high as 15%. The disease may occur epidemically or sporadically and usually appears in late summer or early fall.

At first, the patient experiences diarrhea, anorexia, malaise, diffuse myalgias, generalized weakness,

Spotting carriers of Lyme disease

The illustrations show the two ticks that carry Lyme disease—*Ixodes dammini,* which is prevalent in the northeastern United States, and *I. pacificus,* prevalent in the western United States. Note their shapes and relative sizes.

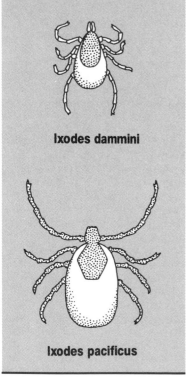

Ixodes dammini

Ixodes pacificus

headache, recurrent chills, cough, and an unremitting fever, possibly as high as 105° F (40.5° C). Other characteristic findings include nausea, vomiting, disorientation, mental sluggishness, confusion, mild temporary amnesia, pleuritic chest pain, tachypnea, dyspnea, fine crackles, and bradycardia.

Leukemia

The malignant proliferation of white blood cells, leukemia ranks 20th in causes of cancer-related deaths among people of all ages. Among children, however, it's the most common form of cancer.

Leukemia is classified according to the type and maturation of aberrant white blood cells. In acute lymphocytic leukemia, the aberrant cells are lymphoblasts; in acute nonlymphocytic leukemia, the cells are myeloblasts, monoblasts, erythroblasts, or, rarely, megakaryoblasts, produced in the bone marrow. Chronic lymphocytic leukemia is characterized by abnormal proliferation of early B-cell lymphocytes or occasionally T-cell lymphocytes in lymphoid tissue. Chronic myelogenous leukemia (CML) is characterized by the abnormal proliferation of granulocytic precursors in bone marrow, peripheral blood, and body tissues.

The patient with *acute leukemia* experiences sudden onset of high fever accompanied by thrombocytopenia and abnormal bleeding such as nosebleeds, gingival bleeding, purpura, ecchymoses, petechiae, easy bruising after minor trauma, and prolonged menses. Other insidious signs include pallor, chills, and recurrent infection. Untreated, acute leukemia is invariably fatal. With treatment, prognosis varies. In acute lymphocytic leukemia, for example, treatment induces remissions in 90% of children and in 65% of adults. In acute nonlymphocytic leukemia, prognosis is poor, even in children and adults who receive treatment.

Chronic myelogenous leukemia proceeds in two distinct phases: the insidious chronic phase, with anemia and bleeding abnormalities and, eventually, the acute phase, marked by the rapid proliferation of myeloblasts. The disease is invariably fatal; most patients die within 6 months of the onset of the acute phase.

Chronic lymphocytic leukemia is the most benign and most slowly progressive form of leukemia. Nearly all patients are men over age 50. In early stages, patients usually develop fatigue, malaise, fever, infection, and nodal enlargement. In advanced stages, patients may experience extreme fatigue and weight loss, with liver or spleen enlargement, bone tenderness, and edema from lymph node obstruction. Later signs and symptoms include anemia, pallor, dyspnea, tachycardia, palpitations, bleeding, and opportunistic fungal, viral, and bacterial infections. Gross bone marrow replacement is the most common cause of death, which usually takes place within 4 to 5 years after diagnosis.

Lyme disease

First identified in a group of children in Lyme, Connecticut, this multisystemic disease results from the spirochete *Borrelia burgdorferi,* which is carried by the minute tick *Ixodes dammini* or another tick in the Ixodidae family. It often begins in the summer with the classic skin lesion called erythema chronicum migrans. Without antibiotic treatment, cardiac or neurologic abnormalities sometimes develop weeks or months later, possibly followed by arthritis.

Lymphoma

This heterogeneous group of malignant neoplasms originate in the lymph glands and other lymphoid tissue. Usually, the patient first develops swelling of the lymph glands, enlarged tonsils and adenoids, and painless rubbery nodes in the cervical supraclavicular area. As the lymphoma progresses, he experiences symptoms specific to the area involved and systemic complaints of fatigue, malaise, weight loss, fever, and night sweats. In children, the disease causes dyspnea and coughing.

Lymphomas are categorized according to the degree of cellular differentiation and the presence or absence of nodularity. Nodular lymphomas yield a better prognosis than diffuse forms of the disease. Overall, malignant lymphomas offer a less favorable outcome than Hodgkin's disease.

Mastoiditis
In this bacterial infection and inflammation of the air cells of the mastoid process, primary clinical features include a dull ache and tenderness in the area of the mastoid process, low-grade fever, and a thick purulent discharge that gradually becomes more profuse, leading to otitis externa. Postauricular erythema and edema may push the auricle out from the head; pressure within the edematous mastoid antrum may produce swelling and obstruction of the external ear canal, causing conductive hearing loss. Although prognosis is good with early treatment, possible complications include meningitis, facial paralysis, brain abscess, and suppurative labyrinthitis.

Ménière's disease
This labyrinthine dysfunction produces fullness or blocked feeling in the ear, severe tinnitus, and sensorineural hearing loss. The patient experiences violent paroxysmal attacks that last from 10 minutes to several hours. During an acute attack, he may also develop severe nausea, vomiting, sweating, giddiness, or nystagmus. Vertigo may cause loss of balance and falling to the affected side.

Frequently, the patient will assume a characteristic posture—lying on the unaffected ear and looking in the direction of the affected ear. Ménière's disease usually affects adults between ages 30 and 60. After multiple attacks over several years, it leads to residual tinnitus and hearing loss.

Meningitis
In meningitis, the brain and spinal cord meninges become inflamed, usually as a result of bacterial infection. Such inflammation may involve all three meningeal membranes—the dura mater, the arachnoid, and the pia mater. The patient exhibits signs of infection (fever, chills, and malaise); signs of increased ICP (headache and vomiting); and signs of meningeal irritation (nuchal rigidity, positive Brudzinski's and Kernig's signs, exaggerated and symmetrical deep tendon reflexes and opisthotonos). Other manifestations include sinus arrhythmias; irritability; photophobia, diplopia, and other visual problems; and delirium, deep stupor, and coma.

If the patient is diagnosed in the early stages of illness and responds well to antibiotics, he stands a good chance of recovery. The disease presents a greater danger to elderly patients and infants.

Multiple sclerosis
This neurologic disorder represents a major cause of chronic disability in young adults. Progressive demyelination of the white matter in various parts of the brain and the spinal cord leads to widely disseminated and varied neurologic dysfunction with exacerbations and remissions of symptoms. Symptoms may last for minutes, hours, or weeks; they may wax and wane with no predictable pattern, varying from day to day. The patient typically first experiences visual problems and sensory impairment, such as

numbness and paresthesia. He may develop ocular disturbances, muscular dysfunction, urinary disturbances, and emotional lability. Clinical effects may be so bizarre that the patient appears hysterical.

MS may progress rapidly, disabling the patient by early adulthood or causing death within months of onset. Prolonged remissions, however, along with drug therapy to shorten exacerbations and relieve neurologic deficits, enable 70% of patients to lead active, productive lives.

Mumps
Children between ages 5 and 9 are most vulnerable to this acute illness. Carried in the saliva of a infected person, the mumps paramyxovirus is transmitted by droplets or direct contact. Usually, the patient experiences prodromal syndromes for 24 hours: these include myalgia, anorexia, malaise, headache, and low-grade fever. Then, the patient develops an earache that's aggravated by chewing; parotid gland tenderness and swelling; a temperature of 101° F to 104° F (38.3° C to 40° C); and pain when chewing or when drinking sour or acidic liquids. Simultaneously with the swelling of the parotid gland, or several days later, one or more of the other salivary glands may become swollen.

Most patients recover completely, although complications, including epididymo-orchitis and mumps meningitis, may develop.

Muscular dystrophy
This group of congenital disorders is characterized by progressive systemic wasting of skeletal muscles without neural or sensory defects. Paradoxically, these wasted muscles tend to enlarge because of connective tissue and fat deposits, giving a false impression of muscle strength. Four main types of muscular dystrophy occur. *Duchenne's muscular dystrophy* accounts for 50% of all cases. It

usually strikes during early childhood and results in death within 10 to 15 years of onset. *Facioscapulohumeral* and *limb girdle* dystrophies usually don't shorten life expectancy. Both types are slowly progressive and often relatively benign. The *mixed type* progresses rapidly; usually the patient dies within 5 years after onset.

Myasthenia gravis

This disorder causes a failure of transmission of nerve impulses at the neuromuscular junction. It produces sporadic but progressive weakness and abnormal fatigability of striated (skeletal) muscles. Exercise and repeated movement exacerbate the patient's symptoms. Usually this disorder affects muscles innervated by the cranial nerves (face, lips, tongue, neck, and throat), but it can affect any muscle group.

Myasthenia gravis follows an unpredictable course of recurring exacerbations and periodic remissions. There's no known cure, but anticholinesterase and corticosteroid drug therapy may allow the patient to lead a relatively normal life, except in times of exacerbation. If the disease affects the respiratory system, it may become life-threatening.

Myocardial infarction

An occlusion of a coronary artery leads to myocardial ischemia and necrosis. The patient experiences persistent crushing substernal pain that may radiate to the left arm, jaw, neck, or shoulder blades. Other signs and symptoms include a feeling of impending doom, fatigue, nausea, vomiting, and shortness of breath. A history of CAD, persistent chest pain, changes in ECG, and elevated serum enzyme (CPK-MB) levels over a 72-hour period support a diagnosis of MI.

Treatment includes narcotic analgesics to relieve pain and provide sedation, and oxygen therapy

to ease dyspnea. The patient may also receive lidocaine to correct dysrhythmias, atropine to correct heart block, and nitroglycerin, calcium channel blockers, or isosorbide dinitrate to reduce cardiac work load. If treatment begins within six hours of MI onset, the doctor may order infusion of thrombolytic drugs. Other interventions include insertion of an intra-aortic balloon pump to help correct cardiogenic shock, dobutamine to reduce cardiac contractility, beta-adrenergic blockers to prevent another infarction, and percutaneous transluminal coronary angioplasty to open an occluded artery.

Myocarditis

This focal or diffuse inflammation of the cardiac muscle most frequently results from bacterial or viral infections. It may also follow hypersensitive immune reactions, radiation therapy, chemical poisoning, or parasitic or helminthic infections. Mild myocarditis often fails to produce specific cardiovascular symptoms or ECG abnormalities; the patient may recover spontaneously without experiencing residual effects. Alternatively, the patient may experience continuous pressure or soreness in the chest. The patient may also experience nonspecific symptoms such as fatigue, dyspnea, palpitations, and fever, which reflect an accompanying systemic infection. Occasionally, complications — CHF and, rarely, cardiomyopathy — develop.

Neurofibromatosis

A congenital condition that may be transmitted as an autosomal dominant trait or occur as a new genetic mutation, neurofibromatosis is characterized by numerous neurofibromas of the nerves and skin and by cafe-au-lait spots on the skin. Effects vary with the location and size of tumors. Some patients

develop a mild form that frequently goes unnoticed while others may suffer numerous anomalies of the muscles, bones, and viscera. Some patients (like the 19th century's so-called "Elephant Man") develop large, pedunculated soft tissue tumors. Bone changes may result in skeletal deformities, especially curvature of the spine. Neurofibromas may appear in the alimentary tract, bladder, endocrine glands, and cranial nerves.

Osgood-Schlatter disease

The patient with this disease, most often an active adolescent boy, experiences a painful, incomplete separation of the epiphysis of the tibial tubercle from the tibial shaft in one or both knees. He feels aching and pain below the kneecap when performing activities that cause forceful contraction of the patellar tendon on the tubercle; for example, ascending and descending stairs. He may also develop soft-tissue swelling, tenderness, and localized heat. Most often the disease results from trauma, but it may also be the consequence of a deficient blood supply or genetic factors. Severe disease may cause permanent tubercle enlargement.

Otitis media

Otitis media, inflammation of the middle ear, may be suppurative or secretory, acute or chronic. Children frequently develop acute otitis media, especially during the winter months. *Acute suppurative otitis media* produces deep, throbbing pain. *Acute secretory otitis media* produces severe conductive hearing loss and, possibly, a sensation of fullness in the ear and popping, crackling, or clicking sounds on swallowing or with jaw movement. With treatment, most patients recover from acute otitis media. However, prolonged accumulation of fluid in the middle ear cavity causes chronic otitis media, with possible perforation of the tympanic membrane. *Chronic suppurative otitis media* may lead to scarring, adhesions, and severe structural or functional ear damage; *chronic secretory otitis media,* with its persistent inflammation and pressure, may cause conductive hearing loss.

Otosclerosis

Patients with this disorder experience slowly progressive unilateral hearing loss which may advance to bilateral deafness. Spongy bone slowly forms in the otic capsule, particularly at the oval window, disrupting the conduction of vibrations from the tympanic membrane to the cochlea.

The most common cause of conductive deafness, otosclerosis occurs in at least 10% of all Caucasians, with an especially high prevalence among females between ages 15 and 30. Treatment may consist of stapedectomy or a hearing aid.

Paget's disease

A slowly progressive metabolic bone disease, Paget's disease consists of an initial phase of excessive bone resorption (osteoclastic phase) followed by a reactive phase of excessive abnormal bone formation (osteoblastic phase). Chaotic, fragile, and weak, the new bone structure causes painful deformities of both external contour and internal structure. Paget's disease usually localizes in one or several areas of the skeleton (most frequently the lower torso), but occasionally the patient develops widely distributed skeletal deformity. He may develop cranial enlargement over frontal and occipital areas or kyphosis and asymmetric bowing of the tibia and femur.

Paget's disease can prove fatal, particularly if associated with CHF (widespread disease creates a continuous need for high cardiac output), bone sarcoma, or giant cell tumors.

Pancreatitis

Pancreatic inflammation occurs in acute and chronic forms. In both, the enzymes normally excreted by the pancreas digest pancreatic tissue. In men, the disease is commonly associated with alcoholism, trauma, or peptic ulcer; in women, with biliary tract disease. Mild pancreatitis may cause only steady epigastric pain unrelieved by vomiting. A severe attack causes extreme pain, persistent vomiting, abdominal rigidity, diminished bowel activity, crackles at lung bases, and left pleural effusion. Severe pancreatitis also produces extreme malaise and restlessness, with mottled skin, tachycardia, low-grade fever, and cold, sweaty extremities. Proximity of the inflamed pancreas to the bowel may cause ileus. If pancreatitis follows biliary tract disease, the patient stands a good chance of recovery. If it follows alcoholism, the outlook appears less hopeful. Mortality rises as high as 60% if pancreatitis is associated with necrosis and hemorrhage.

Parkinson's disease

A patient with this neurological disorder commonly experiences muscle rigidity and akinesia, along with an insidious tremor that begins in the fingers (unilateral pill-roll tremor), increases during stress, or anxiety, and decreases with purposeful movement and sleep. Other signs and symptoms include bradykinesia; cogwheel rigidity; masked facies; excessive perspiration; and gait, posture, and equilibrium disturbances. Deterioration progresses for an average of 10 years. Death usually results from aspiration pneumonia or other infection. Treatment aims to relieve symptoms and keep the patient functional as long as possible; measures include drugs, physical therapy, and, in severe cases, stereotactic neurosurgery.

Pelvic inflammatory disease

An acute, subacute, recurrent, or chronic infection of the oviducts and ovaries with adjacent tissue involvement, pelvic inflammatory disease (PID) usually results from infection with the aerobic organism *Neisseria gonorrhoeae.* However, it may follow infection with other aerobic or anaerobic organisms. PID may involve inflammation of the cervix (cervicitis), uterus (endometritis), fallopian tubes (salpingitis), and ovaries (oophoritis). Inflammation may extend to the connective tissue lying between broad ligaments (parametritis).

Usually the patient develops a profuse, purulent vaginal discharge, sometimes accompanied by low-grade fever and malaise. She experiences lower abdominal pain. Movement of the cervix or palpation of the adnexa may become extremely painful. Early treatment with antibiotic drugs prevents damage to the reproductive system. Untreated PID may cause infertility and may lead to potentially fatal septicemia, pulmonary emboli, and shock.

Pericarditis

This inflammation of the thin layer of muscle tissue that forms the pericardial sac occurs in acute and chronic forms. *Acute pericarditis* can be fibrinous or effusive, with purulent serous or hemorrhagic exudate; *chronic constrictive pericarditis* leads to dense fibrous pericardial thickening. Possible causes include bacterial, viral, or fungal infection; neoplasms; high-dose radiation to the chest; uremia; hypersensitivity or autoimmune disease; postcardiac injury; drugs such as hydralazine or procainamide; and idiopathic factors.

Typically, the patient experiences a sharp and often sudden pain that usually starts over the sternum and radiates to the neck, shoulders, back, and arms. However, unlike the pain of MI, pericardial pain is often pleuritic, increasing with deep inspiration and decreasing when the patient sits up and leans forward.

Treatment deals with the underlying cause of inflammation. Early treatment can help to avoid constrictive pericarditis and symptoms of CHF.

Personality disorders
Personality disorder refers to a chronic pattern of inflexible, maladaptive personality traits that influence a patient's affect, cognition, behavior, and style of interacting with others. It causes severe personal distress and impairs social and occupational function. Typically, the patient has had difficulty with emotional development during early childhood. Symptoms often appear by childhood or adolescence and make it difficult to cope with demands of everyday life. The disorder may result from ineffective or absent early childhood experiences, temperament at birth, or genetic and biochemical factors. Categories of personality disorder include paranoid, avoidant, compulsive, schizoid, dependent, passive-aggressive, histrionic, antisocial, narcissistic, and borderline.

Pertussis
This highly contagious respiratory infection produces an irritating cough that becomes paroxysmal and often ends in a high-pitched inspiratory whoop. Usually, it's caused by the nonmotile, gram-negative coccobacillus *Bordetella pertussis*, and occasionally the related similar bacteria *Bordetella parapertussis* and *Bordetella bronchiseptica*.

Since the 1940s, immunization and aggressive diagnosis and treatment have significantly reduced mortality from pertussis in the United States. Children under age 1, however, may die from complications such as pneumonia, and elderly patients face a greater risk than older children and adults.

Phenylketonuria
Infants born with this disorder have insufficient phenylalanine hydroxylase, an enzyme that acts as a catalyst in the conversion of phenylalanine to tyrosine. As a result, phenylalanine and its metabolites accumulate in the blood, causing mental retardation.

The infant appears normal at birth, but by 4 months of age begins to show signs of arrested brain development, including personality disturbances such as uncontrollable temper. Other symptoms include macrocephaly; eczematous skin lesions; dry, rough skin; a musty odor; abnormal EEG patterns; and seizures. In his first year the patient will show a precipitous decrease in IQ, and usually behave hyperactively and irritably and show purposeless, repetitive motions, increased muscle tone, and an awkward gait. Restricting dietary intake of phenylalanine can prevent mental retardation and neurologic damage.

Pneumonia
An acute infection of the lung parenchyma, pneumonia commonly impairs gas exchange. It can be viral, bacterial, fungal, protozoal, mycobacterial, mycoplasmal, or rickettsial in origin. *Bronchopneumonia* involves distal airways and alveoli; *lobular pneumonia* involves part of a lobe; *lobar pneumonia* involves an entire lobe. *Primary pneumonia* results from inhalation or aspiration of a pathogen. *Secondary pneumonia* may follow initial lung damage from noxious chemicals or other insult, or may result from hematogenous spread of bacteria of distant focus.

Patients with early bacterial pneumonia exhibit five cardinal signs: coughing, sputum production, pleuritic chest pain, shaking, chills, and fever. Physical signs vary widely, ranging from diffuse, fine crackles to signs of localized or extensive consolidation and pleural effusion. Patients with normal lungs and an intact immune system before the onset of pneumonia enjoy a good chance for recovery; for debilitated patients, however, bacterial pneumonia can prove fatal.

Progressive systemic sclerosis
Also known as scleroderma, progressive systemic sclerosis (PSS) produces diffuse fibrosis in skin and internal organs accompanied by proliferative arterial occlusions. It most often afflicts women between ages 20 and 30, and usually leads to chronic disability. Scientists suspect that an autoimmune dysfunction causes this disorder.

In more than half of affected patients, PSS begins with Raynaud's phenomenon. In the *edematous phase*, symmetrical nonpitting edema develops in the hands and may progress to the arms, upper chest, abdomen, back, and face. In the *sclerotic phase*, skin becomes tight, smooth, and waxy; skin folds and wrinkles disappear. The patient's face takes on a stretched, mask-like appearance, her lips become thin, and her nose becomes "pinched." Pigment changes and telangiectasis also may appear during this phase. The skin may stabilize, then may either return to normal or progress to the final *atrophic phase*.

The patient may also experience joint pain, swelling, and stiffness. Muscle wasting and inflammatory myopathy may also develop. GI involvement produces dysphagia, gastroesophageal reflux, and heartburn. Other complaints include abdominal cramps, bloating, and alternating diarrhea and constipation. Slowed GI motility commonly occurs. Lung fibrosis with dyspnea on exertion is also common, as is cor pulmonale.

Some PSS patients develop the CREST syndrome: calcinosis, Raynaud's phenomenon, esophageal dysfunction, sclerodactyly, and telangiectasia. This syndrome typically evolves slowly, with gradually worsening skin and visceral involvement.

Prostate cancer

The second most common neoplasm in men over age 50 and the third leading cause of male cancer death, prostate cancer usually occurs as an adenocarcinoma. Only rarely does a sarcoma arise in the prostate. About 85% of prostate carcinomas originate in the posterior part of the prostate gland; the rest originate near the urethra. Malignant prostatic tumors seldom result from the benign hyperplastic enlargement that commonly develops around the prostatic urethra in elderly men.

Seventy percent of patients with prostatic cancer survive at least 5 years if they receive treatment while their condition is localized; after metastasis the 5-year survival rate falls to under 35%. Death commonly results from widespread bone metastases. Prostate carcinoma seldom produces symptoms until well advanced. A rectal examination that reveals a small, hard nodule may help diagnose prostatic cancer before symptoms develop. Therefore, a routine physical examination of men over age 40 should always include a rectal examination.

Prostatic hypertrophy, benign

Although most men over age 50 experience some prostatic enlargement, in benign prostatic hypertrophy or hyperplasia (BPH), the prostate gland enlarges sufficiently to compress the urethra and cause overt urinary obstruction. The patient may first experience a group of symptoms known as "prostatism": reduced urine stream caliber and force, straining during micturition, feeling of incomplete voiding, and, occasionally, urine retention. As obstruction increases, he urinates more frequently and develops nocturia, incontinence, and, possibly, hematuria. As BPH worsens, complete urinary obstruction may follow infection or ingestion of decongestants, tranquilizers, alcohol, antidepressants, or anticholinergics.

Proper treatment depends on the size of the enlarged prostate, the patient's age and health, and the extent of obstruction. Patients may receive symptomatic treatment (measures include prostatic massages, sitz baths, short-term fluid restriction, and encouraging regular sexual intercourse) or undergo surgery (procedures include transurethral resection and open surgical removal of the prostate).

Pseudomembranous enterocolitis

This rare disorder causes an acute inflammation and necrosis of the small and large intestines. It usually affects the mucosa but may extend into submucosa and, rarely, other layers. Its cause remains unknown, but *Clostridium difficile* may produce a toxin that contributes to its development. The patient with pseudomembranous enterocolitis experiences sudden onset of symptoms including copious watery or bloody diarrhea, abdominal pain, and fever. In 1 to 7 days, he may die from severe dehydration and from toxicity, peritonitis, or perforation.

Pulmonary edema

This fluid accumulation in the lung's extravascular spaces initially causes dyspnea on exertion, paroxysmal nocturnal dyspnea, orthopnea, and coughing. Over time, the patient may develop tachycardia, tachypnea, dependent crackles, neck vein distention, and a diastolic gallop. If the alveoli and bronchioles fill with fluid, symptoms intensify. Respiration becomes labored and rapid, with more diffuse crackles and coughing producing frothy, bloody sputum. Tachycardia increases and dysrhythmias may occur. Skin becomes cold, clammy, diaphoretic, and cyanotic. Blood pressure falls and pulse becomes thready as cardiac output falls.

A common complication of CHF and other cardiac disorders, pulmonary edema may also result from barbiturate and opiate poisoning, diffuse infections, hemorrhagic pancreatitis, and renal failure. It may follow near-drowning, the inhalation of irritating gases, or the rapid administration of whole blood or plasma. Pulmonary edema can occur as a chronic condition or develop quickly and rapidly become fatal. Treatment of acute pulmonary edema includes cardiotonic agents (digitalis), bronchodilators, a fast-acting diuretic, and the administration of oxygen.

Reye's syndrome

This acute disorder primarily affects infants, children and adolescents. It causes fatty infiltration of the liver with concurrent hyperammonemia, encephalopathy, and increased ICP. Fatty infiltration of the kidneys, brain, and myocardium may occur as well.

Reye's syndrome develops in five stages. After an initial viral infection, a brief recovery period follows when the child doesn't seem seriously ill. A few days later he develops intractable vomiting; lethargy; rapidly changing mental status (mild to severe agitation, confusion, irritability, and delirium); rising blood pressure, respiratory rate, and pulse rate; and hyperactive reflexes. Reye's syndrome often progresses to coma. As coma deepens, seizures develop, followed by decreased tendon reflexes and, frequently, respiratory failure. Cerebral edema may lead to ICP.

Prognosis depends on the severity of CNS depression. Because of ICP monitoring, early treatment of increased ICP, and other measures, about 80% of children with Reye's syndrome survive. Comatose patients who survive may have residual brain damage. Death usually results from cerebral edema or respiratory arrest.

Rheumatic heart disease

This disease results from damage to the heart muscle or heart valves caused by episodes of rheumatic fever. After an individual acquires a group A beta-hemolytic streptococcal infection, an autoimmune reaction occurs in heart tissue, resulting in permanent deformities of heart valve or chordae tendineae. During acute rheumatic fever, heart involvement may become evident or symptoms may not appear until long after the acute disease has subsided.

Compensatory alterations take place in the size of the chambers of the heart and the thickness of their walls. Stenosis, or insufficiency of the valves, may cause the patient to develop a heart murmur. He may also develop abnormalities of pulse rate and rhythm, heart block, and CHF. Fatalities usually result from heart failure or bacterial endocarditis.

Episodes of acute rheumatic fever require vigorous treatment with supportive therapy for heart failure. Chronic rheumatic heart disease may require no immediate treatment except for close observation. Some patients require surgical commissurotomy or valve replacement.

Rocky Mountain spotted fever

Prolonged tick bites transmit *Rickettsia rickettsii,* the microorganism that causes this febrile, rash-producing illness. After an incubation period of 2 to 14 days, the patient develops a persistent temperature of 102° F to 104° F (38.9° C to 40° C) as well as aching in the bones, muscles, joints, and back. A thick white coating covers his tongue. Within 2 days, eruptions cover the entire body including the scalp, palms, and soles.

Partly because of the growing popularity of hiking and backpacking, Rocky Moutain spotted fever is now endemic throughout the continental United States and particularly prevalent in the southeast and southwest. Incidence rises in the spring and summer. Fatalities occur in about 5% of patients. Treatment includes antibiotic therapy; delaying treatment increases mortality risk.

Rubella

Also called German measles, this acute, mildly contagious viral disease produces a distinctive 3-day rash and lymphadenopathy. It occurs most often among children ages 5 to 9, adolescents, and young adults. An individual may acquire the rubella virus through contact with the blood, urine, stools, or nasopharyngeal secretions of infected persons and possibly by contaminated articles of clothing. Transplacental transmission, especially in the first trimester of pregnancy, can cause serious birth defects.

After an incubation period of from 16 to 18 days, the child abruptly develops an exanthematous, maculopapular rash. In adolescents and adults, prodromal symptoms—headache, malaise, anorexia, low-grade fever, coryza, lymphadenopathy, and sometimes conjunctivitis—appear first. Suboccipital, postauricular and postcervical lymph node enlargement are hallmark signs of the disease.

Rubeola

One of the most common and serious childhood diseases, rubeola or measles is an acute, highly contagious paramyxovirus infection. It spreads through direct contact or through contaminated airborne respiratory droplets.

After an incubation period, the patient experiences prodromal symptoms: fever, photophobia, malaise, anorexia, conjunctivitis, coryza, hoarseness, and a hacking cough. Next, Koplik's spots, the hallmark of the disease, appear. These spots look like tiny, bluish gray specks surrounded by a red halo. After Koplik's spots slough off, a slight, pruritic rash appears, which becomes papular and erythematous and spreads over the entire face, neck, eyelids, arms, chest, back, abdomen, and thighs. After about 3 days, a temperature of 103° F to 105° F (39.4° C to 40.6° C), severe cough, puffy red eyes, and rhinorrhea develop. In a few more days, symptoms begin to disappear and communicability ends.

The measles vaccine has reduced incidence of the disease among young children, but cases among adolescents and young adults are increasing. In the United States, most patients fully recover; in developing countries, many children still die from rubeola.

Sickle cell anemia

A congenital hemolytic anemia that occurs primarily but not exclusively in blacks, sickle cell anemia results from a defective hemoglobin molecule that causes red blood cells to roughen and become sickle-shaped. Such cells impair circulation, resulting in chronic ill health, periodic crises, long-term complications, and premature death.

Common sexually transmitted diseases

A patient with a sexually transmitted disease (STD) can show up for treatment anywhere, not just in a venereal disease clinic. A 10-year-old girl brought to a pediatrician's office with vaginal discharge may be suffering from an STD. So might a 65-year old man who complains of urinary frequency and dysuria.

Wherever you work, you're much more likely to encounter a patient with gonorrhea or syphilis than one with acquired immunodeficiency syndrome (AIDS), which, despite all its publicity, is less common than other STDs. As you interview and examine patients, be alert for signs and symptoms that could indicate an STD.

Disease and causative organism	Transmission	Incubation period	Signs and symptoms
Gonorrhea *Neisseria gonorrhoeae* (bacterium)	• Sexual contact with person infected with *N. gonorrhoeae* organism • May be contracted by newborn during delivery	• Typically, 3-10 days (rarely, up to 30 days)	In men, early signs and symptoms usually severe; in women, usually mild or asymptomatic. They include: • purulent yellowish to greenish discharge • dysuria • urinary frequency. *In men —* • penile pain, redness, or swelling *In women —* • cervical tenderness • swollen, painful labia majora from enlarged Bartholin's glands • inflamed, swollen vulva; inflamed vagina (usually in children) *Note:* In men, untreated infection may spread throughout reproductive system; scarring of vas deferens may lead to sterility. In women, untreated infection may spread throughout reproductive system and to abdomen; fallopian tube scarring may cause ectopic pregnancy or sterility. In men and women, systemic infections can develop.
Syphilis *Treponema pallidum* (bacterium)	• Sexual contact with person who has infective lesion • Transfusion of contaminated blood • May be contracted transplacentally by fetus	• Typically, 3-90 days (initial chancres appear in 2-4 weeks)	Untreated syphilis progresses through four stages: *primary, secondary, latent,* and *late.* *Primary stage.* Chancres at infection site appear as red maculae that become papular, then erode. They have raised, indurated edges and granular tissue in center; a yellowish or grayish scab may form. Chancres are painless (unless secondarily infected) and may be accompanied by local, bilateral, painless lymphadenopathy. If left untreated, chancres disappear in 2-8 weeks. *Secondary stage:* Lesions are infectious: if untreated, they disappear in 2-6 weeks. Typically, secondary effects appear 2-6 months after disease contraction. They include: • generalized or localized bilateral, symmetrical rash (macular, papular, papulosquamous, pustular, or nodular) • generalized painless lymphadenopathy • patchy alopecia of scalp, eyelashes, eyebrows, or beard • fever; malaise; anorexia; nausea; vomiting; weight loss; headache; sore throat; muscle, joint, or bone pain

(continued)

Common sexually transmitted diseases (continued)

Disease and causative organism	Transmission	Incubation period	Signs and symptoms
Syphilis (continued)			• mucous patch (gray-white lesion with red edges) on mucous membranes in mouth, vagina, penis, or rectum • condyloma lata (pink to gray, flat, wartlike papules) in moist area, such as genital region or skin folds. *Latent stage:* In early latent stage, signs and symptoms usually cease. Secondary lesions may recur for up to 2 years after infection is contracted. Late latent stage begins about 2 years after infection is contracted and may last for rest of patient's life. Usually, patient has no signs or symptoms. *Late stage:* Usually, this stage lasts 3-10 years after infection is contracted, though it may occur later. Not all patients experience this stage, however. Signs and symptoms include: • cardiovascular lesions that can cause scarring, destruction, and fibrosis of blood vessels, especially the aorta; aneurysm may develop; aortic valves may be destroyed • nervous system lesions that may affect spinal cord, meninges, and brain tissue, causing symptoms such as headache and mental changes • endarteritis obliterans (destruction of blood vessels) • gummas (nodular or ulcerative lesions) that affect skin, mucous membranes, bones, muscles, joints, and organs • periostitis, irregular deposits of new bone.
Nongonococcal urethritis (NGU) Several organisms. One of the most common — *Chlamydia trachomatis* (modified bacterium)	• Sexual contact with infected person • May be contracted by newborn during delivery	• Typically, 1-3 weeks (can be up to several months)	Similar to signs and symptoms of gonorrhea but milder. Patients, especially women, may be asymptomatic. *In men —* • mild to severe dysuria • urethral itching and discharge • inflamed urethral meatus *In women —* • urethritis and cystitis • cervicitis, possibly with edema and erosions • small amounts of thin, mucopurulent vaginal discharge.
Genital herpes *Herpesvirus hominis* Type 2 (virus)	• Sexual contact with person who has infection • May be contracted by newborn during delivery	• Typically, primary lesions appear 3-7 days after infection is contracted	• fever and lymphadenopathy • burning, tingling, or itching at infection site (before lesions appear) • lesions at infection site (usually groin, rectum, or abdomen) — clusters of small, painful vesicles that burst and form reddened ulcerous lesions. (These lesions may coalesce into larger ulcerous lesions, which form crusts and heal in up to 3 weeks. Recurring lesions follow same pattern but heal in 1-2 weeks. When lesions heal, virus migrates to nerve sites and becomes dormant.) • edema and urine retention (with lesions).

Syndrome of inappropriate antidiuretic hormone secretion

This disorder causes excessive release of antidiuretic hormone (ADH). Inability to excrete dilute urine, retention of free water, expansion of intracellular fluid volume, and hyponatremia lead to severely disturbed fluid and electrolyte balances. Most commonly, syndrome of inappropriate antidiuretic hormone secretion (SIADH) results from oat cell carcinoma of the lung. Other neoplastic diseases — for example, pancreatic and prostatic cancer, Hodgkin's disease, and thymoma — may also trigger SIADH. Less commonly, it occurs secondary to drug therapy, CNS disorders, pulmonary disorders, myxedema or psychosis. SIADH may produce weight gain (despite anorexia), nausea and vomiting and, possibly, coma and convulsions. Treatment is symptomatic and prognosis depends largely on the underlying disorder.

Systemic lupus erythematosus

A chronic, inflammatory disorder, systemic lupus erythematosus (SLE) causes structural changes in the patient's connective tissue. SLE may produce only mild effects. However, its effects on the heart, blood vessels, kidneys, lungs, and central nervous system may be life-threatening. It strikes women 8 times as often as men.

Patients experience a variety of signs and symptoms. The most common include a butterfly rash on the face (facial erythema), hair loss, stiff and aching joints, musculoskeletal deformity, and photosensitivity. Fatigue, weight loss, chills, fever, sensitivity to heat and cold, and musculoskeletal pain may also occur.

The cause of SLE remains uncertain; researchers suspect that an autoimmune response generates immune complexes, which damage connective tissue and cause inflammation. SLE's unpredictable course includes exacerbations interspersed with long periods of complete or near-complete remission. Because immune complexes may reside in any part of the body, different symptoms may appear at different times, with varying severity.

Tay-Sachs disease

This disease results from a congenital deficiency of an enzyme, hexosaminidase A, required for the metabolism of certain lipids. An autosomal recessive disorder, it occurs rarely but strikes Ashkenazic Jews about 100 times more often than the general population.

By age 3 to 6 months, a child born with Tay-Sachs becomes apathetic and responds to loud sounds only. Increasing physical and mental deterioration follows. Soon he can't sit up or lift his head. He has difficulty turning over, can't grasp objects, and has progressive vision loss. By 18 months, he's usually deaf and suffers from seizures and generalized paralysis and spasticity. His pupils are always dilated and don't react to light. Decerebrate rigidity and a complete vegetative state follow. After age 2 the child suffers recurrent bronchopneumonia. Tay-Sachs invariably proves fatal, usually before age 5.

Thrombocytopenia

The most common cause of hemorrhagic disorders, thrombocytopenia occurs in patients who lack a sufficient number of circulating platelets. It poses a serious threat to hemostasis.

Thrombocytopenia may result from decreased or defective production of platelets in the bone marrow (for example, in leukemia, aplastic anemia, and certain drug toxicities). Alternatively, it may result from increased destruction outside the marrow caused by an underlying disorder (for example, in cirrhosis of the liver, disseminated intravascular coagulation, or severe infection).

Thrombocytopenia may produce a sudden onset of petechiae or ecchymoses in the skin or bleeding into any mucous membrane (gastrointestinal, urinary, vaginal, or respiratory). Because of internal bleeding, the patient suffers malaise, fatigue, general weakness, and lethargy. In adults, large blood-filled bullae appear in the mouth. In severe thrombocytopenia, hemorrhage may lead to tachycardia, shortness of breath, loss of consciousness, and eventually, death.

Prognosis depends on treatment of the underlying cause. In drug-induced thrombocytopenia, the patient may experience immediate recovery upon withdrawal of the offending agent.

Tic douloureux

Also called trigeminal neuralgia, this painful disorder affects one or more branches of the fifth cranial (trigeminal) nerve. Following a light touch to a trigger zone (a hypersensitive area, such as the tip of the nose, the cheeks, or the gums), the patient experiences paroxysmal attacks of excruciating facial pain. Pain probably results from an interaction or short-circuiting of touch and pain fibers.

The patient often reports a searing or burning pain that occurs in lightning-like jabs and lasts 1 to 2 minutes. Pain occurs in one side of the face, primarily in the maxillary or mandibular divisions of the trigeminal nerve. Frequency of attacks varies from many times a day to several times a month or year.

To relieve pain, the doctor may order carbamazepine, phenytoin, or narcotics. Neurosurgical procedures may provide permanent relief. Occasionally, the disorder goes into spontaneous remission for several months or years.

Tourette's syndrome
The most severe of the stereotyped movement disorders, Tourette's syndrome is marked by violent twitching or convulsive movements of the face, arms, and other body parts. The patient may also emit bizarre vocalizations — explosive sounds; a loud, barking cough; or compulsive shouting of obscene words. The condition probably reflects a neurologic abnormality. Treatment includes psychotropic drugs as well as psychotherapy.

Toxic shock syndrome
This acute bacterial infection, caused by penicillin resistant *Staphylococcus aureus*, is strongly associated with the continuous use of tampons, especially super-absorbent tampons, during the menstrual period. Incidence is rising and the recurrence rate is about 30%.

Toxic shock syndrome (TSS) produces intense myalgias, temperature over 104° F (40° C), vomiting, diarrhea, headache, decreased level of consciousness, rigors, conjunctival hyperemia, and vaginal hyperemia and discharge. The patient suffers severe hypotension and hypovolemic shock. Within a few hours of onset, a deep red rash develops — especially on the palms and soles — and later desquamates. Treatment consists of I.V. antistaphylococcal antibiotics and fluid replacement.

Tuberculosis
This acute or chronic infection results from *Mycobacterium tuberculosis* and sometimes other strains of *Mycobacteria*. The disorder spreads through aerosolized droplets and is characterized by for-mation of tubercles and caseous necrosis in the tissues. Bacilli usually enter the lungs, multiply and invade the lymphatic system and bloodstream, thereby spreading to other organs. Individuals living in crowded, poorly ventilated conditions face the greatest risk of becoming infected.

In primary infection, after an incubation of 4 to 8 weeks, patients remain asymptomatic or experience nonspecific symptoms such as fatigue, weakness, anorexia, weight loss, night sweats, and low-grade fever. In most people, bacilli lie dormant for months or years, becoming active with lowered resistance. In reactivation, symptoms may include a cough that produces mucopurulent sputum, occasional hemoptysis, and chest pains. Combination drug therapy provides the most effective treatment.

Ulcerative colitis
This inflammatory, chronic disease affects the mucosa and submucosa of the colon. It produces congestion, edema (leading to mucosal friability), and ulcerations that eventually develop into abscesses. Ulcerative colitis usually begins in the rectum and sigmoid colon, and often extends upward into the entire colon; it rarely affects the small intestine, except for the terminal ileum.

The patient develops recurrent attacks of bloody diarrhea, often containing pus and mucus, interspersed with remissions. The severity of these attacks varies with the extent of inflammation. Other symptoms include spastic rectum and anus, abdominal pain, irritability, weight loss, weakness, anorexia, nausea, and vomiting.

Ulcerative colitis ranges from a mild, localized disorder to a fulminant disease that may cause a perforated colon, progressing to potentially fatal peritonitis and toxemia.

Ulcers
Peptic ulcers — circumscribed lesions in the gastric mucosal membrane — can develop in the lower esophagus, stomach, pylorus, duodenum, or jejunum from contact with gastric juice (especially hydrochloric acid and pepsin). About 80% of all peptic ulcers are duodenal ulcers, which affect the proximal part of the small intestine and occur most often in men between ages 20 and 50. Gastric ulcers, which affect the stomach mucosa, are most common in both middle-aged and elderly men, especially among the poor and undernourished, and in chronic users of aspirin or alcohol.

Uterine cancer
The most common gynecologic cancer, this disorder usually affects postmenopausal women between ages 50 and 60. Typically, it occurs as an adenocarcinoma of the endometrium that late in the course of illness metastasizes to the cervix, ovaries, fallopian tubes, and other peritoneal structures. Through the blood or lymphatic system, it may spread to distant organs such as the lungs and the brain. Lymph node involvement can also occur.

Common indications of uterine cancer include uterine enlargement, persistent and unusual premenopausal bleeding, or any postmenopausal bleeding. Discharge may at first appear watery and blood-streaked; gradually it becomes more bloody. Other symptoms such as pain and weight loss don't appear until advanced stages of cancer. Depending on the stage of illness, treatment may include surgery, radiation therapy, or hormonal therapy.

Valvular heart disease
Valvular heart disease prevents efficient blood flow through the heart. Depending on the disease's severity and the number of valves

involved, heart failure, dysrhythmias, and other life-threatening complications may occur.

The two main types of valvular disease include *stenosis* (valvular tissue thickening that narrows the valvular opening) and *insufficiency* (valvular incompetence that prevents complete valve closure). Stenosis limits blood flow through the heart, increasing afterload (pressure overload). Valvular insufficiency (also called regurgitation) permits blood backflow, which increases preload (volume overload). Thus, both stenosis and insufficiency increase the heart's work load.

A third valvular disease, *mitral valve prolapse,* occurs when valve leaflets protrude into the left atrium during systole. Although usually benign, this condition may lead to mitral insufficiency in some patients.

Medical interventions focus on preventing the disease from worsening and minimizing the risk of complications. If medical interventions fail, however, the doctor may recommend surgery. Repair procedures include *valvuloplasty* to repair the valve and suture torn leaflets; *catheter balloon valvuloplasty* to open stenotic valves; *annuloplasty* to tighten and suture the malfunctioning valve annulus (ring); and *commissurotomy or valvotomy* to enlarge the valve opening by mechanically dilating the valve's commissures.

In some cases, the doctor may remove the valve and replace it with a prosthetic device.

Zollinger-Ellison syndrome
This sydrome is characterized by severe peptic ulceration, gastric hypersecretion, and pancreatic or duodenal gastrinoma. Two-thirds of the tumors are malignant. Although the syndrome occurs in early childhood, it's more common in patients between ages 20 and 50.

Reportable disorders

Where do scientists obtain statistical data to help fight the battle against infectious disease? From reports given by doctors, researchers, and health care workers to state health departments, which in turn submit the information to the Centers for Disease Control (CDC). The chart below lists diseases reportable to the CDC, beginning with the most common.

Disorder	Reported cases, 1989
Gonorrhea	
Civilian	547,104
Military	9,194
Hepatitis	
Hepatitis A	27,869
Hepatitis B	18,276
Hepatitis C	1,912
Hepatitis (unspecified)	1,847
Syphilis, primary and secondary	
Civilian	32,176
Military	197
Acquired immunodeficiency syndrome (AIDS)	28,104
Tuberculosis	17,001
Measles (indigenous and imported)	12,593
Aseptic meningitis	7,663
Mumps	4,416
Rabies, animal	3,789
Pertussis	2,778
Meningococcal infections	2,142
Malaria	1,040

Disorder	Reported cases, 1989
Legionellosis	858
Encephalitis	
Primary	681
Infectious	70
Rocky Mountain spotted fever	572
Typhoid fever	403
Rubella (German measles)	375
Toxic shock syndrome	300
Congenital syphilis (ages under 1 year)	165
Leprosy	136
Tularemia	130
Psittacosis	84
Leptospirosis	75
Brucellosis	71
Botulism	
Foodborne	21
Infant	15
Other	4
Tetanus	36
Trichinosis	15
Plague	4
Diphtheria	3
Congenital rubella syndrome	2
Rabies, human	1

Most common causes of death in U.S.

Death rate/100,000

Cause	Rate
Ischemic heart disease	207.9
Malignant neoplasms, all forms	198.6
Chronic ischemic heart disease	104.3
Acute MI	101.7
Cerebrovascular disease	61.1
Malignant respiratory and intrathoracic neoplasms	57.3
Malignant digestive system neoplasms	47.4
COPD	33.3
Pneumonia and influenza	31.5
Malignant neoplasms of genital organs	21.8
Motor vehicle accidents	20.4
Malignant neoplasms of the breast	17.5
Diabetes mellitus	16.1
Suicide	12.3
Cirrhosis and chronic liver disease	10.6
Other neoplasms of lymphatic and hematopoietic tissue	11.5
Atherosclerosis	9.6
Homicide	9.0
Nephritis, nephrotic syndrome, and nephrosis	8.9
Septicemia	8.5
Hypertensive heart disease	8.3
Malignant neoplasms of urinary organs	7.9
Neonatal-perinatal causes	7.5
Leukemia	7.1
Acquired immunodeficiency syndrome	6.6

Cancer watch: Trends and numbers

The statistics on cancer are indeed bewildering. About 1,375 people in the U.S. die of cancer each day. (That's 1 person every 3 seconds.) If current trends prevail, according to the American Cancer Society, 76 million Americans (about 30% of the population) now living will eventually develop cancer. Over the years, cancer will strike 3 out of 4 families.

But there's another side to the story. Not long ago, people believed cancer was incurable. Yet today, there are 3 million survivors: people who fought cancer and won. And of patients diagnosed with cancer this year, 40% will be alive 5 years from now.

The battle against cancer is far from over, though. Consider this: Last year, about 178,000 people died from cancer who could have been saved by earlier diagnosis and prompt treatment.

Cancer by site and sex

These figures provide a breakdown by site and sex for the major types of cancer. As you can see, the most prevalent cancers for men are cancer of the lung, prostate, colon, and rectum. For women, the most prevalent cancers are of the breast, colon, rectum, lungs, and uterus.

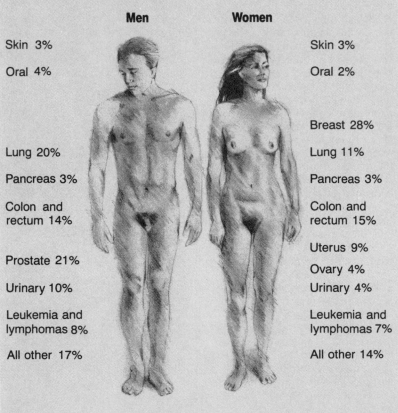

Men

Skin 3%

Oral 4%

Lung 20%

Pancreas 3%

Colon and rectum 14%

Prostate 21%

Urinary 10%

Leukemia and lymphomas 8%

All other 17%

Women

Skin 3%

Oral 2%

Breast 28%

Lung 11%

Pancreas 3%

Colon and rectum 15%

Uterus 9%

Ovary 4%

Urinary 4%

Leukemia and lymphomas 7%

All other 14%

Cancer death rates by organ site

In the U.S., death rates from the most major forms of cancer have either declined or leveled off in the past 50 years. Lung cancer is the one exception: death rates continue to soar.

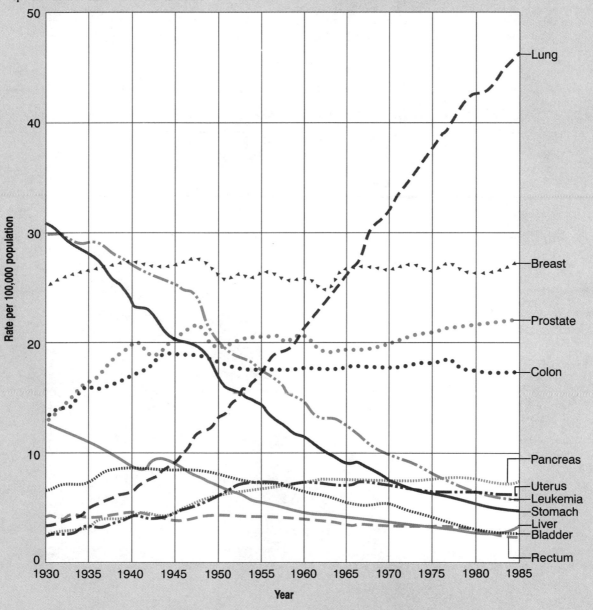

AIDS forecast

Even if researchers develop an HIV vaccine in the next 5 years, the AIDS epidemic will go on, fueled by people who already have become infected by HIV. The World Health Organization estimates that between 5 and 10 million people now carry HIV worldwide.

Public health officials estimate that 1 million people in the United States are infected with HIV. As of May 1, 1991, a total of 174,893 AIDS cases and 110,530 deaths in the U.S. had been reported to the Centers for Disease Control.

Not long ago, a typical patient who developed AIDS symptoms usually died within 28 months of diagnosis. But with aggressive treatment and drug therapy, many now live longer. Besides homosexual males, AIDS victims include increasing numbers of females, heterosexual I.V. drug abusers, and newborns.

AIDS in the U.S.: A state-by-state breakdown

The map below shows AIDS cases reported by each state to the Centers for Disease Control (CDC) in 1990. States with more than 500 reported AIDS cases appear in color.

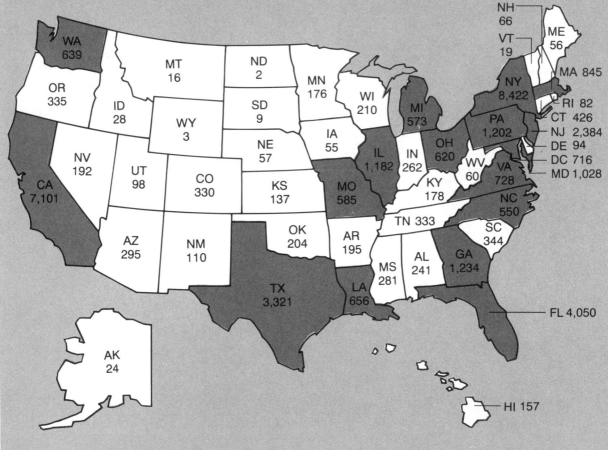

AIDS: An epidemic in progress

The chart below shows a year-by-year breakdown of the number of AIDS cases and deaths in the U.S. from 1981 through 1990, as reported to the CDC. (*Note:* 1990 death figure is projected.)

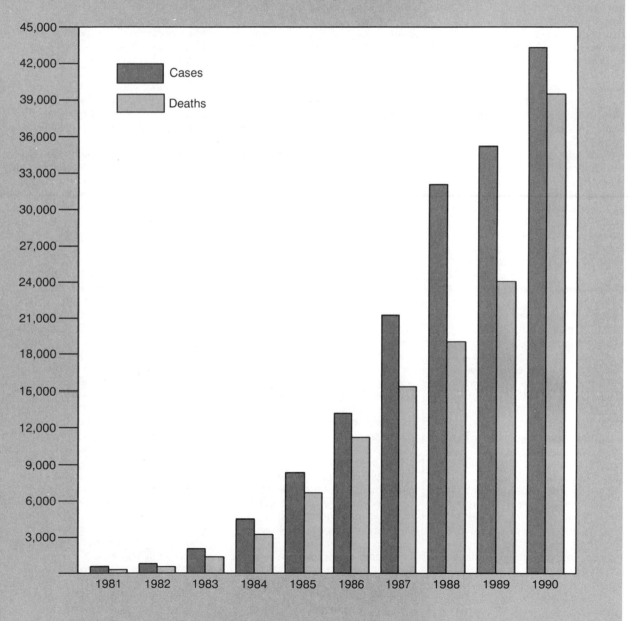

Preventing HIV infection on the job

As the number of HIV-infected patients continues to climb, your risk of exposure to infected blood grows. To reduce the infection risk, the Centers for Disease Control (CDC) urges you to treat all patients as if they were HIV-positive, even if you have no diagnostic information to support that premise. This approach is referred to as "universal blood and body-fluid precautions," or simply "universal precautions."

Following universal precautions eliminates the need for adhering to isolation precautions previously recommended by the CDC for use with patients with known or suspected infections from blood-borne pathogens. However, if the patient also has an associated condition, such as infectious diarrhea or tuberculosis, you may have to revert to disease-specific isolation precautions.

Universal precautions
Use appropriate barrier precautions routinely to keep from exposing your skin or mucous membranes to patients' blood and certain body fluids. Blood is the single most important source of HIV in an occupational setting. Universal precautions also apply to tissues and to semen; vaginal secretions; and cerebrospinal, synovial, pleural, peritoneal, pericardial, and amniotic fluids.

Universal precautions don't apply to feces, nasal secretions, sputum, sweat, tears, urine, and vomitus unless they contain visible blood. Nor do universal precautions apply to breast milk or saliva. Health care workers frequently exposed to breast milk may choose to wear gloves. Current infection control practices should minimize the minute risk of salivary transmission of HIV.

Use your judgment in deciding which specific types of barriers (gloves, gowns, masks, and protective eyewear) are needed for each clinical situation:
• Wear gloves when touching blood and indicated body fluids, mucous membranes, or broken skin; when handling items or surfaces soiled with blood or related body fluids; and when performing venipuncture and other vascular access procedures. Change gloves after contact with each patient. Also, be sure to wear a gown or apron and shield your face and eyes during procedures likely to generate droplets of blood or body fluids.
• Discard used surgical or examination gloves; don't wash or disinfect them for reuse. Washing with surfactants may enhance the penetration of liquids through undetected holes in the glove. Disinfecting agents may cause deterioration. Use general purpose utility gloves for instrument cleaning, decontamination procedures, and housekeeping chores involving potential blood contact. You may decontaminate and reuse utility gloves, but discard gloves that are peeling, cracked, discolored, torn, or show any other evidence of deterioration.
• Wash your hands and other skin surfaces immediately and thoroughly if they're contaminated by blood or body fluids. Wash your hands immediately after removing your gloves.
• Take precautions to prevent injuries caused by needles, scalpels, and other sharp instruments during procedures. Also take precautions when cleaning used instruments, disposing of used needles, and handling sharp instruments after procedures. To prevent needlestick injuries, don't recap needles, bend or break them by hand, or remove them from disposable syringes. After use, place disposable syringes and nee-

dles, scalpel blades, and other sharp items in puncture-resistant containers for disposal. Keep containers nearby. Place large-bore, reusable needles in a puncture-resistant container for transport to the reprocessing area.
• You need not wear gloves when feeding patients and when wiping saliva from skin. However, consider minimizing the need for emergency mouth-to-mouth resuscitation by keeping mouthpieces, resuscitation bags, and other ventilation devices nearby.
• If you have exudative lesions or weeping dermatitis, don't give direct patient care or handle patient care equipment until the condition resolves.
• If you're pregnant, you're probably at no greater risk for contracting HIV infection than if you weren't pregnant. However, because you can transfer the virus to the fetus, you should be especially familiar with precautions and follow them closely.

Invasive procedure precautions
According to the CDC, an invasive procedure includes:
• surgical entry into tissues, cavities, or organs, or repair of major traumatic injuries, in a operating or delivery room, emergency department, or outpatient setting (including a dentist's office)
• cardiac catheterization or angiography
• vaginal or cesarean delivery or other obstetrical procedure where bleeding occurs
• manipulation, cutting, or removal of any oral or perioral tissues, including teeth, where bleeding occurs or the potential for bleeding exists.

For invasive procedures, follow the universal precautions as well as those listed below.
• Take barrier precautions with all patients. Always wear gloves and a surgical mask. For procedures that could cause splashing blood or body fluids, or flying bone chips,

wear an apron or gown, and protective eyewear or a face shield.
• Wear gloves and a gown when handling the placenta or an infant during vaginal or cesarean delivery until blood and amniotic fluid have been removed from the infant's skin. Wear gloves while caring for the umbilical cord after delivery.
• If your glove tears or you get a needlestick or other injury, remove the old glove, and put on a new one as quickly as possible. Remove the needle or instrument from the sterile field.

Environmental precautions
Even though HIV doesn't seem to be transmitted environmentally, take the following precautions with all patients:
• Sterilize and disinfect all patient care equipment. HIV dies quickly after exposure to common chemical germicides, even at concentrations much lower than typically used. Besides commercial germicides, sodium hypochlorite (household bleach) is effective in concentrations of 1:100 to 1:10, depending on the amount of blood, mucus, or other material that needs to be removed from the surface being disinfected. Povidone-iodine is also effective.
• Clean the walls, floor, and other surfaces as usual; extraordinary measures aren't necessary.
• Clean and disinfect surfaces contaminated with blood and body fluids with chemical germicides approved for use as "hospital disinfectants." In patient care areas, remove visible material first, then decontaminate the area. Always wear gloves during cleaning and decontamination.
• When storing and processing soiled linen, handle it gently and as little as possible. Bag all soiled linen at the location where it was used; don't sort or rinse it in patient care areas. Put linen soiled with blood or body fluids in leak-proof bags.

Dialysis precautions
HIV-infected patients with end-stage renal disease who are undergoing maintenance dialysis can be dialyzed using conventional infection-control precautions. Use universal precautions when dialyzing all patients.

Specimen collection and handling precautions
Consider blood and body fluids from all patients to be infectious. (This eliminates the need for warning labels on specimens; all specimens are considered infectious.)
Besides adhering to the universal precautions, follow these safeguards:
• Consider wearing gloves whenever you perform a phlebotomy. You must wear gloves if you have cuts, scratches, or other breaks in your skin; if you believe contamination is likely to occur (for example, when drawing blood from an uncooperative patient); when performing finger or heel sticks on infants and children; or if you're receiving training in phlebotomy.
• When collecting a specimen, avoid contaminating the outside of the container or the laboratory form accompanying the specimen. Put all specimens in a sturdy container with a tight lid to prevent leakage during transport.
• Wear gloves when processing blood and body-fluid specimens. Wear a mask and protective eyewear if your mucous membranes might contact blood or body fluids. Change gloves and wash your hands after processing each specimen.
• Use a Class I or II biological safety cabinet for procedures likely to produce droplets, such as blending, sonicating, or vigorous mixing. A biological safety cabinet isn't necessary for routine procedures.
• Use a mechanical pipetting device for manipulating all liquids. Never pipette by mouth.

• Don't use needles and syringes unless absolutely necessary, and follow the recommendations for preventing accidental needlesticks.
• Clean work surfaces with an appropriate chemical germicide after spills of blood or body fluids and after work is finished.
• Decontaminate test materials before reprocessing them, or place them in bags and dispose of them following your hospital policy.
• Clean and decontaminate equipment contaminated with blood and body fluids before repairing it in the laboratory or transporting it to the manufacturer.
• Wash your hands and remove protective clothing before leaving the laboratory.

If you're exposed
If you sustain parenteral exposure (such as a needlestick or cut), mucous membrane exposure (such as a splash to the eye or mouth), or cutaneous exposure involving large amounts of blood or prolonged contact (especially if the exposed skin is chapped, abraded, or has dermatitis), notify the patient of your exposure and request his consent for HIV testing. Consult hospital policy for testing patients who can't give consent, such as unconscious patients.
If the patient has AIDS, tests positive for HIV antibody, or refuses to be tested, you should seek counseling about the risk of infection and should undergo HIV testing as soon as possible. You should also report and seek medical attention for any acute, febrile illness occurring within 12 weeks of exposure. Such an illness can indicate recent HIV infection.
If initial test results are negative, have follow-up tests performed 6 weeks after exposure and at intervals thereafter, such as 12 weeks after exposure, and 6 months after exposure. Most people seroconvert during the first 6 to 12 weeks after exposure. Dur-

ing that period, assume that you may have the virus and take measures to prevent transmission.

If the patient is seronegative, you'll need no follow-up unless the patient is at high risk for HIV infection. In this case, you should be retested later (12 weeks after exposure, for example).

If the patient's exposed

If the patient has parenteral or mucous membrane exposure to blood or body fluids from a health-care worker, inform him of the incident. Then follow the precautions outlined above.

Isolation precautions

If your patient's illness may be contagious, you'll need to take isolation precautions. These precautions seek to interrupt the route of transmission whereby an infectious organism reaches a susceptible host.

Placing a patient in isolation intensifies the loneliness of the hospital environment. Take time to explain to the patient why he's been placed in isolation. Encourage him to ask questions so you can clear up any misconceptions he may have.

Most infectious diseases are transmitted in one of four ways: contact transmission (the susceptible host comes in direct or indirect contact with the source); airborne transmission (inhalation of contaminated, evaporated saliva droplets); enteric transmission (oral-fecal transmission through direct or indirect contact with feces or objects heavily contaminated by feces); or vectorborne transmission (an intermediate carrier, such as a flea or mosquito transfers an organism).

The chart below describes six levels of isolation and lists the diseases associated with each level. Keep in mind that the Centers for Disease Control now recommends treating *all* patients as if they were HIV positive. This approach is called "universal blood and body-fluid precautions."

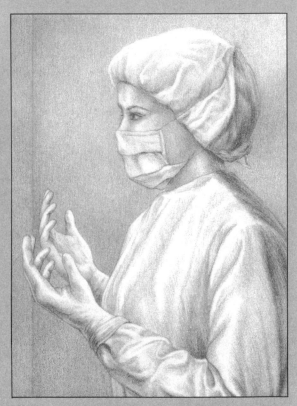

Diseases that require isolation	Private room	Mask	Gown	Gloves	Special handling of waste or contaminated articles
Strict isolation (may require room with special ventilation) Pharyngeal diphtheria, viral hemorrhagic fevers, pneumonic plague, smallpox, varicella (chicken pox), and herpes zoster (localized in immunocompromised patient or disseminated).	X with door closed	X	X	X	X

Isolation precautions (continued)

Diseases that require isolation	Private room	Mask	Gown	Gloves	Special handling of waste or contaminated articles
Contact isolation Group A *Streptococcus* endometritis; impetigo; pediculosis; *Staphylococcus aureus*, or pneumonia; rabies; rubella; scabies; scalded skin syndrome; major skin, wound, or burn infection; vaccinia; primary disseminated herpes simplex; and infection or colonization with multiply resistant bacteria. In infants and young children: acute respiratory infections, influenza, infectious pharyngitis, and viral pneumonia. In newborns: gonococcal conjunctivitis, staphylococcal furunculosis, and neonatal disseminated herpes simplex.	X	O	⊗	⊗	X
Respiratory isolation *Haemophilus influenzae* epiglottitis, erythema infectiosum, measles, *H. influenzae* or meningococcal meningitis, meningococcal pneumonia, meningococcemia; mumps, pertussis, and *H. influenzae* pneumonia in children.	X with door closed	O	—	—	X
Acid-fast bacillus isolation (requires room with special ventilation) Tuberculosis	X with door closed	O	⊗	—	X
Enteric precautions Amebic dysentery; cholera; coxsackievirus disease; acute diarrhea with suspected infection; echovirus disease; encephalitis caused by enteroviruses; *Clostridium difficile* or *Staphylococcus* enterocolitis; enteroviral infection; gastroenteritis caused by *Campylobacter* species, *Cryptosporidum* species, *Dientamoeba fragilis, Escherichia coli, Giardia lamblia, Salmonella* species, *Shigella* species, *Vibrio parahaemolyticus,* viruses, *Yersinia enterocolitica;* hand, foot, and mouth disease; hepatitis A; herpangina; viral meningitis caused by enteroviruses; necrotizing enterocolitis; pleurodynia; poliomyelitis; typhoid fever; viral pericarditis, myocarditis, or enteroviral meningitis.	D	—	⊗	⊗	X
Drainage and secretion precautions Conjunctivitis; minor or limited abscess; minor or limited burn, skin, wound, or pressure sore infection.	—	—	⊗	⊗	X

KEY: X = Always necessary
      ⊗ = Necessary if soiling of hands or clothing is likely
      O = Necessary for close contact or if patient is coughing and doesn't reliably cover mouth
      D = Desirable but optional; necessary only if patient has poor hygiene
      — = Unnecessary

Diagnostic-related groups: A complete listing

Diagnostic-related groups (DRGs), the patient classification system established by Medicare, has dramatically changed the nation's health care system. When you care for a Medicare patient, the total amount of money the federal government will pay for the patient's hospital care is based on the DRG into which the patient's condition falls. If the hospital bill exceeds this predetermined amount, the hospital must absorb the difference. Hospitals that are able to provide care at a cost below the Medicare amount, however, are rewarded for their efficiency—they can pocket the difference.

Restricted hospital stays have caused many patients to wait longer before seeking medical attention. As a result, patients are more acutely ill when they enter the hospital and when they leave. Many are choosing

alternatives to prolonged hospital stays, such as ambulatory care, extended care, home health care, or treatment in hospices or self-care units.

As patient advocates, nurses need an understanding of the DRG system to help guard against inappropriate dismissals and incorrect DRG code assignments.

The following table lists all conditions for which a patient is entitled to receive Medicare reimbursement under the DRG system. Reimbursement covers in-hospital costs for doctors' and nurses' services and some costs for other care related to a patient's hospitalization. Keep in mind that the length of stay allowed under each DRG will vary depending on the size of the hospital, complications, the doctor's expertise, and other factors.

DRG number	Major diagnostic code*	General diagnostic classification	Description
1	1	•	Craniotomy, age > 17, except for trauma
2	1	•	Craniotomy for trauma, age > 17
3	1	•	Craniotomy, age < 18
4	1	•	Spinal procedures
5	1	•	Extracranial vascular procedures
6	1	•	Carpal tunnel release
7	1	•	Peripheral, cranial nerve, and other nervous system procedure, age > 69, with complications or comorbidity (CC)
8	1	•	Peripheral, cranial nerve, and other nervous system procedure, age < 70, without CC
9	1	†	Spinal disorders and injuries
10	1	†	Nervous system neoplasms, age > 69, with CC
11	1	†	Nervous system neoplasms, age < 70, without CC
12	1	†	Degenerative nervous system disorders
13	1	†	Multiple sclerosis and cerebellar ataxia
14	1	†	Specific cerebrovascular disorders except transient ischemic attacks
15	1	†	Transient ischemic attacks
16	1	†	Nonspecific cerebrovascular disorders with CC
17	1	†	Nonspecific cerebrovascular disorders without CC
18	1	†	Cranial and peripheral nerve disorders, age > 69, with CC
19	1	†	Cranial and peripheral nerve disorders, age < 70 without CC
20	1	†	Nervous system infection except viral meningitis
21	1	†	Viral meningitis
22	1	†	Hypertensive encephalopathy
23	1	†	Nontraumatic stupor and coma
24	1	†	Seizure and headache, age > 69 with CC
25	1	†	Seizure and headache, age 18 to 69 without CC

*grouped by body systems   • surgical   † medical

Diagnostic-related groups: A complete listing (continued)

DRG number	Major diagnostic code*	General diagnostic classification	Description
26	1	†	Seizure and headache, age 0 to 17
27	1	†	Traumatic stupor and coma, coma > 1 hour
28	1	†	Traumatic stupor and coma, coma < 1 hour, age > 69 with CC
29	1	†	Traumatic stupor and coma, coma < 1 hour, age 18 to 69 without CC
30	1	†	Traumatic stupor and coma, coma < 1 hour age 0 to 17
31	1	†	Concussion, age > 69 with CC
32	1	†	Concussion, age 18 to 69 without CC
33	1	†	Concussion, age 0 to 17
34	1	†	Other disorders of nervous system, age > 69 with CC
35	1	†	Other disorders of nervous system, age < 70 without CC
36	2	•	Retinal procedures
37	2	•	Orbital procedures
38	2	•	Primary iris procedures
39	2	•	Lens procedures
40	2	•	Extraocular procedures except orbit, age > 17
41	2	•	Extraocular procedures except orbit, age 0 to 17
42	2	•	Intraocular procedures except retina, iris, and lens
43	2	†	Hyphema
44	2	†	Acute major eye infections
45	2	†	Neurological eye disorders
46	2	†	Other disorders of the eye, age > 17 with CC
47	2	†	Other disorders of the eye, age > 17 without CC
48	2	†	Other disorders of the eye, age 0 to 17
49	3	•	Major head and neck procedures
50	3	•	Sialoadenectomy
51	3	•	Salivary gland procedures except sialoadenectomy
52	3	•	Cleft lip and palate repair
53	3	•	Sinus and mastoid procedures, age > 17
54	3	•	Sinus and mastoid procedures, age 0 to 17
55	3	•	Miscellaneous ear, nose, and throat procedures
56	3	•	Rhinoplasty
57	3	•	Tonsil and adenoid procedure except tonsillectomy and adenoidectomy, age > 17
58	3	•	Tonsil and adenoid procedure except tonsillectomy and adenoidectomy, age 0 to 17
59	3	•	Tonsillectomy and adenoidectomy, age > 17
60	3	•	Tonsillectomy and adenoidectomy, age 0 to 17
61	3	•	Myringotomy, age > 17
62	3	•	Myringotomy, age 0 to 17
63	3	•	Other ear, nose, and throat O.R. procedures
64	3	†	Ear, nose, and throat malignancy
65	3	†	Dysequilibrium
66	3	†	Epistaxis
67	3	†	Epiglottitis
68	3	†	Otitis media and upper respiratory infection (URI), age > 69 with CC

*grouped by body systems   • surgical   † medical

(continued)

Diagnostic-related groups: A complete listing *(continued)*

DRG number	Major diagnostic code*	General diagnostic classification	Description
69	3	†	Otitis media and URI, age 18 to 69 without CC
70	3	†	Otitis media and URI, age 0 to 17
71	3	†	Laryngotracheitis
72	3	†	Nasal trauma and deformity
73	3	†	Other ear, nose, and throat diagnoses, age > 17
74	3	†	Other ear, nose, and throat diagnoses, age 0 to 17
75	4	•	Major chest procedures
76	4	•	O.R. procedure on respiratory system except major chest with CC
77	4	•	O.R. procedure on respiratory system except major chest without CC
78	4	†	Pulmonary embolism
79	4	†	Respiratory infections and inflammations, age > 69 with CC
80	4	†	Respiratory infections and inflammations, age 18 to 69 without CC
81	4	†	Respiratory infections and inflammations, age 0 to 17
82	4	†	Respiratory neoplasms
83	4	†	Major chest trauma, age > 69 with CC
84	4	†	Major chest trauma, age < 70 without CC
85	4	†	Pleural effusion, age > 69 with CC
86	4	†	Pleural effusion, age > 70 without CC
87	4	†	Pulmonary edema and respiratory failure
88	4	†	Chronic obstructive pulmonary disease
89	4	†	Simple pneumonia and pleurisy, age > 69 with CC
90	4	†	Simple pneumonia and pleurisy, age 18 to 69 without CC
91	4	†	Simple pneumonia and pleurisy, age 0 to 17
92	4	†	Interstitial lung disease, age > 69 with CC
93	4	†	Interstitial lung disease, age < 70 without CC
94	4	†	Pneumothorax, age > 69 with CC
95	4	†	Pneumothorax, age < 70 without CC
96	4	†	Bronchitis and asthma, age > 69 with CC
97	4	†	Bronchitis and asthma, age 18 to 69 without CC
98	4	†	Bronchitis and asthma, age 0 to 17
99	4	†	Respiratory signs and symptoms, age > 69 with CC
100	4	†	Respiratory signs and symptoms, age < 70 without CC
101	4	†	Other respiratory diagnoses, age > 69 with CC
102	4	†	Other respiratory diagnoses, age < 70 without CC
103	5	•	Heart transplant
104	5	•	Cardiac valve procedure with pump and catheterization
105	5	•	Cardiac valve procedure with pump, no catheterization
106	5	•	Coronary bypass with catheterization
107	5	•	Coronary bypass, no catheterization
108	5	•	Cardiothoracic procedure except valve and coronary bypass with pump
109	5	•	Cardiothoracic procedures, no pump
110	5	•	Major reconstructive vascular procedures, age > 69 with CC
111	5	•	Major reconstructive vascular procedures, age < 70 without CC
112	5	•	Vascular procedures except major reconstruction
113	5	•	Amputation for circulatory disorders except upper limb and toe

*grouped by body systems   • surgical   † medical

Diagnostic-related groups: A complete listing *(continued)*

DRG number	Major diagnostic code*	General diagnostic classification	Description
114	5	•	Upper limb and toe amputation for circulatory disorders
115	5	•	Permanent cardiac pacemaker implant with acute myocardial infarction (AMI) or congestive heart failure (CHF)
116	5	•	Permanent cardiac pacemaker implant, no AMI or CHF
117	5	•	Cardiac pacemaker replacement and revision except pulse generator replacement only
118	5	•	Cardiac pacemaker pulse generator replacement only
119	5	•	Vein ligation and stripping
120	5	•	Other O.R. procedures on the circulatory system
121	5	†	Circulatory disorders with AMI with cardiovascular complications, discharged alive
122	5	†	Circulatory disorders with AMI without cardiovascular complications, discharged alive
123	5	†	Circulatory disorders with AMI, expired
124	5	†	Circulatory disorders except AMI with cardiac catheterization and complex diagnosis
125	5	†	Circulatory disorders except AMI with cardiac catheterization, without complex diagnosis
126	5	†	Acute and subacute endocarditis
127	5	†	Heart failure and shock
128	5	†	Deep vein thrombophlebitis
129	5	†	Cardiac arrest
130	5	†	Peripheral vascular disorders, age > 69 with CC
131	5	†	Peripheral vascular disorders, age < 70 without CC
132	5	†	Atherosclerosis, age > 69 with CC
133	5	†	Atherosclerosis, age < 70 without CC
134	5	†	Hypertension
135	5	†	Cardiac congenital and valvular disorders, age > 69 with CC
136	5	†	Cardiac congenital and valvular disorders, age 18 to 69 without CC
137	5	†	Cardiac congenital and valvular disorders, age 0 to 17
138	5	†	Cardiac dysrhythmia and conduction disorders, age > 69 with CC
139	5	†	Cardiac dysrhythmia and conduction disorders, age < 70 without CC
140	5	†	Angina pectoris
141	5	†	Syncope and collapse, age > 69 with CC
142	5	†	Syncope and collapse, age < 70 without CC
143	5	†	Chest pain
144	5	†	Other circulatory diagnoses with CC
145	5	†	Other circulatory diagnoses without CC
146	6	•	Rectal resection, age > 69 with CC
147	6	•	Rectal resection, age < 70 without CC
148	6	•	Major small and large bowel procedures, age > 69 with CC
149	6	•	Major small and large bowel procedures, age < 70 without CC
150	6	•	Peritoneal adhesiolysis, age > 69 with CC
151	6	•	Peritoneal adhesiolysis, age < 70 without CC
152	6	•	Minor small and large bowel procedures, age > 69 with CC

*grouped by body systems   • surgical   † medical

(continued)

Diagnostic-related groups: A complete listing (continued)

DRG number	Major diagnostic code*	General diagnostic classification	Description
153	6	•	Minor small and large bowel procedures, age < 70 without CC
154	6	•	Stomach, esophageal, and duodenal procedures, age > 69 with CC
155	6	•	Stomach, esophageal, and duodenal procedures, age 18 to 69 without CC
156	6	•	Stomach, esophageal, and duodenal procedures, age 0 to 17
157	6	•	Anal procedures, age > 69 with CC
158	6	•	Anal procedures, age < 70 without CC
159	6	•	Hernia procedures except inguinal and femoral, age > 69 with CC
160	6	•	Hernia procedures except inguinal and femoral, age 18 to 69 without CC
161	6	•	Inguinal and femoral hernia procedures, age > 69 with CC
162	6	•	Inguinal and femoral hernia procedures, age 18 to 69 without CC
163	6	•	Hernia procedures, age 0 to 17
164	6	•	Appendectomy with complicated principal diagnosis, age > 69 with CC
165	6	•	Appendectomy with complicated principal diagnosis, age < 70 without CC
166	6	•	Appendectomy without complicated principal diagnosis, age > 69 with CC
167	6	•	Appendectomy without complicated principal diagnosis, age < 70 without CC
168	6	•	Procedures on the mouth, age > 69 with CC
169	6	•	Procedures on the mouth, age < 70 without CC
170	6	•	Other digestive system procedures, age > 69 with CC
171	6	•	Other digestive system procedures, age < 70 without CC
172	6	†	Digestive malignancy, age > 69 with CC
173	6	†	Digestive malignancy, age < 70 without CC
174	6	†	GI hemorrhage, age > 69 with CC
175	6	†	GI hemorrhage, age < 70 without CC
176	6	†	Complicated peptic ulcer
177	6	†	Uncomplicated peptic ulcer, age > 69 with CC
178	6	†	Uncomplicated peptic ulcer, age < 70 without CC
179	6	†	Inflammatory bowel disease
180	6	†	GI obstruction, age > 69 with CC
181	6	†	GI obstruction, age > 70 without CC
182	6	†	Esophagitis, gastroenteritis, and miscellaneous digestive disease, age > 69 with CC
183	6	†	Esophagitis, gastroenteritis, and miscellaneous digestive disease, age 18 to 69 without CC
184	6	†	Esophagitis, gastroenteritis, and miscellaneous digestive disease disorders, age 0 to 17
185	6	†	Dental and oral disease except extractions and restorations, age > 17
186	6	†	Dental and oral disease except extractions and restorations, age 0 to 17
187	6	†	Dental extractions and restorations
188	6	†	Other digestive system diagnoses, age > 69 with CC
189	6	†	Other digestive system diagnoses, age 18 to 69 without CC
190	6	†	Other digestive system diagnoses, age 0 to 17
191	7	•	Major pancreas, liver, and shunt procedures
192	7	•	Minor pancreas, liver, and shunt procedures
193	7	•	Biliary tract procedures except total cholecystectomy, age > 69 with CC

*grouped by body systems   • surgical   † medical

Diagnostic-related groups: A complete listing *(continued)*

DRG number	Major diagnostic code*	General diagnostic classification	Description
194	7	•	Biliary tract procedures except total cholecystectomy, age < 70 without CC
195	7	•	Total cholecystectomy with common duct exploration (CDE), age > 69 with CC
196	7	•	Total cholecystectomy with CDE, age < 70 without CC
197	7	•	Total cholecystectomy without CDE, age > 69 with CC
198	7	•	Total cholecystectomy without CDE, age < 70 without CC
199	7	•	Hepatobiliary diagnostic procedure for malignancy
200	7	•	Hepatobiliary diagnostic procedure for nonmalignancy
201	7	•	Other hepatobiliary or pancreas O.R. procedures
202	7	†	Cirrhosis and alcoholic hepatitis
203	7	†	Malignancy of hepatobiliary system or pancreas
204	7	†	Disorders of pancreas except malignancy
205	7	†	Disorders of liver except malignancy, cirrhosis, alcoholism, and hepatitis, age > 69 with CC
206	7	†	Disorders of liver except malignancy, cirrhosis, alcoholism, and hepatitis, age < 70 without CC
207	7	†	Disorders of the biliary tract, age > 69 with CC
208	7	†	Disorders of the biliary tract, age < 70 without CC
209	8	•	Major joint procedures
210	8	•	Hip and femur procedures except major joint, age > 69 with CC
211	8	•	Hip and femur procedures except major joint, age 18 to 69 without CC
212	8	•	Hip and femur procedures except major joint, age 0 to 17
213	8	•	Amputations for musculoskeletal system and connective tissue disorders
214	8	•	Back and neck procedures, age > 69 with CC
215	8	•	Back and neck procedures, age < 70 without CC
216	8	•	Biopsies of musculoskeletal system and connective tissue
217	8	•	Wound debridement and skin graft except hand, for musculoskeletal and connective tissue disorders
218	8	•	Lower extremity and humerus procedures except hip, foot, and femur, age > 69 with CC
219	8	•	Lower extremity and humerus procedures except hip, foot, and femur, age 18 to 69 without CC
220	8	•	Lower extremity and humerus procedures except hip, foot, and femur, age 0 to 17
221	8	•	Knee procedures, age > 69 with CC
222	8	•	Knee procedures, age < 70 without CC
223	8	•	Upper extremity procedures except humerus and hand, age > 69 with CC
224	8	•	Upper extremity procedures except humerus and hand, age < 70 without CC
225	8	•	Foot procedures
226	8	•	Soft tissue procedures, age > 69 with CC
227	8	•	Soft tissue procedures, age < 70 without CC
228	8	•	Ganglion hand procedures
229	8	•	Hand procedures except ganglion

*grouped by body systems   • surgical   † medical

(continued)

Diagnostic-related groups: A complete listing *(continued)*

DRG number	Major diagnostic code*	General diagnostic classification	Description
230	8	•	Local excision and removal of internal fixation devices of hip and femur
231	8	•	Local excision and removal of internal fixation devices except hip and femur
232	8	•	Arthroscopy
233	8	•	Other musculoskeletal system and connective tissue O.R. procedures, age > 69 with CC
234	8	•	Other musculoskeletal system and connective tissue O.R. procedures, age < 70 without CC
235	8	†	Fractures of femur
236	8	†	Fractures of hip and pelvis
237	8	†	Sprains, strains, and dislocations of hip, pelvis and thigh
238	8	†	Osteomyelitis
239	8	†	Pathological fractures and musculoskeletal and connective tissue malignancy
240	8	†	Connective tissue disorders, age > 69 with CC
241	8	†	Connective tissue disorders, age < 70 without CC
242	8	†	Septic arthritis
243	8	†	Medical back problems
244	8	†	Bone diseases and septic arthropathy, age > 69 with CC
245	8	†	Bone diseases and septic arthropathy, age < 70 without CC
246	8	†	Nonspecific arthropathies
247	8	†	Signs and symptoms of musculoskeletal system and connective tissue
248	8	†	Tendinitis, myositis, and bursitis
249	8	†	Aftercare, musculoskeletal system and connective tissue
250	8	†	Fractures, sprains, strains, and dislocations of forearm, hand, and foot, age > 69 with CC
251	8	†	Fractures, sprains, strains, and dislocations of forearm, hand, and foot, age 18 to 69 without CC
252	8	†	Fractures, sprains, strains, and dislocations of forearm, hand, and foot, age 0 to 17
253	8	†	Fractures, sprains, strains, and dislocations of upper arm and lower leg except foot, age > 69 with CC
254	8	†	Fractures, sprains, strains, and dislocations of upper arm and lower leg except foot, age 18 to 69 without CC
255	8	†	Fractures, sprains, strains, and dislocations of upper arm and lower leg except foot, age 0 to 17
256	8	†	Other diagnoses of musculoskeletal system and connective tissue
257	9	•	Total mastectomy for malignancy, age > 69 with CC
258	9	•	Total mastectomy for malignancy, age < 70 without CC
259	9	•	Subtotal mastectomy for malignancy, age > 69 with CC
260	9	•	Subtotal mastectomy for malignancy, age < 70
261	9	•	Breast procedures for nonmalignancy except biopsy and local excision
262	9	•	Breast biopsy and local excision for nonmalignancy
263	9	•	Skin grafts for skin ulcer or cellulitis, age > 69 with CC
264	9	•	Skin grafts for skin ulcer or cellulitis, age < 70 without CC

*grouped by body systems   • surgical   † medical

Diagnostic-related groups: A complete listing (continued)

DRG number	Major diagnostic code*	General diagnostic classification	Description
265	9	•	Skin grafts except for skin ulcer or cellulitis with CC
266	9	•	Skin grafts except for skin ulcer or cellulitis without CC
267	9	•	Perianal + pilonidal procedures
268	9	•	Skin, subcutaneous tissue, and breast plastic procedures
269	9	•	Other skin, subcutaneous tissue and breast O.R. procedures, age > 69 with CC
270	9	•	Other skin, subcutaneous tissue and breast O.R. procedures, age < 70 without CC
271	9	†	Skin ulcers
272	9	†	Major skin disorders, age > 69 with CC
273	9	†	Major skin disorders, age < 70 without CC
274	9	†	Malignant breast disorders, age > 69 with CC
275	9	†	Malignant breast disorders, age < 70 without CC
276	9	†	Nonmalignant breast disorders
277	9	†	Cellulitis, age > 69 with CC
278	9	†	Cellulitis, age 18 to 69 without CC
279	9	†	Cellulitis, age 0 to 17
280	9	†	Trauma to the skin, subcutaneous tissue, and breast, age > 69 with CC
281	9	†	Trauma to the skin, subcutaneous tissue, and breast, age 18 to 69 without CC
282	9	†	Trauma to the skin, subcutaneous tissue, and breast, age 0 to 17
283	9	†	Minor skin disorders, age > 69 with CC
284	10	†	Minor skin disorders, age < 70 without CC
285	10	•	Amputations for endocrine, nutritional, and metabolic disorders
286	10	•	Adrenal and pituitary procedures
287	10	•	Skin grafts and wound debridement for endocrine, nutritional, and metabolic disorders
288	10	•	O.R. procedures for obesity
289	10	•	Parathyroid procedures
290	10	•	Thyroid procedures
291	10	•	Thyroglossal procedures
292	10	•	Other endocrine, nutritional, and metabolic O.R. procedures, age > 69 with CC
293	10	•	Other endocrine, nutritional, and metabolic O.R. procedures, age < 70 without CC
294	10	†	Diabetes, age > 36
295	10	†	Diabetes, age 0 to 35
296	10	†	Nutritional and miscellaneous metabolic disorders, age > 69 with CC
297	10	†	Nutritional and miscellaneous metabolic disorders, age 18 to 69 without CC
298	10	†	Nutritional and miscellaneous metabolic disorders, age 0 to 17
299	10	†	Inborn errors of metabolism
300	10	†	Endocrine disorders, age > 69 with CC
301	10	†	Endocrine disorders, age < 70 without CC
302	11	•	Kidney transplant

*grouped by body systems   • surgical   † medical

(continued)

Diagnostic-related groups: A complete listing *(continued)*

DRG number	Major diagnostic code*	General diagnostic classification	Description
303	11	•	Kidney, ureter, and major bladder procedure for neoplasm
304	11	•	Kidney, ureter, and major bladder procedures for nonmalignancy, age > 69 with CC
305	11	•	Kidney, ureter, and major bladder procedures for nonmalignancy, age < 70 without CC
306	11	•	Prostatectomy, age > 69 with CC
307	11	•	Prostatectomy, age < 70 without CC
308	11	•	Minor bladder procedures, age > 69 with CC
309	11	•	Minor bladder procedures, age < 70 without CC
310	11	•	Transurethral procedures, age > 69 with CC
311	11	•	Transurethral procedures, age < 70 without CC
312	11	•	Urethral procedures, age > 69 with CC
313	11	•	Urethral procedures, age 18 to 69 without CC
314	11	•	Urethral procedures, age 0 to 17
315	11	•	Other kidney and urinary tract O.R. procedures
316	11	†	Renal failure without dialysis
317	11	†	Renal failure with dialysis
318	11	†	Kidney and urinary tract neoplasms, age > 69 with CC
319	11	†	Kidney and urinary tract neoplasms, age < 70 without CC
320	11	†	Kidney and urinary tract infections, age > 69 with CC
321	11	†	Kidney and urinary tract infections, age 18 to 69 without CC
322	11	†	Kidney and urinary tract infections, age 0 to 17
323	11	†	Urinary stones, age > 69 with CC
324	11	†	Urinary stones, age < 70 without CC
325	11	†	Kidney and urinary tract signs and symptoms, age > 69 with CC
326	11	†	Kidney and urinary tract signs and symptoms, age 18 to 69 without CC
327	11	†	Kidney and urinary tract signs + symptoms, age 0 to 17
328	11	†	Urethral stricture, age > 69 with CC
329	11	†	Urethral stricture, age 18 to 69 without CC
330	11	†	Urethral stricture, age 0 to 17
331	11	†	Other kidney and urinary tract diagnoses, age > 69 with CC
332	11	†	Other kidney and urinary tract diagnoses, age 18 to 69 without CC
333	11	†	Other kidney and urinary tract diagnoses, age 0 to 17
334	12	•	Major male pelvic procedures with CC
335	12	•	Major male pelvic procedures without CC
336	12	•	Transurethral prostatectomy, age > 69 with CC
337	12	•	Transurethral prostatectomy, age < 70 without CC
338	12	•	Testes procedures for malignancy
339	12	•	Testes procedures for nonmalignancy, age > 17
340	12	•	Testes procedures, nonmalignant, age 0 to 17
341	12	•	Penis procedures
342	12	•	Circumcision, age > 17
343	12	•	Circumcision, age 0 to 17
344	12	•	Other male reproductive system O.R. procedures for malignancy
345	12	•	Other male reproductive system O.R. procedures except for malignancy

*grouped by body systems   • surgical   † medical

Diagnostic-related groups: A complete listing *(continued)*

DRG number	Major diagnostic code*	General diagnostic classification	Description
346	13	†	Malignancy, male reproductive system, age > 69 with CC
347	13	†	Malignancy, male reproductive system, age < 70 without CC
348	13	†	Benign prostatic hypertrophy, age > 69 with CC
349	13	†	Benign prostatic hypertrophy, age < 70 without CC
350	13	†	Inflammation of the male reproductive system
351	13	†	Sterilization, male
352	13	†	Other male reproductive system diagnoses
353	13	•	Pelvic evisceration, radical hysterectomy, and vulvectomy
354	13	•	Nonradical hysterectomy, age > 69 with CC
355	13	•	Nonradical hysterectomy, age < 70 without CC
356	13	•	Female reproductive system reconstructive procedures
357	13	•	Uterus and adenexa procedures for malignancy
358	13	•	Uterus and adenexa procedures for nonmalignancy except tubal interruption
359	13	•	Tubal interruption for nonmalignancy
360	13	•	Vagina, cervix, and vulva procedures
361	13	•	Laparoscopy and endoscopy female except tubal interruption
362	13	•	Laparoscopic tubal interruption
363	13	•	D & C, conization, and radio-implant for malignancy
364	13	•	D & C, conization except for malignancy
365	13	•	Other female reproductive system O.R. procedures
366	13	†	Malignancy, female reproductive system, age > 69 with CC
367	13	†	Malignancy, female reproductive system, age < 70 without CC
368	13	†	Infections, female reproductive system
369	13	•	Menstrual and other female reproductive system disorders
370	14	•	Cesarean section with CC
371	14	•	Cesarean section without CC
372	14	†	Vaginal delivery with complicating diagnoses
373	14	†	Vaginal delivery without complicating diagnoses
374	14	•	Vaginal delivery with sterilization or D & C
375	14	•	Vaginal delivery with O.R. procedures except sterilization and D & C
376	14	†	Postpartum diagnoses without O.R. procedure
377	14	•	Postpartum diagnoses with O.R. procedure
378	14	†	Ectopic pregnancy
379	14	†	Threatened abortion
380	14	†	Abortion without D & C
381	14	†	Abortion with D & C
382	14	†	False labor
383	14	†	Other antepartum diagnoses with medical complications
384	14	†	Other antepartum diagnoses without medical complications
385	15	•	Neonates, died or transferred
386	15	•	Extreme immaturity, neonate
387	15	•	Prematurity with major problems
388	15	•	Prematurity without major problems
389	15	•	Full-term neonate with major problems

*grouped by body systems   • surgical   † medical

(continued)

Diagnostic-related groups: A complete listing (continued)

DRG number	Major diagnostic code*	General diagnostic classification	Description
390	15	•	Neonates with other significant problems
391	15	•	Normal newborns
392	16	•	Splenectomy, age > 17
393	16	•	Splenectomy, age 0 to 17
394	16	•	Other O.R. procedures of the blood and blood-forming organs
395	16	†	Red blood cell disorders, age > 17
396	16	†	Red blood cell disorders, age 0 to 17
397	16	†	Coagulation disorders
398	16	†	Reticuloendothelial and immunity disorders, age > 69 with CC
399	16	†	Reticuloendothelial and immunity disorders, age < 70 without CC
400	17	•	Lymphoma or leukemia with major O.R. procedure
401	17	•	Lymphoma or leukemia with minor O.R. procedure, age > 69 with CC
402	17	•	Lymphoma or leukemia with minor O.R. procedure, age < 70 without CC
403	17	†	Lymphoma or leukemia, age > 69 with CC
404	17	†	Lymphoma or leukemia, age 18 to 69 without CC
405	17	†	Lymphoma or leukemia, age 0 to 17
406	17	•	Myeloproliferating disorder or poorly differentiated neoplasm with major O.R. procedure and CC
407	17	•	Myeloproliferating disorder or poorly differentiated neoplasm with major O.R. procedure without CC
408	17	•	Myeloproliferating disorder or poorly differentiated neoplasm with minor O.R. procedure
409	17	†	Radiotherapy
410	17	†	Chemotherapy
411	17	†	History of malignancy without endoscopy
412	17	†	History of malignancy with endoscopy
413	17	†	Other myeloproliferating disorder or poorly differentiated neoplasm diagnosis, age > 69 with CC
414	17	†	Other myeloproliferating disorder or poorly differentiated neoplasm diagnosis, age < 70 without CC
415	18	•	O.R. procedure for infections and parasitic diseases
416	18	†	Septicemia, age > 17
417	18	†	Septicemia, age 0 to 17
418	18	†	Postoperative and posttraumatic infections
419	18	†	Fever of unknown origin, age > 69 with CC
420	18	†	Fever of unknown origin, age 18 to 69 without CC
421	18	†	Viral illness, age > 17
422	18	†	Viral illness and fever of unknown origin, age 0 to 17
423	18	†	Other infectious and parasitic diseases diagnoses
424	19	•	O.R. procedures with principal diagnosis of mental illness
425	19	†	Acute adjustment reaction and disturbances of psychosocial dysfunction
426	19	†	Depressive neuroses
427	19	†	Neuroses except depressive
428	19	†	Disorders of personality and impulse control
429	19	†	Organic disturbances and mental retardation

*grouped by body systems   • surgical   † medical

Diagnostic-related groups: A complete listing *(continued)*

DRG number	Major diagnostic code*	General diagnostic classification	Description
430	19	†	Psychoses
431	19	†	Childhood mental disorders
432	19	†	Other diagnoses of mental disorders
433	20	†	Substance use and substance-induced organic mental disorders, left against medical advice
434	20	†	Drug dependence
435	20	†	Drug use except dependence
436	20	†	Alcohol dependence
437	20	†	Alcohol use except dependence
438	20	†	Alcohol and substance-induced organic mental syndrome
439	21	•	Skin grafts for injuries
440	21	•	Wound debridements for injuries
441	21	•	Hand procedures for injuries
442	21	•	Other O.R. procedures for injuries, age > 69 with CC
443	21	•	Other O.R. procedures for injuries, age < 70 without CC
444	21	†	Multiple trauma, age > 69 with CC
445	21	†	Multiple trauma, age 18 to 69 without CC
446	21	†	Multiple trauma, age 0 to 17
447	21	†	Allergic reactions, age > 17
448	21	†	Allergic reactions, age 0 to 17
449	21	†	Toxic effects of drugs, age > 69 with CC
450	21	†	Toxic effects of drugs, age 18 to 69 without CC
451	21	†	Toxic effects of drugs, age 0 to 17
452	21	†	Complications of treatment, age > 69 with CC
453	21	†	Complications of treatment, age < 70 without CC
454	21	†	Other injuries, poisonings, and toxic effects diagnosis, age > 69 with CC
455	21	†	Other injuries, poisonings, and toxic effects diagnosis, age < 70 without CC
456	22	•	Burns, transferred to another acute care facility
457	22	•	Extensive burns
458	22	•	Nonextensive burns with skin grafts
459	22	•	Nonextensive burns with wound debridement and other O.R. procedures
460	22	†	Nonextensive burns without O.R. procedure
461	23	•	O.R. procedures with diagnoses of other contact with health services
462	23	†	Rehabilitation
463	23	•	Signs and symptoms with CC
464	23	•	Signs and symptoms without CC
465	23	•	Aftercare with history of malignancy as secondary diagnosis
466	23	•	Aftercare without history of malignancy as secondary diagnosis
467	23	•	Other factors influencing health status
468			Unrelated O.R. procedure
469			PDX invalid as discharge diagnosis
470			Ungroupable: Record does not meet criteria for any DRG

*grouped by body systems   • surgical   † medical

7 Treatments: Choices and patient care

Profiles of common surgeries

Almost everyone can expect to be wheeled into the operating room at some point in life. As a nurse, you'll have to care for patients undergoing a vast range of surgeries: correction of broken bones, bowel resections, hernia repairs, hysterectomies, appendectomies, and so on.

Appendectomy

The surgical removal of an inflamed vermiform appendix, this procedure is commonly performed as an emergency procedure with the patient under general anesthesia. The surgeon makes an incision in the lower right abdominal quadrant to expose the appendix. After dividing and ligating the appendicular blood vessels, he divides the appendix from the cecum and removes it. He ligates the base of the appendix and places a purse-string suture in the cecum. Before closing the incision, he removes any fluid or tissue debris from the abdominal cavity.

Therapeutic benefit: Appendectomy prevents imminent rupture or perforation of the appendix.

Arthroplasty

In this reconstruction or replacement of a joint, the surgeon either reshapes the bones of the joint and places soft tissue or a metal disc between the reshaped ends, or uses a metal or polyethylene prosthesis to totally or partially replace the joint. Prostheses available today can replace all joints except the spine.

Therapeutic benefit: Successful arthroplasty restores mobility and stability and relieves pain for patients with diseased or damaged joints. It may help them achieve an increased sense of independence and self-worth. Recent improvements in techniques and prosthetic devices have made arthoplasty increasingly common for patients with severe chronic arthritis, degenerative joint disorders, extensive joint trauma, and congenital deformities. Elderly patients commonly undergo total hip or knee replacement.

Arthroscopy

After inserting a large-bore needle into the suprapatellar pouch, the doctor injects sterile saline solution to distend the joint. Then he passes a fiber-optic scope through puncture sites lateral or medial to the tibial plateau, allowing direct visualization.

Therapeutic benefit: With a large arthroscope, the surgeon can remove articular debris, including small fragments of bone, muscle tissue, ligaments, and cartilage, and repair a torn meniscus.

Bowel resection

This surgery involves resection of diseased intestinal tissue and anastomosis of the remaining segments. The incision site varies depending on the location of pathology. The surgeon may use end-to-end or side-to-side anastomosis to restore patency. Unlike the patient who undergoes total colectomy or more extensive surgery, the patient who undergoes this treatment usually retains normal bowel function.

Therapeutic benefit: This surgery treats localized obstructive disorders, including diverticulosis, intestinal polyps, adhesions that cause bowel dysfunction, and malignant or benign intestinal lesions. While effective against localized bowel cancer, bowel resection isn't indicated for widespread carcinoma, which usually requires massive resection with creation of a temporary or permanent colostomy or ileostomy.

Cataract removal

To perform cataract removal, the

surgeon may choose intracapsular or extracapsular techniques.

In intracapsular cataract extraction, the surgeon makes a partial incision at the superior limbus arc. He then removes the lens, using specially designed forceps or a cryoprobe which freezes and adheres to the lens, facilitating its removal.

In extracapsular cataract extraction, the surgeon may make an incision at the limbus, open the anterior lens capsule with a cystotome and exert pressure from below to express the lens. He then irrigates and suctions the remaining lens cortex. Alternatively, he may use an ultrasonic probe to break the lens into minute particles, which are then aspirated by the probe.

Therapeutic benefit: This procedure removes a cloudy, cataractal lens that prevents light rays from reaching the retina. A surgeon may also perform the procedure to correct aphakia by implanting an intraocular lens.

Cholecystectomy
Removal of the gallbladder, usually performed with the patient under general anesthesia, relieves symptoms in over 95% of patients. The surgeon excises the entire gallbladder and ligates the cystic duct and artery. The body responds by increasing bile flow into the duodenum. During the procedure, the surgeon may explore the common bile duct for additional stones or perform a cholangiogram. He'll remove stones using a Fogarty catheter, Dormia basket, or stone forceps. He usually inserts a T-tube in the common bile duct to permit bile drainage during healing.

Therapeutic benefit: Successful surgery will correct biliary tract obstruction and restore biliary flow from the liver to the small intestine. Candidates for cholecys-

tectomy include patients with gallstone disease (cholecystitis or cholelithiasis) and widespread carcinoma.

Circumcision
The surgeon performing a circumcision may choose from several procedures.

When using a *circumcision bell*, he slides the device between the foreskin and the glans penis and then tightly ties a length of suture around the foreskin at the glans' coronal edge. The foreskin atrophies and drops off in 5 to 8 days.

Alternatively, the surgeon may stretch the foreskin forward over the glans and apply a *Gomco clamp* on the penis distal to the glans. He then excises the foreskin, removes the clamp, and sutures around the base of the glans.

Most adult patients undergo a *sleeve resection.* In this procedure, the surgeon incises and excises the inner and outer surfaces of the foreskin, then puts sutures in place to approximate the skin edges.

Therapeutic benefit: An adult may undergo circumcision to treat phimosis (abnormal tightening of the foreskin around the glans), or paraphimosis (inability to return the foreskin to its normal position after retraction).

Most commonly, circumcision is performed on neonates 2 or 3 days after birth. Considerable disagreement exists regarding the medical value of routine circumcision. Nevertheless, it remains the most commonly performed of all pediatric surgeries—largely because of its religious significance. The religions of approximately one-sixth of the world's population require circumcision. In Judaism, it's performed by a *mohel* on the 8th day after birth.

Coronary artery bypass grafting (CABG)
This surgery restores blood flow to the myocardium by circumventing an occluded coronary artery with an autogenous graft (usually a segment of the saphenous vein or the internal mammarian artery). The most common technique, aortocoronary bypass, involves suturing one end of the autogenous graft to the ascending aorta and the other end to a coronary artery distal to the occlusion. Other techniques may be employed depending on the patient's condition and the number of arteries being bypassed.

Therapeutic benefit: CABG may benefit patients with severe angina from atherosclerosis and those at high risk for myocardial infarction (MI) because of coronary artery disease. The goal is to relieve anginal pain, improve cardiac function, and enhance the patient's quality of life. Its long-term effectiveness in preventing recurrence of atherosclerosis or reducing the risk of MI remains uncertain.

Craniotomy
After the patient receives a general anesthetic, the surgeon marks an incision line and cuts through the scalp to the cranium, forming a scalp flap that he turns to one side. He then bores two or more holes through the skull in the corner of the cranial incision, using an air-driven or electric drill, and cuts out a bone flap with a small saw. After pulling aside or removing the bone flap, he incises and retracts the dura, exposing the brain. After proceeding with surgery, the surgeon reverses the incision procedure and covers the site with a sterile dressing.

Therapeutic benefit: Craniotomy exposes the brain for a number of treatments including ventricular shunting, excision of tumor or abscess, hematoma aspiration, and aneurysm clipping.

Dilatation and curettage (D&C)
The most commonly performed gynecologic surgery, D&C involves cervical dilatation to allow access to the endocervix and uterus. The surgeon begins by performing a preliminary bimanual pelvic examination, with the patient in the dorsal lithotomy position. He then exposes the cervix and checks the depth and direction of the uterine cavity.

Next, the surgeon explores the uterine cavity, removing any polyps. If he suspects any cervical or uterine malignancy, he obtains biopsy specimens from the endocervical canal. Then he performs standard curettage to remove the superficial layer of the endometrium, taking biopsy specimens from the four quadrants of the cervix. When treating an incomplete abortion, he removes the remaining products of conception.

Therapeutic benefit: A D&C may treat an incomplete abortion, control abnormal uterine bleeding, and provide an endometrial or endocervical sample for cytologic study.

Hemorrhoidectomy
After administering a local anesthetic, the surgeon digitally dilates the rectal sphincter and removes hemorrhoidal varicosities, either by clamping and cauterization or by ligation and excision. The surgeon may place a small lubricated tube in the patient's anus to drain air, fluid, blood, and flatus, or he may elect to pack the area with petrolatum gauze.

Therapeutic benefit: Hemorrhoidectomy offers the most effective treatment for intolerable hemorrhoidal pain, excessive bleeding, or large prolapse. It's used when diet,

drugs, sitz baths, and compresses fail to provide effective relief.

Herniorrhaphy
The surgeon makes an incision over the area of herniation. He manipulates the herniated tissue back to its proper position and then repairs the defect in the muscle or fascia. If necessary, he reinforces the area of defect with wire, mesh, or another material. Then he closes the incision and applies a dressing. Herniorrhaphy requires general anesthesia.

Therapeutic benefit: Successful surgery returns a protruding intestine to the abdominal cavity and repairs the abdominal wall defect. It's the surgery of choice for inguinal and other abdominal hernias.

Hysterectomy
During this excision of the uterus, the doctor uses either a vaginal or abdominal approach and places the patient under general or spinal anesthesia. A *total* hysterectomy involves removal of the entire uterus. A *subtotal* hysterectomy removes only a portion of the uterus, leaving the cervical stump intact. A *radical* hysterectomy involves removal of all the reproductive organs.

Therapeutic benefit: Both total and subtotal hysterectomy are commonly performed for myomas or endometrial disease. They may also be performed postpartum if the placenta fails to separate from the uterus after a cesarean delivery or in cases of amnionitis. Patients with cervical carcinoma may undergo radical hysterectomy.

Incision and drainage (I&D)
The surgeon begins by anesthetizing the area surrounding a suppurative infection. If the infected area is superficial and appears ready to rupture, he may aspirate the pus with needle and syringe.

If the area's large, he may make an incision directly over the suppurative area, spreading its edges to allow drainage of the pus.

After pus drains, the surgeon leaves the cavity open to promote healing. With a large cavity, he may pack it with gauze to provide further drainage and assist debridement.

Therapeutic benefit: A patient may undergo I&D when an infection fails to resolve spontaneously. For example, I&D may treat a furuncle or carbuncle, in which inflammation traps bacteria in a small localized area.

Laminectomy
With the patient under general anesthesia and placed in a prone position, the surgeon makes a midline vertical incision and strips the fascia and muscles off the bony laminae. He then removes one or more sections of the laminae to expose the spinal defect. For a herniated disk, the surgeon removes part or all of the disk. For a spinal cord tumor, he incises the dura and explores the cord for metastasis. Then he dissects the tumor and removes it, using suction, forceps, or dissecting scissors.

Therapeutic benefit: Most commonly, laminectomy relieves pressure on the spinal cord or spinal nerve roots resulting from a herniated disk. It may also treat compression fracture, dislocation of the vertebrae, or a spinal cord tumor.

Laparoscopy
The laparoscope, a type of endoscope consisting of an illuminated tube with a fiber-optic tip, allows visualization of pelvic and upper abdominal organs. By passing a laser beam, a probe, or a cryosurgical or electrocautery device through the laparoscope, the doctor may perform surgery.

Therapeutic benefit: Various laparoscopic procedures remove endometrial implants. The surgeon may use an argon laser beam to destroy widespread, deep-seated endometrial implants or a CO_2 laser to remove shallow endometrial implants. Local freezing or extreme heat will also destroy endometrial tissue.

Mastectomy
Until recently, radical mastectomy was the treatment of choice for breast cancer. Now, doctors and patients may choose from six mastectomy options:

In *partial mastectomy* (lumpectomy), the surgeon removes the entire tumor mass along with at least 1" (2.5 cm) of the surrounding healthy tissue.

In *subcutaneous mastectomy*, he removes all breast tissue but preserves the overlying skin and nipple. In a *simple mastectomy,* he removes the entire breast without dissecting the lymph nodes and may apply a skin graft if necessary.

Modified radical mastectomy involves removal of the entire breast. The surgeon also resects all the axillary nodes while leaving the pectoralis major intact. He may or may not remove the pectoralis minor. If the patient has small lesions and no metastases, the surgeon may perform breast reconstruction immediately or a few days later.

In *radical mastectomy,* the surgeon removes the entire breast, the axillary lymph nodes, the underlying pectoral muscles, and adjacent tissues.

In *extended radical mastectomy,* the surgeon removes the breast, underlying pectoral muscles, axillary contents, and the upper internal lymph node chain.

Therapeutic benefit: A *partial mastectomy* treats stage I malignant breast lesions. This approach leaves a cosmetically satisfactory breast but may fail to remove all malignant tissue in axillary lymph nodes.

The surgeon may perform *subcutaneous mastectomy* on a patient with a central, noninvasive tumor, chronic cystic mastitis, multiple fibroadenomas, or hyperplastic duct changes.

The patient may undergo *simple mastectomy* if her tumor is confined to breast tissue. It's also used palliatively for advanced ulcerative malignancy and as treatment for extensive benign disease.

A *modified radical mastectomy,* the standard surgery for Stage I and II lesions, removes small, localized tumors. Besides causing less disfigurement than a radical mastectomy, it reduces postoperative arm edema and shoulder complications.

A *radical mastectomy* controls the spread of larger, metastatic lesions. The surgeon may perform breast reconstruction later.

Rarely, an *extended radical mastectomy* may treat malignancy in the medial quadrant of the breast or in subareolar tissue. It's used to prevent possible metastasis to the internal mammary lymph nodes.

Myringotomy
In this procedure, the surgeon visualizes the tympanic membrane. If the middle ear contains serous fluid, he makes a radial incision — a small slit in the membrane. After making this incision, he inserts a plastic tube or Teflon grommet.

If the middle ear contains pus or thick drainage, the surgeon makes an circumferential incision. A circumferential incision involves a larger, U-shaped cup that permits more drainage. The surgeon may irrigate the middle ear or apply gentle suction to remove tenacious drainage. If drainage is copious, he may apply a dressing over the ear.

Therapeutic benefit: This surgery relieves pain and treats membrane rupture by allowing drainage of pus or fluid from the middle ear. Children with acute otitis media commonly undergo myringotomy.

Open reduction of fractures
With the patient under general anesthesia, the surgeon makes an incision through the skin and soft tissue and spreads the muscle to expose the fracture or dislocation. He realigns the fractured fragments or dislocated joint segments. He then inserts one or more screws or other fixation device to immobilize the fragments. After closing the incision, he applies a cast, splint, or traction to protect the surgical site and maintain alignment.

Therapeutic benefit: Open reduction attempts to restore the normal position and alignment of fragmented bones or dislocated joints. It's indicated for patients with compound fractures, comminuted fractures, and impacted fractures, and for fractures or dislocations that cause serious nerve or circulatory impairment.

Radioactive implant
A radioactive implant is a form of locally delivered internal radiation. The doctor places radioactive substances into the tissue surrounding the tumor or into the tumor itself. This may involve placing special radioactive guides or needles within the tumor mass or surgically placing radioactive gold grains into cancerous tissue. Radioactive sources include radium, radon, iridium, cesium, cobalt, or iodine 125.

Therapeutic benefit: Radiation deters the proliferation of malignant cells by decreasing the rate of mitosis or impairing synthesis of DNA and RNA. Indications for interstitial implantation include cancer of the buccal mucosa, head, tongue, neck and chest, prostate, uterus, and cervix.

Rhinoplasty
The surgeon fractures the nasal bones, removes excess tissue, and then repositions the bones. He makes an incision in the groove between the upper and lower nasal cartilages and trims the soft tissue to reshape the tip of the nose. This surgery requires topical and local anesthetics.

Therapeutic benefit: Successful rhinoplasty enhances the nose's external appearance, correcting congenital or traumatic deformity.

Sclerosing of esophageal varices
Injection of a sclerosing agent through a fiber-optic endoscope causes the varix to collapse, leading to thrombosis and sclerosis.

Therapeutic benefit: This technique provides prophylactic and therapeutic treatment of bleeding esophageal varices.

Tonsillectomy and adenoidectomy
For tonsillectomy, a child usually receives a general anesthetic, an adult a local anesthetic. The surgeon removes tonsillar tissue by dissection and snare.

An adenoidectomy also requires general anesthesia for children. With the child's head tilted far back, the surgeon removes adenoidal tissue with a gentle sweeping motion. An adenoidectomy is usually performed before tonsillectomy. The combination of the two procedures is called adenotonsillectomy.

Therapeutic benefit: The use of antibiotics to treat tonsils and adenoids enlarged by bacterial infection has significantly reduced the number of patients who undergo these two procedures. However, either or both of these surgeries may treat obstruction of the upper airway caused by tonsillar tissue enlargement. Tonsillectomy remains the preferred treatment for peritonsillar abscess. The patient with chronic tonsillitis who suffers seven acute attacks within two years may also require surgery. Adenoidectomy may prevent recurrent otitis media, although some experts dispute its effectiveness.

Transurethral resection of the prostate (TURP)
In this procedure, the patient is placed in lithotomy position and anesthetized. The surgeon then introduces a resectoscope into the urethra and advances it to the prostate. After instilling a clear irrigating solution and visualizing the obstruction, he uses the resectoscope's cutting loop to resect prostatic tissue and restore the urethral opening.

Therapeutic benefit: TURP is the most common surgical approach for treating benign prostatic hypertrophy, chronic prostatitis, and prostate cancer.

Urinary diversion
Several types of urinary diversion surgery exist. The two most commonly performed are cutaneous ureterostomy and ileal conduit. In *cutaneous ureterostomy,* the surgeon dissects one or both ureters from the bladder and brings it out through the skin surface on the flank or the abdominal wall to form one or two stomas.

To construct an *ileal conduit,* the surgeon excises a segment of the ileum and then anastomoses the remaining ileal ends to maintain intestinal integrity. Next, he dissects the ureters from the bladder and implants them in the ileal segment. He then sutures one end of the ileal segment closed and brings the other through the abdominal wall to form a stoma.

Therapeutic benefit: Urinary diversion provides an alternate route for urine excretion when bladder dysfunction or removal doesn't allow normal drainage. Candidates for diversion surgery include patients who've undergone total or partial cystectomy, and patients with a congenital urinary tract defect; a severe urinary tract infection that threatens renal function; an injury to the ureters, bladder, or urethra; an obstructive malignancy; or a neurogenic bladder.

What do you tell the preoperative patient?

Regardless of whether he's had surgery before, your patient will enter the operating room with many fears and questions.

Unfortunately, he's likely to absorb only limited information during the short time he's in your care. Concentrate on providing a general overview of what he can expect before, during, and after surgery. Use the following list of teaching points as a guide.

Preop preparation
Discuss preoperative routines to help alleviate the patient's anxiety.
• Urge the patient to read the surgical consent form carefully and to ask any questions before signing it.
• Explain that a large area of his skin will be cleaned. Discuss the rationale behind shaving or depilatory hair removal—to prevent surgical wound infection by cleaning the skin of microorganisms found in body hair.
• Tell the patient that once food and fluids are withheld, he mustn't eat anything (including hard candy), drink anything (including water), or chew gum.
• Inform him that once he's completed all preoperative routines, including dressing in a surgical cap and gown, he'll receive pre-

anesthetic medication. You'll then raise his side rails and ask him to remain in bed. Tell him that this medication will help him relax, although he probably won't fall asleep. Advise him that his mouth will feel dry, because the medication helps dry up secretions.
• Tell the patient that he will receive an I.V. line either before he goes to surgery or after he gets to the operating room. Explain that fluids and nutrients, given during surgery, help prevent postoperative complications.
• Help the patient deal with fears about anesthesia. Tell him the name of his anesthesiologist and explain that this person is responsible for his care until he leaves the recovery room. The patient can expect a visit from the anesthesiologist before surgery; during this visit he will have the opportunity to ask questions. Encourage the patient to jot down his questions beforehand.

Your patient may harbor fears that he's reluctant to admit. He may fear awakening in the middle of the operation or never awakening at all. Assure your patient that the anesthesiologist will monitor his condition carefully throughout surgery and provide just the right amount of anesthetic.

An overview of the operation
Counsel the patient on operating room procedure.
• Warn the patient that he may have to wait a short time in the holding area. Explain that the doctors and nurses will wear surgical dress and that even though they'll be observing him closely, they probably won't talk to him. Tell him that this will allow the medication to take effect.
• When discussing transfer procedures and techniques, describe sensations the patient will experience. Advise the patient that he'll be taken to the operating room on a stretcher and transferred from the stretcher to the operating ta-

ble. For his own safety, he'll be strapped securely to the table. The operating room nurses will check his vital signs frequently.
• Warn the patient that the operating room may feel cool. Electrodes may be put on his chest to monitor his heart rate during surgery.
• Describe the drowsy, floating sensation he'll feel as the anesthetic takes effect. Tell him it's important that he relax at this time.

Getting ready for recovery
Prepare the patient for his eventual stay in the recovery room.
• Briefly describe the sensations the patient will experience when the anesthetic wears off. Tell him that the recovery room nurse will call his name, then ask him to answer questions and follow simple commands, such as wiggling his toes. He may feel pain at the surgical site, but the nurse will try to minimize it.
• Describe the oxygen delivery device, such as the nasal cannula, that he'll need after surgery.
• Tell the patient that once he's recovered from the anesthesia, he'll return to his room. He'll be able to see his family, but will probably feel drowsy and wish to nap.
• Make sure he's aware that you'll be taking his blood pressure and pulse frequently. That way, he won't be alarmed by these routine precautions.

How to conduct a preoperative assessment

A thorough preoperative assessment is the foundation of good surgical care. It provides a baseline for comparison throughout nursing care and medical treatment. It can also help to identify conditions that impair the patient's ability to tolerate stress or surgery

or to comply with postoperative routines.

Initial steps
• Focus on problem areas suggested by the patient's history, and on any body system directly affected by the surgical procedure.
• Note your patient's general appearance. Does he look healthy and well-nourished, or does he appear ill?
• Record the patient's height, weight, and vital signs measurements. For accuracy, take blood pressure readings in both arms and document the patient's position during the procedure. Update vital signs measurements at least twice a day throughout the preoperative period. Use these measurements to establish a baseline for your patient.
• Next, systematically examine your patient from head to toe. Use the following as a guide:

Head and neck
• Check the patient's scalp for lesions or parasitic infection.
• Check the jugular veins for distention.
• Note the color of his sclerae. A yellowish color suggests jaundice.
• Evert his lower eyelid and note the color of the conjunctivae. If this tissue looks pale, suspect anemia.
• Check his nose and throat for signs of respiratory infection.
• Assess his mouth for sores, ulcerations, or bleeding of tongue, gums, and cheeks. Check his lips for a bluish or gray color which may suggest cyanosis.
• Check his neck for stiffness or cervical node enlargement.

Neurologic system
• Assess the patient's level of consciousness and orientation.
• Assess his gross motor movements (for example, while standing or walking), and his fine motor movements (for example, while writing).

• If you know or suspect that your patient has a neurologic problem, conduct a complete neurologic exam.

Extremities and skin
• Look for changes in the skin color or temperature that suggest impaired circulation. Check for cyanotic nailbeds and finger clubbing.
• Note skin lesions.
• Assess skin turgor for signs of dehydration.
• Check extremities for edema. Ask the patient if his feet, ankles, or fingers ever swell.
• Note hair distribution on the patient's extremities. Uneven hair distribution suggests poor peripheral circulation.
• Carefully palpate leg veins for varicosity.
• Check all peripheral pulses (radial, pedal, femoral, and popliteal). Remember to check them bilaterally.

Respiratory system
• Document the patient's respiratory rate.
• Assess his breathing pattern. Inspect his chest wall for symmetry; look for use of accessory muscles.
• Auscultate his anterior and posterior chest for breath sounds. Listen for wheezing, coughing, and crackles. Note dyspnea.

Cardiovascular system
• Assess the patient's apical pulse for rate and regularity.
• Auscultate his heart sounds.
• Palpate his chest to find the point of maximal impulse.

GI system
• Note the contour and symmetry of his abdomen; check for distention.
• Note the position and color of his umbilicus; look for herniation.
• Auscultate his bowel sounds. Ask the patient if his bowel movements are regular.
• Percuss his abdomen for air and fluid.

• Palpate his abdomen for softness, firmness, and bladder height. Note any tenderness.
• Assess the six Fs: fat, fluid, flatus, feces, fetus (possibility of pregnancy), and fibroid tissue (or any unusual mass).

Genitourinary system
• Obtain a urine sample, if ordered; note its color and clearness.
• Ask the patient if he ever experiences any pain, burning, or bleeding during urination. Does he frequently feel the need to urinate? Is he ever incontinent? Is he able to empty his bladder completely? Does he awaken at night to urinate?
• Note the general appearance of the patient's genitalia.
• If your patient's female, ask when her last menstrual period occurred, and find out if her cycle is regular. In addition, ask if she could possibly be pregnant.

How to care for the postoperative patient

Keep in mind that the early postoperative period is the most critical phase of the patient's convalescence. Successful recovery from surgery depends largely on the quality of care delivered during this phase. When receiving a patient from the recovery room, follow these steps to ensure his well-being.

Before the patient returns
Before he returns to the medical-surgical unit, make sure you get appropriate information from the recovery room nurse. This includes the patient's name; the surgical procedure performed; the type of anesthetic used; his vital signs, level of consciousness, and general condition; and whether

any I.V. lines, catheters, or drainage tubes are present.

Based upon your conversation with the recovery room nurse, anticipate any special patient needs and obtain appropriate equipment.

When the patient arrives
Make sure equipment, such as an indwelling (Foley) catheter or I.V. tubing, doesn't become entangled in the bed frame or side rails as you assist with transfer from stretcher to bed.

As you help with the transfer, begin assessing your patient. For example, note his overall muscle coordination, his general level of consciousness, and his skin color.

After he's in bed, complete your assessment. Watch for any change in your patient's status, whether it's an obvious skin color change, or a more subtle indicator such as mild confusion.

Repeat assessment as often as your hospital policy requires. Usually, you'll assess your patient at least every 15 minutes the first hour, every 30 minutes for the next 2 hours, once an hour for 4 hours, and then every 4 hours.

Keep in mind that the patient's appearance can be dangerously deceptive. When he seems to be sleeping peacefully, the patient could actually be going into shock. Be vigilant in your assessment.

If your patient shows any signs or symptoms of a postoperative complication (no matter how subtle), increase the frequency of your assessments. Document all assessment findings in your nurses' notes.

Be sure to assess your patient for pain, nausea, or vomiting, ability to assume a comfortable position, and sensations of coldness or warmth. Take any steps necessary to decrease the discomfort he's feeling—for example, by providing medication or blankets.

When you compare your patient's vital signs with his previous values, keep in mind that minor variations sometimes occur after transport. For example, he may have an increase in blood pressure, pulse rate, and respiratory rate. However, report any significant changes to the doctor immediately.

Encourage your patient to cough and deep breathe frequently, as taught preoperatively.

Before leaving your patient
Help ensure his safety by lowering the bed to its lowest position, rais-

ing the side rails, and placing a call bell within his reach.

Notify family members of your patient's return from surgery and his general condition.

How to manage postoperative complications

Despite your best efforts to prepare the patient for surgery and its aftermath, complications may still occur. By knowing how to recognize and manage these complications, you can limit their effect. This chart provides a quick reference for managing common postoperative complications.

Hypovolemia This complication develops when the patient loses from 15% to 25% of his total blood volume. It may result from blood loss, severe dehydration, or third-space fluid sequestration caused by burns, peritonitis, intestinal obstruction, or acute pancreatitis. Abnormal fluid loss caused by excessive vomiting or diarrhea may also lead to hypovolemia.	*Check for:* • hypotension and a rapid, feeble pulse • cool, clammy, and perhaps slightly mottled skin • rapid, shallow respirations • oliguria or anuria • lethargy.	*To treat hypovolemia:* • Administer I.V. crystalloids, such as normal saline solution or lactated Ringer's, to increase blood pressure. • To restore urinary output and fluid volume, administer colloids, such as plasma, albumin, or dextran.
Septicemia and septic shock Septicemia, a severe systemic infection, may result from a break in asepsis during surgery or wound care. In ruptured appendix or ectopic pregnancy, peritonitis may lead to septicemia. The most common causative organism in postoperative septicemia is *Escherichia coli.* Septic shock occurs when bacteria release endotoxins into the bloodstream. The endotoxins decrease vascular resistance, resulting in dramatic hypotension.	*To detect septicemia, check for:* • fever • chills • rash • abdominal distention • prostration • pain • headache • nausea • diarrhea. *To detect septic shock, watch for these additional symptoms:* • a drastic fall in blood pressure • tachycardia • tachypnea • flushed skin • confusion • coma • an elevated white blood cell count.	*To treat septicemia and septic shock:* • Obtain specimens (blood, wound, and urine) for culture and sensitivity tests to verify the cause of septicemia and guide treatment. • Monitor vital signs and level of consciousness to detect septic shock. • Administer I.V. antibiotics, as ordered. Monitor serum peak and trough levels to help ensure effective therapy. • Give I.V. fluids and blood or blood products to restore circulating blood volume.
Atelectasis and pneumonia In atelectasis, incomplete lung expansion causes the distal alveoli to collapse. After surgery, this	*To detect atelectasis:* • auscultate for diminished or absent breath sounds over the affected area and note flatness on	*To treat atelectasis or pneumonia:* • Encourage the patient to cough and deep breathe every 1 to 2 hours while he's awake.

(continued)

How to manage postoperative complications *(continued)*

Atelectasis and pneumonia
(continued)
complication usually results from excessive retained secretions, which provide an excellent medium for bacterial growth and set the stage for stasis pneumonia.

In pneumonia, the alveoli and bronchioles become plugged with a fibrous exudate, making them firm and inelastic.

percussion
- observe for decreased chest expansion and mediastinal shift toward the side of collapse
- assess for fever, restlessness or confusion, worsening dyspnea, and increased blood pressure, pulse, and respiratory rate.

To detect pneumonia:
- watch for sudden onset of shaking chills with high fever and headache
- again, auscultate for diminished breath sounds or for telltale crackles over the affected lung area
- assess the patient for dyspnea; tachypnea; sharp chest pain that's exacerbated by inspiration; and a productive cough with pinkish or rust-colored sputum
- observe for cyanosis with hypoxemia, confirmed by arterial blood gas measurement
- look for patchy infiltrates or areas of consolidation appearing in chest X-rays.

- Show him how to use an incentive spirometer to facilitate deep breathing.
- Perform chest physiotherapy, if ordered.
- Administer antibiotics, if ordered.
- Administer humidified air or oxygen to loosen secretions, as ordered.
- Elevate the head of the patient's bed to reduce pressure on the diaphragm and to encourage optimal lung expansion.
- Reposition the patient at least every 2 hours to prevent pooling of secretions.

Thrombophlebitis and pulmonary embolism
Postoperative venous stasis associated with immobility predisposes the patient to thrombophlebitis — an inflammation of a vein, usually in the leg, accompanied by clot formation. If a clot breaks away, it may become lodged in the lung, causing a pulmonary embolism. This obstruction of a pulmonary artery interrupts blood flow, thereby decreasing gas exchange in the lungs.

To detect thrombophlebitis:
- watch for telltale signs along the length of a superficial vein. For example, the vessel will feel hard and thready or cordlike and will be extremely sensitive to pressure; the surrounding area may be red, swollen, and warm
- note any swelling along the affected leg, especially at the ankle, as well as pale, cold skin
- observe for aching or cramping pain, especially in the calf, when the patient walks or dorsiflexes the foot (Homans' sign).

To detect a pulmonary embolism:
- assess for sudden anginal or pleuritic chest pain; dyspnea; rapid, shallow respirations; cyanosis; restlessness; and possibly a thready pulse
- auscultate for fine to coarse crackles over the affected lung area.

To treat thrombophlebitis:
- Elevate the affected leg and apply warm compresses and antiembolism stockings.
- Offer analgesics, as ordered.
- Administer I.V. heparin, if ordered, to hinder clot formation. During this therapy, monitor prothrombin and partial thromboplastin times regularly, as ordered.

To treat a pulmonary embolism:
- Administer oxygen by face mask or nasal cannula, as ordered, to improve tissue perfusion.
- Administer an analgesic and I.V. heparin, as ordered.
- Elevate the head of the patient's bed to relieve dyspnea.

Where patients report pain

Pain is a universal phenomenon that everyone experiences at some point in life. Yet it's also a personal phenomenon—each individual's experience is unique. The sufferer is the only truly qualified expert on his pain. Physiology and perception are so completely intertwined that distinguishing one from the other often becomes impossible. Yet relieving pain is the oldest and most important nursing responsibility.

Leading temporary pain sites
In one study, patients identified the locations illustrated below as the five most common pain sites. The head, face, and lower extremities ranked highest as the sites of pain.

Leading persistent pain sites
In the same study, the back ranked highest among sites for persistent pain.

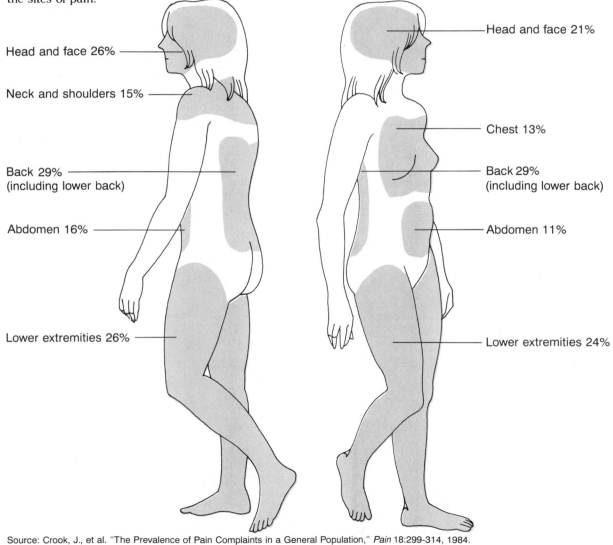

Head and face 26%

Neck and shoulders 15%

Back 29%
(including lower back)

Abdomen 16%

Lower extremities 26%

Head and face 21%

Chest 13%

Back 29%
(including lower back)

Abdomen 11%

Lower extremities 24%

Source: Crook, J., et al. "The Prevalence of Pain Complaints in a General Population," *Pain* 18:299-314, 1984.

Comparing cognitive pain control techniques

Teaching your patient mind-over-matter techniques will allow him to participate in treatment and achieve a degree of control over pain. However, the success of these techniques depends largely on the patient's motivation and commitment, and on your ability to convince him that they do indeed work. Use the following chart to determine which cognitive pain control techniques suit your patient best.

Technique	Advantages	Disadvantages
Behavior modification Reinforces behavior to increase activity level, reduce concentration on pain, and enhance a healthy life-style.	• Improved self-esteem. • Increased activity and productivity. • Decreased preoccupation with pain, suffering, and disability.	• Requires trained personnel and the cooperation of everyone involved, especially the family. Personnel unfamiliar with treatment plan may inadvertently undo its beneficial effects. • May be best suited for pain clinics. • Requires exploration of environmental and social problems that cause or worsen pain. Otherwise, relief may be short-term.
Biofeedback Gives immediate feedback on biological processes affected by relaxation, such as temperature and muscle tension.	• Enhances control over muscle tension. • Some people benefit most from immediate feedback.	• Patient may become dependent on biofeedback machine to achieve relaxation. • Patient may "fight" the machine, becoming more tense.
Distraction Removes attention from pain, focusing instead on some other activity, such as knitting or reading. Most effective when multiple senses are involved.	• Easily taught.	• Difficult if pain is unrelenting, unpredictable, and severe.
Guided imagery Encourages the imagining of a peaceful, pleasant scene, thereby providing a substitute for pain sensations.	• Patient can relive or experience peaceful, comfortable feelings to the exclusion of pain and suffering.	• Requires a vivid imagination and excellent concentration.
Hypnosis Concentrates the patient's attention on something other than pain. Since the mind can truly concentrate on only one thing at a time, pain is no longer the center of attention.	• May change the patient's perception of pain, create a sense of control, and provide long-lasting relief. • Posthypnotic suggestion can maintain pain relief.	• If hypnosis triggers a traumatic memory, it may increase the patient's anxiety and pain. • Patient tends to become dependent on the therapist.
Meditation Focuses concentration on the art of breathing and on a single number, object, or phrase to produce relaxation.	• Does not require a vivid imagination. • Focuses attention away from pain. • May be especially useful while waiting for an analgesic to work.	• Immediate results unlikely.

How to distinguish between acute and chronic pain

By definition, chronic pain lasts for a prolonged period; acute pain is of shorter duration. But at what point does acute pain become chronic? Use the chart below to better distinguish between acute and chronic pain.

	Acute	Chronic
Location	Often highly localized	Often poorly localized
Characteristics	Usually sharp, may radiate. Generally arises from an acute injury or disease process and passes quickly.	Dull, aching, diffuse, constant, nagging; may be intractable. Possibly associated with chronic pathology or recovery from a disease or injury.
Signs and symptoms	Associated with autonomic nervous system (ANS) response: increased blood pressure, tachycardia, diaphoresis, pallor, mydriasis, restlessness, grimacing, facial expression, anxiety.	ANS signs and symptoms may be absent; patient may appear exhausted, listless, depressed, and withdrawn.
Expectations	Patient often expects intervention to relieve pain.	Patient may expect intervention to reduce pain but may also expect pain to continue.

Therapeutic alternatives to common surgeries

Alternative treatments frequently offer significant advantages over surgery: reduced cost, at-home patient management, and decreased interruption of the patient's life-style.

Disorder	Surgery	Alternatives	Comments
Herniated disk	Laminectomy and spinal fusion	Bed rest, traction, moist heat, muscle relaxants, chemonucleolysis (with chymopapain)	Moist heat penetrates deeper and produces less perspiration than dry heat, but it carries a higher risk of burns. Apply with caution to heat-sensitive areas such as scar tissue or stomas. Muscle relaxants may cause drowsiness and impaired cognitive and motor function; avoid mixing with alcohol or other central nervous system depressants.
Gallstones (cholelithiasis)	Cholecystectomy	Drug therapy with chenodiol or ursodeoxycholic acid, extracorporeal shock wave lithotripsy (ESWL)	ESWL may be contraindicated in pregnancy or in a patient with a pacemaker. It requires administration of an anesthetic and may have to be repeated for large or multiple calculi.

(continued)

Therapeutic alternatives to common surgeries (continued)

Disorder	Surgery	Alternatives	Comments
Carpal tunnel syndrome	Surgical decompression	Hydrotherapy, splinting, corticosteroid injections	Splinting will usually prove successful in relieving early unilateral symptoms. Corticosteroids will usually provide temporary relief of symptoms, especially if strenuous use of hands continues.
Renal calculi	Pyelolithotomy, nephrolithotomy, calculi basketing	ESWL, percutaneous ultrasonic lithotripsy	Percutaneous ultrasonic lithotripsy greatly reduces recovery time compared with conventional surgery. It may also help remove residual fragments following ESWL.
Coronary artery disease	Coronary artery bypass grafting (CABG)	Thrombolytic agents (streptokinase, alteplase, urokinase), percutaneous transluminal coronary angioplasty (PTCA), drug therapy with anticoagulants, antilipemic agents, vasodilators	PTCA allows for shorter hospital stays with fewer complications. However, it's appropriate for only about 10% of CABG patients.
Aneurysms	Excision, wrapping, clipping	Embolization, antihypertensive therapy, steroids, rest, altering life-style to decrease stress	Embolization proves useful when an arteriovenous malformation is inaccessible to surgery.
Burns, skin ulcer	Skin graft	Drug therapy with silver sulfadiazine, wet dressing, dry dressing, biological dressing	Biological dressings may be made from cadavers, amniotic membranes, or animals. They provide protection against infection and fluid loss without the discomfort of autologous grafting.
Peptic or duodenal ulcer	Gastrectomy	Antacids, histamine receptor antagonists (cimetidine), anticholinergics, rest, exercise	Drug therapy usually proves successful with early, uncomplicated disease.
Ulcerative colitis	Colectomy with ileostomy	Anti-inflammatory agents (sulfasalazine), adrenal corticosteroids, and antidiarrheal drugs	Drug therapy demands fewer life-style changes and does less harm to body image than colectomy.
Endometriosis	Hysterectomy with bilateral salpingo-oophorectomy	Hormones (danazol), high-dose oral contraceptives	Hormone therapy may preserve child-bearing capabilities and causes less damage to sexual identity than surgery.

Profiles of common therapeutic procedures

Therapeutic procedures may require highly specialized training or simply the application of basic nursing skills. Becoming familiar with them can diminish your anxiety about new nursing assignments and ensure good patient care.

Arthrocentesis
During this procedure, the doctor inserts a needle into the joint space to aspirate synovial fluid or blood, to instill corticosteroids or other anti-inflammatory drugs, or to obtain a specimen for diagnostic testing. Most commonly performed on the knee, arthrocentesis may also be done on the elbow, shoulder, or other joints.

Purpose: Arthrocentesis commonly provides adjunctive treatment for orthopedic disorders, such as joint trauma or septic arthritis.

Autotransfusion
This procedure collects, filtrates, and reinfuses a patient's own blood. Because autotransfused blood is autologous, it eliminates disease transmission, transfusion reactions, and isoimmunization.

During autotransfusion, a vacuum system sucks shed blood through a sterile chest tube and into a sterile canister liner. The canister contains citrate phosphate dextrose to prevent clotting of the collected blood, and a fine-screen filter to remove microaggregated platelets, air bubbles, fat, and debris. Upon reinfusion, the liner is removed from the canister and the blood is transfused back to the patient.

Purpose: Autotransfusion retrieves blood for patients suffering from massive blood loss. Blood loss may result from hemothorax or primary injuries of the lungs; liver; chest wall; heart; pulmonary vessels; spleen; kidneys; inferior vena cava; and iliac, portal, and subclavian veins.

Barbiturate coma
In this treatment, the patient receives high I.V. doses of a short-acting barbiturate (such as pentobarbital or phenobarbital) to produce coma.

Purpose: When conventional treatments—such as fluid restriction, diuretic or corticosteroid therapy, or ventricular shunting—fail to correct sustained or acute episodes of increased intracranial pressure (ICP), the doctor may order barbiturate coma to reduce the patient's metabolic rate and cerebral blood flow, thereby relieving increased ICP and preventing brain tissue damage.

Blood transfusion
Transfusion may deliver whole blood or such blood components as packed red cells (blood in which 80% of the plasma has been removed), platelets (the smallest cells of the blood necessary for coagulation), fresh frozen plasma (the liquid portion of blood frozen within a few hours of collection), or granulocytes (blood cells that help fight bacterial infection).

Purpose: Transfusions help treat massive hemorrhage as well as a range of hematologic disorders. *Whole blood transfusion replenishes* both the volume and oxygen-carrying capacity of the circulatory system. *Packed cells* restore the patient's oxygen-carrying capacity, but they don't replenish lost blood volume. They're used to treat symptomatic anemia. *Platelets* may be administered prophylactically or therapeutically. Candidates for platelet transfusion include patients with aplastic anemia or leukemia or those who are receiving antineoplastic chemotherapy. *Fresh frozen plasma* contains all of the blood's liquid protein factors and primarily provides treatment for clotting factor deficiencies. Granulocytopenic patients who have an infection that doesn't respond to antibiotics require a transfusion of *granulocytes.*

Cerebrospinal fluid drainage: ventricular catheter and the subarachnoid screw
To drain cerebrospinal fluid (CSF), the surgeon inserts a ventricular catheter or a subarachnoid screw through a twist drill hole created in the skull. The ventricular catheter consists of a small polyethylene cannula and reservoir; the surgeon introduces it into a lateral ventricle. The subarachnoid screw, a small hollow steel screw with a sensor tip, is inserted into the subarachnoid space. Both devices possess a built-in transducer to convert ICP to electrical impulses that create visible wave forms and a drain system.

Purpose: Besides monitoring increased ICP, the ventricular catheter and the subarachnoid screw allow periodic drainage of the CSF from the brain, thereby reducing ICP. The ventricular catheter may provide a continuous CSF drainage system.

Continuous passive motion
This treatment uses a electrically powered or manually operated machine attached to the patient's bed to automatically move a joint through its normal range of motion for an extended time. The nurse sets the machine to the degree of flexion and extension prescribed.

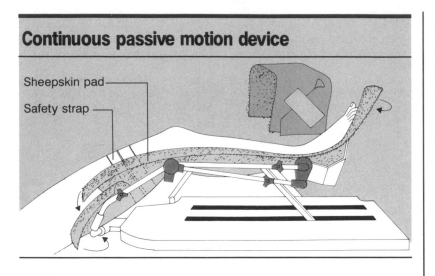

Continuous passive motion device

Sheepskin pad

Safety strap

Purpose: An alternative to nurse-assisted passive range-of-motion exercises, continuous passive motion may help patients recover from total hip or knee replacement; internal fixation of the knee; ankle fractures; or removal of the synovial membrane in the knee or other major joints.

Defibrillation
Defibrillation delivers a strong burst of electric current to the heart through paddles applied to the patient's chest. It completely depolarizes the myocardium, allowing the heart's natural pacemaker to regain control of cardiac rhythm. The procedure is successful about 40% of the time.

Purpose: Defibrillation is the treatment of choice for ventricular fibrillation and pulseless ventricular tachycardia. It may also benefit patients in asystole who show signs of ventricular fibrillation. Because ventricular fibrillation can lead to irreparable brain damage, you must perform defibrillation as soon as possible, even before intubating the patient or administering drugs.

Esophagogastric tamponade
In this emergency treatment, the doctor inserts a multilumen esophageal tube through the patient's nostril or sometimes through his mouth, and then passes it through the esophagus into the stomach. Inflation of the tube's esophageal and gastric balloons exerts pressure on varices and stops bleeding, while a suction lumen allows esophageal and gastric contents to be aspirated.

Purpose: Esophagogastric tamponade provides temporary control of esophageal or gastric hemorrhage from ruptured varices and prevents excessive blood loss.

Extracorporeal shock wave lithotripsy (ESWL)
A revolutionary noninvasive technique, ESWL uses high-energy shock waves to break up renal calculi. After being anesthetized, the patient is placed in a water tank with his affected kidney positioned over an electric spark generator. This generator creates high-energy shock waves that shatter calculi without damaging surrounding tissue.

Purpose: ESWL breaks obstructive renal calculi into fine particles that the patient can easily excrete. The doctor may order ESWL as a preventive measure in a patient with potentially obstructive calculi, or as emergency treatment for acute obstruction.

Gastric lavage (iced)
This procedure involves intubating the patient with a large bore single or double lumen tube and then instilling an irrigating fluid. The nurse advances the tube into the patient's mouth or nostril. After making sure the tube is correctly placed, she instills a total of about 250 ml of irrigating fluid, which has been chilled in a basin of ice. After waiting about 30 seconds, she begins aspirating the fluid into a syringe. Lavage may continue until aspirated fluid becomes clear.

Purpose: Iced fluid causes vasoconstriction of GI vessels, and can effectively control upper GI hemorrhage. The doctor may order addition of a vasoconstrictor to the irrigating fluid to enhance this effect.

Hemodialysis
This form of dialysis removes toxic wastes and other impurities from the blood of a patient with renal failure. In this technique, the blood is removed through a surgically created access site, pumped through a dialyzing unit to remove toxins, and then returned to the body. By extracting byproducts of protein metabolism (notably urea and uric acid), as well as creatinine and excess water, hemodialysis helps restore or maintain acid-base and electrolyte balance and prevent uremic complications.

Purpose: Hemodialysis removes toxic wastes from the blood until renal failure resolves, kidney transplant can be performed, or the patient dies.

Immobilization

Immobilization devices come in many different forms. *Braces* are support devices of metal, leather and hard plastic, usually worn externally. A patient may wear a *cast* made of plaster or synthetic material just about anywhere, from a single finger to full body coverage. Made of soft foam or metal and plastic components, *collars* fit around the neck and under the chin. *Skeletal traction* involves placing a pin through a bone and attaching a traction apparatus. *Skin traction* consists of weights, ropes, pulleys, and slings applied to the skin and soft tissue, thereby pulling on the skeletal system. *Slings* are composed of a soft material or Elastoplast fabric. *Splints* are made of leather, metal, and hard plastic components.

Purpose: These devices help heal injured bones, joints, and surrounding soft tissue by maintaining proper alignment, limiting movement, and relieving pressure and pain. Besides enhancing the stability of an injured or weakened joint, *braces* may help correct neuromuscular defects in cerebral palsy, other spastic disorders, and scoliosis. *Casts* help to heal traumatic injuries and to correct congenital deformities. *Collars* support and align an injured or weakened cervical spine. *Skeletal traction* may enhance healing of fractures, help correct congenital abnormalities, or help stabilize spinal degeneration. *Skin traction* relieves muscle spasms and restricts movement and provides for proper alignment in cervical disk disease, pelvic fractures of the extremities, and spinal deformities. *Slings* may support an injured hand or wrist, or help treat other upper extremity problems such as fractures of

the scapula or clavicle and shoulder dislocation. *Splints* provide support for injured or weakened limbs or digits. They may also help correct deformities, such as mallet finger, and help treat spinal tuberculosis; inflammatory lesions of the hip, spine, or shoulder; hip dislocation or dysplasia; long-bone fractures; scoliosis; and foot drop.

Incentive spirometry

A *flow incentive spirometer* measures the patient's inspiratory effort or flow rate, in cubic centimeters per second. A *volume incentive spirometer* does this as well. In addition, it calculates the volume of air the patient inhales.

Purpose: Primarily used postoperatively, incentive spirometry encourages the patient to produce deep, sustained inspiratory efforts that normally occur as yawns or sighs. As the patient steadily strives to meet his target flow and volume, he prevents or reverses atelectasis that occurs secondary to shallow respirations. Incentive spirometry also improves clearance of secretions by increasing the respiratory volume available for coughing.

Intra-aortic balloon counterpulsation (IABC)

In this procedure, the doctor threads a balloon catheter through the femoral artery into the descending thoracic aorta. Once the catheter's in place, he connects its external end to a pump that automatically inflates the balloon in early diastole and deflates it just before systole.

Purpose: IABC temporarily reduces left ventricular work load and improves coronary perfusion. It's used to treat cardiogenic shock from acute MI; septic shock; intractable angina pectoris before surgery; intractable ventricular dysrhythmias; and ventricular,

septal, or papillary muscle ruptures. Patients who suffer pump failure before or after cardiac surgery may also undergo IABC.

This procedure may help sustain a patient's life in the operating room as well as during bedside emergencies. For example, IABC may augment cardiac function in a operating room patient who can't be weaned from a cardiac bypass machine.

Mechanical ventilation

Mechanical ventilation artificially controls or assists a patient's respirations. Typically requiring an endotracheal tube or tracheostomy tube, it can deliver room air under positive pressure or oxygen-enriched air in concentrations of up to 100%.

Major types of mechanical ventilation systems include positive-pressure, negative-pressure, and high-frequency ventilation (HFV). Positive pressure systems can be volume-cycled or pressure-cycled and may deliver positive-end expiratory pressure or continuous positive airway pressure. Negative-pressure systems provide ventilation for patients unable to generate adequate inspiratory pressure. HFV systems provide high ventilation rates with low peak airway pressures.

Purpose: Mechanical ventilation decreases the work of breathing and provides supporting ventilation to patients with profoundly impaired gas exchange. Signs of inadequate respiration include hypoxia, hypercapnia, and increased work of breathing (nasal flaring, intercostal retraction, decreased blood pressure, and diaphoresis).

Nasal balloon catheter

This treatment provides an alternative for posterior nasal packing. The doctor lubricates the nasal balloon catheter with an antibiotic ointment and inserts it through the patient's nostril. He then inflates the balloon by inserting sterile saline solution into the appropriate valve.

The *single cuffed nasal balloon catheter* consists of two parts: a cuff that, when inflated, compresses the blood vessels; and a soft, collapsible outside bulb that prevents the catheter from slipping out of place posteriorly. The *double cuffed catheter* consists of a posterior cuff that, when installed, secures the catheter in the nasopharynx; an anterior cuff that, when inflated, compresses the blood vessels; and a central airway that helps the patient breathe more comfortably.

Purpose: Single and double cuffed catheters control posterior epistaxis.

Nasal packing
If a patient has severe bleeding from the anterior nose, the doctor applies an anterior nasal pack. He uses forceps to layer petrolatum or iodoform gauze strips horizontally in the patient's anterior nostrils, usually near the turbinates. Horizontal layers ensure uniform packing and prevent displacement of the pack into the patient's throat.

If the patient bleeds from the posterior nose, the doctor inserts a lubricated catheter into the nose and advances it into the nasopharynx. When the catheter appears in the nasopharynx, the doctor pulls it out through the mouth and secures it to the sutures of the posterior pack. Then he withdraws the catheter through the nose, pulling the pack into its proper position behind the soft palate and against the posterior part of the septum. Insertion of a posterior pack requires sedation and hospitalization.

Purpose: To control severe epistaxis that doesn't respond to direct pressure or cautery.

Nasoenteric decompression
This treatment involves inserting a long, weighted nasoenteric tube through the patient's stomach and into the intestinal tract. The tube is then propelled by peristalsis through the intestine to, and possibly through, an obstruction.

Purpose: Along with fluid and electrolyte replacement, nasoenteric decompression helps relieve acute intestinal obstruction resulting from polyps, adhesions, fecal impaction, volvulus, or localized carcinoma. It may also be performed to aspirate gastric contents for examination or to prevent nausea, vomiting, and abdominal distention after GI surgery.

Peritoneal dialysis
Peritoneal dialysis uses the patient's own peritoneal membrane as semipermeable dialyzing membrane to remove toxins from the blood. In this procedure, the nurse instills a hypertonic dialyzing solution through a catheter inserted into the peritoneal cavity. Then, by diffusion, excessive concentrates of electrolytes and uremic toxins in the blood move across the peritoneal membrane into the dialysis solution. Next, by osmosis, excessive water in the blood does the same. After an appropriate dwelling time, the nurse allows the dialysis solution to drain from the peritoneal cavity, taking toxins and wastes with it. Peritoneal dialysis may be performed manually, by an automatic or semiautomatic cycler machine, or as continuous ambulatory peritoneal dialysis.

Purpose: Peritoneal dialysis removes toxic wastes from the blood of a patient with renal failure. It's simpler, less costly, safer, and less stressful than hemodialysis, and nearly as effective. A patient may undergo peritoneal dialysis until his disease resolves, or he receives a kidney transplant, or until he requires hemodialysis.

Plasmapheresis
Also called therapeutic plasma exchange or TPE, plasmapheresis involves withdrawing blood from a patient and dividing it into plasma and formed elements (red cells, white cells, platelets). The plasma is collected in a container for disposal, while the formed elements are mixed with a plasma replacement solution and returned to the patient through another vein. Alternatively, the plasma is separated, filtered to remove a specific disease mediator, and then returned to the patient.

Purpose: By removing and replacing the plasma, plasmapheresis cleans the blood of harmful substances such as toxins, and of disease mediators, such as immune complexes and autoantibodies. It has several neurologic applications, including Guillain-Barré syndrome, multiple sclerosis, and especially myasthenia gravis.

Radioactive iodine therapy
This procedure takes place in the nuclear medicine or radiation therapy department. The patient receives an oral dose of the isotope iodine 131 (^{131}I) in solution. ^{131}I is rapidly absorbed and concentrated in the thyroid as if it were normal iodine. Effective dosage depends on thyroid uptake, the length of time ^{131}I remains within the gland, and the sensitivity of thyroid cells to radiation.

Purpose: An alternative to thyroidectomy or drug therapy, ^{131}I treats hyperthyroidism and provides adjunctive treatment for thyroid cancer. Absorption of ^{131}I by the thyroid causes acute radiation thyroiditis and gradual thyroid atrophy, eventually leading to reduced thyroid hormone levels.

Sitz bath

A sitz bath is a bath in which the patient immerses only his hips or buttocks in water or saline solution. For heat application, water temperature should be 110° F to 115° F (43° C to 46° C). Water temperature should be 94° F to 98° F (34° C to 37° C). Most institutions have sitz bath basins that fit into toilet seats.

Purpose: Sitz baths may benefit patients who've undergone rectal or perineal surgery. They help promote healing of a perineal wound, decrease edema, and relieve perineal pain.

Transcutaneous electrical nerve stimulation (TENS)

This technique requires a portable battery-powered generator that sends a mild current through skin points related to the patient's pain. A physical therapist or specially trained nurse may perform TENS. After placing gelled electrodes on the patient's skin, she turns the generator unit on, with the pulse width and rate set as recommended, and adjusts the intensity until she achieves the desired effect.

Purpose: This approach helps relieve both acute and chronic pain. Electrical impulses sent through peripheral nerves block transmission of pain impulses to the brain. Indications include back pain, and pain after knee, hip, or lower back surgery, as well as any other postoperative pain. Patients with dental pain, labor pain, peripheral neuropathy, nerve injury, postherpetic neuralgia, reflex sympathetic dystrophy, musculoskeletal trauma, arthritis, and phantom limb pain also may benefit.

Ultraviolet light treatments

A patient may undergo this procedure in the hospital or doctor's of-

fice, or at home. A bank of high-intensity fluorescent bulbs set into a reflective cabinet may emit therapeutic light. Alternatively, the patient may use a small sunlamp at home.

Therapy with ultraviolet light uses one of two possible wavelengths: ultraviolet light B (UVB), the component of sunlight that causes sunburn, or ultraviolet light A (UVA). UVA has no effect on normal skin, but use of the drug psoralen creates an artificial sensitivity to UVA by binding with the DNA in epidermal basal cells. The combination of UVA with psoralen is called photochemotherapy or PUVA therapy.

Purpose: Ultraviolet light therapy decreases epidermal cell proliferation, probably by inhibiting DNA synthesis. It helps treat psoriasis, mycosis fungoides, atopic dermatitis, and uremic pruritus.

Vaginal dilation

The patient begins vaginal dilation by inserting one lubricated finger, or the smallest in a series of graduated plastic dilators, into her vagina and holding it there for a few minutes. After she successfully completes this exercise, she next introduces two fingers or the next size dilator into her vagina. She continues to gradually increase the size of the dilator introduced until it approximates the size of the penis.

Purpose: Dilation treats vaginismus by reducing the patient's anxiety about vaginal penetration.

Ventricular shunting

This treatment involves inserting a catheter into the ventricular system to drain CSF into another body sac (usually the peritoneal sac) for absorption. The shunt extends from the cerebral ventricle to the scalp, where it's tunneled under the skin to the appropriate

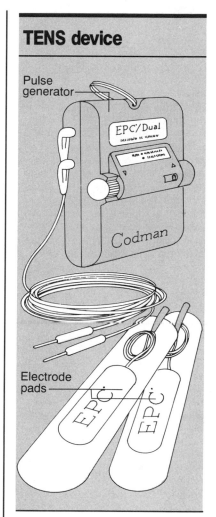

TENS device

Pulse generator

EPC/Dual

Codman

Electrode pads

EPC   EPC

cavity. Implantation of the shunt may require a craniotomy.

Purpose: Both adult and pediatric patients may undergo shunt implantation. Ventricular shunts treat both communicating and noncommunicating hydrocephalus. By draining excessive CSF or relieving blockage, shunting can lower ICP and prevent brain damage caused by persistently elevated ICP.

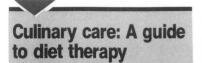

Culinary care: A guide to diet therapy

Calorie-modified diet for obese patients

Say the word "diet" to most patients and they'll think of a low-calorie diet. These diets are among the most popular—and most abused—forms of self-treatment. A large part of your job with obese patients will be to counter popular misconceptions about dieting. Explain that a balanced low-calorie diet that results in a weight loss of a pound or so a week is the most effective means of long-term weight loss.

Depending on the obese patient's sex, weight, and activity level, the doctor may prescribe a diet providing 1,000 to 1,800 calories a day, with about 20% of them coming from protein. For the patient whose obesity presents an immediate threat to life, the doctor will probably recommend an extremely low-calorie diet—about 300 to 700 calories a day—that includes high-quality protein and few carbohydrates.

A weight-reduction diet includes foods from all four groups. Besides limiting carbohydrates, it restricts fats and alcohol and includes fiber to reduce caloric density and slow digestion.

Nursing considerations

• Encourage the patient to join a weight-loss support group.
• Help him set reasonable weight-loss goals, and stress that gradual reduction helps keep weight from returning.
• Weigh the patient weekly to chart his progress. Because he'll ideally be losing only 1 lb per week, explain to him that more frequent weighings aren't necessary. In fact, daily fluctuations result primarily from fluid retention

and are likely to be misleading.
• Have the patient keep a food diary and bring it in when he's weighed. Review with him the choices and amounts of foods that he eats. Be sure that the patient is drinking sufficient fluids to prevent orthostatic hypotension.
• Monitor urine nitrogen levels in an overweight patient. The reason? Nitrogen imbalance and loss of lean tissue mass are especially prevalent in a patient on an extremely low-calorie diet.
• Enlist the support of the patient's family. Their encouragement and cooperation are vital to help the patient maintain his diet.
• Suggest that the overweight patient plan menus and shopping lists for the week to prevent impulse-buying and eating. Encourage him to have fish and poultry instead of red meat, to substitute polyunsaturated fats for saturated ones, and to eat vegetables and fruits instead of sweets.
• Warn the patient to expect setbacks, and explore ways of overcoming them. Encourage the patient not to abandon his diet simply because he sometimes "cheats"; explain that occasional noncompliance matters little to long-term success. Help him use behavior modification techniques to reduce noncompliance; for example, set a goal of slowly reducing the number of "cheating" episodes per week.
• Tell the patient on a reducing diet to avoid alcohol since it can cause a hypoglycemic response.
• Tell the female patient who's losing weight to watch for menstrual disorders and to report them to her doctor. Prolonged dieting can cause amenorrhea.
• Be sure that the patient regulates his energy expenditure. The overweight person should develop an exercise program.
• Tell the patient that he can eat several small meals throughout the day instead of three regular ones (but tell him not to eat too

heavily in the evening hours, since these calories will tend to be converted into fat as he sleeps).
• Above all, be positive; tell the patient that although change may come slowly and painfully, the benefits are well worth the struggle.

Calorie-modified diet for underweight patients

For some patients, a calorie-modified diet means *increased* caloric intake. Patients may be underweight because of poor eating patterns; excessive activity (for example, athletic training); improper food absorption; wasting diseases, such as cancer or hyperthyroidism; or anorexia nervosa. For these patients, the goal of therapy is to add 500 to 1,000 calories a day through a diet that's high in protein and carbohydrates, with moderate amounts of fat.

Gradually increase caloric intake over time so that he can adjust to the added amounts. Recommend a hearty breakfast and regular meals. Use extra helpings, snacks, and concentrated supplements to increase caloric intake.

Nursing considerations

• Suggest to the underweight patient that he eat dried fruits and nuts for between-meal snacks, as

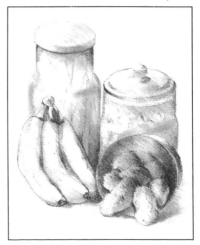

they're high in calories and nutritious.

• Recommend that the patient eat bananas with breakfast and that he have potatoes, pasta, noodles, or rice at least twice a day.

• Enlist the support of the patient's family. Their encouragement and cooperation are vital to help the patient maintain his diet.

• Weigh the patient weekly to chart his progress. Since he will ideally be gaining only 1 lb per week, explain to him that more frequent weighings aren't necessary. In fact, daily fluctuations primarily result from fluid retention and are likely to be misleading.

• Have the patient keep a food diary and bring it in when he's weighed. Review with him the choices and amounts of foods that he eats. Be sure that the patient drinks sufficient fluids to prevent orthostatic hypotension.

• Be sure that the patient regulates his energy expenditure. The underweight patient may need to cut down on his activities.

High-fiber diet

Fiber promotes peristalsis, reduces intestinal transit time, and increases stool volume and weight. A high-fiber diet can help prevent diverticulitis by distending the colon and relieving pressure on the intestinal wall. It can help treat obesity by decreasing caloric density and promoting a feeling of fullness. Water-soluble fibers, such as pectin, can lower serum cholesterol levels and help prevent coronary artery disease. A high-fiber, low-cholesterol diet can help diabetic patients reduce — and in some cases, eliminate — their need for insulin and oral hypoglycemic drugs, apparently by promoting a moderate blood glucose response to ingested food and enhancing tissue sensitivity to insulin. Some researchers even believe that a high-fiber diet can prevent bowel cancer by reducing the concentration of carcinogens in fecal matter.

Diabetic patients on a high-fiber diet should consume 30 to 50 g of fiber a day; for other patients, the diet is more flexible and should simply include as much fiber as practical.

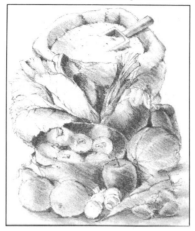

Nursing considerations

• A high-fiber diet should include breads and baked goods made from 100% whole wheat or whole rye flour instead of white flour. Other sources of high fiber include granola, oatmeal, unpeeled apples and other fruits, and raw and leafy vegetables, such as carrots and lettuce. Coarsely ground bran can be added to cereals, muffins, or bread as a further fiber supplement. Fiber supplements made from guar gums or methylcellulose may also be added.

• With the dietitian, help the patient and his family identify foods that are high in fiber. Explain that mineral and vitamin deficiencies may occur because of reduced absorption. Mention that the patient needs to eat a variety of foods and may have to take vitamin and mineral supplements.

• Tell the patient that side effects, such as a bloated feeling and diarrhea, can be minimized by adding fiber to his diet gradually.

• If the patient on a high-fiber diet doesn't have at least one soft stool per day, tell him to add a bran supplement to his diet.

• Advise the female patient to increase her calcium intake to prevent osteoporosis. Tell her to drink at least two glasses of milk a day and to eat cheese and yogurt. If she's trying to lose weight or suffers from diabetes, recommend skim milk and low-fat cheese.

• Tell the patient to eat plenty of iron-rich foods, such as liver. To increase his zinc intake, recommend meat, nuts, beans, wheat germ, and cheese.

• Instruct him to take a list of high-fiber foods with him when he grocery shops to remind him of which foods to buy.

• Remind the patient to schedule follow-up appointments to evaluate his progress and assess his nutritional status.

Low-fiber diet

Although dietary fiber is usually beneficial, its use may need to be restricted in patients who are suffering from indigestion, gastric reflux, or diarrhea. In addition, a low-fiber diet is normally ordered both before and after GI surgery. In all of these instances, the diet aims to eliminate mechanical stimulation of an inflamed or irritated GI tract.

Because low-fiber diets lack sufficient vitamins and minerals, they can be used for only a limited time.

Nursing considerations

• A low-fiber diet consists of soft, mild food. It excludes raw vegetables and fruits, nuts, seeds, coarse breads, and strong seasonings. Fried foods and fats are limited, since they can increase gastric reflux. The patient may eat milk and dairy products and should cook meats and vegetables until they're quite tender.

• Explain that mineral and vitamin deficiencies may occur with a low-fiber diet. Mention that the patient needs to eat a variety of foods

and may have to take vitamin and mineral supplements.
• Remind the patient to schedule follow-up appointments to evaluate his progress and assess his nutritional status.

High-protein diet
A high-protein diet may be necessary for those with increased body-building needs, such as growing children, athletes, and pregnant women. In addition, a high-protein diet can benefit patients with increased tissue breakdown or with nitrogen depletion caused by stress or increased secretions of thyroid or glucocorticoid hormones. And it's often used in patients who've suffered protein loss because of immobilization, dietary deficiency, advanced age, infection, alcoholism, drug addiction, or chronic disease.

The beneficial effects of a high-protein diet can be striking. In just a few weeks the patient's general health and well-being begin to improve. He gains weight and feels stronger; his resistance to infection increases and wounds heal more quickly.

The goal of a high-protein diet is to provide approximately 125 g of protein and 2,500 calories each day.
• Tell the patient to select one-half to two-thirds of the day's protein allowance from complete-protein foods and to divide his protein allowance as evenly as possible among the meals of the day.
• Suggest that he add nonfat dry milk to regular milk and to casseroles to increase their protein content.
• Tell the patient who requires a high-protein diet that he also needs to eat plenty of carbohydrates; otherwise, the body simply burns protein as fuel.
• If the patient on a high-protein diet is hospitalized, weigh him daily; if he's an outpatient, weigh him weekly. Expect to see a weight gain of 1 to 2 lb per week.

• Monitor him for signs of protein deficiency, such as weakness, decreased resistance to infection, and low hemoglobin levels. In severe protein deficiency, monitor serum albumin levels. Also check for edema, a sign of albumin deficiency.
• Encourage the patient to return for frequent checkups.
• Remind the patient to increase his protein and calorie consumption gradually.

Low-protein diet
Some patients suffer an *excess* of protein and must adhere to a low-protein regimen. Typically, these patients have illnesses that impair the body's ability to eliminate the products of protein catabolism — for example, end-stage renal disease or severe hepatic disease.

A *low-protein diet* should provide 75% of the dietary protein allowance in the form of high-value protein, such as that found in eggs. As with high-protein regimens, the protein allowance should be distributed as evenly as possible among meals. To minimize protein catabolism, be sure the diet includes enough calories to meet the patient's energy requirements. The prescribed diet may also include supplements to prevent amino acid deficiencies.

Nursing considerations
• Emphasize to the patient that he'll need to limit the size of portions as well as the types of foods that he eats; using the food on his hospital tray or plastic models, show him the correct portion size for various foods.
• Show him how to use a food scale, and have him give you a return demonstration.
• If the patient on a low-protein diet has end-stage renal disease, monitor his blood urea nitrogen and serum creatinine levels; these levels reflect the clearance of the end products of protein metabolism. Also monitor the glomerular

filtration rate (GFR); it can serve as a guide for the degree to which proteins need to be restricted. For example, a patient with a GFR of 10 to 15 ml/minute should restrict protein intake to 40 to 55 g/day. Similarly, monitor urine flow to determine how much fluid the patient should be consuming; daily fluid intake should be 500 to 600 ml more than urine output.
• If the patient's receiving a low-protein diet because of liver disease, monitor his serum ammonia levels daily and watch for signs of ammonia intoxication, such as flapping hand motions or tremors. Elevated levels will require further dietary restrictions.
• Encourage the patient to return for frequent checkups.
• Recommend a vegetarian cookbook.

Low-cholesterol diet
Dietary therapy represents the first line of defense in the fight against high serum cholesterol levels and associated cardiovascular complications. However, this diet isn't curative, so most patients must remain on it permanently. Typically, results don't become apparent for at least 3 months.

Explain to the patient that not all fats are the same; saturated fats (which are often solid, such as butter or animal fat) tend to be converted to cholesterol. Serum cholesterol levels can be significantly reduced by using monounsaturated and polyunsaturated fats (such as olive oil, safflower oil, and corn oil). Tell him to strive toward a diet in which the ratio of polyunsaturated to saturated fats is about 1:1 (in the typical American diet, it's about 1:3).

Also explain the role of low-density lipoprotein (LDL) in cardiovascular disease. Tell the patient that LDL carries cholesterol to the cells and that high LDL levels can therefore promote the accumulation of cholesterol in arterial walls. Explain that high-density lipoprotein (HDL), by contrast, is desirable, since it helps remove cholesterol from the blood and transport it to the liver for elimination.

Nursing considerations
• The low-cholesterol diet doesn't usually produce side effects. However, if the patient's dietary cholesterol intake is very low, he may require vitamin A supplements. He may also require mineral supplements, since large amounts of dietary fiber may interfere with absorption of calcium, iron, and zinc.
• Monitor serum cholesterol level and HDL, LDL, and VLDL (very low-density lipoprotein) fractions to evaluate treatment. Have the patient keep a chart of these values to provide positive reinforcement of the diet.
• To promote compliance, encourage the patient to master one part of the diet at a time. For example, he may choose to limit his consumption of red meat before reducing the number of eggs that he eats.
• When the patient eats out, recommend that he select salads and vegetables, that he choose poultry over red meat, and that he have simply prepared dishes (but not fried food) rather than those that come with rich sauces or dressings. Pasta and Chinese dishes especially vegetarian ones — are often good choices; however, tell the patient to avoid pasta dishes that contain large amounts of whole-milk cheeses.
• High-fiber foods such as whole grain cereal and bread, fruits, and raw vegetables may reduce cholesterol levels. Oat cereals, apples, leafy and root vegetables may also help to reduce cholesterol levels. Suggest beans as an alternate source of protein.
• Be sure the patient ingests enough dairy products to make up for impaired calcium absorption. He should eat beans and leafy

vegetables to obtain iron and zinc, which may be poorly absorbed with high amounts of fiber.
• Recommend a cooking spray for frying and baking.
• Tell the patient to use tub margarines rather than the stick form and to select a type that's high in polyunsaturated or monounsaturated fat. Tell him to buy a brand that shows vegetable oils first in the list of ingredients.
• Suggest that he make soups or stews a day ahead of time and refrigerate them; he can then skim off the hardened fat before reheating.
• Recommend to the patient that he use egg substitutes or egg whites in recipes calling for eggs. Advise him that low-cholesterol substitutes may replace mayonnaise, salad dressings, hot dogs, egg noodles, ice cream, and many other foods.

Low-fat diet
A low-fat diet benefits a variety of patients. For instance, in patients with malabsorption disorders secondary to hepatic or pancreatic disease, it reduces problems caused by impaired fat digestion and absorption. In those with gallbladder disease, it can diminish fat-induced contractions of the gallbladder; and while it can't dissolve gallstones or prevent attacks, it can provide symptomatic relief. In patients with gout, the diet can help prevent uric acid retention. Many researchers believe that it can also help patients with multiple sclerosis, slowing the progression of disease and reducing the incidence of new attacks. And in patients with hyperlipoproteinemia, a low-fat diet can sometimes reduce serum levels of lipoproteins and, if it's started early in life, can help prevent atherosclerosis in patients with hereditary hyperlipoproteinemia.

Most Americans eat about 160 g of fat per day, accounting for some 40% of their caloric intake. Nutri-

tionists recommend limiting fat to no more than 30% of total caloric intake — that is, about 120 g/day. Patients with certain disorders may require a diet that's even lower in fat: either one containing only 50 g of fat per day or an extremely low-fat diet containing only 25 to 30 g of fat per day.

Nursing considerations
• A diet of 30 to 40 g of fat per day excludes whole milk and its products. However, the patient may use skim milk and products made from it and have 1 tbsp of oil, lard, butter, or mayonnaise and 4 oz of lean meat daily. Eggs are limited to three a week. The patient should avoid such high-fat snacks as chocolate, nuts, cheese crackers, and chips. Substitutes include vegetables, fruits, bread, cereals, rice, and pasta. If necessary, this basic diet can be modified further; for example, by eliminating eggs and reducing intake of other high-fat foods.
• Make sure the patient receives a vitamin supplement to compensate for reduction in the intake of fat-soluble vitamins. In addition, watch for signs that he's deficient in these vitamins.
• Monitor the patient's protein intake since a low-fat diet tends to restrict high-protein foods. Also keep an eye on his weight, since a low-fat diet also tends to be low in calories. For many patients, weight loss may be beneficial; others may have to increase caloric intake if weight loss becomes excessive.
• Teach the patient how to shop for low-fat foods. For example, tell him to look for dairy products made with skim milk and for pasta that doesn't contain eggs. Suggest that the patient explore ethnic foods, such as Italian, Japanese, and Chinese dishes; they're often low in fat and offer some variety to his diet. However, tell him to watch the amount of cheese in Italian dishes.

• Explain that the patient should remove visible fat and skin from meat and should broil or bake foods rather than fry them. Tell him to put baked meats or poultry on a rack away from the drippings. Point out that fat is often invisible—for example, when it's a component in cream, milk, eggs, or some meat. Recommend that he use egg substitutes or egg whites for cooking.

• Counsel the patient about eating out. Suggest that he order juice for an appetizer and use lemon juice or vinegar on salads. Remind him that he must limit portions of meat, and should order foods that are broiled, baked, or poached. Tell him to omit sauces and gravies and to select ices, fruit, or a liqueur for dessert.

• Check with the doctor to see if the patient's diet can include medium-chain triglycerides. These synthetic substances, which are absorbed directly into the portal vein, may be used in place of cooking oil. Although they're expensive, they can improve the patient's compliance with fat restrictions and increase his caloric intake.

Low-sodium diet

Patients with congestive heart failure, hypertension, chronic renal failure with edema, and cirrhosis with ascites may benefit from limiting their sodium intake, which helps to correct excess water retention.

Most Americans typically consume 3,000 to 5,000 mg of sodium daily. Typically, the doctor restricts sodium in the patient's diet to one of five levels: 2,000 to 3,000 mg; 1,000 mg; 800 mg; 500 mg; or 200 mg. Many patients find the low-sodium diet tasteless and bland and have difficulty accepting it.

Nursing considerations

• Help the patient identify all dietary sources of sodium. Sodium occurs naturally in all foodstuffs, not just table salt (sodium chloride). In general, meat, poultry, fish, milk, cheese, and eggs contain more sodium than whole grain cereals, fruits, and most vegetables (although celery, carrots, and spinach have a high sodium content). What's more, food additives, such as monosodium glutamate (MSG) and baking soda (sodium bicarbonate), can significantly increase the sodium content of his diet. Chocolate milk and ice cream contain high sodium additives. Point out that many of these additives don't give food a salty taste.

• On a 200-mg sodium diet, distilled water must be used for drinking and for making beverages, such as coffee and tea. All other diets contain an allowance of 100 mg of sodium for 1 qt of tap water.

• Usually, the patient on a sharply restricted sodium diet (500 mg or less of sodium) is hospitalized. You'll need to monitor him carefully—especially when sodium restriction is prolonged—to avoid hyponatremia, hypochloremia, and, eventually, sodium-depletion azotemia. Watch for complaints of weakness, lassitude, anorexia and vomiting, confusion, abdominal cramps, and aching skeletal muscles. To detect fluid retention, weigh the patient daily and report any sudden increase. Also watch for diminished fluid output, which may signal renal failure.

• Teach the patient how to read food labels when grocery shopping to determine an item's sodium content. The sodium content is noted on the label (200 mg of salt equals 80 mg of sodium). Also, inform him that additives are listed in order of greatest quantity. Tell him to avoid a product if one of these additives is among the first five listed: salt, sodium benzoate, sodium nitrate, or MSG.

• Warn him that many over-the-counter medications contain sodium.

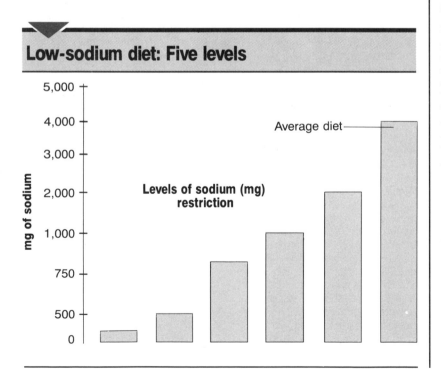

Low-sodium diet: Five levels

mg of sodium

5,000
4,000
3,000
2,000
1,000
750
500
0

Levels of sodium (mg) restriction

Average diet

Some examples include Alka-Seltzer, Di-Gel, Maalox Plus, Metamucil, Rolaids, and Vicks Formula 44 Cough Mixture. Have him consult his doctor or pharmacist about the sodium content of any unprescribed medicine that he wishes to take.

• To help make the sodium-restricted diet more palatable, suggest seasoning foods with herbs and spices instead of salt.

• Tell the patient to avoid salt substitutes, unless his doctor approves. Explain that some products advertised as low-sodium salt substitutes contain another salt and sodium chloride, giving them half as much sodium as regular table salt. They may contain potassium or ammonium salt, which could be harmful if the patient has kidney or liver disease. Vegetized salts use powdered dehydrated vegetables as a base and may contain considerable sodium.

• At restaurants, advise the patient to order baked, broiled, or roasted foods and to skip gravies, juices, soups, and cheesy dressings.

• Teach the patient how to modify ethnic food practices:

— Advise the patient who likes Southern cuisine or "soul food" not to cook with bacon or salt pork.

— To be kosher, freshly slaughtered meat and poultry must be salted for 1 hour to remove the blood. A Jewish patient who follows kosher dietary laws may want to boil meat and discard the broth before serving.

— Advise the patient who likes Italian food to use fresh tomatoes whenever possible for soups and sauces or to use unsalted canned tomatoes, tomato paste, or tomato juice. Have him avoid or restrict his intake of olives, Italian cheese, and Italian bread.

— Caution the patient who likes Japanese or Chinese foods not to season his food with MSG or soy sauce. He can purchase low-sodium soy sauce.

• Inform the patient about the availability of specially prepared low-sodium products, such as low-sodium milk, unsalted canned vegetables, unsalted butter and margarine, low-sodium soups, and low-sodium baking powder.

• Recommend using a system similar to counting calories for counting the milligrams of sodium eaten. The patient can eat small portions of sodium-containing food as part of the daily sodium allotment. Suggest low-sodium recipes to keep his diet varied and enjoyable.

• Explain that bottled soft drinks may be high in sodium, depending on the sodium content of the water in the area where they're manufactured. In low-caloric beverages, substituting sodium saccharin for sugar increases the sodium content even more.

• Eliminating salt from his diet may place the patient at risk for iodine deficiency if his iodine intake depends mainly on the use of iodized salt. Teach him about other dietary sources of iodine, such as seafood and vegetables grown in iodine-rich soil. Explain that he can have the iodine content of his garden soil analyzed. Advise him to take supplemental iodine tablets, as ordered, if the iodine content of his diet and local drinking water is inadequate. Tell him to contact his water authority or have his well water tested for its iodine content.

Gluten-free diet
For patients with celiac disease, a gluten-free diet prevents bloating, projectile vomiting, and poor growth patterns. In this disease, which is usually first diagnosed in infancy or early childhood, the glutamine-bound fraction of protein found in many grain products damages the intestinal lining.

A gluten-free diet can't reverse the intestinal damage of celiac disease. However, it can prevent further damage, improve symptoms, and correct malabsorption of nutrients. Children placed on a gluten-free diet may improve within 2 weeks; in adults, results take a little longer — usually a month or two.

Initially, the patient's diet excludes sources of gluten and includes foods high in protein, calories, vitamins, and minerals to correct previous dietary deficiencies. Once deficiencies are corrected, the patient adheres to a diet that's normal except for the gluten content. He must follow this diet scrupulously for the rest of his life; those who go on and off the diet repeatedly may eventually fail to respond to it.

Nursing considerations
• A gluten-free diet eliminates all products containing wheat, rye, oats, barley, malt, and buckwheat. In their place, the patient may eat cereals and breads made from rice, corn, soy, and potatoes. Initially, the patient refrains from consuming milk and milk products, since intestinal damage often causes an intolerance to lactose. As symptoms improve, these dairy products can be gradually reintroduced.

• The patient may initially require hospitalization to stabilize his condition and provide nutritional supplementation. While he's in the hospital, monitor hemoglobin and hematocrit values for signs of anemia, and administer iron, folate, or vitamin B_{12}, as ordered. Bleeding may result from vitamin K deficiency; monitor prothrombin time. Osteomalacia may develop because of vitamin D and calcium deficiencies; watch for rheumatic-type pain in the pelvis and limbs. In addition, monitor intake and output carefully.

• Explain that gluten is hidden in many foods — for example, in chocolate syrup (where it's used as a stabilizing and thickening agent); in sausages, hot dogs, and turkey injected with hydrolyzed vegetable protein; and in distilled

white vinegar and whiskeys.
• Inform the patient or his parents about foods specially made for the patient with celiac disease; the dietitian can recommend brands. Suggest that they look for them in health-food stores or gourmet shops.
• Suggest shopping at an Asian food store, which carries many products made entirely from rice and rice flour.
• Explain that mixing special gluten-free flour with liquid in a recipe may make foods less grainy. The patient or his parents should boil the flour with the liquid and cool this mixture before adding it to other ingredients.
• For older children and adults, discuss selecting foods in restaurants. Suggest broiled or baked meat or fish; tell the patient to avoid sauces, gravies, and breaded foods.
• Emphasize the need for frequent checkups.

Low-purine diet

This diet restricts foods with preformed purines — for example, liver, eggs, and sardines — which the body breaks down into uric acids. It's primarily used to control gout and prevent renal calculi, two conditions caused by high uric acid levels. In addition, a low-purine diet can be used for patients with increased uric acid levels secondary to obesity, hypertension, hypertriglyceridemia, fasting, alcoholism, lead toxicity, toxemia of pregnancy, leukemia, polycythemia, psoriasis, or diuretic therapy.

Since the body synthesizes purines, dietary measures alone won't always control these conditions. For that reason, the diet's usually supplemented with drugs, such as allopurinol and probenecid, that reduce uric acid levels, as well as an exercise and weight-control program.

Nursing considerations

• The low-purine diet contains limited amounts of fats, moderate amounts of protein, and plentiful amounts of complex carbohydrates. In addition, it includes about 2 qt of fluid a day to help promote uric acid excretion, as well as vegetables and fruit to increase the alkalinity of the urine and thereby increase the solubility of uric acid.
• The diet limits the patient's weekly intake of animal protein to about 15 oz of lean beef, veal, lamb, poultry, or fish — in other words, about five servings of no more than 3 oz. The patient should limit consumption of dairy products to 4 cups of skim milk and 2 oz of cheese daily.
• The patient must avoid all high-purine foods, such as organ meats (kidney, liver, brain), meat extracts, bouillon, gravies, fish eggs, shrimp, mackerel, herring, anchovies, mussels, and sardines. In addition, he should avoid alcohol or at least limit it to one drink daily, preferably diluted with water.
• The patient can have three to four daily servings of vegetables, including potatoes and most kinds of green, leafy vegetables. (However, dried beans, peas, spinach, and lentils have moderate amounts of purine and should be restricted to one serving a day.) He can also eat two to three servings of fruit a day, one serving of enriched cereal, and four to six slices of enriched bread with 2 tbsp of margarine or butter. The patient may drink moderate amounts of coffee and tea; the purines that they contain break down to methyl uric acid, which isn't deposited in body tissues.
• If the patient's on an exceedingly strict diet — for example, during an acute attack of gout — he may need to eliminate animal protein, eggs, and cheese altogether. He should drink skim milk and eat cottage cheese to get enough protein and

should avoid alcohol entirely.
• If the patient's hospitalized, closely monitor his serum uric acid levels. Notify the doctor if levels begin to rise sharply.
• Assess the patient regularly for diffuse swelling in the joints and for nodular deposits of sodium urate crystals. In addition, closely monitor his intake and output, and encourage fluids.
• Check urine pH. If ordered, administer sodium bicarbonate or potassium carbonate to increase urine alkalinity.
• Antigout drugs can decrease absorption of sodium, potassium, carotene, riboflavin, and vitamin B_{12}, so watch for deficiencies. If ordered, administer vitamin and mineral supplements.
• Emphasize the need for follow-up visits to monitor his progress and detect dietary deficiencies. Suggest that the patient keep a food diary.
• Tell the patient not to diet during an acute gout attack since the breakdown of adipose tissue decreases uric acid excretion. If he wishes to lose weight, tell him to do so gradually and to avoid fasting, which can precipitate a gout attack.
• Suggest ways that the patient can add fluids to his diet — for example, by eating soup or drinking a glass of water before each meal and at bedtime.

Low-phenylalanine diet

For a child born with phenylketonuria, the low-phenylalanine diet can prevent the mental retardation and neurologic damage that are otherwise inevitable. The diet reduces phenylalanine intake while providing sufficient amino acids and nutrients for normal growth and development. The child begins the diet shortly after birth and must adhere to it scrupulously until adolescence.

Enforcing this diet is a challenge. The child must begin to take responsibility for his eating habits early on and may not understand the consequences of non-compliance. As he leaves the sheltered home environment, he often finds that the diet sets him apart from his friends.

Some controversy exists over how long the patient must follow his diet. Although children have been taken off it at age 7 or 8, reports of learning and behavior problems have prompted researchers to recommend that the diet be observed into adolescence. At that time the patient requires no special dietary restrictions—with one important exception: female patients who want to become pregnant must return to the diet before and for the duration of the pregnancy, since excess phenylalanine can be transmitted to the fetus and cause congenital defects.

Nursing considerations
• The infant receives a special formula made of enzymatic hydrolysate of casein, which contains exceedingly low levels of phenylalanine, normal amounts of other amino acids, and added amounts of carbohydrate and fat. Since he requires some phenylalanine for normal development, he also receives small supplements of evaporated milk or regular infant formula.

As the child grows older, the diet restricts foods to those with a low or moderate phenylalanine content. Since most natural proteins contain phenylalanine, the diet is similar to the low-protein diet.
• Stress to the parents that their child will be physically and psychologically normal *only if he carefully adheres to the diet*. Warn the parents against overemphasizing food intake or overprotecting their child; tell them to treat him as normally as possible. Suggest that they seek family counseling to help them adjust to the dietary regimen.
• Check serum phenylalanine levels weekly in early infancy and

monthly as the child matures to determine his response to therapy. Serum levels should be kept between 2 and 10 mg/dl.
• Assess the child's height, weight, and head circumference regularly to ensure that the diet provides adequate nutrition. In addition, monitor hemoglobin levels, since the diet is low in protein and in magnesium and zinc levels. If deficiencies develop, the doctor will order vitamin and mineral supplements.
• Overzealous adherence to the diet may result in excessively low phenylalanine levels. In addition to monitoring blood values, watch for signs of phenylalanine deficiency: listlessness, anorexia, or stunted growth.
• Instruct the parents to keep a daily food diary. When they come in for follow-up visits, review the diary with them to assess both phenylalanine intake and overall nutrition.
• Tell them that supplemental milk should be mixed with the low-phenylalanine formula so that the infant doesn't develop a taste for regular milk.
• Explain that during illness, tissue breakdown can cause an accumulation of phenylalanine in the blood; during this time, the child may be restricted to clear liquids. Tell parents to reintroduce the formula or diet as soon as possible after the child recovers.
• Parents need additional support and guidance as they introduce new foods to an infant. Have them demonstrate their ability to weigh and measure food properly and to make appropriate choices from the exchange lists.
• Stress to the parents that as the child matures, he must become responsible for his own diet. Help them develop this responsibility early; for example, explain that by age 3 or 4, children can learn that some foods are "no" foods and others are "yes" foods, and they can be taught to count out the

number of crackers that they're allowed to eat.
• Help the parents find sources of low-protein foods, such as specialty shops and mail-order firms, and suggest that they use cookbooks designed for a low-phenylalanine diet and vegetarian cookbooks that include dairy products.

Lactose-reduced diet
This diet constitutes the only treatment for lactose intolerance, a common disorder in which patients have difficulty digesting dairy products.

Some degree of lactose intolerance develops in most people after the age of 5. But for reasons that aren't entirely understood, it's usually more pronounced among Blacks, Asians, Orientals, and South Americans. And in a few cases, the patient has complete lactose intolerance from birth. Secondary lactose intolerance may occur in patients with celiac disease, sprue, colitis, enteritis, cystic fibrosis, or malnutrition and in patients who've undergone a gastrectomy or small-bowel resection.

Few patients require a diet that's totally free of lactose; most can tolerate some milk if it's carefully spaced throughout the day. In addition, many patients may consume cheese, yogurt, or sweet acidophilus milk. Because the diet has some flexibility, it's one of the easiest to follow. In addition, many patients can gradually add dairy products without suffering ill effects.

Nursing considerations
• The patient should limit or eliminate his consumption of ordinary milk and milk products. As a guideline, suggest that he drink no more than half a cup of ordinary milk per day; recommend that he substitute sweet acidophilus milk. If he wishes, he can try eating small quantities of cheese or drinking small amounts of butter-

milk or yogurt, since they contain bacteria that break down lactose. He should avoid baked goods made with milk, sausages that contain milk solids, creamy sauces and gravies, and processed foods that contain lactose. He should also avoid other, less obvious sources of lactose, such as chocolate; caramel; cocoa mixes; certain nondairy creamers, vitamins, and medications; instant potatoes; and frozen french fries.
• Monitor the patient's intake of calcium and riboflavin; both are usually supplied by milk. Provide dietary supplements, if ordered. Also assess his diet to be sure that he's taking in sufficient protein and calories.
• Tell the patient to carefully read food labels to detect the presence of milk, milk solids, whey, lactose, or casein.
• Suggest that he substitute water or fruit juices for milk in recipes.
• Explain that if he eats out, he should avoid foods prepared with sauces, gravies, or breading.
• Tell the patient that if his symptoms improve, he can try adding small amounts of dairy products at one meal; if he tolerates them well, he may gradually increase his intake of them. Inform him that sometimes chocolate milk is tolerated better than regular milk. If he wants to try adding cottage cheese to his diet, tell him to experiment with different brands; the amount of lactose they contain varies widely.

Diabetic diet

Dietary therapy serves as a cornerstone of diabetes treatment. The patient requires a carefully regulated, balanced diet that meets nutritional requirements, achieves weight control, and lowers blood glucose levels without causing hypoglycemia, hyperglycemia, or ketosis.

The patient with Type II (noninsulin-dependent) diabetes commonly needs to lose weight to lower his blood glucose levels. If

he has mild hyperglycemia, he may only need to restrict calories since weight loss usually reduces both hepatic glucose production and insulin resistance. However, if the patient has severe hyperglycemia, he may need to use an exchange system to balance intake of dietary protein, carbohydrate, fat, and calories, distributing them carefully throughout the day.

The patient with Type I (insulin-dependent) diabetes has the additional concern of scheduling his meals and snacks to offset peak insulin action and avoid hypoglycemia. He also needs to follow an exchange system to balance dietary protein, carbohydrate, and fat.

Nursing considerations

• Base the target caloric allowance on the doctor's prescription or calculate it from the patient's ideal body weight. The American Diabetes Association recommends an adult basal caloric need of 10 kcal/lb of ideal body weight, modified for activity according to these formulas:
— ideal body weight muliplied by 3 for a sedentary patient
— ideal weight multiplied by 5 for a patient who exercises moderately
— ideal weight multiplied by 10 for a patient who exercises vigorously.

If the patient needs to lose weight, subtract 500 kcal/day to achieve a weekly decrease of 1 lb.

Once you've determined the patient's daily caloric allowance, divide this between meals and snacks and select foods that meet suggested requirements. Typically, 50% to 60% of his calories should come from carbohydrates, 30% from fat, and the remainder from protein.
• If your patient is a newly diagnosed diabetic with extremely high blood glucose levels, he'll usually require hospitalization while his blood glucose levels are monitored and his insulin requirements are determined. Monitor

him for signs of hypoglycemia, such as nervousness, dizziness, diaphoresis, fatigue, faintness, and, possibly, seizures or coma. Also watch for signs of hyperglycemia, such as polyuria, polydipsia, and dehydration. Finally, be on guard for signs of ketoacidosis, such as a fruity breath odor, dehydration, weak and rapid pulse, and Kussmaul's respirations.
• Once you've prepared a diet that takes into account the doctor's prescription, the patient's caloric needs, and the food proportions to be used, work closely with the patient to help him understand it. If he'll be using food exchanges, review these carefully with him. (Teaching materials are readily available from the American Diabetes Association.) Explain to him that foods are broken down into meat exchanges (including high-, medium-, and low-fat groups); fat exchanges; milk exchanges; vegetable exchanges; fruit exchanges; and bread exchanges (including cereal and starchy vegetables). Show the patient how each exchange category lists the foods that fall within that group; the grams of carbohydrate, fat, and protein included in one exchange; and the quantity of food (1 cup, 1 oz, 1 slice, and so forth) that counts as one exchange.
• Discuss restrictions on sugar intake. Although sugar was formerly forbidden, some doctors now allow their diabetic patients to have modest amounts of sucrose (table sugar) if taken with a meal—up to 5% of the daily carbohydrate allowance if spaced throughout the day. However, other doctors prefer that their patients use fructose or sorbitol, which are metabolized more slowly than sucrose, or aspartame, which is sweeter than sugar but low in calories. Explain that aspartame can be used as a "free" food: one that has few or no calories and can be used as often as desired. Fructose and sorbitol, in contrast, have more calories

and may need to be counted as exchanges.

• Advise the patient about any alcohol restrictions. Typically, the patient can drink limited amounts of alcohol if his doctor approves and his diabetes is well controlled. The Type-II diabetic patient should count alcohol as a fat exchange because the body metabolizes alcohol like fat. In contrast, the Type-I diabetic patient should count alcohol as extra calories but should *not* substitute it for an exchange because of the risk of causing hypoglycemia. He should eat all his regular exchanges when he drinks alcohol.

• Encourage the patient to eat foods that contain unrefined carbohydrates and large amounts of fiber. Daily intake of 10 to 15 g of fiber delays gastric emptying and slows carbohydrate absorption, which can lower blood glucose levels and reduce insulin requirements.

• If your patient is insulin-dependent (Type I), stress the importance of eating on schedule to balance his insulin therapy. If he has to delay a meal, instruct him to eat hard candy or drink a nondietetic soft drink. Tell him he should always carry hard candy, fruit juice, or another source of simple sugar with him to counteract possible hypoglycemia. Also advise him that he needs to eat even if he becomes sick, to prevent hypoglycemia. Suggest that he substitute soft or liquid foods for his exchanges, as necessary.

Quack appeal: Why patients turn to unproven remedies

What makes a patient turn to an unproven remedy? If he suffers a disabling or fatal illness, he may feel he has nothing to lose by trying an unproven treatment. Some people instinctively mistrust doctors and organized medicine, preferring instead herbs, fruits, vegetables, and other "natural remedies." Other patients may become frustrated with the modern emphasis on cure over care: Doctors may project an impatient or unsympathetic attitude and show little interest in supportive measures like nutrition therapy. In addition, unproven remedies are usually cheaper than orthodox therapy, though insurance won't cover the expense.

Arthritis

Most arthritis patients will try one or more unproven remedies.

Some remedies for arthritis are considered harmless. These include:
• acupuncture
• copper bracelets
• mineral springs
• topical creams
• vibrators
• vinegar and honey.

Other remedies, however, have proved to be harmful. These include:
• large doses of vitamins
• snake venom.

Still other remedies haven't had their safety established. These include:
• bee venom
• biofeedback
• dimethyl sulfoxide (DMSO)
• dietary changes
• fish oil
• laser treatments
• vaccines
• yucca.

Cancer

Each year thousands of cancer patients seek out unproven treatments such as the following:

Laetrile. Also known as nitriloside or Vitamin B_{17}, this substance is made from the anogenetic glycoside amygdalin, which comes from apricot pits. Amygdalin has a cyanide component which supposedly kills cancer cells. In fact, many people have poisoned themselves with laetrile. No evidence exists to support the use of laetrile against cancer. Nonetheless, each year 50,000 to 75,000 Americans ask for treatment with it.

Nutritional treatments. Many patients rely on the use of diets and nutritional supplements to cure cancer. The diet may call for prescribed amounts of vegetable juice and perhaps large doses of vitamins, minerals and other compounds. One of the century's most eminent scientists, Linus Pauling, claims that vitamin C can control or cure cancer in patients whose white blood cells haven't been affected by radiation or chemotherapy. Tests of Vitamin C on patients with colon cancer who hadn't been treated with radiation or chemotherapy do not support this claim.

Metabolic therapy. This remedy combines special diets, internal irrigation, and spiritual attitudes to purify the body. Proponents believe cancer comes from inadequate elimination of wastes.

Detoxification. Proponents of this remedy claim that cancer is caused by toxins in the body. To be cured, the patient must detoxify himself with special diets, sweat baths, enemas, and other remedies.

Contraptions. Devices that allegedly cure cancer include charms, necklaces and bracelets, and the orgone box—a zinc-lined box that emits orgone energy to destroy the patient's tumor.

Acquired immunodeficiency syndrome (AIDS)

Partly because of the slow pace of drug testing and approval at the federal level, many patients with the human immunodeficiency virus (HIV) have taken up self-medication. Many use drugs obtained out of the country or through "buyer's clubs." Often patients choose these medications based on anecdotal reports.

Ribavirin. This antiviral medication obtained from Mexico costs about $5,000-$6,000 per year. Controlled studies indicate it has no in vivo action against HIV.

Dried cucumber roots. An experimental drug extracted from Chinese cucumber root, GLQ223 (Compound Q, trichosanthin), may inhibit HIV action when given intravenously. It has received considerable media attention. Many health food stores and herbal shops have begun selling dried roots purportedly containing Compound Q. These roots (when they are, in fact, Chinese cucumber roots, which is not always the case) contain lectins that cause agglutination of blood cells when administered intravenously. Extracting Compound Q from the root is difficult and most dried preparations don't contain enough of the substance to make it feasible.

Other forms of self-medication. Many people with AIDS use more familiar drugs such as cimetidine (which may affect the activity of other medications), dipyridamole (which may interfere with platelet activity), and disulfiram (which causes severe reactions to ethyl alcohol).

Counseling a patient who's using unproven remedies

If a seriously ill patient loses faith in conventional medical treatment and contemplates turning to alternative remedies, you need to keep the lines of communication open. Encourage the patient to share his hopes and fears with you and the doctor. The patient may fear losing your approval if he reveals his interest in alternative remedies, so provide reassurance and encourage the patient to ask questions.

Suppose, for example, you know a cancer patient who is considering discontinuing chemotherapy in favor of a diet therapy. You might say to this patient, "Your concern about diet and therapy tells me you want to make wise choices. We can talk about the pros and cons of the diet and I'll try to answer your questions."

Perhaps you can avoid an either-or situation. If elements of an alternative treatment (such as nutritional therapy) can safely be incorporated into your care plan, offer to discuss it with the doctor. But if you believe the alternative therapy is potentially harmful, offer to help the patient find objective research on both sides of the issue.

What if you suspect a patient is self-administering potentially harmful medication in secret? When confronting him, keep your tone matter-of-fact and non-threatening. You might bring the topic up during a routine assessment. For example, when taking a drug history of an AIDS patient, you may want to ask, "Are you taking any other medications, homeopathic remedies, herbal medicines or over-the-counter drugs?"

Identify the people your patient trusts: family members, friends, a minister, or a therapist. Tell them what you suspect and give them the facts about the dangers of self-treatment. Then ask them to back you up when you talk with the patient.

Remember to document your conversations with the patient and keep the doctor informed of the patient's intentions.

Keep in mind that any unproven remedy, no matter how seemingly benign, can cause harm if it provides an excuse to neglect prescribed therapy. Ultimately, you must help the patient realize that most unorthodox remedies don't stand up to scientific study. Many, in fact, are known to be unsafe. If the patient stubbornly refuses to heed your warnings, though, the best you can do for him is to keep the lines of communication open.

Qualities of a quack

Today's charlatans are vastly different from the hawkers of snake oil who used to peddle their wares in small towns and at country fairs. Today they wear white coats, work in clinics and have offices with walls containing rows of impressive-looking diplomas. They may use conventional and unconventional methods.

Teach the gullible patient to be alert for the qualities of a quack. Be aware of any doctor who:
• Has an unusual degree after his name, such as D.N. for doctor of naturopathy. These degrees come from mail-order diploma mills or unaccredited universities
• Claims his research was too imaginative or avant-garde to be conducted at a well-known laboratory, so it was done at an independent laboratory instead
• Relies on anecdotes and testimonials, often from famous people who know nothing about medicine, instead of publishing in peer-reviewed professional journals or attending recognized scientific meetings
• Guarantees recovery from serious illness without adverse effects from treatment
• Relies on unorthodox tests
• Has a flamboyant personality and uses emotional or pseudoscientific language
• Accuses the medical establishment of persecuting him and compares himself to famous scientists of the past who suffered persecution
• Claims that a conspiracy of doctors, drug companies, and the government runs the medical establishment
• Keeps poor records, if any, so that no one can verify his data.

Vitamin supplements

Most people know that vitamins are essential for growth and development. But how they're stored and given can greatly influence their intended effects. And how they act can depend on the patient's condition, his use of prescription or over-the-counter drugs, and other factors. When you're administering a vitamin supplement, review the appropriate section below for important nursing concerns.

Vitamin C
• Give I.V. doses of vitamin C slowly; rapid injection can cause dizziness and syncope. Administer cautiously in renal insufficiency since excess amounts are excreted in urine.
• Protect parenteral solution from light.
• Avoid giving sodium-containing preparations of vitamin C to patients on a sodium-restricted diet. Similarly, avoid giving preparations containing calcium to patients who are receiving digitalis since cardiac disturbances may result.

Thiamine (vitamin B₁)
• Perform sensitivity tests before giving large I.V. doses. During administration, keep epinephrine readily available to treat anaphylaxis.
• Keep in mind that B vitamins act together; an excess amount of one can cause an increased need for the others.
• Don't add thiamine to alkaline I.V. solutions; it will decompose.
• Rotate I.M. injection sites to reduce discomfort.

Riboflavin (vitamin B₂)
• Before riboflavin is absorbed, it must be combined with phosphorus. Give with dairy products.
• Because riboflavin supplements are sensitive to light, keep them in an opaque container.
• Don't give riboflavin with alkaline substances.

Niacin (vitamin B₃)
• Give I.V. only for severe niacin deficiency. Use slow injection.
• Begin therapy with small doses to minimize side effects; increase dosage gradually. Initial therapeutic response usually occurs within 48 hours.
• Administer niacin supplements with meals to reduce GI upset. Tell the patient to avoid taking niacin with hot beverages because of increased vasodilation.
• Inform the patient that tingling, itching, headache, or a sensation of warmth—especially around the head, neck, and ears—can occur shortly after administration but that these effects usually subside with continued therapy. Niacinamide or timed-release niacin may be given to minimize them.
• Monitor hepatic function and blood glucose levels frequently.
• Caution the patient against prolonged exposure to bright sunlight. Also warn him against engaging in hazardous activities because he may experience dizziness or weakness—particularly early in the course of therapy.

Pyridoxine (vitamin B₆)
• Give the vitamin cautiously during lactation since it blocks prolactin.

Cyanocobalamin (vitamin B₁₂)
• Because I.V. administration may cause an anaphylactic reaction, give by this route only when other routes are ruled out.
• Protect it from light and heat.
• Closely monitor serum potassium levels for first 48 hours. Give potassium, if necessary.

Vitamin A
• Never give any form of vitamin A by I.V. push since *death may occur*.
• Adequate vitamin A absorption requires suitable protein intake, bile, concurrent recommended-daily-allowance doses of vitamin E, and zinc.
• Absorption is fastest and most complete with water-miscible preparations, intermediate with emulsions, and slowest with oil suspensions.
• Watch for symptoms of hypervitaminosis, such as bone pain and irritability. Closely monitor for skin disorders, since high doses may induce chronic toxicity.
• Carefully evaluate vitamin A intake from fortified foods, dietary supplements, and drugs to help avoid toxicity. Discourage self-administration of megadoses.
• In pregnant women, avoid doses exceeding recommended daily allowance.
• Liquid preparations are available if nasogastric administration is necessary. This vitamin may be mixed with cereal or fruit juice.
• Record eating and bowel habits. Report abnormalities to the doctor.
• Protect from light and heat.

Vitamin D
• Monitor eating and bowel habits; dry mouth, nausea, vomiting, metallic taste, and constipation can herald toxicity.
• If the patient has hyperphosphatemia, enforce dietary phosphate restrictions and give binding agents to avoid metastatic calcification and renal calculi.
• When high doses are used, monitor serum and urine calcium, potassium, and urea levels. Doses of 60,000 units/day can cause hypercalcemia.
• Malabsorption due to inadequate bile or to hepatic dysfunction may require addition of exogenous bile salts to oral vitamin D. Space doses. Use together cautiously.
• I.M. injection of vitamin D dispersed in oil is preferable in patients who are unable to absorb oral form.
• This vitamin is fat-soluble. Warn patient against increasing dosage on his own.

• Tell the patient to restrict his intake of magnesium-containing antacids.

Vitamin E
• Water-miscible forms are more completely absorbed in GI tract than other forms.
• Adequate bile is essential for absorption.
• Requirements increase with rise in dietary polyunsaturated acids.
• Vitamin E may protect other vitamins against oxidation.

Folic acid
• If the patient has a sore mouth and tongue, provide soft bland foods or liquids.
• Don't mix folic acid with other medications when administering intramuscularly.
• Protect it from light and heat.

Vitamin K
• Administer I.V. over 2 to 3 hours. Mix in normal saline solution, dextrose 5% in water, or dextrose 5% in normal saline solution. Observe patient closely for flushing, weakness, tachycardia, and hypotension.
• Failure to respond to vitamin K may indicate coagulation defects.
• Protect parenteral products from light. Wrap infusion container with aluminum foil.
• Effects of I.V. injections are more rapid but shorter-lived than S.C. or I.M. injections.
• Monitor prothrombin time to determine dosage effectiveness.

Mineral supplements

Minerals help build bone and soft tissue and form hair, nails, and skin. They also help regulate muscle contraction and relaxation, blood clotting, and acid-base balance.

When administering a mineral supplement, keep in mind these important considerations.

Calcium
• Don't give calcium with dairy products, bran cereal, spinach, rhubarb, or corticosteroids to prevent impaired absorption.
• If the patient's receiving a calcium supplement, tell him to take it 1 hour after meals to reduce GI upset.
• Monitor serum and urine calcium levels.

Phosphorus
• Dilute phosphorus in a large amount of fluid and infuse slowly to prevent vessel irritation. Monitor sodium or potassium levels, depending on which salt is used.
• Be alert for symptoms of tetany.

Sodium
• Monitor serum electrolyte levels frequently since imbalances can occur during therapy.
• Check intake and output daily since excessive sodium can cause fluid retention.
• Weigh the patient daily.

Potassium
• Keep in mind that the parenteral form must be diluted in large amounts of fluid and given slowly. *Direct injection of undiluted potassium can cause death.*
• Monitor intake and output to check kidney function. Check ECG for possible dysrhythmias; if they occur, notify the doctor.
• Tell the patient to take potassium supplements immediately after meals to help prevent GI upset.

Magnesium
• I.V. bolus dose must be injected slowly to avoid respiratory or cardiac arrest.
• If available, use an infusion pump for I.V. administration. Maximum rate is 150 ml/minute.
• Monitor vital signs every 15 minutes when giving I.V. for severe hypomagnesemia. Watch for respiratory depression and signs of heart block. Respirations should exceed 16/minute before administration.
• Monitor intake and output. Output should be 100 ml or more during 4-hour period before dose.
• Test knee jerk and patellar reflexes before each additional dose. If absent, give no more magnesium until reflexes return.
• Check magnesium levels after repeated doses. Keep I.V. calcium available to reverse magnesium intoxication.

Copper and zinc
• Monitor serum levels.
• Tell the patient to take zinc with meals. However, warn him not to take it with dairy products, which can decrease absorption.

Oral iron
• Tell the patient that GI upset is related to dose. Instruct him to take iron between meals since food may decrease absorption; however, if he experiences nausea, he may take iron with food.
• Advise him not to take iron supplements for at least 2 hours after eating dairy products, eggs, coffee, tea, or whole-grain bread or cereals since these foods interfere with absorption.
• If he's taking a liquid iron preparation, instruct him to dilute it in juice (preferably orange juice) or water. If he's taking tablets, tell him to take them with orange juice to promote absorption.
• Warn the patient that iron is toxic and that such symptoms as vomiting, upper abdominal pain, pallor, cyanosis, diarrhea, and drowsiness indicate toxicity.
• Let the patient know that his stools may turn black because of unabsorbed iron. Reassure him that this effect is harmless.
• Check for constipation and record stool color and amount.
• To avoid staining teeth, give iron elixir with a glass straw.
• Monitor hemoglobin and reticulocyte counts during therapy.

8 Drug therapy: What you need to do

Ten tips for giving drugs safely

1. Give the correct drug
Check the name and spelling of each drug against the patient's medication administration record at least twice: once when you remove the drug from the unit dose cart and again before administration. If the container label is blurred or the instructions are unclear, consult the pharmacist, your fellow nurses, or an attending doctor.

2. Identify your patient
Before administering a drug, always check the patient's ID band. Ask him to tell you his name. Remember that elderly or pediatric patients may be confused by the question. You can also verify a patient's identity by consulting with the other unit nurses.

3. Give the right dose
Double check the drug dose that was ordered against the dose you're about to administer. If the prescribed dose seems inappropriate, consult your colleagues. This is particularly important when giving drugs that have minimal differences between therapeutic and toxic levels.

4. Administer the drug by the appropriate route
The choice of route for drugs is determined by their chemical properties, where the drug is supposed to take effect, and the desired onset of action, among other things. Carefully observe the patient for any adverse reactions. Parenteral drugs, for instance, are injected directly into body tissue or fluids and act so rapidly that a drug error may be harmful, or even fatal. Make sure that patients on oral medications are taking them properly.

5. Follow the schedule
Never administer a drug more than a half hour before or after its scheduled time.

6. Document administration
Accurate documentation is time-consuming but essential, both for proper care of the patient and for your own legal protection. List the name of the drug; the date and time you gave it to the patient; and the dose, site, and route used in the patient's medication record. Write down the patient's reaction to the drug, and whether you encountered any problems. If he had an adverse reaction to the drug, note what steps you took. Also note when you withhold a drug from a patient and why, or if you stop administering a drug.

7. Teach your patient well
The time you invest in educating a patient usually pays off. Explain to the patient and his family the importance of taking both prescribed and over-the-counter drugs as directed.

8. Compile a complete drug history
You should know all the drugs your patient is taking, including over-the-counter products. Ask the patient if he's taking any drugs prescribed by dentists and psychiatrists. Ask about alcohol intake and smoking habits, too.

9. Watch for allergies
Any drug may cause an unpredictable reaction. Assess your patient's reactions to drugs you have administered. Note on his chart if he has any allergies.

10. Be aware of interactions
Whenever two or more drugs are given together, their combination can enhance or diminish a drug's effect or absorption. Nutrients can also effect drug action. Take a complete patient history, carefully monitor reactions, and consult with colleagues when necessary.

How to read a drug label

One of the best ways to prevent medication errors is by reading the drug label carefully. Knowing the right dosage, any special instructions, and the drug's expiration date is critical to administering medication correctly. Be sure and check the product name twice before administration.

Unfortunately, labels do not tell you everything. For instance, they don't provide directions for treating an overdose, identify possible adverse reactions, or indicate foods or other drugs to avoid. As a result, consult a reliable drug reference or a pharmacist before administration of a new or unfamiliar drug.

Code number for drug

Storage instructions

Precautions

Drug classification

Recommended use

Store at room temperature, between 15° C and 30° C (59° F and 86° F).

WARNINGS: If you are pregnant or nursing a baby, seek the advice of a health professional before using this product.

CAUTION: Consult your doctor if cough has persisted for 10 or more days or is accompanied by a high fever.

85 98765
EXP 1/94

NDC 0012-3456-78   4 FL.OZ.

DECONGESTANT COUGH MEDICINE

NONNARCOTIC

Each 5 ml (1 teaspoon) contains:
Guaifenesin, USP 100 mg
Alcohol 3.5 percent

KEEP THIS AND ALL MEDICINES
OUT OF REACH OF CHILDREN

**TAMPER-EVIDENT BOTTLE CAP
IF BREAKABLE RING IS
SEPARATED, DO NOT USE**

FOR THE TEMPORARY RELIEF OF COUGHS DUE TO COLDS

DOSAGE: Adults and children 12 years of age and over: 2 teaspoonfuls every four hours, not to exceed 12 teaspoonfuls in a 24-hour period; children 6 to under 12 years: 1 teaspoonful every four hours, not to exceed 6 teaspoonfuls in a 24-hour period; children 2 to under 6 years: ½ teaspoonful every four hours, not to exceed 3 teaspoonfuls in a 24-hour period; children under 2 years: use as directed by physician.

X.Y.Z. Company   Anywhere, PA 12345

Batch
identification number

Ingredients

Manufacturer's
name and address

Dosage

Most common drug errors

A Michigan study showed that the wrong dose, the wrong drug, and four other problems constituted the most common drug errors.

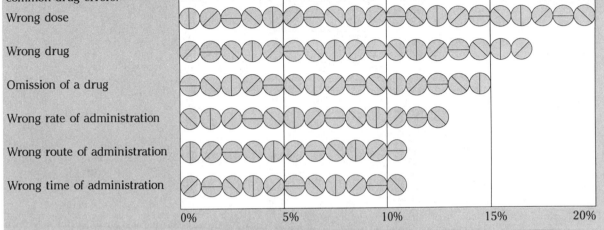

Selected drug levels in conventional and S.I. units

S.I. units are a simplified international system of measurement that eliminates confusion by providing a coherent system of units, ensuring that quantities and units are uniform in concept and style, and minimizing multiples and submultiples in use.

Drug	Conventional values	Conversion factor (Conventional→S.I.)	S.I. units
acetaminophen (P), toxic	> 5 mg/dl	66.16	> 330 µmol/L
carbamazepine (P) therapeutic	4 to 10 mg/liter	4.233	17 to 42 µmol/L

chlordiazepoxide (P)
    therapeutic
    toxic
	0.5 to 5 mg/liter
	> 10 mg/liter
		3.336
		3.336
			2 to 17 µmol/L
			> 33 µmol/L

chlorpromazine (P) therapeutic	50 to 300 ng/ml	3.136	150 to 950 nmol/L
chlorpropamide (P) therapeutic	75 to 250 mg/liter	3.613	270 to 900 µmol/L

diazepam (P)
    therapeutic
    toxic
	0.10 to 0.25 mg/liter
	> 1.0 mg/L
		3,512.0
		3,512.0
			350 to 900 nmol/L
			> 3,510 nmol/L

KEY:	(B) Blood	(P) Plasma	(S) Serum	(U) Urine

(continued)

Selected drug levels in conventional and S.I. units (continued)

Drug	Conventional values	Conversion factor (Conventional→S.I.)	S.I. units
dicumarol (P) therapeutic	8 to 30 mg/liter	2.974	25 to 90 µmol/L

digoxin (P)
  therapeutic
  toxic
	0.5 to 2.2 ng/ml
	> 2.5 ng/ml
		1.281
		1.281
			0.6 to 2.8 nmol/L
			> 3.2 nmol/L

disopyramide (P) therapeutic	2 to 6 ng/liter	2.946	6 to 18 µmol/L
epinephrine (P) therapeutic	31 to 95 pg/ml (at rest for 15 min)	5.458	170 to 520 pmol/L
epinephrine (U)	<10 µg/24 hr	5.458	< 55 nmol/d

ethanol (P)
  legal limit (driving)
  toxic
	< 80 mg/dl
	> 100 mg/dl
		0.2171
		0.2171
			< 17 mmol/L
			> 22 mmol/L

ethosuximide (P) therapeutic	40 to 110 mg/liter	7.084	280 to 780 µmol/L
gold (S) therapeutic	300 to 800 µg/dl	0.05077	15 to 40 µmol/L
insulin (P, S) therapeutic	(P) 5 to 20 µU/ml (S) 0.20 to 0.84 µg/ml	7.175 172.2	35 to 145 pmol/L 35 to 145 pmol/L

isoniazid (P)
  therapeutic
  toxic
	< 2 mg/liter
	> 3 mg/liter
		7.291
		7.291
			< 15 µmol/L
			> 22 µmol/L

lidocaine (P) therapeutic	1 to 5 mg/liter	4.267	4.5 to 21.5 µmol/L
lithium ion (S) therapeutic	0.5 to 1.5 mEq/liter	1.0	0.5 to 1.5 mmol/L

meprobamate (P)
  therapeutic
  toxic
	< 20 mg/liter
	> 40 mg/liter
		4.582
		4.582
			< 90 µmol/L
			> 180 µmol/L

methotrexate (S) toxic	> 2.3 mg/liter	2.2	> 5.0 µmol/L
methsuximide (as desmethylsuximide) (P) therapeutic	10 to 40 mg/liter	5.285	50 to 210 µmol/L
nitroprusside (as thiocyanate) (P) toxic	10 mg/dl	0.1722	1.7 mmol/L

KEY: (B) Blood   (P) Plasma   (S) Serum   (U) Urine

Selected drug levels in conventional and S.I. units *(continued)*

Drug	Conventional values	Conversion factor (Conventional→S.I.)	S.I. units
nortriptyline (P) therapeutic	25 to 200 ng/ml	3.797	90 to 760 nmol/L
pentobarbital (P) therapeutic	20 to 40 mg/liter	4.419	90 to 170 μmol/L
phenobarbital (P) therapeutic	2 to 5 mg/dl	43.06	85 to 215 μmol/L
phensuximide (P) therapeutic	4 to 8 mg/liter	5.285	20 to 40 μmol/L
phenytoin (P) therapeutic toxic	10 to 20 mg/liter > 30 mg/liter	3.964 3.964	40 to 80 μmol/L > 120 μmol/L
primidone (P) therapeutic toxic	6 to 10 mg/liter > 10 mg/liter	4.582 4.582	25 to 46 μmol/L 46 μmol/L
procainamide (P) therapeutic toxic	4 to 8 mg/liter > 12 mg/liter	4.249 4.249	17 to 34 μmol/L > 50 μmol/L
propoxyphene (P) toxic	> 2 mg/liter	2.946	> 5.9 μmol/L
propranolol (P) therapeutic	50 to 200 ng/ml	3.856	190 to 770 nmol/L
quinidine (P) therapeutic toxic	1.5 to 3 mg/liter > 6 mg/liter	3.082 3.082	4.6 to 9.2 μmol/L > 18.5 μmol/L
salicylate (salicylic acid) (S) toxic	> 20 mg/dl	0.0724	> 1.45 mmol/L
sulfonamides (as sulfanilamide) (B) therapeutic	10 to 15 mg/dl	58.07	580 to 870 μmol/L
theophylline (P) therapeutic	10 to 20 mg/liter	5.55	55 to 110 μmol/L
warfarin (P) therapeutic	1 to 3 mg/liter	3.243	3.3 to 9.8 μmol/L

KEY: (B) Blood   (P) Plasma   (S) Serum   (U) Urine

Dangerous drug interactions

Two or more drugs can interact to produce effects that are often undesirable and sometimes hazardous. Such interactions can decrease therapeutic efficacy or bring on toxicity. If possible, avoid administering the combinations shown here.

Drug	Interacting drug	Possible effect
aminoglycosides amikacin gentamicin kanamycin neomycin netilmicin streptomycin tobramycin	cephalosporins, parenteral • ceftazidime • ceftizoxime • cephalothin	Possible enhanced nephrotoxicity
	loop diuretics • bumetadine • ethacrynic acid • furosemide	Possible enhanced ototoxicity
amphetamines amphetamine benzphetamine dextroamphetamine methamphetamine	urine alkalinizers • potassium citrate • sodium acetate • sodium bicarbonate • sodium citrate • sodium lactate • tromethamine	Decreased urinary excretion of amphetamine
angiotensin-converting enzyme (ACE) inhibitors captopril enalapril lisinopril	indomethacin	Decreased or abolished effectiveness of antihypertensive action of ACE inhibitors
barbiturate anesthetics methohexital thiamylal thiopental	opiate analgesics	Enhanced central nervous system and respiratory depression
barbiturates amobarbital aprobarbital butabarbital mephobarbital metharbital pentobarbital phenobarbital primidone secobarbital	valproic acid	Increased serum barbiturate levels
benzodiazepines alprazolam chlordiazepoxide clonazepam clorazepate diazepam	probenecid	Increased pharmacologic effect of benzodiazepines

Dangerous drug interactions *(continued)*

Drug	Interacting drug	Possible effect
benzodiazepines *(continued)* flurazepam halazepam lorazepam midazolam oxazepam prazepam temazepam triazolam	probenecid	Increased pharmacologic effect of benzodiazepines
beta-adrenergic blockers acebutolol atenolol betaxolol carteolol esmolol levobunolol metoprolol nadolol penbutolol pindolol propranolol timolol	verapamil	Enhanced pharmacologic effects of both beta-adrenergic blockers and verapamil
captopril	food	Possible diminished GI absorption
carbamazepine	erythromycin	Increased risk of carbamazepine toxicity
carmustine	cimetidine	Enhanced risk of bone marrow toxicity
ciprofloxacin	antacids containing magnesium or aluminum hydroxide	Decreased plasma levels and effectiveness of ciprofloxacin
clonidine	beta-adrenergic blockers	Enhanced rebound hypertension following rapid clonidine withdrawal
cyclosporine	hydantoins • ethotoin • mephenytoin • phenytoin • rifampin	Reduced plasma levels of cyclosporine
digitalis glycosides	loop and thiazide diuretics • bendroflumethiazide • benzthiazide • chlorothiazide • cyclothiazide • hydrochlorthiazide • hydroflumethiazide	Increased risk of cardiac dysrhythmias because of hypokalemia

(continued)

Dangerous drug interactions (continued)

Drug	Interacting drug	Possible effect

digitalis glycosides (continued)	• methyclothiazide
	• trichlormethiazide
	thiazide-like diuretics
	  • metolazone
	  • polythiazide
	  • quinethazone
	  • trichlormethiazide
		Increased risk of cardiac dysrhythmias because of hypokalemia

	indapamide methimazole propylthiouracil	Increased therapeutic or toxic effects
digitoxin	quinidine	Decreased digitoxin clearance

digoxin	amiodarone
	cyclosporine
	erythromycin
	quinidine
	tetracyclines
	  • demeclocycline
	  • doxycycline
	  • methacycline
	  • minocycline
	  • oxytetracycline
	  • tetracycline
	verapamil
		Elevated serum digoxin levels

dopamine	phenytoin	Hypertension and bradycardia
epinephrine	beta-adrenergic blockers	Increased systolic and diastolic pressures; marked decrease in heart rate
ethanol	disulfiram furazolidone metronidazole	Acute alcohol intolerance reaction

furazolidone	amine-containing foods
	anorexiants
	  • amphetamine
	  • benzphetamine
	  • dextroamphetamine
	  • diethylpropion
	  • fenfluramine
	  • mazindol
	  • methamphetamine
	  • phendimetrazine
	  • phentermine
		Inhibits monoamine oxidase, possibly leading to hypertensive crisis

heparin	salicylates	Enhanced risk of bleeding

Dangerous drug interactions *(continued)*

Drug	Interacting drug	Possible effect
insulin	ethanol	Enhanced hypoglycemic effect
levodopa	furazolidone	Enhanced toxic effects of levodopa
lithium	thiazide diuretics	Decreased lithium excretion
meperidine	monoamine oxidase (MAO) inhibitors	Cardiovascular instability and increased toxicity
methotrexate	probenecid	Decreased methotrexate elimination
	salicylates	Increased risk of methotrexate toxicity

MAO inhibitors
  isocarboxazid
  pargylene
  phenelzine
  tranylcypromine
	amine-containing foods
	anorexiants
		Inhibits monoamine oxidase, possibly leading to hypertensive crisis

nondepolarizing muscle relaxants	aminoglycosides inhalational anesthetics	Enhanced neuromuscular blockade
oral anticoagulants (warfarin)	amiodarone	Decreased hepatic metabolism of warfarin
	androgens • testosterone	Possible enhanced bleeding caused by increased hypoprothrombinemia
	barbiturates carbamazepine	Decreased risk of bleeding because of enhanced hepatic metabolism

	cephalosporins (parenteral, with methyltetrazolthiol chain)
	  • cefamandole
	  • cefoperazone
	  • cefotetan
	  • moxalactam
	chloral hydrate
	cholestyramine
	cimetidine
	clofibrate
	co-trimoxazole
	dextrothyroxine
	disulfiram
	erythromycin
	glucagon
	metronidazole
	phenylbutazone
	quinidine
	quinine
	salicylates
		Increased risk of bleeding

(continued)

Dangerous drug interactions (continued)

Drug	Interacting drug	Possible effect
oral anticoagulants (warfarin) (continued)	sulfinpyrazone thyroid drugs tricyclic antidepressants • amitriptyline • amoxapine • desipramine • doxepin • imipramine • nortriptyline • protriptyline • trimipramine	Increased risk of bleeding
	ethchlorvynol glutethimide griseofulvin	Decreased pharmacologic effect
	rifampin trazadone	Decreased risk of bleeding
	methimazole propylthiouracil	Increased or decreased risk of bleeding
penicillins	tetracyclines	Reduced effectiveness of penicillins
potassium supplements	potassium-sparing diuretics	Increased risk of hyperkalemia
quinidine	amiodarone	Increased risk of quinidine toxicity
sympathomimetics	MAO inhibitors	Increased risk of hypertensive crisis
tetracyclines	antacids containing magnesium, aluminum, or bismuth salts	Decreased plasma levels and effectiveness of tetracyclines

Drugs with sulfite additives

Sulfites, used as drug preservative, can cause allergic reactions in certain patients. The list below identifies sulfite-containing drugs.

amikacin sulfate (Amikin)
aminophylline (Aminophyllin Tablets, Slo-Phyllin 125 Gyrocaps, Slo-Phyllin 250 Gyrocaps)
amphotericin B (Mysteclin-F syrup)

amrinone lactate (Inocor Lactate)
atropine sulfate with meperidine hydrochloride (Atropine and Demerol Injection)
betamethasone sodium phosphate (Celestone Phosphate, Cel-U-Jec, Selestoject)
bupivacaine hydrochloride with epinephrine 1:200,000 (Marcaine Hydrochloride 0.25% with Epinephrine 1:200,000, Marcaine Hydrochloride 0.5% with Epinephrine 1:200,000, Sensorcaine 0.5% with Epinephrine 1:200,000, Marcaine Hydrochloride 0.75% with Epinephrine

1:200,000, Sensorcaine 0.75% with Epinephrine 1:200,000)
carisoprodol, aspirin, and codeine phosphate (Soma Compound with codeine)
chlorpromazine, chlorpromazine hydrochloride (Thorazine, Ormazine, Promaz)
dexamethasone acetate (Dalalone D.P., Dalalone L.A., Decadron-L.A., Decaject-L.A., Dekasol-L.A., Dexacen L.A.-8, Dexone-L.A., Solurex-L.A.)
dexamethasone sodium phosphate (Dalalone, Decadron Phosphate, Dekasol, Dexacen-4, Dexone, Solurex)

dihydroxyacetone (Vitadye)

diphenhydramine hydrochloride (Benadryl, Benadryl 25 Kapseals, Benadryl Kapseals)

dobutamine hydrochloride (Dobutrex Solution)

dopamine hydrochloride (0.08% Dopamine Hydrochloride in 5% Dextrose Injection, 0.16% Dopamine Hydrochloride in 5% Dextrose Injection, 0.32% Dopamine Hydrochloride in 5% Dextrose Injection, 0.64% Dopamine Hydrochloride in 5% Dextrose Injection)

epinephrine, epinephrine bitartrate, epinephrine hydrochloride, racepinephrine hydrochloride (Adrenalin Chloride Solution, Ana-Kit, Asthma-Nefrin, Breatheasy Inhalant, Dey-Dose Racepinephrine Inhalation Solution, Epifrin, Epinephrine Dropperettes, Epinephrine Injection Pediatric, EpiPen Jr, EpiPen Auto-Injector, Glaucon, microNefrin, Nephron Inhalant, S-2 Inhalant, Vaponefrin)

epinephrine bitartrate 1% with pilocarpine hydrochloride 1% (E-Pilo-1, P1E1)

epinephrine bitartrate 1% with pilocarpine hydrochloride 2% (E-Pilo-2, P2E1), epinephrine bitartrate 1% with pilocarpine hydrochloride 3% (E-Pilo-3, P3E1)

epinephrine bitartrate 1% with pilocarpine hydrochloride 4% (E-Pilo-4, P4E1)

epinephrine bitartrate 1% with pilocarpine hydrochloride 6% (E-Pilo-6, P6E1)

etidocaine hydrochloride with epinephrine bitartrate 1:200,000 (Duranest 1% with Epinephrine 1:200,000, Duranest 1.5% with Epinephrine 1:200,000)

heparin calcium, heparin sodium (Heparin Sodium 10,000 units in 5% Dextrose Injection, Heparin Sodium 12,500 units in 5% Dextrose Injection, Heparin Sodium 25,000 units in 5% Dextrose Injection)

hydralazine hydrochloride (Apresazide 25/25, Apresazide 50/50, Apresazide 100/50)

hydrocortisone sodium phosphate (Hydrocortone Phosphate, Prednisolone Sodium Phosphate, Hydeltrasol, Key-Pred SP)

hyoscyamine sulfate (Levsin)

imipramine hydrochloride (Tofranil)

influenza virus vaccine (Fluogen)

isoetharine hydrochloride, isoetharine mesylate (Arm-a-Med Isoetharine Hydrochloride, Dey-Lute Isoetharine Hydrochloride Solution, Isoetharine Hydrochloride Inhalation, Isoetharine Hydrochloride Inhalation, Bronkosol Unit Dose, Isoetharine Hydrochloride Inhalation, Dispos-a-Med Isoetharine Hydrochloride, Beta-2, Bronkosol, Dey-Dose Isoetharine Hydrochloride Solution, Bronkometer, Isoetharine Mesylate Aerosol Solution)

isoproterenol hydrochloride, isoproterenol sulfate (Dispos-A-Med Isoproterenol Hydrochloride, Dey-Dose Isoproterenol Hydrochloride, Dispos-A-Med Isoproterenol Hydrochloride, Isuprel Hydrochloride Solution 1:200, Vapo-Iso, Isuprel Hydrochloride Solution 1:100, Isoproterenol Hydrochloride Injection 1:50,000, Isoproterenol Hydrochloride Injection 1:5000, Isuprel Hydrochloride injection 1:5000, Isuprel Hydrochloride Glossets)

lidocaine hydrochloride with epinephrine hydrochloride (Lidocaine Hydrochloride 0.5% and Epinephrine 1:200,000, Injection Xylocaine 0.5% with Epinephrine 1:200,000, Lidocaine Hydrochloride 1% and Epinephrine 1:100,000, Injection Xylocaine 1% with Epinephrine 1:100,000, Lidocaine Hydrochloride 1% and Epinephrine 1:200,000, Xylocaine 1% with Epinephrine 1:200,000, Lidocaine Hydrochloride 1.5% and Epinephrine 1:200,000, Xylocaine 1.5% with Epinephrine 1:200,000, Lidocaine Hydrochloride 2% and Epinephrine 1:100,000, Injection Xylocaine 2% with Epinephrine 1:100,000, Xylocaine 2% with Epinephrine 1:200,000)

mafenide acetate (Sulfamylon)

metaraminol bitartrate (Aramine, Metaraminol Bitartrate Injection

methotrimeprazine hydrochloride (Levoprome)

methyldopa, methyldopate hydrochloride (Aldomet, Methyldopa Suspension, Aldomet Ester Hydrochloride, Methyldopate Hydrochloride Injection)

metoclopramide hydrochloride (Metoclopramide Hydrochloride Injection)

orphenadrine citrate, orphenadrine hydrochloride (Banflex, Flexoject, Flexon, Myolin, Myotrol, Neocyten, O-Flex, Orphenate)

oxycodone hydrochloride with acetaminophen (Tylox)

pentazocine hydrochloride, pentazocine hydrochloride with acetaminophen (Talwin, Talacen)

perphenazine (Trilafon)

phenylephrine hydrochloride (AK-Dilate, Neo-Synephrine Hydrochloride, Neo-Synephrine, Prefrin-A Murocoll-2)

procainamide hydrochloride (Pronestyl)

procaine hydrochloride (Novocain)

prochlorperazine (Compazine)

prochlorperazine edisylate, prochlorperazine maleate (Compazine Prochlorperazine Edisylate Injection)

promazine hydrochloride (Sparine)

propoxycaine hydrochloride with procaine hydrochloride 2% and levonordefrin 1:20,000 (Ravocaine Hydrochloride 0.4% and Novocain 2% with Neo-Cobefrin 1:20,000) propoxycaine hydrochloride with procaine hydrochloride 2% and norepinephrine bitartrate 1:30,000 (Ravocaine Hydrochloride 0.4% and Novocain 2% with Levophed 1:30,000, with acetone sodium bisulfite)

ritodrine hydrochloride (Yutopar, Ritodrine Hydrochloride injection)

scopolamine hydrobromide with phenylephrine hydrochloride 10% (Murocoll-2)

tetracycline hydrochloride 0.22% topical (Topicycline, Eaton)

thiethylperazine maleate (Torecan)

trifluoperazine hydrochloride (Stelazine Oral Concentrate)

tubocurarine chloride (Tubocurarine Chloride Injection)

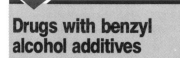

Drugs with benzyl alcohol additives

Used as a preservative in certain parenteral drugs, benzyl alcohol has reportedly caused neonatal kernicterus when given in large amounts. The list below identifies drugs containing benzyl alcohol.

aminocaproic acid (Amicar)
atracurium (Tracrium)
chlordiazepoxide (Librium, supplied diluent)
chlorpheniramine injection (Chlor-100, Chlor-Pro)
chlorpromazine (Ormazine, Promaz, and Thorazine injections)
clindamycin (Cleocin phosphate)
co-trimoxazole (Bactrim I.V. Infusion, Cotrim I.V. Infusion, Septra I.V.)
cytarabine (Cytosar injection)
diazepam (Valium, Zetran injections)
doxapram (Dopram)
erythromycin (Erythrocin, Erythrocin Lactobionate I.V.)

etoposide (Vepesid)
fluphenazine decanoate injection (Prolixin decanoate)
fluphenazine enanthate (Prolixin enanthate)
glycopyrrolate (Robinul)
heparin (Liquaemin)
hydromorphone injection (Dilaudid)
hyoscyamine injection (Levsin)
leuprolide (Leupron)
lincomycin (Lincocin)
lorazepam (Ativan injection)
methotrexate (Mexate)
netilmicin (Netromycin)
pancuronium (Pavulon)
penicillin G procaine (Duracillin A.S.)
phenobarbital sodium injection (Luminal sodium)
phenoxybenzamine (Dibenzylene oral caps)
physostigmine salicylate (Antilerium)
procainamide (Pronestyl)
prochlorperazine edisylate injection (Compazine)
promethazine (Anergan 25, Phenazine 25, Prorex)
pyridostigmine (Regonal, Rexolate)
sodium tetradecyl sulfate (Sotradecol)
sodium thiosalicylate injection (Asproject, Tusal)
spectinomycin (Trobicin, supplied diluent)
succinylcholine
trifluoperazine (Stelazine injection)
tubocurarine (Metubine)
vecuronium (Norcuron)
vinblastine sulfate (Velban)
vincristine sulfate (Oncovin)

Drugs with tartrazine additives

Also known as FD&C Yellow No. 5, tartrazine is a common agent in some drugs. It's usually harmless,

but can provoke a severe allergic reaction in some people. The list below identifies drugs containing tartrazine.

benzphetamine hydrochloride (Didrex tablets)
butabarbital sodium (Butisol sodium elixir, tablets)
carisoprodol (Rela)
chlorphenesin (Maolate)
chlorprothixene (Taractan)
clindamycin (Cleocin hydrochloride caps)
desipramine hydrochloride (Norpramin)
dextroamphetamine sulfate (Dexedrine elixir, spansule, and tablets)
dextrothyroxine (Choloxin)
fluphenazine hydrochloride (Prolixin)
haloperidol (Haldol tablets)
hexocyclium (Trol Filmtab)
hydralazine (Apresoline)
hydromorphone hydrochloride (Dilaudid cough syrup)
imipramine (Janimine, Tofranil PM)
mepenzolate (Cantril)
methamphetamine hydrochloride (Desoxyn Gradumet)
methenamine hippurate (Hiprex)
methysergide maleate (Sansert)
niacin (Nicolar)
paramethadione (Paradione)
penicillin G potassium (Pentids syrup, Pentids 400 syrup, Pentids 800)
penicillin G benzathine (Bicillin)
penicillin V potassium (Veetids 125 oral solution)
pentobarbital sodium (Nembutal sodium)
phenmetrazine (Preludin Endurets)
procainamide (Pronestyl)
promazine hydrochloride (Sparine)
rauwolfia serpentina (Raudixin)
uracil mustard

Drugs with ethanol additives

Many liquid drug preparations for oral use contain ethanol, which produces a slight sedative effect but isn't harmful to most patients and can in fact be beneficial. But ingesting ethanol can be undesirable and even dangerous in some circumstances. The list below identifies drugs containing ethanol.

acetaminophen (Aceta, Dolanex, Tylenol, and Valadol elixirs)
acetaminophen with codeine elixir (Myapap with codeine, Ty-pap elixir, Tylenol Alurate elixir, Aventyl solution, Pamelor solution)
belladonna tincture
bitolterol (Tornalate inhalant)
brompheniramine elixir (Bromphen, Dimetane, Myphetane Butisol Sodium Elixir)
chlorpheniramine elixir (Allerchlor syrup, Chloridamine, Chlor-Trimeton Syrup, Phenetron syrup)
chlorpromazine hydrochloride (Chlorpromazine Intensol [<0.1%])
clemastine fumarate (Tavist syrup)
co-trimoxazole (<1%) (Bactrim Pediatric Suspension, Bactrim suspension, Cotrim Congespirin for Children)
cyproheptadine (Periactin syrup)
dexchlorpheniramine maleate (Polaramine syrup)
dextroamphetamine (Dexedrine elixir)
diazepam (Valium, Zetran injections)
diphenhydramine (Beldin Cough Syrup, Benadryl Cough Syrup, Benadryl elixir, Diphen, Genahist, Hydramine, Hydramine Cough Syrup, Tusstat, Valdrene)
diazoxide (Proglycem suspension)
dihydroergotamine mesylate injection (D.H.E. 45)

digoxin (Lanoxin elixir, Lanoxicaps)
encainide (Brevibloc)
epinephrine (Epinephrine mist inhalant generic, Primatene mist, Bronkaid mist)
ergoloid mesylates (Hydergine oral solution)
ferrous sulfate elixirs
fluphenazine hydrochloride (Permitil oral concentrate, Prolixin elixir, oral concentrate)
hydromorphone cough syrup (Dilaudid cough syrup)
hyoscyamine (Levsin drops)
indomethacin suspension (Indocin)
isoproterenol (Norisodrine Aerotrol, Isuprel Mistometer)
isoetharine (Bronkometer oral inhalant)
mesoridazine besylate (Serentil oral concentrate)
methyldopa suspension (Aldomet, generic)
methdilazine (Tacaryl Syrup)
methadone hydrochloride oral solution (Dolophine hydrochloride)
minocycline (Minocin oral suspension)
molindone hydrochloride (Moban oral concentrate)
nitroglycerin infusion
nystatin (Mycostatin oral suspension, Nilstat oral suspension)
opium alkaloid hydrochlorides (Pantopon injection)
oxycodone hydrochloride (Roxicet, Roxicodone)
paramethadione (paradione solution)
pentobarbital injection (Nembutal sodium solution for injection, Pedric elixir)
perphenazine (Trialfon oral concentrate)
phenobarbital injection
phenytoin sodium injection (Dilantin parenteral suspension)
promethazine (Phenergan syrup plain, Phenergan syrup Fortis)
pyridostigmine (Mestinon syrup)
sodium butabarbital (Butalan elixir)
thioridazine (Mellaril concentrate)
thiothixene (Navane oral solution)

trimethoprim (Septra, Sulfatrim suspensions)
triprolidine (Actidil syrup, Myidyl syrup)
tripellenamine citrate (PBZ Elixir)
trimeprazine (Temaril Syrup)

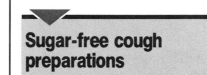

Sugar-free cough preparations

For some patients, such as diabetics, sugar-free cough preparations are desirable. The list below identifies sugar-free cough preparations; an asterisk indicates availability of the drug without a prescription.

Anamine HD Syrup
*Anatuss Syrup (alcohol-free)
Anatuss with Codeine Syrup (alcohol-free)
*Cerose-DM Liquid
Codiclear DH Syrup (alcohol- and dye-free)
*Codimal DM Syrup
Colrex Compound Elixir
*Colrex Cough Syrup
*Conar Expectorant Syrup
*Conar Syrup
*Dexafed Cough Syrup (alcohol-free)
Entuss Expectorant Liquid (alcohol-free)
Entuss Tablets
Entuss-D Liquid (alcohol- and dye-free)
Entuss-D Tablets (dye-free)
Kwelcof Liquid (alcohol- and dye-free)
*Lanatuss Expectorant
*Naldecon DX Adult Liquid (alcohol-free)
Naldecon DX Pediatric Drops
*Naldecon EX Syrup
*Naldecon Senior DX Liquid (alcohol-free)
*Noratuss II Expectorant (alcohol-free)
*Noratuss II Liquid (alcohol- and sodium-free)

*Phanatuss Syrup
Ryna-C Liquid (alcohol- and dye-free)
Ryna-CX Liquid (alcohol- and dye-free)
*Scot-tussin DM Liquid (alcohol-free)
*Silexin Cough Syrup (alcohol-free)

Tolu-Sed Cough Syrup
*Tolu-Sed DM Liquid
Torganic-DM Liquid (alcohol-free)
*Tricodene Liquid
*Trimedine Liquid
*Trind-DM Liquid
Tussadon Liquid (dye-free)
Tussar SF Cough Syrup

Tussirex Sugar Free (alcohol-and dye-free)
Tussi-Organidin Liquid
Tussi-R-Gen DM Liquid (alcohol-free)
Tussi-R-Gen Expectorant (alcohol-free)

Dialyzable drugs

The amount of a drug removed by dialysis differs among patients and depends on several factors, including the patient's condition, the drug's own properties, the length of dialysis and the dialysate used, the rate of blood flow or the dwell time, and the purpose of the dialysis. Below is a chart with general guidelines about dialyzable drugs. Even if a drug is listed as dialyzable, don't assume a dosage adjustment should be made until you consult with the patient's doctor.

Drug	Reduced by hemodialysis	Drug	Reduced by hemodialysis
acetaminophen	Yes (Hemodialysis may not influence toxicity)	atenolol	Yes
		azathioprine	Yes
acyclovir	Yes	azlocillin	Yes
allopurinol	Yes	aztreonam	Yes
alprazolam	No	bretylium	Yes
amdinocillin	Yes	captopril	Yes
amikacin	Yes	carbamazepine	No
aminoglutethimide	Yes	carbenicillin	Yes
amiodarone	No	carmustine	No
amitriptyline	No	carprofen	No
amoxicillin	Yes	cefaclor	Yes
amoxicillin/clavulanate potassium	Yes	cefadroxil	Yes
		cefamandole	Yes
amphotericin B	No	cefazolin	Yes
ampicillin	Yes	cefonicid	Yes (Drug is only slightly dialyzed [20%])
ampicillin/clavulanate potassium	Yes		
aspirin	Yes	cefoperazone	Yes

Dialyzable drugs *(continued)*

Drug	Reduced by hemodialysis	Drug	Reduced by hemodialysis
ceforanide	Yes	cisplatin	Maybe (Drug can be dialyzed within 3 hours after administration)
cefotaxime	Yes		
cefotetan	Yes (Drug is only slightly dialyzed [20%])	clindamycin	No
		clofibrate	No
cefoxitin	Yes	clonazepam	No
ceftazidime	Yes	clonidine	No
ceftizoxime	Yes	clorazepate	No
ceftriaxone	No	cloxacillin	No
cefuroxime	Yes	colchicine	No
cephalexin	Yes	cortisone	No
cephalothin	Yes	co-trimoxazole	Yes
cephapirin	Yes	cyclophosphamide	Yes
cephradine	Yes	diazepam	No
chloral hydrate	Yes	diazoxide	No
chlorambucil	No	diclofenac	No
chloramphenicol	Yes	dicloxacillin	No
chlordiazepoxide	No	digitoxin	No
chloroquine	No	digoxin	No
chlorpheniramine	No	diphenhydramine	No
chlorpromazine	No	dipyridamole	Yes
chlorprothixene	No	disopyramide	Yes
chlorthalidone	No	doxepin	No
cimetidine	Yes	doxorubicin	No
ciprofloxacin	Yes (Drug is only slightly dialyzed [20%])	doxycycline	No
		enalapril	Yes

(continued)

Dialyzable drugs (continued)

Drug	Reduced by hemodialysis	Drug	Reduced by hemodialysis
erythromycin	No	insulin	No
ethacrynic acid	No	isoniazid	Yes
ethambutol	Yes (Drug is only slightly dialyzed [20%])	isosorbide	No
		kanamycin	Yes
ethchlorvynol	Yes	ketoconazole	No
ethosuximide	Yes	ketoprofen	Maybe (Specific data are unavailable. However, substantial removal of the drug by dialysis is unlikely because this drug is highly [99%] protein bound.)
famotidine	No		
fenoprofen	No		
flecainide	No		
flucytosine	Yes	labetalol	No
fluorouracil	Yes	lidocaine	No
flurazepam	No	lithium	Yes
furosemide	No	lomustine	No
ganciclovir	Yes	lorazepam	No
gentamicin	Yes	mechlorethamine	No
glutethimide	Yes	mefenamic acid	No
glyburide	No	mercaptopurine	Yes
haloperidol	No	methadone	No
heparin	No	methicillin	No
hydralazine	No	methotrexate	Yes
hydrochlorothiazide	No	methyldopa	Yes
hydroxyzine	No	methylprednisolone	Yes
ibuprofen	No	metoclopramide	No
imipenem/cilastatin	Yes	metolazone	No
imipramine	No	metoprolol	No
indomethacin	No	metronidazole	Yes

Dialyzable drugs (continued)

Drug	Reduced by hemodialysis	Drug	Reduced by hemodialysis
mexiletine	No	procainamide	Yes
mezlocillin	Yes	propoxyphene	No
miconazole	No	propranolol	No
minocycline	No	protriptyline	No
minoxidil	Yes	quinidine	No
morphine	No	ranitidine	Yes
moxalactam	Yes	reserpine	No
nadolol	Yes	rifampin	No
nafcillin	No	streptomycin	Yes
naproxen	No	sucralfate	No
netilmicin	Yes	sulbactam	Yes
nifedipine	No	sulfamethoxazole	Yes
nitroglycerin	No	temazepam	No
nitroprusside	Yes	terfenadine	No
nortriptyline	No	theophylline	Yes
oxacillin	No	ticarcillin	Yes
oxazepam	No	timolol	No
penicillin G	Yes	tobramycin	Yes
pentazocine	Yes	tocainide	Yes
phenobarbital	Yes	tolbutamide	No
phenylbutazone	No	triazolam	No
phenytoin	No	trimethoprim	Yes
piperacillin	Yes	valproic acid	No
prazepam	No	vancomycin	No
prazosin	No	verapamil	No
prednisone	No	vidarabine	Yes
primidone	Yes		

Drug-smoking interactions

Smoking—or living and working in a smoke-filled environment—can affect a patient's drug therapy, especially if he's taking one of the drugs listed here. If your patient is using any of these drugs, monitor plasma drug levels closely and watch for possible adverse reactions.

Ascorbic acid

Possible effects
• Low serum vitamin C levels
• Decreased oral absorption of vitamin C

Nursing considerations
• Tell the patient to increase his vitamin C intake.

Chlordiazepoxide hydrochloride, chlorpromazine hydrochloride, diazepam

Possible effects
• Increased drug metabolism, which results in reduced plasma levels
• Decreased sedative effects

Nursing considerations
• Watch for a decrease in the drug's effectiveness.
• Adjust the patient's drug dosage, if ordered.

Propoxyphene hydrochloride

Possible effects
• Increased drug metabolism, which results in diminished analgesic effects
• Reduced adverse reactions in some smokers

Nursing considerations
• Watch for a decrease in the drug's effectiveness.
• Increase the dosage, if ordered.

Drug-alcohol interactions

Drug	Effects
• Analgesics • Antianxiety drugs • Antidepressants • Antihistamines • Antipsychotics • Hypnotics	Deepened central nervous system (CNS) depression
• Monoamine oxidase inhibitors	Deepened CNS depression; possible hypertensive crisis with certain types of beer and wine containing tyramine (Chianti, Alicante)
• Oral hypoglycemics • Sulfonylurea	Disulfiram-like effects (facial flushing, headache), especially with chlorpropamide; inadequate food intake may trigger increased hypoglycemic activity
• Cephalosporins • Metronidazole • Some antibacterial agents	Disulfiram-like effects

Drugs whose forms can't be altered

Patients who have trouble ingesting tablets or capsules often prefer that their medication be crushed or altered in some way. But this isn't always possible. Certain drugs, because of their release rates, unusual dosages, or other peculiarities, require them to be swallowed whole, and their forms can't be altered.

Sustained-release tablets and capsules
Medications that come in these forms release a drug at a constant rate or in pulses over time, and have two advantages: they are long-lasting and cause few adverse effects. Crushing them, however, releases too much of the drug too

Propranolol hydrochloride

Possible effects
• Increased metabolism, decreasing drug's effectiveness
• Propranolol's effectiveness hampered by increasing heart rate, stimulating catecholamine release from the adrenal medulla, raising arterial blood pressure and increasing myocardial oxygen consumption

Nursing considerations
• Monitor the patient's blood pressure and heart rate.
• Propranolol's drug-smoking effects may diminish as the patient ages.
• To reduce drug-smoking interaction, the doctor may order a selective beta blocker, such as atenolol.

Oral contraceptives containing estrogen and progestogen

Possible effects
• Increased adverse reactions, such as headache, dizziness, depression, libido changes, migraine, hypertension, edema, worsening of astigmatism or myopia, nausea, vomiting, and gallbladder disease

Nursing considerations
• Inform the patient of increased risk of myocardial infarction and cerebrovascular accident.
• Suggest that the patient stop smoking or use a different birth control method.

Theophylline

Possible effects
• Increased theophylline metabolism (from induction of liver microsomal enzymes) from smoking
• Lower plasma theophylline levels

Nursing considerations
• Monitor plasma theophylline levels and watch for decreased therapeutic effect.
• Increase theophylline dosage, if ordered.

---

quickly, which may in turn cause adverse effects. Moreover, the positive effects of the drug may not last as long, and the patient's symptoms may recur before his next scheduled dose.

You *can* open sustained-release capsules and mix their contents carefully with a liquid or soft food. But don't mix the beads too vigorously or they'll break, causing the same undesirable effects as tablet crushing. Common designations for sustained-release drugs include: Dura-Tab, Extentabs, Gradumets, Gyrocaps, Repetabs, Sequels, Spansules, and Tembids. Similarly, the following abbreviations indicate that drugs are sustained-release: Bid, CR, Dur, LA, Plateau Cap, SA, Span, and SR. Here are some examples of sustained-release tablets and capsules: Artane Sequels, Compazine Spansules, Desoxyn Gradumets, and Dimetane Extentabs.

Enteric-coated tablets
This type of medication is specially treated so that it releases in the small intestine. If the outer coating of the tablet is destroyed, the drug is absorbed in the stomach and may be inactivated or cause adverse effects.

Not all covered tablets are enteric. For example, sugar- and film-coated tablets can be crushed. Here are some examples of enteric-coated tablets: Azulfidine En-tabs, Dulcolax, Ecotrin, and E-Mycin.

Sublingual and buccal tablets
These tablets are placed under the patient's tongue to dissolve. Crushing them causes the drug to inactivate as most of it is rapidly metabolized elsewhere, such as in the liver.

Miscellaneous drugs
Some drugs can't be altered because of their active properties or peculiar dosages. Depakane, for example, comes in liquid-filled capsules which, when opened, irritate the lining of the mouth. Here are some drugs that can't be altered: Ery-Tab, Inderal LA, Nitrospan, and Ritalin-SR.

Administration guidelines. To determine whether a drug can or can't be altered, read the package labeling or the instructions inside. Then ask your pharmacist, who will know whether a drug can be crushed, or if it is available in a liquid. He can also suggest transdermal patches or rectal suppositories, but if you substitute them, you may have to change the dosage. If no alternatives are available, the patient's doctor may prescribe a different drug.

I.V. therapy devices

Direct injection

Winged infusion set

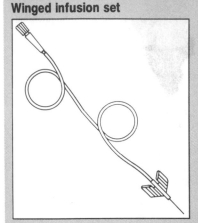

Short hubless steel needle with wings and extension tubing can be attached to a syringe or I.V. tubing. Used for I.V. push, short-term I.V. drug or fluid therapy, and for withdrawing blood specimens from small veins.

How to use
After flushing the tubing to eliminate air, insert the needle into any accessible vein, aspirate blood, and slowly inject the drug.

Special considerations
• With this device, blood return is clearly visible, wings allow easy needle grip, and sharp, thin needle is easy to insert. Also, tubing changes are easily made at extension tubing hub, vein wall damage is less, and infusion rate is more easily controlled than with syringe and needle.
• However, extravasation occurs easily because needle is nonflexible. Tape in place without obscuring needle tip to observe for extravasation.
• Stabilize on arm board for long-term use.

Intermittent injection device (heparin lock)

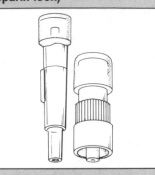

Latex cap with locking connection can be attached to any peripheral or central catheter for intermittent injection or infusion.

How to use
Prime injection cap with sterile fluid, then attach cap to venous access device. (Some needles and cannulas have preattached injection caps.) Inject saline or heparin flush to maintain patency. Before use, flush with normal saline if heparin is incompatible with primary infusion. Clean latex cap with alcohol or povidone-iodine before each use. Attach I.V. tubing to 1" 20G (or smaller) needle, insert into cap, then tape in place.

Special considerations
• If not routinely used, flush at least once daily to prevent clogging.
• Change I.V. site according to hospital policy.
• Cap is resealable with multiple injections.
• Heparin lock can be used instead of keep-vein-open I.V.
• Because of less drug-vein contact, heparin lock is less likely to cause phlebitis.
• Allows patient freedom of movement between infusions.

Intermittent infusion

Piggyback Continuflo-add-a-line system

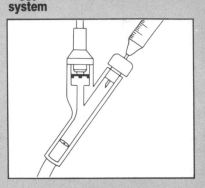

Tubing with backcheck valve and Y injection port uses existing peripheral I.V. line for intermittent delivery of drugs or solution in minibottles or bags.

How to use
Attach 19G or 20G needle to distal end of secondary tubing affixed to piggyback container. Then clean Y injection port of primary line with alcohol or povidone-iodine. Next, insert needle of secondary tubing into piggyback port, and suspend primary container lower than secondary container. Open the clamp on the primary line to regulate flow. Primary I.V. infusion will stop during secondary administration, then resume after drug delivery. Backcheck valve prevents backflow into primary container.

Special considerations
• Permits infusion of most drugs with primary solutions because of minimal mixing of primary and secondary solutions. Before next dose, backflow primary fluid into secondary tubing to remove any air.
• Change tubings according to hospital policy.

• Rate of primary I.V. may need adjustment after secondary container empties.

Click-Lock I.V. system

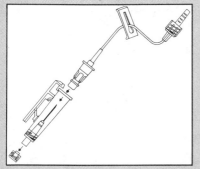

This device has two components: a transparent housing that contains a recessed needle and a diaphragm-covered port that fits into the needle housing. It can be used to piggyback an existing I.V. line into a heparin lock, central line, or an existing peripheral line with regular tubing.

How to use
To use with a regular I.V. line, first attach the Click-Lock extension tubing to the tubing from the I.V. container. Fill the extension tubing with solution, expel the air, and attach it to the I.V. catheter. Next, attach the piggyback I.V. set tubing to the Click-Lock housing unit. Run solution through the set. Then slide the needle housing over the injection port in the extension tubing until they lock.

Special considerations
• This system helps to minimize accidental disconnection, prevent contamination, and avoid needle sticks.
• With a Click-Lock in place, you can draw blood samples from a central line using a Vacutainer set-

up. After drawing blood, flush the central line with 0.9% sodium chloride solution. Next instill 2.5 ml of heparin flush solution (10 units/ml).
• Aseptic technique is critical when handling this equipment.

Volume control set

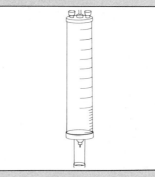

In-line graduated fluid chamber uses existing peripheral I.V. line for administration of drugs or fluids in a small volume of diluent; this device is especially suitable for children.

How to use
Prime set with I.V. fluid and clean the injection port on top of chamber with alcohol or povidone-iodine. Inject drug into port. Agitate chamber gently to disperse the medication. Next, fasten tubing below chamber to 20G needle and into primary line injection port. Open clamp on primary line to regulate infusion rate. Infusion stops when delivery is complete. Refill volume chamber for each dose.

Special considerations
• Volume control set may be attached in piggyback manner to primary I.V. set or connected directly onto I.V. cannula.
• Set is available with or without

in-line filter.
• May be used as continually flowing device by clamping air vent tubing on volume control set.
• Check for incompatibilities if piggybacked into other fluids. Avoid simultaneous infusion if primary infusion of I.V. solution or drugs (or both) is incompatible with piggyback drug.
• Flush entire set after administration to remove drug in distal tubing.

Controlled release infusion system (CRIS)

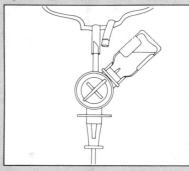

Secondary administration system administers drugs via a reconstituted vial.

How to use
Spike reconstituted vial directly onto a CRIS adapter attached to primary I.V. tubing. Valve on the adapter allows primary solution to enter and flush out the vial, which then delivers drug and solution into tubing.

Special considerations
• Requires minimal amount of diluent to prepare solution (good for fluid-restricted patients).
• Some drugs require transfer to an empty sterile vial with additional diluent.

(continued)

I.V. therapy devices *(continued)*

*Controlled release infusion system (CRIS)**(continued)*
• Check for compatibility with primary infusion.
• System eliminates need for minibags, minibottles, and secondary tubing.

Central venous line catheters
(Hickman, Groshong, multiple lumen)

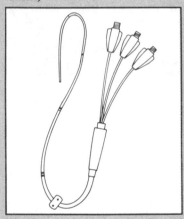

Silastic or polyurethane catheter is inserted into jugular or subclavian vein and terminated in superior vena cava. Used for intermittent infusion of drugs and withdrawal of blood specimens. Drugs and solutions may be simultaneously delivered in double- and triple-lumen catheters; especially suited for long-term and multiple therapies.

How to use
Clean injection cap attached to hub of lumen with alcohol or povidone-iodine. To deliver drug, insert needle with I.V. tubing into cap. After direct injection or infusion, flush line with saline or heparin.

Special considerations
• These catheters must be inserted by doctor, have a greater risk of infection than peripheral line catheters, and require heparin or saline flushes after each use. Also, initial cost is higher than for peripheral catheters.
• Catheters may cause life-threatening complications, such as air embolism and cardiac tamponade.
• Air elimination filtration may be needed to minimize risk of air emboli.
• Sterile technique is critical because of proximity to heart.
• Hickman and Groshong catheters may be tunneled under skin, don't dislodge easily, and are comfortable. However, they may require surgical insertion and removal if used long-term.
• Central venous line catheters allow administration of highly osmolar fluids and irritating drugs because of high volume blood flow in vena cava.
• On multiple lumen tubes, mark lumen used for drug delivery.
• Teach the patient site care and how to administer medication.
• If no complications occur, catheter may stay in place for weeks, months, or even years.

Syringe pump

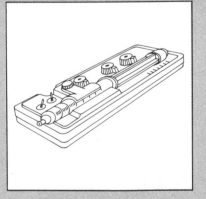

Prefitted and labeled in the pharmacy, syringe (5 to 60 ml) is used for intermittent infusion. A microbore tubing is attached to the syringe and a needle to the distal end.

How to use
After removing air by automatic pump priming, insert needle into a continuous I.V. or a heparin lock. Then start pump to mechanically deliver drug over ordered time interval. If ordered, place multiple doses in syringe. An alarm sounds when dose is infused or syringe is empty.

Special considerations
• Syringe pumps are portable and lightweight. They easily attach to clothing of ambulatory patients.
• A disadvantage is the pump's inability to accept more than 60 ml of drug with solution.
• Small drug volumes increase risk of phlebitis.

Implanted access device
(Chemo-Cath, Infuse-a-Port, Life Port, MediPort, Port-a-Cath, Q-Port, Strato-Port, and others)

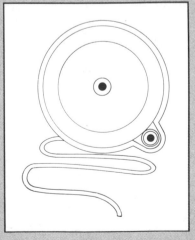

Totally implanted port with self-sealing septum is attached to a silastic catheter that terminates in the superior vena cava or other body cavity. Most commonly used for chemotherapy or other long-term therapies. Injections are made into portal through skin.

How to use
Using sterile gloves and aseptic technique, clean skin over the portal with alcohol or povidone-iodine. Insert 21G or 22G Huber needle (noncoring) attached to syringe or tubing into middle of portal until rigid back of port is palpable. Aspirate blood return to confirm needle placement, then infuse drug. Afterward, flush port with saline and heparin and remove needle.

Special considerations
• May be difficult to palpate portal when entering system (especially if patient is obese).
• Requires sterile techniques.
• Leave capped extension tubing and Huber needle in place for repeated injections.
• Life-threatening complications, such as air embolism and cardiac tamponade, are less common than with central venous lines.
• Risk of infection is low because device is sealed inside body.
• Device requires only once-monthly heparin flush between treatments; dressing changes not required.
• Sealed under the skin, this device is cosmetically acceptable because body image and activity aren't affected. However, acceptance is poor if patient is averse to needles.
• Device requires surgical insertion. More expensive than other central lines.
• Teach patient how to give medication.

Continuous infusion
Existing peripheral I.V.

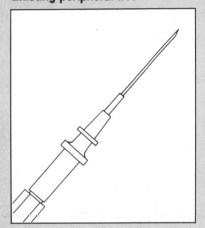

An indwelling plastic cannula can be placed in any accessible peripheral vein to maintain peripheral I.V. line.

How to use
After cleaning the site with povidone-iodine or alcohol, perform a venipuncture. Then place the cannula and stylet into the vein. Blood return indicates correct placement. Remove the stylet and attach I.V. tubing that's been flushed with fluid to remove any air. Tape the tubing in place, and regulate the flow of infusion.

Special considerations
• A peripheral I.V. line is easy to insert and causes less vein trauma than a winged infusion set. It also involves less risk of thrombophlebitis and infiltration.
• If possible, establish I.V. line in large arm veins. Hand veins are more easily irritated by continuous drug therapy. Leg and feet veins aren't usually used because of the potential for thrombophlebitis.

Multiple-lumen peripheral catheter (Arrow Twin-Cath)

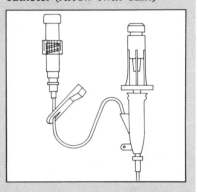

This multiple-lumen over-the-needle catheter is designed for peripheral placement. It has two separate lumens which do not allow mixing of infusates within the catheter. You may also use this catheter for blood sampling.

How to use
After readying the puncture site, prepare the catheter by flushing the proximal port through the injection cap. After performing a venipuncture, remove the introducer needle and attach a stop-cock, injection cap, or connecting tubing to the distal hub. Then check the proximal lumen hub. Aspirate for blood from the proximal port, then flush and attach the proximal hub to the desired connecting line.

Special considerations
• You may use this catheter to infuse incompatible drugs.
• Do not allow the flush solution to go beyond the tip of the catheter when flushing the proximal port.
• When using the proximal port for blood sampling, temporarily shut off the distal port.
• Acetone solution may weaken the catheter and cause leakage.

I.V. drug compatibility

Use this chart only as a guide to drug compatibilities. Compatibility varies with the type, temperature, and volume of diluting solutions. Never combine two drugs if you're uncertain of their compatibility. Check appropriate references or ask a pharmacist to be sure.

KEY:

▨ , ⁨2⁩ = Compatible (Numbers indicate compatibility only for hours indicated)

■ = Incompatible

☐ = Data unavailable

◺ = Identical drug

	albumin	amikacin	aminophylline	amino acid injection	ampicillin	bretylium	calcium gluconate	carbenicillin	cefamandole	cefazolin	cefoxitin	cephalothin	chloramphenicol	cimetidine	clindamycin	corticotropin (ACTH)	dexamethasone	dextrose 5% in water	dextrose 5% in R.L.	dextrose 5% in 0.45% NSS	dextrose 5% in 0.9% NSS	diphenhydramine	dobutamine	dopamine
albumin	◺																							
amikacin			8		24	8		8					24	24	24		4	24	24	24	24	24	24	
aminophylline	8			24		48											24	24			24			
amino acid injection		24			24	24		24		24			24	24										24
ampicillin												1	24				2	4	4					
bretylium		48			48													48	48	48	48			48
calcium gluconate	24		24		48												24	24		24				
carbenicillin	8		24									24					24	24		24			24	
cefamandole														24				24		48				
cefazolin	8		24								24	24					24							
cefoxitin																	24	24	24	24				
cephalothin			24										24	24			24	24		24			6	
chloramphenicol	24			1			24										24	24		24			24	
cimetidine	24		24	24				24		24			24		24			24						
clindamycin	24		24				24			24		24						24		24	24			
corticotropin (ACTH)																								
dexamethasone	4	24											24											
dextrose 5% in water	24	24		2	48	24	24	24	24	24	24	24		24								48	24	
dextrose 5% in R.L.	24		4	48	24	24		24	24	24												48	48	
dextrose 5% in 0.45% NSS	24		4	48		48	24		24			24										48	48	
dextrose 5% in 0.9% NSS	24	24		48	24	24		24	24	24		24										48	48	
diphenhydramine	24								24															
dobutamine																	48	48	48	48				24
dopamine			24		48		24			6	24					24	48	48	48		24			
epinephrine	24								24				24	24		24		24						
erythromycin lactobionate (I.V.)		24	24							24			6			6	24							
gentamicin			24						24			24	24			24								
heparin sodium			24						24		48	24		4		24	24				24			

	epinephrine	erythromycin lactobionate (I.V.)	gentamicin	heparin sodium	hydrocortisone Na succinate	insulin (regular)	isoproterenol	kanamycin	lactated Ringer's	lidocaine	metaraminol	methicillin	methylprednisolone	mezlocillin	moxalactam	multiple vitamin infusion	nafcillin	netilmicin	norepinephrine	0.9% NSS	oxacillin	oxytocin	penicillin G potassium	phytonadione	piperacillin	polymyxin B sulfate	potassium chloride	procainamide	sodium bicarbonate	tetracycline	thiamine	ticarcillin	tobramycin	vancomycin	verapamil	vitamin B complex with C
	24				24					24									24	24	8		8	24	24	4			24	4				24	24	
		24			24					24								24		24									24						48	
			24	24	24		24	24		24	24	24	24						24		24		24	24			24		24						24	
				6					8										24							1			24						24	
				48						24									48								24	48							48	
										24									24																48	
			24		24														24							1	24		24						24	
																			24																24	
																24			24																24	
			24					48							24				24									24				24	24	24	
			24	24														24									24		24					24	
																			24															24	
	24	24	24	48		24	24		24	24		24			48	24	24		24	24	24	24				24		24	24	48
		24	24	24		24	24			24		24		24		24		24		24		24	24	24	24
			4	4																			4						4
	24	6	24		24	24	24		24	6	6	24	24	24	24		6	6	24	24	24	24	24	24	24	24
	24		24	24	24		24	24	24		24	24	24	24		24	24	24	24	24
			24					24	24	24													24
	24	6	24	24	24	24	24	24	24	24	12	24	24	24	24	24	48	24
		24												24						24
	24	24	24	48	24	24	24	24	24	24	24	24
		24	18	24	48	24	18	48	24	24	24	24
		24	2	24	24	24
	18	24	24	24
	24	24	24
	24	24	24	6	24	24	24

(continued)

I.V. drug compatibility (continued)

KEY:

▨ , 2	= Compatible (Numbers indicate compatibility only for hours indicated)
■	= Incompatible
☐	= Data unavailable
◩	= Identical drug

	albumin	amikacin	aminophylline	amino acid injection	ampicillin	bretylium	calcium gluconate	carbenicillin	cefamandole	cefazolin	cefoxitin	cephalothin	chloramphenicol	cimetidine	clindamycin	corticotropin (ACTH)	dexamethasone	dextrose 5% in water	dextrose 5% in R.L.	dextrose 5% in 0.45% NSS	dextrose 5% in 0.9% NSS	diphenhydramine	dobutamine	dopamine
hydrocortisone Na succinate		24	24		6			24				24			24		4	24	24		24			18
insulin (regular)			24		48										24									
isoproterenol			24												24			24	24		24		24	
kanamycin										48					24			24			24			24
lactated Ringer's					8										24								48	48
lidocaine		24	24		24	24									24				24		24		24	24
metaraminol	24		24												24		24	24		24		24		
methicillin			24														6	24	24	24				
methylprednisolone			24											24	24		6							18
mezlocillin																	24							
moxalactam																	24	24	24	24				
multiple vitamin infusion									24					24			24	24		24				
nafcillin			24											48				24	24	24	24			
netilmicin																								
norepinephrine	24		24											24									24	
0.9% NSS	24	24		24	48	24	24	24	24	24	24	24	24	24	24								24	48
oxacillin	8		24														6	24		12				24
oxytocin																	6							
penicillin G potassium	8		24				24							24	24			24	24		24	24		
phytonadione	24		24											24										
piperacillin																	24			24				
polymyxin B sulfate	24			1			1							24										
potassium chloride	4		24				24							24	24		4	24	24		24			24
procainamide				24																			24	
sodium bicarbonate	24	24		24	48		24			24	24			24			24		24				
tetracycline	4		24											24			24	24		24			24
thiamine																								
ticarcillin					6												24							
tobramycin								24									24			48				
vancomycin		24												24				24						
verapamil	■	24	48		24	48	48	24	24	24	24	24	24	24	24			24	24	24	24		24	
vitamin B complex with C									24					48	24		4	24						

	epinephrine	erythromycin lactobionate (I.V.)	gentamicin	heparin sodium	hydrocortisone Na succinate	insulin (regular)	isoproterenol	kanamycin	lactated Ringer's	lidocaine	metaraminol	methicillin	methylprednisolone	mezlocillin	moxalactam	multiple vitamin infusion	nafcillin	netilmicin	norepinephrine	0.9% NSS	oxacillin	oxytocin	penicillin G potassium	phytonadione	piperacillin	polymyxin B sulfate	potassium chloride	procainamide	sodium bicarbonate	tetracycline	thiamine	ticarcillin	tobramycin	vancomycin	verapamil	vitamin B complex with C
						8			24				4							24					24				24						24	
				8					24											24																48
			24						24											24																24
									24											24																24
	24	18		24			24	24		24		24			24	24	24			24		24		24		24			24		24		48	24		24	24
	2		24		24				24											24									24	24						48
									24											24										24						24
			24						24											6																24
			24	4																6																24
																				6																
									24											24																
									24									24		24			4							24	24					
									24											24						24										
														24						24																
																																				24
	24	24	24	6	24		24	24		24	24	6	6	6	24	24	24			8		24		24		24	24	24	24	24		24	48		24	
									24							8												24						24	
																												24						24	
			24						24		24		24		4				24										24					24	
																													24						
			24						24										24								24									
									24									24		24						24								24		
									24											24																
		24		24	24					24	24					24			24	24	24		24			24						24			24	
									24							24			24		24						24								24	
									48										24																24	
									24											48															24	
																																			24	
	24	24	24	24	24	24	48	24		24	48	24	24	24						24	24	24	24	24					24		24		24	24	24	24
									24																											24

Compatibility of drugs combined in a syringe

Combining drugs in one syringe avoids the discomfort of two separate injections. Generally, drugs can be mixed in a syringe in one of three ways: from two multidose vials (regular and long-acting insulin, for example); from one multidose vial and one ampul; or from two ampuls. You can't combine drugs that are not compatible, or when the combined doses exceed the amount of solution that can be absorbed from a single injection site.

KEY:
- ■ = Compatible
- ■ = Not compatible
- ■ = Provisionally compatible; use within 15 minutes of preparation
- ? = Conflicting reports on compatibility; mixing not recommended
- □ = Data unavailable
- ◨ = Identical drug

The following drugs form both the row and column headers of the compatibility matrix:

atropine, butorphanol, chlorpromazine, codeine, diazepam, glycopyrrolate, hydromorphone, hydroxyzine, meperidine, morphine, nalbuphine, pentobarbital, phenobarbital, promethazine, scopolamine, secobarbital, sodium bicarbonate, thiopental

(Cell values are indicated by color coding per the key above. Conflicting-report "?" markers appear at the morphine × promethazine and promethazine × morphine intersections.)

Extravasation: Prevention and treatment

Extravasation, the penetration of a drug into surrounding tissue, stems from a punctured vein or leakage at a venipuncture site. When vesicant drugs or fluid extravasate, local tissue damage can occur. The net result can be prolonged healing, infection, multiple debridements, cosmetic disfigurement, loss of function, and possible amputation.

You can prevent extravasation by following a few simple guidelines.
• Use an existing I.V. line only when patent. Perform a new venipuncture to ensure correct needle placement and vein patency.
• Select the site carefully. Use a distal vein to allow successive venipuncture. Areas to avoid include the hand's dorsum, wrist, and digits and previously damaged areas. Don't attempt venipuncture on an area with poor circulation.
• Avoid probing for a vein. Instead, stop and begin again at another spot.
• Start the infusion with D_5W or

Antidotes for extravasation

Extravasation antidotes are usually administered through existing I.V.s to infiltrate the area, or with a 1-ml tuberculin syringe to inject directly into the affected site.

Antidote	Dose	Extravasated drug
Hyaluronidase 15 units/ml Mix a 150-unit vial with 1 ml normal saline for injection. Withdraw 0.1 ml and dilute with 0.9 ml saline to get 15 units/ml.	0.2 ml × 5 subcutaneous injections around site	aminophylline calcium solutions contrast media dextrose solutions (concentrations of 10% or more) hyperalimentation solutions nafcillin potassium solutions vinblastine vincristine vindesine
Sodium bicarbonate 8.4%	5 ml	carmustine daunorubicin doxorubicin vinblastine vincristine
Phentolamine Dilute 5 to 10 mg with 10 ml of sterile saline for injection.	5 to 10 ml	dobutamine dopamine epinephrine metaraminol bitartrate norepinephrine
Sodium thiosulfate 10% Dilute 4 ml with 6 ml sterile water for injection.	10 ml	dactinomycin mechlorethamine mitomycin
Hydrocortisone sodium succinate 100 mg/ml Usually followed by topical application of hydrocortisone cream 1%.	50 to 200 mg 25 to 50 mg/ml of extravasate	doxorubicin vincristine
Ascorbic acid injection	50 mg	dactinomycin
Sodium edetate	150 mg	plicamycin

normal saline solution.
• Transparent dressings are best to allow for inspection.
• Check for extravasation before starting an infusion. Apply a tourniquet above the needle to occlude the vein and see if the flow continues. If not, the solution isn't infiltrating. You can also lower the I.V. container and check for blood backflow. Bear in mind that the needle may have punctured the opposite vein wall but still rests in the vein. Flush the needle to ensure patency. If swelling occurs at the I.V. site, infiltration has occurred. Give by slow I.V. push through a free-flowing I.V. line or by small-volume infusion (50 to 100 ml).

• During infusion, observe for signs of erythema or infiltration.
• Patients should be instructed to report any burning, stinging, pain, or temperature changes.
• After administering the drug, use several milliliters of D₅W or normal saline solution to flush the vein and prevent leakage when the needle is taken out.

Locating I.M. injection sites

Intramuscular (I.M.) injections deposit medication deep into muscle tissue, where a large network of blood vessels can absorb it readily and quickly. You should choose the site for an I.M. injection carefully, taking into account the patient's physical status and the purpose of the injection. Don't administer I.M. injections at in-

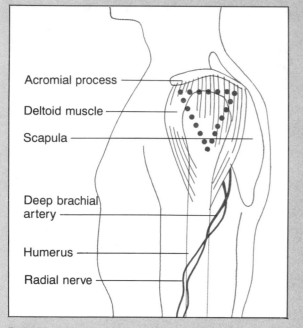

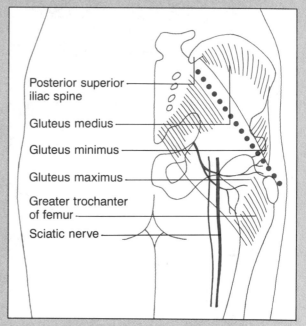

Deltoid. To locate the densest area of muscle and avoid major nerves and blood vessels, find the lower edge of the acromial process and the point on the lateral arm in line with the axilla. Insert the needle 1″ to 2″ (2.5 to 5 cm) below the acromial process, usually 2 to 3 fingerbreadths, at a 90° angle or angled slightly toward the process.

Standard ml injected: 0.5 to 2

Dorsogluteal (upper outer corner of the gluteus maximus). Restrict injections to the area above and outside the diagonal line drawn from the posterior superior iliac spine to the greater trochanter of the femur. Or divide the buttock into quadrants and inject in the upper outer quadrant, about 2″ to 3″ (5 to 7.6 cm) below the iliac crest. Insert the needle at a 90° angle to the muscle.

Standard ml injected: 1 to 5

• Vesicants should be administered last when giving multiple drugs. If possible, they should not be administered using an infusion pump.

If extravasation occurs:
1. Stop the I.V. and remove its line, unless the needle is necessary to administer an antidote.

2. Estimate the amount of extravasation solution and tell the doctor.
3. Follow hospital procedure for administering an antidote.
4. Elevate the extremity.
5. Note the extravasation site, amount of extravasated solution, the patient's symptoms and treatment. Document the time you called the doctor and keep an on-

going record of extravasation symptoms.
6. Apply ice packs or warm compresses to site as determined by hospital procedure.
7. Use silver sulfadiazine cream and gauze dressings or wet-to-dry iodine dressings on damaged skin, as ordered.

flamed, edematous, or irritated areas, or those containing moles, birthmarks, scar tissue, or other lesions. I.M. injections may also be contraindicated for patients with impaired coagulation mechanisms, occlusive peripheral vascular disease, edema, and shock—conditions that impair absorption.

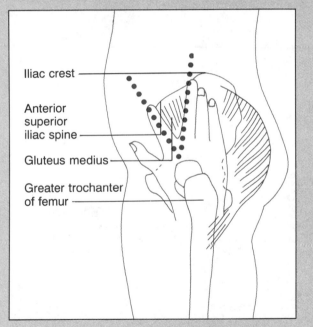

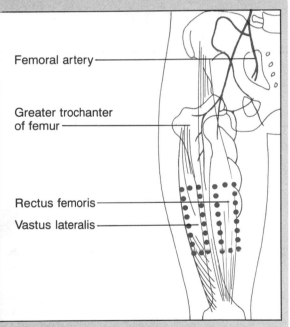

Ventrogluteal (gluteus medius and gluteus minimus). Locate the greater trochanter of the femur with the heel of your hand. Then spread your index and middle fingers to form a V from the anterior superior iliac spine to the farthest point along the iliac crest that you can reach. Insert the needle into the area between the two fingers at a 90° angle to the muscle. Remove your hand before inserting the needle.

Standard ml injected: 1 to 5

Vastus lateralis. Use the lateral muscle of the quadriceps group, along that length of the muscle from a handbreadth below the greater trochanter to a handbreadth above the knee. Insert the needle into the middle third of the muscle on a plane parallel to the surface on which the patient is lying. You may have to bunch the muscle before inserting the needle.

Standard ml injected: 1 to 5; 1 to 3 for infants

Identifying and treating toxic drug reactions

Toxic reaction	Clinical effects	Interventions	Selected causative drugs
Anaphylaxis Sudden, severe, and sometimes fatal systemic hypersensitivity	• Abdominal cramps, nausea, diarrhea • Angioedema • Change or loss of voice resulting from laryngeal edema • Continuous sneezing • Cough • Dilated pupils • Dyspnea, stridor • Edema and pruritus at injection site • Faintness • Feeling of impending doom or fright • Flushing, pallor, or cyanosis • Hypotension • Loss of consciousness • Nasal pruritus • Pounding headache • Seizures • Sweating • Urinary urgency and incontinence • Urticaria • Weak, rapid, thready pulse • Weakness	• Immediately notify doctor. • Inject epinephrine 1:1,000 aqueous solution, 0.1 to 0.5 ml. Repeat q 5 to 20 min as ordered. • Maintain airway patency (a tracheostomy or endotracheal tube may be required if laryngeal edema occurs). • Assess for hypotension and shock. Maintain circulatory volume with volume expanders (plasma, plasma expanders, saline, and albumin) as needed. • If cardiac arrest occurs, begin cardiopulmonary resuscitation. • After completing emergency measures, give corticosteroids, diphenhydramine, or aminophylline, as ordered.	• Antibiotics, especially penicillin and its derivatives • Almost any drug, if patient is hypersensitive to it
Hepatotoxicity Damage to or destruction of liver cells	• Abnormal SGPT (ALT), SGOT (AST), serum bilirubin, and lactic dehydrogenase levels • Jaundice • Abdominal pain, hepatomegaly • Bleeding, low-grade fever, mental changes, weight loss • Dry skin, pruritus, rash	• Reduce dosage or discontinue drug. • Monitor vital signs, blood levels, weight, intake and output, and fluid and electrolyte balance. • Promote rest. • Assist with hemodialysis, if needed. • Provide symptomatic care: Vitamins A, B complex, D, and K; potassium supplements to correct alkalosis; salt-poor albumin to maintain fluid and electrolyte balance; neomycin to suppress bacterial flora in GI tract; aspiration of blood from stomach, reduction of dietary protein, and administration of lactulose to reduce blood ammonia levels.	• Chlorpromazine • Erythromycin estolate • Methotrexate • Methyldopa

Identifying and treating toxic drug reactions *(continued)*

Toxic reaction	Clinical effects	Interventions	Selected causative drugs
Nephrotoxicity Damage to kidney cells	• Casts, albumin, or red or white blood cells in urine • Altered creatinine clearance • Electrolyte imbalance • Elevated blood urea nitrogen • Oliguria • Blurred vision, dehydration (depending on part of kidney affected), edema, mild headache, pallor • Dizziness, fatigue, irritability, slowed mental processes	• Reduce dosage or discontinue drug. • Assist with hemodialysis, if needed. • Monitor vital signs, weight changes, and urine volume. • Provide symptomatic care: fluid restriction and loop diuretics to reduce fluid retention, I.V. solutions to maintain electrolyte imbalance.	• Aminoglycosides • Antineoplastics • Corticosteroids • Diuretics • Narcotics • Tetracyclines • Vasopressors or vasoconstrictors
Neurotoxicity Damage to or destruction of cells in any part of the nervous system	• Akathisia • Apnea, depressed respirations • Bilateral or unilateral palsies • Cerebral infarction • Dystonia • Hypertensive crisis • Fasciculation • Intracerebral or subarachnoid hemorrhage • Muscle twitching, tremors • Paresthesias • Strokelike syndrome • Unsteady gait • Weakness	• Notify doctor as soon as changes appear. • Reduce dosage or discontinue drug. • Monitor carefully for any changes in patient's condition. • Provide symptomatic care: remain with patient, reassure him, and protect him during seizures. Provide a quiet environment, draw shades, speak in soft tones. Maintain airway and ventilate the patient as needed.	• Analeptics • Antibacterials • Anticonvulsants • Antihistamines • Central nervous system depressants • Phenothiazines • Pressor amines, such as epinephrine • Rauwolfia alkaloids • Tricyclic antidepressants
Oculotoxicity Damage to or destruction of cells of the eye	• Acute glaucoma • Blurred, colored, or flickering vision • Diplopia • Miosis • Mydriasis • Optic neuritis • Scotomata • Vision loss	• Notify doctor as soon as changes appear. • Stop drug, as ordered. (Some oculotoxic drugs used to treat serious conditions may be given again at a lower dosage after the eyes return to near-normal state.) • Monitor carefully for changes in symptoms. • Treat effects symptomatically.	• Antibiotics, such as chloramphenicol • Cardiac glycosides • Phenothiazines
Ototoxicity Damage to the eighth cranial nerve or to the organs of hearing and balance	• Ataxia • Hearing loss • Tinnitus • Vertigo	• Notify doctor as soon as changes appear. • Discontinue drug or reduce dosage, as ordered. • Monitor carefully for symptomatic changes.	• Aminoglycosides • Antibiotics, such as sodium colistimethate, gentamicin, kanamycin, streptomycin • Quinine • Salicylates • Ethacrynic acid

(continued)

Identifying and treating toxic drug reactions (continued)

Toxic reaction	Clinical effects	Interventions	Selected causative drugs
Pseudomem-branous colitis Acute inflammation and necrosis of the small and large intestine, which usually affects the mucosa but may extend into the submucosa and, rarely, other layers	• Abdominal pain • Colonic perforation • Fever • Hypotension • Severe dehydration • Shock • Sudden, copious diarrhea (watery or bloody)	• Notify doctor as soon as changes appear. • Immediately discontinue drug, as ordered. • Give another antibiotic, such as vancomycin, metronidazole, or bacitracin. • Maintain fluid and electrolyte balance. Check serum electrolytes daily. If pseudomembranous colitis is mild, give an ion exchange resin as ordered. • Record intake and output. • Monitor vital signs, skin color and turgor, urine output, and consciousness level. • Immediately report signs of shock. • Observe for signs of hypokalemia, especially malaise and weak, rapid, irregular pulse.	• Broad-spectrum antibiotics

Reversing anaphylaxis

Anaphylaxis is the sudden, extreme reaction to a foreign antigen and should be treated immediately. As a general rule, the faster the symptoms' onset, the more severe the reaction. Here is a chart of drugs useful in reversing anaphylactic reactions.

Drug and classification	Indication and dosage	Action	Nursing considerations
diphenhydramine (Benadryl) Antihistamine	*Mild anaphylaxis* *P.O.:* 25 to 100 mg t.i.d. *I.V.:* 25 to 50 mg q.i.d.	• Competes with histamine for H_1 receptor sites • Prevents laryngeal edema • Controls localized itching	• Administer I.V. doses slowly to avoid hypotension. • Monitor patient for hypotension. • Caution patient about driving; drug causes drowsiness and slows reflexes. • Give fluids as needed. Drug causes dry mouth.
epinephrine (Adrenalin) Adrenergic	*Severe anaphylaxis* (drug of choice) *Initial infusion:* 0.2 to 0.5 mg of epinephrine (0.2 to 0.5 ml of 1:1,000	*Alpha-adrenergic effects:* • Increases blood pressure • Reverses peripheral vasodilation and systemic hypotension	• Select large vein for infusion. • Use infusion controller to regulate drip. • Check blood pressure and

Reversing anaphylaxis (continued)

Drug and classification	Indication and dosage	Action	Nursing considerations
epinephrine (continued)	strength diluted in 10 ml normal saline) given I.V. slowly over 5 to 10 min, followed by continuous infusion. *Continuous infusion:* 1 to 4 mcg/min (mix 1 ml of 1:1,000 epinephrine in 250 ml of dextrose 5% in water [D₅W] to get concentration of 4 mcg/ml).	•Decreases angioedema and urticaria •Improves coronary blood flow by raising diastolic pressure •Causes peripheral vasoconstriction *Beta-adrenergic effects:* •Causes bronchodilation •Causes positive inotropic and chronotropic cardiac activity •Decreases synthesis and release of chemical mediator	heart rate. •Monitor patient for dysrhythmias. •Check solution strength, dosage, and label before administering. •Watch for signs of extravasation at infusion site. •Monitor intake and output. •Assess color and temperature of extremities.
hydrocortisone (Solu-Cortef) Corticosteroid	*Severe anaphylaxis* *I.V.:* 100 to 200 mg q 4 hr to q 6 hr.	•Prevents neutrophil and platelet aggregation •Inhibits synthesis of mediators •Decreases capillary permeability	•Monitor fluid and electrolyte balance, intake and output, and blood pressure closely. •Maintain patient on ulcer and antacid regimen prophylactically.
aminophylline (Aminophyllin) Methylxanthine bronchodilator	*Severe anaphylaxis* *I.V.:* 5 to 6 mg/kg loading dose, followed by 0.4 to 0.9 mg/kg/min infusion.	•Causes bronchodilation •Stimulates respiratory drive •Dilates constricted pulmonary arteries •Causes diuresis •Strengthens cardiac contractions •Increases vital capacity •Causes coronary vasodilation	•Monitor blood pressure, pulse, and respirations. •Monitor intake and output, hydration status, and aminophylline and electrolyte levels. •Monitor patient for dysrhythmias. •Use I.V. controller to reduce risk of overdose. •Maintain serum levels at 10 to 20 mcg/ml.
cimetidine (Tagamet) Antihistamine	*Severe anaphylaxis* (experimental use in refractory cases) *I.V.:* 600 mg diluted in D₅W and administered over 20 min.	•Competes with histamine for H₂ receptor sites •Prevents laryngeal edema	•Be aware that Tagamet is incompatible with aminophylline. •Reduce dosage for patients with impaired renal or hepatic function.

▼
Drugs and pregnancy: Rating the risks

Some drugs are riskier than others for patients who are pregnant. The FDA has established five categories (A, B, C, D, and X) that indicate a drug's potential for causing birth defects.

Categories:
A: Controlled studies show no risks to pregnant patients. Adequate studies in pregnant patients failed to demonstrate risks to the fetus.
B: There is no evidence of risk in humans. Either animal studies show risk and human studies do not; or, if no adequate human studies have been done, animal findings are negative.
C: Risk cannot be ruled out. Human studies are lacking, and animal studies are either positive for fetal risk, or are also lacking. However, potential benefits may justify the potential risk.
D: Positive evidence of risk to the fetus. Nevertheless, potential benefits may outweigh potential risks.
X: Contraindicated in pregnancy. Studies in animals or humans have shown fetal risk that clearly outweighs any benefits.

▼
Controlled substance schedule

Many drugs are potentially habit-forming and addictive. But some drugs have a higher potential for abuse than others, and these are administered through Food and Drug Administration (FDA) guidelines in the United States. Controlled substances are divided into five groups, Schedules I to V. Canada's Health Protection Branch classifies all controlled drugs in one group, Schedule G (see chart below).
   If you must administer a controlled drug, follow these guidelines.
• Consult your hospital's procedures for special handling instructions.
• Document on the sign-out sheet any drugs removed from the narcotics stock.
• If there is a leftover drug, dispose of it properly.
• Don't leave any drug unattended. Lock the narcotics cabinet after use.

Schedule	Examples
United States	
I	heroin, lysergic acid diethylamide (LSD), marijuana derivatives, mescaline, peyote, and psilocybin
II	amobarbital, amphetamine, cocaine, codeine, hydromorphone, meperidine, methadone, methamphetamine, methaqualone, methylphenidate, morphine, opium, oxycodone, oxymorphone, pentobarbital, phenmetrazine, and secobarbital
III	barbituric acid derivatives (except those listed in another schedule), benzphetamine, glutethimide, mazindol, methylprylon, paregoric, and phendimetrazine
IV	barbital, benzodiazepine derivatives, chloral hydrate, diethylpropion, ethchlorvynol, ethinamate, fenfluramine, meprobamate, methohexital, paraldehyde, phenobarbital, and phentermine
V	diphenoxylate compound and expectorants with codeine
Canada	
G	all salts and derivatives of the following: amphetamine, barbituric acid, benzphetamine, butorphanol, chlorphentermine, diethylpropion, methamphetamine, methaqualone, methylphenidate, pentazocine, phendimetrazine, phenmetrazine, and phentermine

Recognizing and treating acute substance abuse

Substance	Signs and symptoms	Interventions
Alcohol (ethanol) • beer and wine • distilled spirits • other preparations, such as cough syrup, after-shave, or mouthwash	• Ataxia • Seizures • Coma • Hypothermia • Alcohol breath odor • Respiratory depression • Bradycardia • Hypotension • Nausea and vomiting	• Expect to induce vomiting or perform gastric lavage if ingestion occurred in the previous 4 hours. Give activated charcoal and a saline cathartic, as ordered. • Start I.V. fluid replacement and administer dextrose, thiamine, B-complex vitamins, and Vitamin C, as ordered, to prevent dehydration and hypoglycemia and to correct nutritional deficiencies. • Pad bed rails and apply cloth restraints to protect the patient from injury. • Give an anticonvulsant such as diazepam, as ordered, to control seizures. • Watch the patient for signs and symptoms of withdrawal, such as hallucinations and alcohol withdrawal syndrome. If these occur, give chlordiazepoxide (Librium), chloral hydrate, or paraldehyde, as ordered. (Be sure to administer paraldehyde with a glass syringe or glass cup to avoid a chemical reaction with plastic.) • Auscultate the patient's lungs frequently to detect crackles or rhonchi, possibly indicating aspiration pneumonia. If you note these breath sounds, expect to give antibiotics. • Perform neurologic assessments and monitor the patient's vital signs every 15 minutes until he's stable. Assist with dialysis if the patient's vital functions are severely depressed.
Amphetamines • amphetamine sulfate (Benzedrine) — bennies, greenies, cartwheels • methamphetamine (Methadrin) — speed, meth, crystal • dextroamphetamine sulfate (Dexedrine) — dexies, hearts, oranges	• Dilated reactive pupils • Altered mental status (from confusion to paranoia) • Hallucinations • Tremors and seizure activity • Hyperactive deep tendon reflexes • Exhaustion • Coma • Dry mouth • Shallow respirations • Tachycardia • Hypertension • Hyperthermia • Diaphoresis	• If the drug was taken orally, induce vomiting or perform gastric lavage; give activated charcoal and a sodium or magnesium sulfate cathartic, as ordered. • Acidify the patient's urine by adding ammonium chloride or ascorbic acid to his I.V. solution, as ordered, to lower his urine pH to 5. • Force diuresis by giving the patient mannitol, as ordered. • Expect to give a short-acting barbiturate, such as pentobarbital, to control stimulant-induced seizures. • Restrain the patient, especially if he's paranoid or hallucinating, so he won't injure himself and others. • Give haloperidol (Haldol) I.M., as ordered, to treat agitation or assaultive behavior. • Give an alpha-adrenergic blocking agent, such as phentolamine (Regitine), for hypertension, as ordered. • Watch for cardiac dysrhythmias. Notify the doctor if these develop, and expect to give propranolol or lidocaine to treat tachydysrhythmias or ventricular dysrhythmias, respectively. • Treat hyperthermia with tepid sponge baths or a hypothermia blanket, as ordered. • Provide a quiet environment to avoid overstimulation.

(continued)

Recognizing and treating acute substance abuse (continued)

Substance	Signs and symptoms	Interventions
Amphetamines (continued)		• Be alert for signs and symptoms of withdrawal, such as abdominal tenderness, muscle aches, and long periods of sleep. • Observe suicide precautions, especially if the patient shows signs of withdrawal.
Antipsychotics • chlorpromazine (Thorazine) • phenothiazines • thioridazine (Mellaril)	• Constricted pupils • Photosensitivity • Extrapyramidal side effects (dyskinesia, opisthotonos, muscular rigidity, ocular deviation) • Dry mouth • Decreased level of consciousness • Decreased deep tendon reflexes • Seizures • Hypothermia or hyperthermia • Dysphagia • Respiratory depression • Hypotension • Tachycardia	• Expect to perform gastric lavage if the patient ingested the drug within the past 6 hours. (Don't induce vomiting, because phenothiazines have an antiemetic effect.) Give activated charcoal and a cathartic, as ordered. • Give diphenhydramine (Benadryl) or benztropine (Cogentin), as ordered, to treat extrapyramidal side effects. • Give physostigmine salicylate, as ordered, to reverse the drug's anticholinergic effects in severe cases. • Replace fluids I.V., as ordered, to correct hypotension; monitor the patient's vital signs frequently. • Monitor his respiratory rate and give supplemental oxygen to treat respiratory depression. • Give an anticonvulsant, such as diazepam, or a short-acting barbiturate, such as pentobarbital sodium (Nembutal), as ordered, to control seizures. • Keep the patient's room dark to avoid exacerbating his photosensitivity.
Anxiolytic sedative-hypnotics • benzodiazepines (Valium, Librium)	• Confusion • Drowsiness • Stupor • Decreased reflexes • Seizures • Coma • Shallow respirations • Hypotension	• Induce vomiting or perform gastric lavage; give activated charcoal and a cathartic, as ordered. • Give supplemental oxygen to correct hypoxia-induced seizures. • Administer fluids I.V., as ordered, to correct hypotension; monitor the patient's vital signs frequently. • If the patient's severely intoxicated, give physostigmine salicylate (Antilirium), as ordered, to reverse respiratory and CNS depression.
Barbiturate sedative-hypnotics • amobarbital sodium (amytal sodium)—blue angels, blue devils, blue birds • phenobarbital (Luminal)—phennies, purple hearts, goofballs • secobarbital sodium (Seconal)—reds, red devils, seccy	• Poor pupil reaction to light • Nystagmus • Depressed level of consciousness (from confusion to coma) • Flaccid muscles and absent reflexes • Hyperthermia or hypothermia • Cyanosis • Respiratory depression • Hypotension • Blisters or bullous lesions	• Induce vomiting or perform gastric lavage if the patient ingested the drug within 4 hours; give activated charcoal and a saline cathartic, as ordered. • Maintain his blood pressure with I.V. fluid challenges and vasopressors, as ordered. • If the patient's taken a phenobarbital overdose, give sodium bicarbonate I.V., as ordered, to alkalinize his urine and to speed the drug's elimination. • Apply a hyper- or hypothermia blanket, as ordered, to help return the patient's temperature to normal. • Prepare your patient for hemodialysis or hemoperfusion if toxicity is severe. • Perform frequent neurologic assessments and check your patient's pulse rate, temperature, skin color, and reflexes often.

Recognizing and treating acute substance abuse (continued)

Substance	Signs and symptoms	Interventions
Barbiturate sedative-hypnotics (continued)		• Notify the doctor if you see signs of respiratory distress or pulmonary edema. • Watch for signs of withdrawal, such as hyperreflexia, tonic-clonic seizures, and hallucinations. • Protect the patient from injuring himself and provide symptomatic relief of withdrawal symptoms, as ordered.
Cocaine • "free-base" • cocaine hydrochloride • crack	• Dilated pupils • Confusion • Alternating euphoria and apprehension • Hyperexcitability • Visual, auditory, and olfactory hallucinations • Spasms and seizures • Coma • Tachypnea • Hyperpnea • Pallor or cyanosis • Respiratory arrest • Tachycardia • Hypertension or hypotension • Fever • Nausea and vomiting • Abdominal pain • Perforated nasal septum or oral sores	• Calm the patient down by talking to him in a quiet room. • If cocaine was ingested, induce vomiting or perform gastric lavage; give activated charcoal followed by a saline cathartic, as ordered. • Give the patient a tepid sponge bath and administer an antipyretic, as ordered, to reduce fever. • Monitor his blood pressure and heart rate. Expect to give propranolol, for symptomatic tachycardia. • Administer an anticonvulsant, such as diazepam (Valium), as ordered, to control seizures. • Scrape the inside of his nose to remove residual amounts of the drug. • Monitor his cardiac rate and rhythm—ventricular fibrillation and cardiac standstill can occur as a direct cardiotoxic result of cocaine. Defibrillate and initiate cardiopulmonary resuscitation, if indicated.
Glutethimide (Doriden) cibas, CD, blues	• Small, reactive pupils • Nystagmus • Drowsiness • Irritability • Impaired thought processes (memory, judgment, attention span) • Slurred speech • Twitching, spasms, and seizures • Hypothermia • Central nervous system (CNS) depression (unresponsive to deep coma) • Apnea • Respiratory depression • Hypotension • Paralytic ileus • Poor bladder control	• If the drug was taken orally, induce vomiting or perform gastric lavage; give activated charcoal and a cathartic, as ordered. • Maintain the patient's blood pressure with I.V. fluid challenges and vasopressors, as ordered. • Assist with hemodialysis or hemoperfusion if the patient has hepatic or renal failure or prolonged coma. • Administer an anticonvulsant, such as diazepam, for seizures, as ordered. • Perform hourly neurologic assessments: coma may recur because of the drug's slow release from fat deposits. • Be alert for signs of increased intracranial pressure, such as decreasing level of consciousness and widening pulse pressure. Give mannitol I.V., as ordered. • Watch for signs of withdrawal, such as hyperreflexia, tonic-clonic seizures, and hallucinations. • Protect the patient from injuring himself, and provide symptomatic relief of withdrawal symptoms.

(continued)

Recognizing and treating acute substance abuse (continued)

Substance	Signs and symptoms	Interventions
Hallucinogens • lysergic acid diethylamide (LSD) — hawk, acid, sunshine • mescaline (peyote) — mese, cactus, big chief	• Dilated pupils • Intensified perceptions • Agitation and anxiety • Synesthesia • Impaired judgment • Hyperactive movement • Flashback experiences • Hallucinations • Depersonalization • Moderately increased blood pressure • Increased heart rate • Fever	• Reorient the patient repeatedly to time, place, and person. • Restrain the patient to protect him from injuring himself and others. • Calm the patient down by talking to him in a quiet room. • If the drug was taken orally, induce vomiting or perform gastric lavage; give activated charcoal and a cathartic, as ordered. • Give diazepam I.V., as ordered, to control seizures.
Narcotics • codeine • heroin — smack, H, junk, snow • hydromorphone hydrochloride (Dilaudid) — D, lords • morphine — mort, monkey, M, Miss Emma	• Constricted pupils • Depressed level of consciousness (but the patient's usually responsive to persistent verbal or tactile stimuli) • Seizures • Hypothermia • Slow, deep respirations • Hypotension • Bradycardia • Skin changes (pruritus, urticaria, and flushed skin)	• Repeat naloxone (Narcan) administration, as ordered, until the drug's CNS depressant effects are reversed. • Replace fluids I.V., as ordered, to increase circulatory volume. • Correct hypothermia by applying extra blankets; if the patient's body temperature doesn't increase, use a hyperthermia blanket, as ordered. • Reorient the patient frequently. • Auscultate his lungs frequently for crackles, possibly indicating pulmonary edema. (Onset may be delayed.) • Administer oxygen via nasal cannula, mask, or mechanical ventilation to correct hypoxemia from hypoventilation. • Monitor cardiac rate and rhythm, being alert for atrial fibrillation. (This should resolve spontaneously when the hypoxemia's corrected.) • Be alert for signs of withdrawal, such as piloerection (goose flesh), diaphoresis, and hyperactive bowel sounds.
Nonbarbiturate sedative-hypnotics • methaqualone (Quaaludes) — ludes, soapers, love drug	• Dilated pupils • Nystagmus • Disorientation • Slurred speech • Hypertonicity • Ataxia • Twitching and seizures • Coma • Dry mouth • Anorexia • Nausea, vomiting, or diarrhea	• Expect to induce vomiting or perform gastric lavage if the patient ingested the drug within the past 2 to 4 hours. Give activated charcoal and a cathartic, as ordered. • Maintain his blood pressure with I.V. fluids and vasopressors, as ordered. • If the patient has severe toxicity, prepare him for hemodialysis or hemoperfusion. • Give diazepam initially, as ordered, to treat hypertonicity. If hypertonicity doesn't improve, expect the doctor to give curare and to place the patient on a mechanical ventilator. • Give diazepam, phenytoin, or phenobarbital, as ordered, to control seizures.

Recognizing and treating acute substance abuse *(continued)*

Substance	Signs and symptoms	Interventions
Nonbarbiturate sedative-hypnotics *(continued)*		• Auscultate his lungs frequently. Note crackles, rhonchi, or decreased breath sounds, possibly indicating aspiration pneumonia. Give supplemental oxygen and antibiotics, as ordered. • Watch for signs of withdrawal, such as hyperreflexia, tonic-clonic seizures, and hallucinations. • Give pentobarbital or phenobarbital, as ordered, to treat withdrawal signs and symptoms.
Phencyclidine (PCP) angel dust, peace pill, hog	• Blank staring • Nystagmus • Amnesia • Decreased awareness of surroundings • Recurrent coma • Violent behavior • Hyperactivity • Seizures • Gait ataxia • Muscle rigidity • Drooling • Hyperthermia • Hypertensive crisis • Cardiac arrest	• If the drug was taken orally, induce vomiting or perform gastric lavage; instill and remove activated charcoal repeatedly, as ordered. • Force acidic diuresis by acidifying the patient's urine with ascorbic acid, as ordered, to increase excretion of the drug. • Give diazepam and haloperidol, as ordered, to control agitation or psychotic behavior. • Administer diazepam, as ordered, to control seizures. • Expect to continue to acidify his urine for 2 weeks, because signs and symptoms may recur when fat cells release their stores of PCP. • Provide a quiet environment and dimmed light. • Give propranolol, as ordered, to treat hypertension and tachycardia. If the patient's hypertension is severe, give nitroprusside, as ordered. • Closely monitor his urine output and serial renal function tests—rhabdomyolysis, myoglobinuria, and renal failure may occur in severe intoxication. • If the patient develops renal failure, prepare him for hemodialysis.
Tricyclic antidepressants • amitriptyline hydrochloride (Elavil) • imipramine hydrochloride (Tofranil)	• Dilated pupils • Blurred vision • Altered mental status (from agitation to hallucinations) • Loss of deep tendon reflexes • Seizures • Coma • Anticholinergic effects (dry mucous membranes, diminished secretions) • Tachycardia • Hypotension • Nausea and vomiting • Urine retention	• Expect to induce vomiting or perform gastric lavage if the patient ingested the drug within the past 24 hours. (Anticholinergic effects of these drugs decrease gastric emptying.) Give activated charcoal and a magnesium sulfate cathartic, as ordered. • Replace fluids I.V. to correct hypotension, as ordered. • Give sodium bicarbonate and sodium physostigmine I.V., as ordered, to correct hypotension and dysrhythmias; if bifascicular or complete heart block occurs, assist with insertion of a temporary transvenous pacemaker. • Treat seizures with diazepam or phenobarbital I.V., as ordered.

What to do with a patient who abuses drugs or alcohol

A patient who abuses drugs or alcohol presents a liability to you and to the hospital. If he harms himself or someone else, you may be held legally responsible. The guidelines for handling drug and alcohol abusers vary among hospitals, so you should be familiar with the rules of your institution.

Your hospital may require that you confiscate drugs or alcohol and that you take further steps to prevent the patient from obtaining more.

When you suspect a patient is taking drugs
If you think a patient is taking drugs but have no proof, you may be expected to perform a drug search.

If you believe a patient poses a threat to himself or to others, and you can document this, you're probably within your legal rights to search the patient's room and his possessions. Confer with your supervisor and then inform the patient. Bring along a security guard for protection and to act as a witness.

What you can and cannot search
Hospital policy generally spells out what can and cannot be searched. Typically, you can search the patient's room and his belongings, and you're required to confiscate illegal drugs. Alcohol should also be confiscated and returned to the patient when he leaves the hospital.

You may have to report your findings to the police, so you should document your search in your notes and file an incident report. You should also inform the patient's doctor.

Administering code drugs

Drug, route, and dosage	Precautions
atropine sulfate *To treat bradycardia:* 0.5 mg I.V. every 5 min, up to 2 mg total. *To treat asystole:* 1 mg I.V.; repeat after 5 min if asystole persists. *Infusion:* Not recommended. *Intratracheal:* May be used.	• Lower doses (<0.5 mg) may cause bradycardia. • Higher doses (>2 mg) may cause full vagal blockage. • Contraindicated for glaucoma patients (use isoproterenol instead).
bretylium tosylate (Bretylate, Bretylol) *I.V. push:* Rapidly administer 5 mg/kg; can be repeated in 15 to 30 min to total of 30 mg/kg. *Infusion:* 500 mg diluted with at least 50 ml with D_5W or D_5 normal saline solution; infuse at 1 to 2 mg/min.	• Not typically used to treat premature ventricular contractions unless other drugs fail. • May increase digitalis toxicity. • May lower blood pressure.
calcium chloride *I.V. push:* Administer 5 to 10 ml of 10% solution at 1 ml/min; can be repeated every 10 min. *Infusion:* Not generally recommended. Can add to D_5W or normal saline solution; flow rate shouldn't exceed 1.5 mEq/min.	• Contraindicated in patients with hypercalcemia. • Infiltration may produce severe tissue damage. • Use cautiously in patients receiving digoxin; may produce dysrhythmias. • Don't give to patients with high serum phosphate levels; may produce fatal calcium deposits. • Don't mix with other medications.
dobutamine hydrochloride (Dobutrex) *I.V. push:* Not recommended. *Infusion:* Reconstitute with D_5W or normal saline solution, then prepare standard dilution; administer 2.5 to 10 mcg/kg/min.	• Don't use with beta blockers, such as propranolol. • Drug is incompatible with alkaline solutions. • Patients with atrial fibrillation should receive digoxin first, or they may develop rapid ventricular response. • Infiltration may produce severe tissue damage.
dopamine hydrochloride (Intropin) *I.V. push:* Not recommended. *Infusion:* Standard dilution. May use with D_5W, D_5 normal saline solution, or $D_5\frac{1}{2}$ normal saline solution; administer 2 to 5 mcg/kg/min, up to 50 mcg/kg/min.	• Don't use for treating uncorrected tachydysrhythmias or ventricular fibrillation. • May precipitate dysrhythmias. • Drug is incompatible with alkaline solutions. • Infiltration may produce severe tissue damage. • Solution deteriorates after 24 hours.

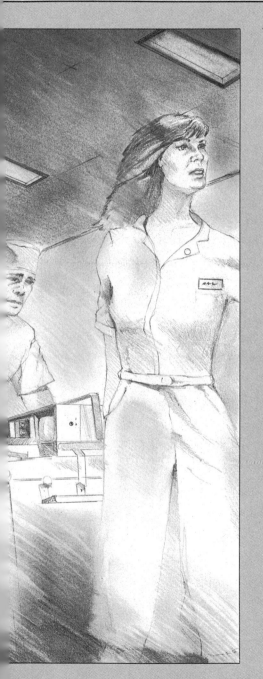

Drug, route, and dosage	Precautions
epinephrine hydrochloride (Adrenalin) *I.V. push:* Administer 5 to 10 ml of 1:10,000 solution (0.5 to 1 mg) over 1 min. *Intracardiac:* Administer 5 ml of 1:10,000 solution. *Infusion:* Not recommended. *Intratracheal:* 0.5 to 1 mg.	• Increases intraocular pressure. • May exacerbate congestive heart failure (CHF), dysrhythmias, angina pectoris, hyperthyroidism, and emphysema. • May cause headaches, tremors, or palpitations.
isoproterenol hydrochloride (Isuprel) *I.V. push:* Administer 0.02 to 0.04 mg initially, then 0.01 to 0.2 mg. *Infusion:* Administer at 0.5 to 5 mcg/min and titrate as needed.	• Don't administer with epinephrine. • Don't mix with barbiturates, sodium bicarbonate, any calcium preparation, or aminophylline.
lidocaine hydrochloride (Xylocaine) *I.V. push:* Administer 50 to 100 mg; can be repeated every 5 min. Total dose should not exceed 300 mg in 1-hr period. *Infusion:* Standard dilution. Administer at 1 to 4 mg/min. *Intratracheal:* May be used.	• Don't mix with sodium bicarbonate. • Don't use if patient has high-grade sinoatrial or atrioventricular (AV) block. • Discontinue if PR interval or QRS complex widens or if dysrhythmias worsen. • May lead to CNS toxicity.
procainamide hydrochloride (Pronestyl) *I.V. push:* Give 20 mg/min, up to 1 g total (in emergency). The usual dosage is 50 mg every 5 min until desired response occurs, up to 1 g. *Infusion:* Infuse at 1 to 4 mg/min.	• Can cause precipitous hypotension; don't use for treating second- or third-degree heart block unless a pacemaker's been inserted. • Can cause AV block.
sodium bicarbonate *I.V. push:* Rapidly administer 44.6 mEq in 50 ml D_5W (1 mEq/kg); give no more than half this dose every 10 min thereafter. *Infusion:* Not recommended.	• Don't mix with epinephrine; causes epinephrine degradation. • Don't mix with calcium salts; forms insoluble precipitates.
verapamil hydrochloride (Calan, Isoptin) *I.V. push:* Give 5 mg initially, then 10 mg 15 to 30 min later if dysrhythmia persists. *Infusion:* For maintenance only; infuse at 0.005 mg/kg/min.	• Contraindicated in patients with hypotension, cardiogenic shock, severe CHF, or second- or third-degree AV block. • High doses or administering too rapidly can cause a significant drop in blood pressure.

Estimating body surface area in children

Pediatric drug dosages should be calculated on the basis of body surface area or body weight. If your pediatric patient is of average size, find his weight and corresponding surface area on the first scale to the left. Otherwise, use the nomogram to the right: Lay a straightedge on the correct height and weight points for your patient, and observe the point where it intersects on the surface area scale at center. *Note:* Don't use drug dosages based on body surface area in premature or full-term newborns. Instead, use body weight.

For children of normal height and weight

Nomogram

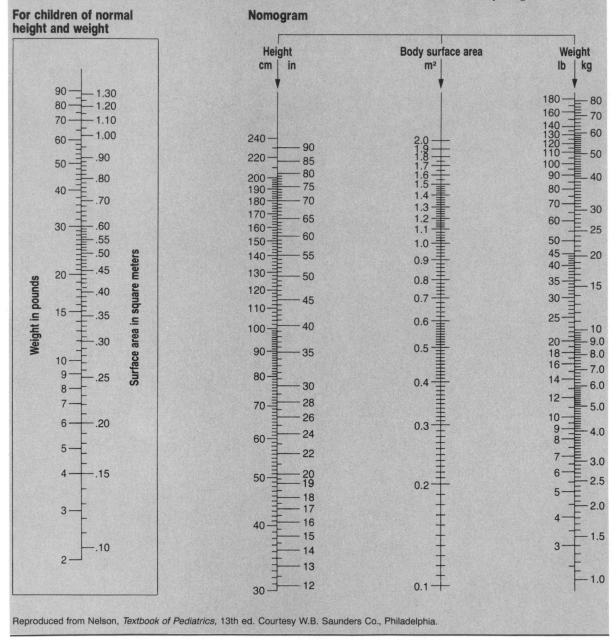

Reproduced from Nelson, *Textbook of Pediatrics,* 13th ed. Courtesy W.B. Saunders Co., Philadelphia.

Estimating body surface area in adults

Place a straightedge from the patient's height in the left-hand column to his weight in the right-hand column. The intersection of this line with the center scale reveals the body surface area. The adult nomogram is especially useful in calculating dosages for chemotherapy.

Height	Body surface area	Weight

Reproduced from Lenter, C., ed. *Geigy Scientific Tables*, 8th ed. Courtesy CIBA-GEIGY, Basle, Switzerland.

Recommended dosage adjustments in renal failure

This table lists recommended dosage adjustments in mild, moderate, and severe renal failure. These adjustments are necessary because impaired renal function may modify a drug's bioavailability, distribution, pharmacologic action, or elimination, thereby predisposing the patient to drug toxicity. For example, digoxin toxicity can follow impaired renal function because digoxin is eliminated from the body almost exclusively by the kidneys (via glomerular filtration).

Drug	Mild renal impairment (glomerular filtration rate [GFR] > 50 ml/min)		Moderate renal impairment (GFR 10 to 50 ml/min)		Severe renal impairment (GFR < 10 ml/min)	
	% of normal dose	Interval	% of normal dose	Interval	% of normal dose	Interval
acetaminophen	100%	q 4 hr	100%	q 6 hr	100%	q 8 hr
acetazolamide	100%	q 6 hr	100%	q 12 hr	Avoid	Avoid
acetohexamide	100%	q 12 hr	Avoid	Avoid	Avoid	Avoid
acyclovir	100%	q 8 hr	100%	q 24 hr	100%	q 48 hr
allopurinol	100%	q 8 hr	75%	q 8 hr	50%	q 8 hr
amantadine	100%	q 12 to 24 hr	100%	q 48 to 72 hr	100%	q 7 days
amikacin	60% to 90%	q 8 to 12 hr	30% to 70%	q 12 hr	20% to 30%	q 24 hr
amoxicillin	100%	q 6 hr	100%	q 6 to 12 hr	100%	q 12 to 16 hr
amphotericin B	100%	q 24 hr	100%	q 24 hr	100%	q 24 to 36 hr
ampicillin	100%	q 6 hr	100%	q 6 to 12 hr	100%	q 12 to 16 hr
aspirin	100%	q 4 hr	100%	q 4 to 6 hr	Avoid	Avoid
atenolol	100%	q 24 hr	100%	q 48 hr	100%	q 96 hr
azathioprine	100%	q 24 hr	100%	q 24 hr	100%	q 36 hr
azlocillin	100%	q 4 to 6 hr	100%	q 6 to 8 hr	100%	q 8 hr
bleomycin	100%	Varies	100%	Varies	50%	Varies
bretylium	100%	Continuous infusion	25% to 50%	Continuous infusion	Avoid	Avoid
captopril	100%	t.i.d.	100%	t.i.d.	50%	t.i.d.
carbamazepine	100%	q 6 to 8 hr	100%	q 6 to 8 hr	75%	q 6 to 8 hr
carbenicillin	100%	q 8 to 12 hr	100%	q 12 to 24 hr	100%	q 24 to 48 hr
cefaclor	100%	q 6 hr	50% to 100%	q 6 hr	33%	q 6 hr
cefadroxil	100%	q 8 hr	100%	q 12 to 24 hr	100%	q 24 to 48 hr

Recommended dosage adjustments in renal failure (continued)

Drug	Mild renal impairment (GFR > 50 ml/min)		Moderate renal impairment (GFR 10 to 50 ml/min)		Severe renal impairment (GFR < 10 ml/min)	
	% of normal dose	Interval	% of normal dose	Interval	% of normal dose	Interval
cefamandole	100%	q 6 hr	100%	q 6 to 8 hr	100%	q 8 hr
cefotaxime	100%	q 6 to 8 hr	100%	q 8 to 12 hr	100%	q 12 to 24 hr
cefoxitin	100%	q 8 hr	100%	q 8 to 12 hr	100%	q 24 to 48 hr
cephalexin	100%	q 6 hr	100%	q 6 to 8 hr	100%	q 12 hr
cephalothin	100%	q 6 hr	100%	q 6 hr	100%	q 8 to 12 hr
cephapirin	100%	q 6 hr	100%	q 6 to 8 hr	100%	q 12 hr
cephradine	100%	q 6 hr	50%	q 6 hr	25%	q 6 hr
chloral hydrate	100%	At bedtime	Avoid	Avoid Avoid	Avoid	
chlorpropamide	100%	q 24 hr	Avoid	Avoid	Avoid	Avoid
chlorthalidone	100%	q 24 hr	100%	q 24 hr	100%	q 48 hr
cimetidine	100%	q 6 hr	100%	q 8 hr	100%	q 12 hr
cisplatin	100%	Varies	75%	Varies	50%	Varies
clofibrate	100%	q 6 to 12 hr	100%	q 12 to 18 hr	100%	q 24 to 48 hr
clonidine	100%	b.i.d.	100%	b.i.d.	50% to 75%	b.i.d.
colchicine	100%	Varies	100%	Varies	50%	Varies
cyclacillin	100%	q 6 hr	100%	q 6 to 12 hr	100%	q 12 to 24 hr
cyclophosphamide	100%	q 12 hr	100%	q 12 hr	100%	q 18 to 24 hr
diflunisal	100%	q 12 hr	100%	q 12 hr	50%	q 12 hr
digitoxin	100%	q 24 hr	100%	q 24 hr	50% to 75%	q 24 hr
digoxin	100%	q 24 hr	100%	q 36 hr	100%	q 48 hr
diphenhydramine	100%	q 6 hr	100%	q 6 to 9 hr	100%	q 9 to 12 hr
disopyramide	100%	q 6 hr	100%	q 12 to 24 hr	100%	q 24 to 40 hr
doxycycline	100%	q 12 hr	100%	q 12 to 18 hr	100%	q 18 to 24 hr
ethacrynic acid	100%	q 6 hr	100%	q 6 hr	Avoid	Avoid

(continued)

Recommended dosage adjustments in renal failure (continued)

Drug	Mild renal impairment (GFR > 50 ml/min)		Moderate renal impairment (GFR 10 to 50 ml/min)		Severe renal impairment (GFR < 10 ml/min)	
	% of normal dose	Interval	% of normal dose	Interval	% of normal dose	Interval
ethambutol	100%	q 24 hr	100%	q 24 to 36 hr	100%	q 48 hr
ethosuximide	100%	q 12 hr	100%	q 12 hr	75%	q 12 hr
flucytosine	100%	q 6 hr	100%	q 12 to 24 hr	100%	q 24 to 48 hr
gemfibrozil	100%	b.i.d.	50%	b.i.d.	25%	b.i.d.
gentamicin	60% to 90%	q 8 to 12 hr	30% to 70%	q 12 hr	20% to 30%	q 24 hr
guanethidine	100%	q 24 hr	100%	q 24 hr	100%	q 24 to 36 hr
hydralazine	100%	q 8 hr	100%	q 8 hr	100%	q 8 to 16 hr (fast acetylators) q 12 to 24 hr (slow acetylators)
hydroxyurea	100%	Varies	100%	Varies	50%	Varies
isoniazid	100%	q 24 hr	100%	q 24 hr	66% to 75%	q 24 hr
kanamycin	60% to 90%	q 8 to 12 hr	30% to 70%	q 12 hr	20% to 30%	q 24 hr
lincomycin	100%	q 6 hr	100%	q 12 hr	100%	q 24 hr
lithium carbonate	100%	t.i.d. to q.i.d.	50% to 75%	t.i.d. to q.i.d.	25% to 50%	t.i.d. to q.i.d.
lorazepam	100%	t.i.d. to q.i.d.	100%	t.i.d. to q.i.d.	50%	t.i.d. to q.i.d.
meprobamate	100%	q 6 hr	100%	q 9 to 12 hr	100%	q 12 to 18 hr
methadone	100%	q 6 to 8 hr	100%	q 6 to 8 hr	50% to 75%	q 6 to 8 hr
methotrexate	100%	Varies	50%	Varies	Avoid	Avoid
methyldopa	100%	q 6 hr	100%	q 9 to 18 hr	100%	q 12 to 24 hr
metoclopramide	100%	Varies	75%	Varies	50%	Varies
metronidazole	100%	q 8 hr	100%	q 8 to 12 hr	100%	q 12 to 24 hr
mezlocillin	100%	q 4 to 6 hr	100%	q 6 to 8 hr	100%	q 8 hr
mithramycin	100%	Varies	75%	Varies	50%	Varies
mitomycin C	100%	Varies	100%	Varies	75%	Varies

Recommended dosage adjustments in renal failure (continued)

Drug	Mild renal impairment (GFR > 50 ml/min)		Moderate renal impairment (GFR 10 to 50 ml/min)		Severe renal impairment (GFR < 10 ml/min)	
	% of normal dose	Interval	% of normal dose	Interval	% of normal dose	Interval
moxalactam	100%	q 8 hr	100%	q 12 hr	100%	q 12 to 24 hr
nadolol	100%	q 24 hr	50%	q 24 hr	25%	q 24 hr
nalidixic acid	100%	q.i.d.	Avoid	Avoid	Avoid	Avoid
neostigmine	100%	q 6 hr	100%	q 6 hr	100%	q 12 to 18 hr
netilmicin	60% to 90%	q 8 to 12 hr	30% to 70%	q 12 hr	20% to 30%	q 24 hr
nicotinic acid	100%	t.i.d.	50%	t.i.d.	25%	t.i.d.
nitrofurantoin	100%	q.i.d.	Avoid	Avoid	Avoid	Avoid
oxazepam	100%	q.i.d.	100%	q.i.d.	75%	q.i.d.
penicillin G	100%	q 6 to 8 hr	100%	q 8 to 12 hr	Avoid over 10 million units/day	q 12 to 16 hr
phenobarbital	100%	t.i.d.	100%	t.i.d.	100%	q 12 to 16 hr
phenylbutazone	100%	t.i.d. to q.i.d.	100%	t.i.d. to q.i.d.	Avoid	Avoid
piperacillin	100%	q 4 to 6 hr	100%	q 6 to 8 hr	100%	q 8 hr
primidone	100%	q 8 hr	100%	q 8 to 12 hr	100%	q 12 to 24 hr
probenecid	100%	q.i.d.	Avoid	Avoid	Avoid	Avoid
procainamide	100%	q 4 hr	100%	q 6 to 12 hr	100%	q 8 to 24 hr
propoxyphene	100%	q 4 hr	100%	q 4 hr	25%	q 4 hr
reserpine	100%	q 24 hr	100%	q 24 hr	Avoid	Avoid
spironolactone	100%	q 6 to 12 hr	100%	q 12 to 24 hr	Avoid	Avoid
streptomycin	100%	q 24 hr	100%	q 24 to 72 hr	100%	q 72 to 96 hr
sulfamethoxazole	100%	q 12 hr	100%	q 18 hr	100%	q 24 hr
sulfisoxazole	100%	q 6 hr	100%	q 8 to 12 hr	100%	q 12 to 24 hr
sulindac	100%	b.i.d.	100%	b.i.d.	50%	b.i.d.
terbutaline	100%	t.i.d.	50%	t.i.d.	Avoid	Avoid

(continued)

Recommended dosage adjustments in renal failure (continued)

Drug	Mild renal impairment (GFR > 50 ml/min)		Moderate renal impairment (GFR 10 to 50 ml/min)		Severe renal impairment (GFR < 10 ml/min)	
	% of normal dose	Interval	% of normal dose	Interval	% of normal dose	Interval
ticarcillin	100%	q 8 to 12 hr	100%	q 12 to 24 hr	100%	q 24 to 48 hr
tobramycin	60% to 90%	q 8 to 12 hr	30% to 70%	q 12 hr	20% to 30%	q 24 hr
triamterene	100%	q 12 hr	100%	q 12 hr	Avoid	Avoid
trimethoprim	100%	q 12 hr	100%	q 18 hr	100%	q 24 hr
vancomycin	100%	q 1 to 3 days	100%	q 3 to 10 days	100%	q 10 days
vidarabine	100%	Continuous infusion	100%	Continuous infusion	75%	Continuous infusion

9 | Emergencies: How to respond

Setting priorities in an emergency

Determining your priorities in an emergency requires making split-second decisions. To help you determine them correctly, remember your ABCs.

Airway
Check the victim's airway immediately. If it's occluded, remove any obstruction, if possible. A swollen tongue, mucus, or secretions may also block the airway. Observe carefully.

Breathing
Look for chest expansion, listen for air flow, and feel for expired breath. If the victim isn't breathing, provide emergency assistance.

Circulation
Locate the carotid pulse in an adult or child older than age 1, or the brachial pulse in an infant. (You may also decide to try locating the femoral pulse.) If you can't detect a pulse, begin cardiac compression immediately.

Categorizing an emergency

On the medical-surgical unit and in the emergency department (ED), your nursing skills and knowledge determine which patients require care first. This kind of sorting process, called triage, uses nursing personnel and their available resources to the best advantage in emergency situations.

Prioritize your patients' needs according to their medical condition. Problems are categorized as emergent, urgent, or nonurgent.

Emergent
This patient has first priority in the ED and on the unit. In the ED, the patient might have:
- cardiac arrest
- airway and breathing problems
- chest pain with acute dyspnea or cyanosis
- active seizures
- obvious or suspected severe bleeding
- severe head injury
- comatose state
- open chest wound
- abdominal wound
- severe shock

- fever over 105° F (40.6° C).
  In the medical-surgical unit, the patient might have:
- cardiac arrest
- airway and breathing problems
- chest pain with acute dyspnea or cyanosis
- active seizures
- obvious or suspected severe bleeding
- a change in level of consciousness
- injury from a fall
- sudden alteration in vital signs
- fever over 105° F (40.6° C).

Urgent
Medical treatment must be given within a few hours or the patient will suffer irreversible injury or death. This patient has second priority in the ED; call the doctor and stay with patient on the unit.
  In the ED, the patient might have:
- cerebrovascular accident or transient ischemic attack
- persistent nausea and vomiting or diarrhea
- severe pain of any type
- fever over 102° F (38.9°C)
- circulatory deficit in limb
- severe or sudden headache.
  In the medical-surgical unit, the patient might have:
- sudden numbness or paralysis

• persistent nausea and vomiting or diarrhea
• severe pain of any type
• sudden fever over 102° F (38.9° C)
• circulatory deficit in limb
• severe or sudden headache.

Nonurgent
This patient doesn't require ED resources. Refer to a private doctor or clinic. He doesn't need constant supervision on the unit.

In the ED, the patient may have sprains or strains, mild headache,

or minor lacerations.

In the medical-surgical unit, the patient would have no acute problem. He might be hospitalized for diagnostic purposes or be waiting for discharge or transfer to an extended-care facility.

Using accident information to predict injuries

When you're assessing an accident victim, every second counts. You simply don't have time to do a complete head-to-toe assessment and to obtain a detailed health history. So how can you make the most of every second? As quickly as you can, find out what type of accident caused the damage. Then, knowing that each major type of accident has a distinctive

mechanism of injury, you can predict the types of injuries your patient's likely to have and focus your assessment accordingly.

This chart shows you the mechanisms of injury and related possible injuries for major accidents and assaults.

Type	Mechanism of injury	Possible injuries
Motor vehicle collisions—occupant injuries		
Head-on	Body travels down and under, striking knees on dashboard, then chest on steering wheel	Knee dislocation, femur fracture, posterior fracture or dislocation of hip, cardiac contusion, aortic tears and dissection
	Body travels up and over, snapping head forward (hitting windshield) and striking lower chest or upper abdomen on steering wheel	Head trauma, hyperflexion or hyperextension, cervical spine injuries, rib fractures, intra-abdominal injuries
Rear-end	Body travels forward as head remains in place, then snaps back across backrest or headrest	Whiplash injuries of third to fourth cervical vertebrae
	If frontal impact's also involved, body travels forward and hits dashboard and steering wheel	Injuries from frontal impact (such as cardiac contusion, rib fractures, intra-abdominal and intrathoracic injuries)
Lateral impact	Body slams into door, injuring chest, pelvis, and neck	Chest injuries with or without humerus fracture, pelvic or femur fractures, contralateral neck injuries (tears or sprain of neck ligaments)
Rotational force	Body reacts to collision as vehicle hits stationary object and rotates around it	Combination of head-on and lateral impact collision injuries
Rollover	Body stays in place (if restrained) or bounces around as vehicle rolls over	Various collision injuries, similar to rotational-force injuries
Seat belt	Body compresses against lap belt worn too high (above anterior superior iliac spine)	Abdominal organ injuries, thoracic or lumbar spine injuries

Using accident information to predict injuries *(continued)*

Type	Mechanism of injury	Possible injuries
Motor vehicle accidents – pedestrian injuries		
Head-on (Waddell's triad)	Body impacts with bumper and hood	Femur and chest injuries
	Force propels victim toward third point of impact (when body comes to rest)	At third point of impact, contralateral skull injuries
Lateral impact	Lower and upper leg impact with bumper and hood	Tibia, fibula, and femur fractures; ligament damage in opposite knee because of excess stress
Motorcycle collisions		
Head-on	Head and chest strike handlebars	Head, chest, and abdominal injuries, bilateral femur fractures
Angular	Motorcycle falls on body	Crush injuries to lower limbs, open fractures
Ejection	Body is thrown from motorcycle into an object	Head and spine injuries, deceleration injuries
Assaults		
Beating	Body—especially head, neck, abdomen—is struck by blunt object or fist	Soft tissue injuries, major organ injuries in specific area of blunt trauma
Stab wound	Body—usually chest or abdomen—is stabbed with sharp weapon	Major blood loss, sucking chest wound, organ penetration, heart or major vessel penetration (location and direction of attack, length and type of weapon, and height and strength of attacker determine severity)
Missile injuries	Projectile from a pistol, rifle, shot gun, or explosion enters and exits body, or enters and lodges in body *and*	Range from minor puncture to life-threatening wound of chest, abdomen, or head
	Projectile follows path of least resistance *and*	Lacerated tissue in bullet's path, possible injury to remote organs
	Projectile forms cavity as it releases energy into tissues in its path *and*	Initial wound, subsequent tissue injury (not necessarily in direct path of bullet), secondary infection
	Energy travels through affected tissues and injures other tissues *and*	Internal tissue and bone damage
	Close contact may cause muzzle blast injury	Internal tissue and bone damage

(continued)

Using accident information to predict injuries *(continued)*

Type	Mechanism of injury	Possible injuries
Jumps and falls		
Compression force (Don Juan syndrome)	Person falls from a height and lands on his heels; forward momentum causes acute flexion of lumbar spine, then continued forward momentum causes person to land on outstretched hands	Bilateral fractures of calcaneus; compression fractures of vertebrae; Colles' fracture of wrists
Indirect force	Person falls backward and lands on back and head	Spine and head injuries, tibia and fibula fractures
Twisting force	Person falls (usually during sports activity) and twists legs	Tibia and fibula fractures

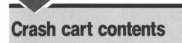

Crash cart contents

Crash carts typically contain drugs and equipment, but their actual contents vary among hospitals and individual units. The standard crash cart stock includes:
- Ambu bag
- Cardiopulmonary resuscitation board
- Defibrillator monitor
- Drugs
- I.V. supplies, syringes, needles
- Intubation equipment
- O_2 cylinder
- Arterial blood gas kits, central venous pressure lines
- Nasogastric tube, suction catheters, indwelling urinary (Foley) catheter
- I.V. solutions and tubing, blood pressure cuff, procedure trays.

You should familiarize yourself with the cart on your floor, as well.

Check the cart's contents during every shift and after every emergency, restocking as necessary.

Assessing a noncommunicative patient

In an emergency, the best way to get a medical history is from the victim himself. But he may be unconscious, or his throat obstructed, in which case you'll exercise other options:
- Question anyone familiar with the victim, such as family, friends, eyewitnesses, or rescue personnel.
- Check for medical indentification. If he's wearing a Medic Alert bracelet or necklace, note what it says about his medical status.
- If he's a transferee from a nursing home, outpatient clinic, or referral agency, call them for an update on his medical history.
- Check to see if he's carrying any prescription medicine. The medicine itself may indicate a preexisting condition; the container label will tell the prescribing doctor and pharmacy. You can call both for a patient history. Most pharmacies maintain patient profile cards containing pertinent medical information.
- If the victim is a former hospital admittee, you may be able to locate the old chart or ED record.

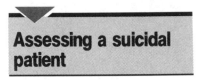

Assessing a suicidal patient

Do you have a suicidal patient in your charge? Given the number of misconceptions that surround suicide, you may not know. These are the facts:
- Eight out of ten people who commit suicide have warned others of their intentions.
- People who attempt suicide are ambivalent about dying. Most of them can't decide whether to live or die; neither wish is stronger.
- People who want to kill themselves can overcome these feelings with professional help and go on to live normal lives.
- A "lift" in a person's depression doesn't necessarily mean he's recovered from suicidal thoughts.

Most persons commit suicide within 3 months after reporting feeling better; this hiatus from depression may be attributed to their decision to commit suicide. Without treatment, suicide-bent patients will make more than one attempt, as well.

How you can recognize a potential suicide

Consider several factors in determining whether your patient is contemplating suicide. Some, like age and sex, are general indicators of the more likely candidates. Others, such as familial and friend relationships, can tell whether he's severed these ties to fulfill his intentions.

• *Age and sex.* Suicide is highest in young people (ages 15 to 24) and in persons over 50. Men are more successful at it than women.

• *Ways and means.* Does the patient have a plan and the resources (such as pills) to carry it out?

• *Behavior.* Patients who seem out of control or have a history of emotional problems are at higher risk.

• *Relationships.* Does your patient have positive relationships with others? Has he suffered any recent losses? One indicator of a potential suicide is if he talks of having made a will and is giving away prized possessions.

• *Medical history.* Patients with chronic illnesses are at a greater risk than those with terminal illnesses. Suicide attempts are also higher after childbirth or surgery, when a person's body image changes.

Preventing an imminent suicide

Suppose a patient on your unit threatens to kill himself. At the very worst, he will. At the very least, you'll need to calm him until the crisis intervention team arrives. The important thing is to remain calm and act quickly.

Immediate interventions

• Tell your patient that you'll stay with him but have to alert others as to your whereabouts. Call the nurses' station or switchboard, identify yourself, and say that you're in a room with a patient who needs someone to talk with right now, and that you can't leave him. This should notify the staff of the situation but not alarm the patient. Carefully edge toward the patient in a nonagitating manner.

• Tell the patient that you want to help. Ask him what's wrong. Such an appeal buys time, helps relax him, and brings a sense of normalcy to the crisis.

• Speak to him in a calm, reassuring voice. Try to make visual and verbal contact. Decrease any excessive noise by turning down TVs, radios, and other stimuli. If the patient seems to be calming down, ask him to have a seat by issuing simple, direct commands. When the intervention team member arrives, introduce him to the patient. By showing a link to this person, you're giving the patient permission to transfer some of his good feeling for you to the team member.

Long-term interventions

• Once the patient is out of danger, make arrangements for a psychiatric consultation and transfer to a mental health unit. If none is available, place the patient in a room next to the nursing station.

• Review and implement the hospital's suicide precautions policy.

• Record your actions on the patient's chart; file an incident report, if required.

• Evaluate your response to the crisis. If appropriate, call a staff meeting to discuss the crisis. Issue reminders to staff to closely observe chronically ill or depressed patients. Encourage staff to pay close attention to patients and use their listening skills to prevent potential suicide attempts.

▼

Emergency assessment: Body system approach

In an emergency, you collect objective assessment data by rapidly assessing the patient's physical condition. Concentrate on both the chief area of complaint, and the key body systems outlined below.

Vital signs

• Auscultate or palpate the patient's blood pressure.

• Note the rate, depth, pattern, and symmetry of his respirations.

• Palpate his radial pulse and note its rate, rhythm, and strength.

• Take his temperature.

Neurologic system

• Determine the patient's level of consciousness.

• Inspect his pupils for size, symmetry, and reaction to light.

• Observe him for abnormal posture (decorticate or decerebrate).

• Inspect and palpate his scalp for trauma or deformities.

• Assess the sensory and motor responses of each affected body part.

• Observe him for facial asymmetry, and listen for slurred speech.

• Assess deep tendon reflexes.

Eyes, ears, nose, and throat

• Inspect the patient's eyes for burns.

• Inspect and palpate his face and his eyes, ears, nose, and throat for trauma or deformities.

• Assess his speech for dysphonia or aphonia.

• Inspect his ears and nose for bleeding, drainage, and foreign objects.

• Inspect his oral mucosa for color, hydration, inflammation, and bleeding.

• Inspect and palpate his thyroid gland for tenderness and enlargement.
• Inspect his oropharynx for signs of burns due to ingestion of caustic agents.
• Assess gross visual acuity and eye movements.

Respiratory system
• Observe the patient for use of accessory muscles, for paradoxical chest movements, and for respiratory distress.
• Inspect his chest for contour, symmetry, and deformities or trauma.
• Auscultate his lungs for adventitious sounds and increased or decreased breath sounds.
• Palpate his chest for tenderness, pain, and crepitation.

Cardiovascular system
• Palpate the patient's peripheral pulses — especially of each affected body part — for rate, rhythm, quality, and symmetry.
• Inspect him for jugular vein distention.
• Inspect and palpate his extremities for edema, mottling and cyanosis, and temperature change.
• Auscultate his heart sounds for timing, intensity, pitch, and quality, and note the presence of murmurs, rubs, or extra sounds.
• Auscultate blood pressure in both arms.

GI system
• Inspect the patient's abdomen for obvious distention or signs of trauma.
• Inspect any vomitus or stool for amount, color, presence of blood, and consistency.
• Auscultate his abdomen for bowel sounds.
• Palpate his abdomen for pain, tenderness, or rigidity.
• Percuss his abdomen for possible ascites.

Genitourinary system
• Inspect the patient's external genitalia for bleeding, ecchymoses, edema, or hematoma.
• Palpate his abdomen for suprapubic pain.
• Palpate his external genitalia for pain or tenderness.

Musculoskeletal system
• Palpate for costovertebral angle tenderness.
• Inspect the patient's body for trauma and deformities.
• Gently palpate his cervical spine for tenderness and deformities.
• Palpate his vertebral spine and percuss his costovertebral areas for tenderness.
• Inspect his skin for color, ecchymoses, pigmentation, and discoloration.
• Palpate pulses distal to any injury.
• Palpate the area of suspected injury for tenderness, pain, and edema.
• Assess motor and sensory responses.
• Observe the range of motion of his injured extremity.
• Inspect his skin for needle marks.
• Assess him for nuchal rigidity.

Emergency assessment: Head-to-toe approach

There's no time in an emergency for a detailed assessment of a patient's physical condition. This head-to-toe checklist is a quick survey to systemically observe every part of the patient's body, concentrating, of course, on the primary area of distress or injury.

Vital signs
• Auscultate or palpate the patient's blood pressure.

• Note the rate, depth, pattern, and symmetry of his respirations.
• Palpate his radial pulse and note its rate and rhythm (regular or irregular).
• Take his temperature.

General survey
• Observe the patient's level of consciousness, behavior, and mental status.
• Inspect his body for obvious deformities due to trauma.
• Observe him for severe, moderate, or mild distress and anxiety.
• Inspect his skin for color, moisture, turgor, temperature, and ecchymoses.
• Note any distinctive odors on his breath, such as alcohol or acetone.
• Note his degree of mobility.

Head
• Inspect the patient's eyes for injuries or burns.
• Inspect his oropharynx for burns.
• Observe him for nasal flaring.
• Inspect and palpate his scalp and face for trauma and deformities.
• Inspect his pupils for size, symmetry, and reaction to light.
• Inspect his ears and nose for bleeding, drainage, and foreign objects.
• Inspect his oral mucosa for color, hydration, inflammation, and bleeding.

Neck
• Gently palpate the patient's cervical spine for tenderness and deformities.
• Inspect him for jugular vein distention.
• Inspect and palpate his thyroid gland for tenderness and enlargement.

Chest
• Inspect the patient's chest for contour, symmetry, and deformities or trauma.
• Palpate his chest for tenderness, pain, and crepitation.

- Auscultate his lungs for increased or decreased breath sounds or the presence of adventitious sounds.
- Auscultate his heart sounds for timing, intensity, pitch, and quality, and note the presence of murmurs, rubs, or extra sounds.

Back
- Inspect the patient's back for deformities or trauma.
- Palpate for tenderness in his vertebral spine and percuss his costovertebral areas.

- Palpate his flanks for tenderness.

Abdomen
- Inspect the patient's abdomen for deformities, trauma, bleeding, and abnormal drainage or pulsations.
- Auscultate for bowel sounds.
- Palpate the four quadrants for pain, tenderness, and rigidity.
- Percuss his abdomen for ascites.

External genitalia
- Inspect the patient's genitalia for bleeding, ecchymoses, edema, or hematoma.

- Palpate the genitalia for pain and tenderness.

Extremities
- Inspect and palpate the patient's extremities for trauma, deformities, and edema.
- Inspect his arms for needle marks.
- Palpate the distal pulses of an injured extremity.
- Assess the motor and sensory responses of an injured extremity.
- Palpate his extremities for pain and tenderness.

Common pitfalls in emergency assessment

After you've assessed the patient and documented your findings, what should you do? Most importantly, avoid drawing hasty—and possibly inaccurate—conclusions about the patient's condition. Never assume that you can immediately identify all your patient's problems. And always keep your eyes and ears open for sudden changes in his condition. Study the chart below to avoid some common assessment pitfalls.

Signs and symptoms	Assumed cause	Other possible causes
Restlessness, agitation, and talkativeness, with alcohol odor on breath	• Alcohol or drug abuse	• Hidden GI bleeding • Psychiatric disorder, such as mania • Subdural hematoma
Unilateral dilated pupil	• Neurologic disorder or injury	• Eye prosthesis • Previous eye injury
Multifocal premature ventricular contractions	• Severe heart disease	• Benign cardiac dysrhythmia (of long-standing duration) • Digitalis toxicity
Restlessness, belligerence, combativeness, urinary or fecal incontinence, poor hygienic habits, disheveled appearance	• Alcohol or drug abuse • Psychiatric disorder	• Brain lesion • Hypoxia
Hallucinations, delusions of grandeur, disorientation, or combativeness	• Psychiatric disorder, such as psychosis • Alcohol or drug abuse	• Atypical reaction to a drug overdose • Organic brain syndrome • Bacterial meningitis

What causes anaphylaxis?

Common causes of anaphylaxis include certain foods, diagnostic agents, antibiotics and other drugs, blood products, and venoms.

Foods
Chocolate, citrus fruits, cottonseed oil, eggs, grains, milk, nuts, seafood, seeds, shellfish, soybeans, spinach, strawberries, and tomatoes

Diagnostic agents
Bromsulphalein dye, dehydrocholic acid, iodinated contrast media, and iopanoic acid

Antibiotics
Aminoglycosides, amphotericin B, cephalosporins, nitrofurantoin, penicillins, and tetracyclines

Chemotherapeutic drugs
Adriamycin, bleomycin, cisplatin, cyclophosphamide, L-asparaginase, and melphalan

Local anesthetics
Bupivacaine, lidocaine, procaine, and tetracaine

Other drugs
Adrenocorticotropic hormone, aspirin, codeine, dextrans (including iron dextran), diuretics, histamine, hydralazine, iodides, meprobamate, morphine, succinylcholine, thiazides, and tubocurarine

Blood products and antisera
Cryoprecipitate, immune globulin, plasma, and whole blood

Venoms
Stings or bites from bees, hornets, jellyfish, snakes, spiders, and wasps

Recognizing anaphylaxis

Anaphylaxis is an extreme reaction to a foreign antigen. In severe cases, it leads to respiratory failure, hypovolemic shock, and death. Typically, the faster the reaction, the greater its severity. Most symptoms occur within seconds or minutes of contact with the antigen, but symptoms from injections may appear within an hour.

Early signs of anaphylaxis include anxiety, dizziness, disorientation, loss of consciousness, and facial swelling, particularly on the lips or tongue. Anaphylaxis victims may also complain of a lump in their throat or experience wheezing.

If your patient experiences anaphylaxis, follow these steps:
• Assess his breathing. Begin resuscitation if needed. If the patient has no pulse, begin CPR. If his airway is blocked, notify the doctor, who will perform an emergency tracheostomy.
• Discontinue any obvious sources for an anaphylactic reaction, such as an I.V. However, time is of the essence and you don't need to know the cause to treat symptoms.
• Insert or maintain an I.V. line. The doctor will commonly order epinephrine to reverse life-threatening situations, but observe closely for possible side effects.
• Anticipate administering normal saline or lactated Ringer's solution to restore fluid, stabilize blood pressure and cardiac output, and allay lactic acidosis.
• Check the patient's vital signs every 15 to 30 minutes for first few hours. After a severe reaction, monitor the patient closely for 24 hours in case another reaction occurs.

Recognizing the stages of shock

Knowing the stages of shock—and their accompanying signs—helps you intervene appropriately.

Early or compensatory stage
• Restlessness, irritability, apprehension
• Slightly increased heart rate
• Normal blood pressure, slightly elevated systolic pressure, or slightly lowered diastolic pressure
• Mild orthostatic blood pressure changes (15 to 25 mm Hg)
• Normal or slightly diminished urine output
• Pale and cool skin in hypovolemic shock; warm and flushed skin in septic, anaphylactic, and neurogenic shock
• Slightly increased respiratory rate
• Slightly lowered body temperature (except in septic shock fever)

Intermediate or progressive stage
• Listlessness, apathy, confusion, slowed speech
• Tachypnea, tachycardia, weak and thready pulse, hypotension, narrowed pulse pressure (except in septic shock)
• Moderate to severe orthostatic blood pressure changes
• Oliguria
• Cold, clammy skin
• Lowered body temperature

Late or decompensatory stage
• Confusion and incoherent, slurred speech; possibly unconsciousness
• Depressed or absent reflexes
• Dilated pupils slow to react
• Slowed, irregular, thready pulse
• Severe hypotension
• Oliguria or anuria
• Cold, clammy, cyanotic skin
• Slow, shallow, irregular respirations
• Sharply lower body temperature

Emergency procedures: When seconds count

In an emergency, you need to assess the patient accurately and intervene quickly and effectively. You'll be in a better position to fulfill this responsibility by reading over the descriptions of the common emergencies you might be called on to handle on the unit or in the ED.

Amputation
Managing a patient with a traumatic amputation involves two priorities. The first is to stabilize the patient, coping with obvious hemorrhaging or occult blood loss, which requires assessing his circulation, and administering analgesics and tetanus prophylaxis. The second priority is to prepare the amputated part for possible replantation.

Prepare the amputated part for possible surgery by flushing it in a normal saline or lactated Ringer's solution. Dry and place in a watertight sealed bag and immerse in ice water.

Arterial hemorrhage control
Arterial bleeding, if not quickly controlled, causes shock and even death. Control bleeding by applying a pressure dressing made from any kind of thick gauze or clean cloth. If dressings are unavailable, apply pressure with your hand.

Exert steady pressure directly over the bleeding vessel and, if bleeding continues, use digital pressure on the arterial pressure point nearest the wound. (See *Identifying arterial pressure points.*) If the procedure is performed correctly, the patient's pulse should be undetectable below the pressure point. Once bleeding is controlled, apply a pressure compress. Tie in place and apply additional bandages atop the dressing as needed.

Identifying arterial pressure points

To quickly control arterial bleeding, apply pressure using your fingers on the arterial pressure point nearest the patient's wound. If you can't pinpoint the exact arterial pressure point, press with the heel of your hand in the approximate locale. These sites include: subclavian (armpit and chest), temporal (scalp and forehead), carotid (head and neck), brachial (arm or hand), facial (bleeding below the eyes), radial and ulnar (hand), and femoral (leg).

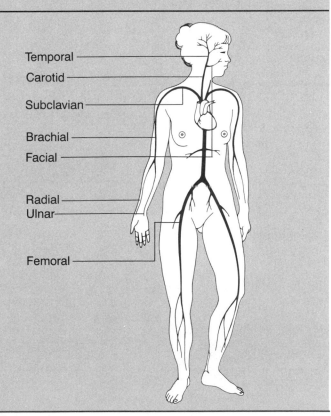

Tourniquet technique

When pressure dressings fail and bleeding persists, your final alternative is to carefully tie a tourniquet. Loose or improperly applied bandaging can increase blood loss. To proceed:

• Position the tourniquet on the limb between the injury site and the heart.

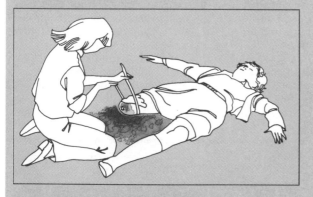

• Wrap the bandage around the limb about 2″ (5 cm) above the wound, tie it with a half knot, then place a stick over the half knot and tie a square knot over it.

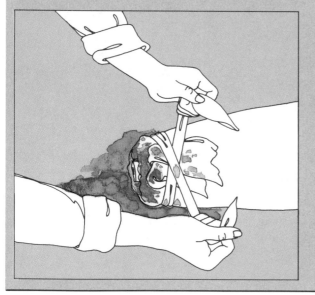

• Secure the stick with the tourniquet ends or a piece of cloth. Twist the stick until bleeding stops.

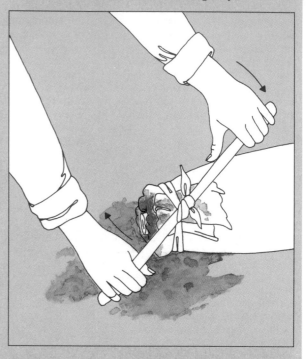

• Write a T on the patient's forehead to call attention to the tourniquet, indicating the time of placement.

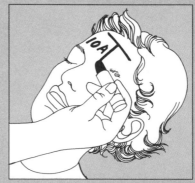

• To avoid possible massive hemorrhaging, don't loosen the tourniquet before reaching the hospital.

Autotransfusion

Autotransfusion is the collection, filtration, and reinfusion of a victim's own blood to treat shock resulting from a massive blood loss from heart or great vessel injuries that allow no time for the typing and cross-matching of blood.

During autotransfusion, a vacuum system sucks blood through a sterile chest tube and into a canister liner. The canister contains a fine-screen filter to remove debris and a solution of citrate phosphate dextrose to prevent clotting. During reinfusion, the canister liner is removed and the blood reinfused through transfusion tubing using a gravity drip or infusion pump for rapid replacement.

The procedure is contraindicated in patients whose chest cavities are contaminated with GI contents stemming from esophageal, stomach, or bowel injuries; when wounds are more than 4 hours old; or when the blood has been hemolyzed.

Blood transfusion

Whole blood is usually transfused during severe hemorrhagic episodes, whereas packed cells are transfused when normal blood volume drops to prevent fluid and circulatory overload, or to patients suffering from severe anemia or congestive heart failure. Hospital policies differ, but transfusions usually require identification of the patient and blood product by two nurses to prevent errors. Possible transfusion reactions may nonetheless result.

Blood components are usually transfused more slowly than whole blood using a standard administration set. An emergency, however, may require rapid transfusion of blood using a pressure cuff or positive-pressure set. These are set up similarly to a standard set in which the filter and tubing are primed to remove all air and the tubing connected to the needle or catheter hub. Observe the patient closely during the procedure to detect possible complications.

Transfusion reactions. During blood transfusion, patients are at risk for developing one of these reactions:
• Hemolytic reaction — chills, low back and chest pain, dyspnea, hypotension, nausea and vomiting
• Plasma protein incompatibility — chills, fever, flushing, abdominal pain, diarrhea, dyspnea, and hypotension
• Blood contamination — abdominal pain, nausea and vomiting, chills, bloody diarrhea, hypotension
• Febrile reaction — symptoms range from mild chills and flushing to symptoms similar to hemolytic reaction
• Allergic reaction — pruritus, urticaria, hives, chills, fever, nausea, vomiting, respiratory distress, and shock.

Transfusion reactions demand quick action to prevent further complications and death:
• Stop the transfusion.
• Change the I.V. tubing to prevent infusing any more blood. Administer a saline solution I.V.
• Take the patient's vital signs and notify the doctor.
• Obtain urine and blood samples, noting on them "possible transfusion reaction" for the laboratory.
• Observe for signs of oliguria or anuria because hemoglobin may deposit in the renal tubules.
• Administer oxygen and emergency drugs, if ordered.

Cardiopulmonary resuscitation (CPR)

CPR aims to revive patients suffering respiratory or circulatory arrest. It must be performed within 3 to 4 minutes of the symptom's onset to prevent permanent brain damage or death.

For an adult, open the airway, providing ventilation to revive breathing. Using both hands, apply steady, rhythmic compressions (about 80 per minute) to the victim's chest. Intersperse by giving the victim 2 quick lung inhalations every 15 chest compressions.

For a child, follow same routine but use the heel of only one hand on chest and give the victim a breath every fifth compression.

For an infant, place the tips of your index and middle fingers of one hand in the middle of the victim's chest, delivering 100 compressions per minute and a breath every fifth compression.

Advanced cardiac life support (ACLS). The second phase of CPR, advanced cardiac life support involves using special equipment and drugs to revive the patient and maintain cardiac and respiratory systems. Besides continuation of CPR, ACLS can include administration of oxygen and cardiac drugs, endotracheal intubation, and defibrillation or cardioversion to restore heart rhythm.

Carotid massage

In this procedure, pressure applied to the carotid sinus slows the heart rate. Manual pressure is applied to the right or left of the carotid sinus located slightly above the branches of the carotid arteries in the neck. Pressure is applied alternately to each sinus for less than 5 seconds. The procedure is accompanied by continuous ECG monitoring and discontinued if the monitor registers a change in rhythm.

Chest tube insertion

Insertion of a chest tube into the pleural space promotes breathing by draining away blood, fluid, and pus. It reestablishes atmospheric and intrathoracic gradients and allows the lungs to fully expand. It's used for patients who have pneumothorax, hemothorax, empyema, pleural effusion, or chylothorax.

Dealing with accidental extubation

If a tube is removed accidentally (or deliberately by a patient), take the following steps immediately:
• Remove any remaining part of the tube.
• Ventilate the patient using common resuscitation techniques or an Ambu bag.
• Notify the doctor.
• Restrain the patient if he's extubated himself.
• Once the tube is reinstated, periodically check its position and the condition of the tape holding it. For a secure fit, anchor the tape from the nape of the patient's neck to and around the tube.

The patient's skin is prepared for insertion of the tube at a site determined by his symptoms. To relieve pneumothorax, for example, the tube is placed in the second intercostal space along the midclavicular line.

Cricothyrotomy
This procedure involves surgical opening of the patient's airway. Used when all other efforts to relieve obstruction have failed, it should only be performed by specially trained personnel.

After palpating the patient's neck to locate the cricothyroid membrane (found between the first and second prominence at the top of the neck), the doctor makes a small incision, inserts a small tube, and attaches it to an Ambu bag or other type of ventilator.

Defibrillation
This procedure delivers a strong burst of electric current to the heart through paddles applied to the patient's chest. It completely depolarizes the myocardium, allowing the heart's natural pacemaker to regain control of cardiac rhythm. The procedure is successful about 40% of the time.

Defibrillation is the treatment of choice for ventricular fibrillation and pulseless ventricular tachycardia. It may also benefit patients in asystole who show signs of ventricular fibrillation. Because ventricular fibrillation can lead to irreparable brain damage, you must perform defibrillation as soon as possible, even before intubating the patient or administering drugs.

Defibrillators vary in their setup and operation, but basically consist of a set of paddles that are applied to the patient's chest or anteroposterior and discharge an electrical shock. After the first discharge, the patient's cardiac monitor should be checked. If ventricular fibrillation continues, defibrillation should be performed again. Sodium bicarbonate or epinephrine may also be given I.V.

Emergency infant delivery
In emergency delivery, you have three priorities: to prevent maternal and fetal infection by cleansing your hands and the patient's perineum, if possible; to keep the delivery slow to prevent infant distress and the mother's tearing and hemorrhaging; and to protect the newborn from the cold.

Don't attempt to deliver an infant whose foot, arm, or shoulder presents first. If the infant's head crowns first, don't apply pressure or pull it out. Keep the delivery at a slow and steady pace to prevent tearing. If the amniotic membrane is unbroken, pinch it. Check for the position of the cord, loosening it around the infant's neck. (If tightly wrapped, tie the cord in two places and cut between the ties.) Ease the infant's shoulders out gently and then deliver the rest of his body. Dry and wrap him securely for warmth. The cord can be tied when it stops pulsating. Don't try to remove the placenta until the patient reaches the hospital.

Endotracheal intubation
Patients needing ventilatory support often require an artificial airway. The endotracheal tube (nasal or oral) has a low-pressure, inflatable cuff and mechanical ventilator that assists breathing.

Endotracheal tubes are inserted through the nose or mouth and passed into the trachea; the cuffs are inflated and deflated by a mechanical device. The tubing is anchored by tape to the skin. (For more information, see *Dealing with accidental extubation*.)

Esophageal airway insertion
The esophageal obturator airway (EOA) tube temporarily (maximum 2 hours) maintains ventilation in a comatose patient during cardiac or respiratory arrest. This tube (and another similar device called the esophageal gastric tube airway) clears the airway and prevents the patient from choking on his stomach contents.

The EOA is particularly useful for patients with suspected spinal injuries, since insertion involves no hyperextension of the neck. It's contraindicated, however, for conscious or semiconscious patients; children under age 16; and patients with facial trauma. Other contraindications include the absence of a gag reflex, the recent ingestion of toxic chemicals, esophageal disease, or a suspected narcotic overdose.

After determining that the patient is a candidate for an EOA, insert the tube using both hands. Use one to hold the patient's jaw and chin while the other guides the airway tube over the tongue, pharynx, and into the esophagus. Then fit the mask snugly over the patient's mouth and inflate it. Discontinue when respirations are steady—about 16 to 20 respirations per minute.

Eye irrigation for chemical burns
Chemical eye burns are caused by acid or alkaline solutions which, depending on their composition, can cause severe or permanent eye damage. The eye must be irrigated immediately using I.V. tubing and a standard saline solution. A less common flushing method involves a special contact lens fitted to the eye and then flushed with saline.

Irrigate the patient's eye and surrounding facial area for about 10 minutes to flush away caustic substances and relieve pain. Ask the patient for the name of the chemical he came into contact with—alkaline solutions can sear the Bowman's membrane, while acidic substances usually affect the cornea. Test the patient's conjunctival pH using litmus paper. If abnormal, continue flushing procedure. Order corticosteroid ointments, if indicated.

Gastric lavage
This suctioning procedure empties the stomach when vomiting is contraindicated or a patient is comatose. It can also be used when a patient is alert, but has consumed a highly toxic substance (not caustic, however) and doesn't vomit after ingesting ipecac. This procedure can also be performed on patients with upper GI bleeding. It isn't appropriate for patients with a depressed gag reflex or those who need activated charcoal instillation as part of treatment.

Gastric lavage requires an irrigating solution, rubber tubing, an inflow and outflow clamp, and a suction machine. After massaging the patient's stomach to break up its contents, anesthetize the throat and insert a Ewald tube or Salem sump tube. Operate the suctioning machine. Inflow is usually 5 to 10 liters of fluid, as ordered. Monitor the patient's vital signs during the procedure.

Manual ventilation
An inflatable device, such as an Ambu bag, allows delivery of oxygen or room air to the lungs. It can be attached to a face mask or directly to an endotracheal or tracheostomy tube, sealed tightly, and compressed by hand. It's used for patients who can't breathe independently as a result of chest trauma, respiratory depression, severe anxiety, neurologic deficits, or metabolic disorders.

Nasoenteric decompression
Along with fluid and electrolyte replacement, nasoenteric decompression helps relieve acute intestinal obstruction resulting from polyps, adhesions, fecal impaction, volvulus, or localized carcinoma. This treatment involves inserting a long, weighted nasoenteric tube through the patient's stomach and into the intestinal tract. The tube is then propelled by peristalsis through the intestine to, and possibly through, an obstruction.

Neonatal airway clearance
A newborn must quickly establish a regular breathing pattern. You can assist him by clearing his airway as soon as his head emerges. Using both hands, rotate his head to one side and gently stroke the infant's nose downward to release fluid and mucus. Stroke his throat from the neck to chin, then use your fingers to clear his mouth.

Obstructed airway management
A patient's airway can either be obstructed partially or completely. First determine if the patient can speak. If he can't speak, cough, or breathe, call for help and then perform abdominal thrusts: Stand behind the patient, wrap your arms around his waist, and place the thumb side of one fist against his abdomen at midline (slightly above the navel, well below the xiphoid tip). Grasp the fist with your other hand and make quick upward thrusts. Repeat until you're successful or the patient loses consciousness.

If the patient becomes unconscious, position him supine and call for help again. Open his mouth with a tongue-jaw lift and sweep deeply into his mouth. Open his airway with the head-tilt, chin-lift maneuver and attempt to ventilate.

If you don't succeed, straddle the patient's thighs and position the heel of one hand against his abdomen at the midline point. Place your other hand on top of it and deliver 6 to 10 abdominal thrusts. Use chest thrusts for obese patients and women in the late stages of pregnancy. (For more information, see *Positions for Heimlich maneuver [Abdominal thrust]*, page 252.)

If unsuccessful, the patient is intubated or may require a tracheostomy or emergency bronchoscopy. Suction airways blocked by blood or vomitus using an endotracheal or tracheostomy tube. Trachea tumors can be bypassed by intubating the right mainstem bronchus. Follow-up is a priority, particularly for patients whose airways were obstructed by a sharp object which, although removed, may have irritated the airway.

Oropharyngeal airway insertion
The oropharyngeal airway is a plastic, rubber, or metal semicircular device inserted into the mouth to the posterior pharynx to ventilate patients experiencing cardiac arrest. Because the tongue usually obstructs the posterior pharynx of unconscious patients, insertion of this airway corrects this obstruction and allows air to pass through and around the tube.

Positions for Heimlich maneuver (abdominal thrust)

Standing or sitting positions

Position your arms around the patient's waist. Then, place your fist against the abdomen, above the navel and below the xiphoid process, as shown. If possible, have the patient bend forward to allow gravity to assist your efforts. Press upward and inward with four quick thrusts.

Position for obese or pregnant person

Place the top of your clenched fist against the middle of the sternum. Then put your hand on top of your clenched fist. Perform chest thrusts until the obstruction is expelled or the victim loses consciousness.

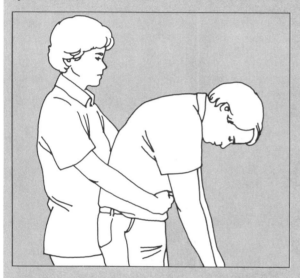

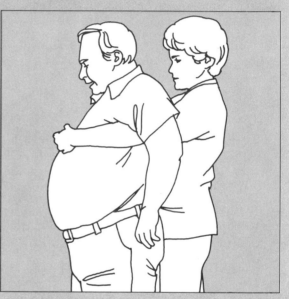

Recumbent position (unconscious patient)

Face the patient and straddle her hips, making sure your shoulders are directly over the abdomen. Place the heel of one hand on top of the other and place both hands on the patient's abdomen, above the navel and below the xiphoid process. Press upward and inward six to ten times.

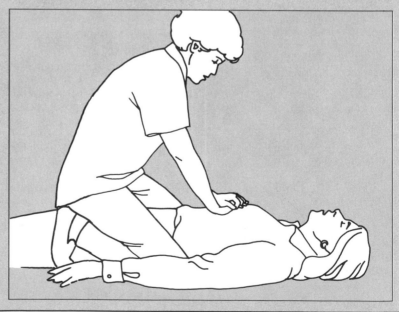

Insert the oropharyngeal airway backward into the patient's mouth, twisting it into proper position at the base of the tongue and the pharynx wall, ensuring the patient's lips and tongue do not obstruct the airway.

Pacemaker insertion

Temporary pacemakers electronically stimulate the heart to maintain an adequate cardiac rate and rhythm in patients suffering from acute dysrhythmias that have failed to respond to antiarrhythmic drugs.

Temporary pacemakers are inserted in an emergency to provide atrial or ventricular pacing. The doctor threads a pacing catheter through the appropriate veins and, once in place at the apex of the right heart, the pacemaker is connected to an external pacemaker that sets the proper rhythm. *Note:* The ECG may signal premature ventricular contractions, ventricular tachycardia, or ventricular fibrillation — lidocaine administration and defibrillation may be necessary.

Pericardiocentesis

Patients suspected of cardiac tamponade, in which fluid accumulates in the heart's pericardial space, may undergo an emergency pericardiocentesis. This procedure involves insertion of a 16G to 18G needle into the pericardial sac to aspirate fluid and relieve pressure.

Although a pericardiocentesis is straightforward — the needle is inserted and its position charted by ECG — its complications are severe. If the needle pierces the myocardium, bleeding can result. The procedure can also cause ventricular dysrhythmias and coronary artery laceration. Your role is to monitor the patient's ECG, blood pressure, and central venous pressure, along with other vital signs.

Pneumatic antishock garment

This garment (known as MAST or Jobst G Antigravity Suit) produces an effect similar to autotransfusion by applying pressure to the lower body and abdomen, and squeezing blood upward. A MAST suit recirculates blood in patients with shock and lower extremity hemorrhage. It also stabilizes and splints pelvic and femoral fractures. Contraindications include congestive heart failure, pulmonary edema, and tension pneumothorax.

The MAST suit is made of inflatable bags sandwiched between fabric. Depending on the injuries, the suit is slid or arranged over the patient and fastened over the lower extremities, with its upper edge resting *below* the rib cage. Inflate the suit slowly and uniformly to prevent irreversible shock from hypovolemia. Don't remove the suit until the patient's condition is stabilized, his blood volume restored, or he is being prepared for surgery.

Skull traction and cervical collars

Spinal injuries vary in severity, but patients suffering neck or back pain, muscle weakness, or paralysis may need immediate immobilization. A Philadelphia collar is positioned to prevent further injury. If the patient sustains minor fractures, he'll need a firm cervical collar. If he has a dislocation, he'll require a halo traction device or skull tongs.

Skull tongs and halo traction devices are required when a patient needs to be immobilized for several months to promote healing and prevent further injury. These units are weighted with traction devices and attached with pins and tongs. The halo traction device allows greater patient mobility of the two and is attached at specific pin sites.

Priorities in cardiac arrest

Victims of cardiac arrest are your first priority for treatment in the ED and on the unit. How you proceed may mean a matter of life and death. Here's a quick checklist to aid your decision-making.
- Alert the resuscitation team and place victim on a firm surface. Use a cardiac board or bedboard. Don't move a patient who's already on the floor.
- Begin CPR.
- Attach patient to a monitoring device, such as an electrocardiograph, and to a defibrillator.
- Defibrillate for ventricular fibrillation (countershock.)
- Start an I.V., if warranted.
- Set up oxygen apparatus correctly. Prepare tracheal suction equipment and catheters.
- Assist with intubation, as indicated. Secure intubation tray from the resuscitation cart. Suction patient, if needed.
- Document events.
- Provide pertinent data to resuscitation team.
- Monitor the victim's vital signs.
- Remove excess furniture, equipment, and personnel from the area.
- Give support to family and friends.
- Assure care for the other patients on the unit. Consult your fellow nurses to remove nearby patients or screen them from the ongoing activity.
- Notify the attending doctor.
- Provide necessary equipment from stock room.

Upon completing successful resuscitation, transfer patient to a monitored area for close observation. If the procedure fails, perform postmortem care (if required) and provide additional support for family.

Giving emergency drugs to children

Many emergency drugs used for adults have special dosage instructions when administered to children. For instance, the pediatric dosage for dopamine is calculated per kilogram of body weight. Calcium chloride, on the other hand, is given slowly in children, particularly those taking digitalis, because it can cause dysrhythmias. The essential drugs for advanced life support are listed below with recommended dosages.

Aminophylline
This drug stimulates the respiratory center in the medulla, prevents diaphraghmatic fatigue, and causes bronchodilation by relaxing smooth muscle. If aminophylline hasn't been given, administer a loading dose of 4 to 6 mg/kg over 15 to 20 minutes. Give the maintenance infusion of 0.9 to 1.25 mg/kg/hr.

Atropine
The initial dose of 0.01 mg/kg I.V. (minimum of 0.2 mg) can be repeated every 5 minutes up to a maximum dose of 2 mg. Atropine may also be given intratracheally.

Bretylium
Give the initial dose of 5 mg/kg I.V. rapidly and then follow by defibrillation. If defibrillation fails to produce conversion, bretylium should be repeated at 10 mg/kg I.V., followed once again by defibrillation.

Calcium chloride
The initial dose is 10 mg/kg administered through a central line access port to avoid sclerosing the child's vein. Repeat the initial dose if necessary. However, additional doses require monitoring through the ionized serum calcium level. Always administer calcium slowly in children, especially in those who are taking digitalis, as it can cause dysrhythmias.

Keep in mind that calcium isn't recommended during initial resuscitation unless hypocalcemia is evident.

Calcium gluconate
Less irritating to children than calcium chloride, calcium gluconate can be administered through peripheral veins in an initial dose of 30 mg/kg. The dosage schedule is similar to that for calcium chloride.

Dopamine
Usually administered by continuous infusion, dopamine may initially be given in varying amounts depending on the desired effects. For a child in shock, prepare an infusion by adding 60 mg of dopamine to 1 dl of D_5W, administering it at the rate of 1 ml/hour for each kilogram of body weight. A more exact calculation of dosage may be needed in a nonemergency.

Epinephrine
For asystole or ventricular fibrillation, initially give 10 mcg/kg I.V. Give successive doses based on dose response; these can be doubled. Therefore, the first dose is 10 mcg/kg; second dose, 20 mcg/kg; third dose, 40 mcg/kg; and fourth dose, 80 mcg/kg. Epinephrine can also be given intratracheally, if necessary.

Furosemide
Initially give 1 mg/kg I.V. to children who have no urine output or for initial management of head injury. If no urine output follows the first dose in 20 to 30 minutes, the dose may be repeated or doubled.

D-Glucose (dextrose)
Dextrose is an essential drug for children because of their inability to store glycogen. Inadequate serum glucose levels may also be related to decreased intake before cardiac arrest. The initial dose for dextrose is 1 g/kg I.V. given in a 25% solution. Additional doses depend on serum glucose levels.

Isoproterenol
Continuous infusion may be given to increase the heart rate, cardiac contractility, and venous return. Prepare an infusion quickly by adding 0.6 mg of isoproterenol to 1 dl of D_5W. Infusing this solution at the rate of 1 ml/minute for each kilogram of body weight delivers the initial dose of 0.1 mcg/kg/minute.

Lidocaine
The initial dose of 1 mg/kg I.V. can be repeated every 5 minutes for 15 minutes. If ventricular fibrillation or premature ventricular beats continue, an infusion of 10 to 20 mcg/kg/minute can be started.

Naloxone
This drug reverses the effects of codeine, morphine, and other narcotics. The initial dose is 0.01 mg/kg I.V. with a rapid onset and short half-life. If the initial dose is beneficial, a repeat dose may be administered.

Sodium bicarbonate
The recommended dose is 1 mEq/kg I.V. The formula for administration is:

$$\text{Amount of bicarbonate} = \frac{\text{Base deficit} \times \text{wt (kg)} \times 0.4}{2}$$

Subsequent administration should be based on the patient's pH and the estimated need to combat acidosis.

Administering antidotes in poisoning or overdose

The chart below summarizes the major uses and dosage recommendations for commonly used antidotes.

Antidote and dosage	Type of poisoning or overdose	Special considerations
amyl nitrite inhalants (Step I) *Adults:* Inhale for 30 sec for every 1 to 2 min. **sodium nitrite** (Step II) *Adults:* 300 mg in 10 ml solution given I.V. over 2 to 4 min (repeat once if symptoms recur). *Children:* Depends on hemoglobin level. **sodium thiosulfate** (Step III) *Adults:* 50 ml of 25% sodium thiosulfate given I.V. at a rate of 2.5 to 5 ml/min (if symptoms recur, give sodium nitrite again in half the original dose). *Children:* Depends on hemoglobin level.	Cyanide	• Nitrites cause vasodilation. Hypotension may result.
atropine sulfate *Adults:* 2 to 5 mg I.V. for pesticides (may repeat every 10 to 30 min until signs of atropinization appear). *Children:* 0.05 mg/kg for pesticides (may repeat every 10 to 30 min until signs of atropinization appear).	Anticholinesterase substances, organophosphate pesticides, carbamate pesticides	• Large doses (2 to 2,000 mg over several hours to several days) may be required to maintain full atropinization. • Sudden cessation of atropine may cause pulmonary edema. • Maintain adequate ventilation to prevent dysrhythmias.
deferoxamine mesylate (Desferal) *Adults and children:* 1,000 mg I.M. or I.V. initially, then 500 mg q 4 hr for 2 doses. Subsequent doses of 500 mg q 4 to 12 hr may be given; maximum dosage 6,000 mg daily.	Heavy metals, iron	• Renal excretion of compound will turn urine pink.
digoxin immune FAB (Digibind) *Adults:* Depends on amount of digoxin or digitoxin to be neutralized. If unable to determine dosage using manufacturer-supplied formulas, infuse 800 mg over 30 min. *Children:* Depends on amount of digoxin or digitoxin to be neutralized. Use formulas supplied by manufacturer.	Digoxin or digitoxin	• Reserve for severe overdose only. • If cardiac arrest seems imminent, administer dose as a bolus injection. • Monitor serum potassium levels carefully to detect hyperkalemia or hypokalemia. • Monitor cardiac rate and rhythm.
dimercaprol (BAL) *Adults:* 3 to 5 mg/kg deep I.M. q 4 hr for 2 days; q 4 to 6 hr for 2 more days; then q 4 to 12 hr up to 12 more days.	Mercury, arsenic, gold	• Give drug promptly to ensure effectiveness. • Don't administer in iron poisoning. • Use requires that patient has adequate renal and hepatic function to excrete toxins.

(continued)

Administering antidotes in poisoning or overdose (continued)

Antidote and dosage	Type of poisoning or overdose	Special considerations
D-penicillamine (Cuprimine) *Adults:* 250 mg by mouth (P.O.) q.i.d. for up to 5 days. Don't exceed 40 mg/kg/day. *Children:* 24 to 50 mg/kg P.O. q.i.d.	Lead, iron, mercury, copper	• D-penicillamine should be used in patients with minimal signs and symptoms and positive serum lead levels.
naloxone hydrochloride (Narcan) *Adults:* 0.4 to 0.8 mg I.V. bolus to reverse the narcotic effect (may need to repeat dose q 20 to 60 min to maintain reversal). *Children:* 0.01 mg/kg I.V. bolus.	Opiates: morphine, heroin, methadone, meperidine, oxycodone	• Time of action is shorter than that of narcotic. As a result, observe patient for recurring narcosis (loss of consciousness or depressed respirations). Repeat doses or a continuous infusion may be necessary.
n-acetylcysteine (Mucomyst) *Adults:* 140 mg/kg P.O. diluted in soft drinks, juice, or water. Follow loading dose with 17 additional doses of 70 mg/kg q 4 hr (repeat if dose is vomited within 1 hr).	Acetaminophen	• Activated charcoal will absorb the antidote if both are present in the gut. If charcoal is used, aspirate it before giving the antidote.
physostigmine salicylate (Antilirium) *Adults:* 2 mg I.V. slowly over 2 to 3 min (repeat with a 1 to 2 mg dose in 20 min if symptoms are still present; repeat with a 1 to 4 mg dose if life-threatening symptoms reappear). *Children:* 0.5 mg slow I.V. over 2 to 3 min (repeat within 5 min if symptoms recur); maximum dosage is 2 mg.	Anticholinergics; tricyclics (amitriptyline, atropine); plants (jimsonweed, some mushroom species, black nightshade); antihistamines	• Reserve for severe poisoning marked by coma, hallucinations, delirium, tachycardia, dysrhythmias, or hypertension. • Rapid I.V. injection may cause bradycardia and hypersalivation with respiratory difficulties and convulsions. • Physostigmine can produce a cholinergic crisis. If so, give atropine as an antidote.
pralidoxime chloride (Protopam Chloride) *Adults:* 1 g I.V. at 0.5 g/min or diluted in 250 ml normal saline solution and given over 30 min (repeat in 3 intervals 8 to 12 hr apart if muscle weakness persists). *Children:* 25 to 50 mg/kg I.V. (may repeat in 8- to 12-hr intervals).	Organophosphate pesticides	• Effective if given up to 36 hr after exposure. • Pesticide absorption is possible through the skin. Wash patient and remove contaminated clothing or symptoms may reappear within 48 to 72 hr. • Drug has no anticholinergic effects.
protamine sulfate *Adults:* 5 ml of a 1% solution slow I.V. over 10 min (give 1 to 1.25 mg protamine for each 100 units of heparin consumed).	Heparin	• Maximum dosage is 50 mg (as a single dose).
vitamin K analogue (AquaMEPHYTON) *Adults:* 10 mg I.M. for large ingestions (can be given P.O. if patient is not vomiting). *Children:* 1 to 5 mg I.M.	Warfarin	• Fresh whole blood may be necessary to stop bleeding.

Helping a rape victim

A victim of rape requires both effective nursing and emotional care to overcome her trauma. When she arrives in the emergency department, you'll first have to assess her physical injuries. If she's not seriously injured, let her remain clothed and take her to a quiet, private, well-protected room, where she can talk with you or a counselor before the necessary physical examination.

Understand the victim's reactions
Immediate reactions to rape differ. Some victims cry, others actually laugh. Some feel hostility and confusion, others withdraw or appear outwardly calm. Often anger and rage don't surface until sometime later.

During the assault, the victim may have felt demeaned, helpless, fearful for her life; afterward, she may feel ashamed, guilty, shocked, vulnerable, disbelieving, or without self-esteem.

It's up to you to offer her support and reassurance and help her explore her feelings by listening to her, conveying trust and respect, remaining nonjudgmental. Don't leave her alone unless she asks you to.

Document the rape
Be careful to upset the victim as little as possible when obtaining an accurate history of the rape, pertinent to physical assessment. (Remember: Your notes may be used as evidence if the rapist is tried.) Record the victim's statements in the first person, using quotation marks. Also document objective information provided by others.

Never speculate as to what may have happened or record subjective impressions or thoughts. Include in your notes the time the victim arrived at the hospital, the date and time of the alleged rape, and the time the victim was examined. Ask the victim about allergies to penicillin and other drugs, if she's had recent illnesses (especially venereal disease), if she was pregnant before the attack, the date of her last menstrual period, and details of her obstetric/gynecologic history.

Prepare the victim for the physical examination
Thoroughly explain the examination the victim will undergo, explaining to her why it's necessary: to rule out internal injuries and obtain a specimen for venereal disease testing. Obtain her informed consent for treatment and for the police report. If you can, allow her some control. For instance, ask her if she's ready to be examined or if she'd rather wait a bit.

Before the examination, ask the victim whether she douched, bathed, or washed before coming to the hospital. Note this on her chart. Have her change into a hospital gown, and place her clothing in paper bags. (*Never* use plastic bags, because secretions and seminal stains will mold, destroying valuable evidence.) Label each bag and its contents.

Tell the victim she may urinate, but warn her not to drink fluids or to wipe or otherwise cleanse the perineal area.

Stay with the victim during the examination
You or counselor should stay with the victim throughout the examination. Even if the victim wasn't beaten, physical examination (including a pelvic examination by a gynecologist) will probably show signs of physical trauma, especially if the assault was prolonged. Depending on specific body areas attacked, a patient may have a sore throat, mouth irritation, difficulty swallowing, ecchymoses, or rectal pain and bleeding.

If additional physical violence accompanied the rape, the victim may have hematomas, lacerations, bleeding, severe internal injuries, and hemorrhage; and if the rape occurred outdoors, she may suffer from exposure. X-rays may reveal fractures. If severe injuries require hospitalization, introduce the victim to her primary nurse, if possible.

Throughout the examination, provide support and reassurance, and carefully label all possible evidence. Before the victim's pelvic area is examined, take vital signs, and if the patient is wearing a tampon, remove it, wrap it, and label it as evidence.

This exam is often very distressing to the rape victim. Reassure her, and allow her as much control as possible.

Help collect specimens
During the exam, assist in specimen collection, including those for semen and gonorrhea. Carefully label all specimens with the patient's name, the doctor's name, and the location from which the specimen was obtained. List all specimens in your notes. If the case comes to trial, specimens will be used for evidence, so accuracy is vital.

Collect and label fingernail scrapings and foreign material obtained by combing the victim's pubic hair; these also provide valuable evidence. Note to whom these specimens are given.

For a male victim, be especially alert for injury to the mouth, perineum, and anus. As ordered, obtain a pharyngeal sample for a gonorrhea culture and rectal aspirate for acid phosphatase or sperm analysis.

Most states require the hospital to report all incidents of rape. The patient may elect not to press charges and not to assist the police investigation.

Helping the family in crisis

When a family member is ill, his relatives assume an additional emotional burden that can be draining. A family, after all, can be thought of as an interacting unit—a group standing together with arms interlocked. When one member is weak, the others attempt to carry him, each person shifting his weight to shoulder additional responsibility. Although all families are unique, most follow predictable stages during this struggle.

Stage I: Denial
This avoidance technique helps to cope with a harsh or painful reality. It's a natural defense mechanism against emotional pain and conflict throughout life. Illness in a family triggers shock and disbelief among its members. This denial leads to various behaviors, such as rationalizing symptoms and resisting treatment. Family members often cling to unrealistic expectations: they may refuse to accept the implications of their loved one's illness. Families in denial can be difficult, refusing to cooperate, comprehend, or respond to your interventions.

Although denial usually is transitory, you can't "push" the family out of denial into the next stage. Acknowledging this defense as a normal part of the adjustment process is crucial. Your empathy and support can then guide the family to a deeper level of understanding.

Stage II: Disorganization
Out of denial comes a sense of disorganization. No longer able to deny the obvious, some family members can display demanding and irrational behavior. Their nor-

mal coping mechanisms may be useless if nothing in their past has prepared them to deal with a serious illness.

This sense of disorganization or floundering may give way to anger and blame usually directed at you or other family members. Try to remember that their anger is displaced and temporary. Acknowledge their feelings, offering support and concrete assistance. One suggestion is that they ask neighbors or friends to help them handle routine chores.

Stage III: Anxiety
A hospital is an alien environment, with unfamiliar procedures, machines, and terminology that intensifies the family's emotional turmoil. Decision-making can be particularly difficult at first. You can help the family by acknowledging their discomfort. Then, explain in layman's terms their loved one's medical treatment. Your sympathetic touch, support, and guidance can help them deal with the crisis, no matter how intimidating their anxiety makes it seem to them.

Stage IV: Adjustment
This final stage represents a gradual emotional evolution. How quickly a family adjusts depends on their emotional strength as individuals and as a family. As an internal dynamic, adjustment doesn't always happen according to the health care system's timetable. As a caregiver, you can ease the family's crisis by communicating with them and doing a quick assessment. Ask yourself:
• How are family members communicating with the health care team? Are they angry, quiet, aggressive?
• How are family members communicating with each other?
• What are family members asking and saying?
• What aren't they asking or saying?

• Is there a family spokesperson?

Easing the crisis
Once you've finished your initial assessment, you can help to ease the crisis by following these steps.

Fine-tune your listening skills. Listen not only to the words spoken but also to the feelings expressed. If they're hostile or confused, don't respond with aggression. This only creates more turmoil for the family and you and fellow caregivers.

Develop a plan of action. What does the family need from you? Be prepared to give specific help, such as information about medical procedures. Pass on new and important information.

Provide a realistic view of hospital life. The family may expect wonderful food, and readily available doctors and nurses. Explain to them the demands on the nursing staff and what's considered a reasonable time frame for consultations.

Enlist support. Call on social workers, psychologists, or clergy available at the hospital to provide additional support for the family. Suggest that the family contact community resources, such as crisis centers or private therapists, as well.

Guarding against lawsuits in an emergency

Responding to an emergency requires immediate decisions. Protect yourself from possible malpractice suits by heeding this advice.

Defining your role

Request a written job description that outlines the responsibilities and limits of your nursing role. Know to whom you report and consult them when involved in a conflict with your patient and his family, doctor, or the police. Your supervisor is the hospital spokesperson; don't act without his approval.

Documenting your actions

Your notes reflect all aspects of the nursing process, including a patient assessment, care plan, implementation, and your evaluation of the care's effectiveness.

Improving your skills

Take courses and seek clinical supervision to enhance your experience.

Insuring yourself

Damages awarded to patients can be steep. So can the legal fees to defend yourself even if a malpractice suit is dropped or settled out of court. Provide your own professional liability insurance, and understand your hospital's policy on legal representation.

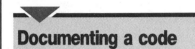

Documenting a code

Your findings and interventions during a code are important. If your hospital has a form for this critical information, use it. If not, document the details in your nurse's notes, including the following information:
• Patient's name and weight
• Time the code was called
• If the patient died, his time of death
• Code team doctors
• Patient's attending doctor: when you notified him and when he arrived
• Airway resuscitation: when was it performed and who did it
• Cardiac compressions: when was it performed and who did it
• Intubation: tube size and who inserted it
• Respiratory therapist
• Nursing supervisor
• I.V. injections: location, solution, and who started them
• Medications: drug names; time, dosage, and route of administration; who administered them
• Defibrillation: time, voltage, who performed the procedure
• Laboratory test values: the time samples were collected, the site, the results (including when you received them)
• Vital signs, including when they were taken
• Procedures, including when they were completed.

After a code, also document the patient's vital signs (if he survived) and the unit to which he was transferred, if any. Date and sign your report.

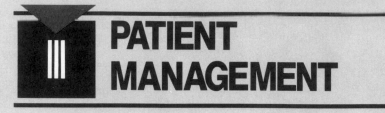

PATIENT MANAGEMENT

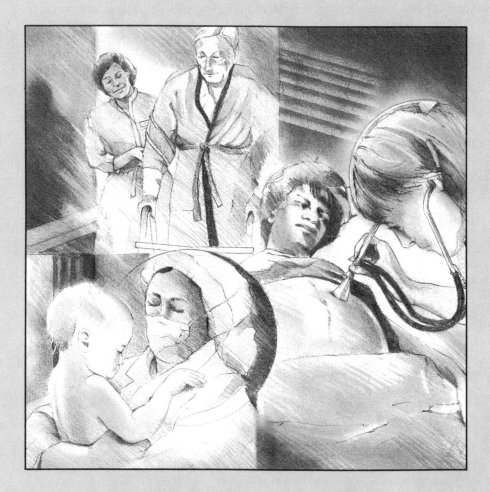

10 Overcoming common problems

Seven steps to securing your patient's trust

One of the most important parts of nursing is winning your patient's trust. By developing a good rapport with the patient, you'll be able to treat him more effectively.

Introduce yourself
During your initial visit with the patient, or during rounds between shifts, have the nurse who is going off-duty introduce you to the patient and briefly summarize his condition. This will help you gain the patient's trust.

Call your patient by name
Hospitals are an alien environment and can easily threaten a person's identity. In calling a patient by his name, you bolster his weakened self-image. Use his name throughout his stay at the hospital. This will make him feel like a human being, not just "the patient in room 409."

Have a positive attitude
Your attitude should foster trust, not negate it. Even with an overly demanding patient, treat him as individual and maintain a positive attitude when taking care of him.

Explain your role
Tell the patient the length of your shift and the nursing procedures you'll be performing on him. Establishing this routine at the start will prevent an overly demanding patient from becoming anxious or unrealistic.

Discuss procedures
Lessen your patient's anxiety by explaining the functions of the equipment you will be using. Tell him what you intend to do and why. Answer his questions and talk to him during the procedure itself, explaining each step.

Keep your appointments
If you have to break an appointment, let the patient know in advance and set up another time. If the patient must break an appointment, try to accommodate his schedule.

Be honest
Keep your promises. Don't tell a patient you'll return if there's a chance that you won't. Avoid bluffing your way through difficult medical questions with double-talk. If the patient has a question, and you say you'll find out the answer and get back to him, do so.

Learning to listen

Chances are, you decided to become a nurse because you wanted to help people, which often means giving them advice. When you think you understand a patient's problem, your instinct probably tells you to give him suggestions or words of encouragement. But you should resist this temptation—at least for awhile.

Instead, you should say nothing: just listen to your patient. Listening, along with interpreting his nonverbal cues, will help you understand not only what the patient is trying to say, but also *why* he's saying it.

For example, if a terminally ill cancer patient asks you, "Do you think there's any hope for me?" he may actually be asking you, "Have you given up on me?" or "Has the doctor given up on me?" or "Has my family given up on me?" or "Am I dying?" Whatever his specific concerns, the patient does not want a "Yes" or "No" answer. Instead, he probably wants to discuss his feelings about the situation, and by listening to him, you can discover his real concerns.

Communicating effectively: The do's and don'ts

During your first interview—and in later conversations with the patient—effective communication is essential. To gain accurate information from a patient, listen to what he has to say and respond appropriately. Below are some communication techniques that will help you learn more about the patient, plus a list of responses to avoid.

Do's

Technique	Purpose or effect	Example
Using open-ended questions	To allow the patient to clarify and elaborate on his thoughts	Patient: "I haven't felt comfortable since I went on this new treatment schedule." Nurse: "How are you handling your new treatment routine?"
Using closed questions	To direct the patient toward providing specific information	Patient: "I had a battery of tests done at my last doctor's appointment." Nurse: "When was your last doctor's appointment?"
Restating	To clarify meanings for you and the patient	Patient: "The day after New Year's, I went in for tests, and they found the cause of my abdominal pain immediately. I followed my medication very carefully, but I had to go back to the hospital again last month because the gastritis had started up again." Nurse: "So this is your third visit this year? You were admitted in January and again in May, each time for gastritis?"
Communicating support (empathy)	To encourage the patient to continue and to show your concern	Patient: "My folks have gone out of their way recently to care for me and I'm grateful to them. But I find myself thinking back to just a month ago when I was completely on my own." Nurse: "It must be hard to depend on your parents after being independent for so long."
Reflecting (echoing)	To allow the patient to evaluate his thoughts and feelings through your restatement	Patient: "I don't know. My family is so upset by my illness that I guess I've tried to ignore other treatment possibilities." Nurse: "So your family has been so upset by your illness that you haven't explored alternative treatments."
Using silence	To allow the patient to collect his thoughts and to reflect on the conversation	Patient: "I guess what it comes down to is that I felt too guilty about being a burden." Nurse: (remain silent)

Don'ts

Changing the topic	Makes the patient think you don't care or aren't listening	Patient: "I think I'm doing all right today." Nurse: "What time does your doctor usually come in?"
Giving false assurances	Misleads the patient	Patient: "I'm afraid the test results will be bad news." Nurse: "Maybe they won't be bad at all."
Interrupting	Forces the patient to reinitiate the conversation	Patient: "You know, the thing I've been—" Nurse: "Would you like to sit up?"

Communicating effectively: The do's and don'ts (continued)

Technique	Purpose or effect	Example
Don'ts (continued)		
Making assumptions	Fails to clarify and creates confusion	Patient: "I haven't felt this way for days." Nurse: "I know what you're saying."
Trivializing feelings	Ignores the patient's feelings	Patient: "I'm not sure I'm doing the right thing, asking my sister to come here." Nurse: "Well, you know what they say, nothing ventured, nothing gained."
Giving advice	Makes the patient more dependent	Patient: "How do you think I should explain this to my children?" Nurse: "Tell them the truth."
Being defensive	Interferes with getting at the root of the problem	Patient: "This hospital isn't very clean." Nurse: "It's as clean as any hospital you'll find."

How to handle an aggressive patient

Aggressive patients can be talkative, restless, agitated, demanding, abusive, and inattentive. Coping with them can be taxing. But you shouldn't try to suppress their behavior. Instead, you should let them express their feelings. Here are some pointers for handling aggressive patients in stressful situations:

• Be attentive to the patient. Don't react to any challenging or unkind remarks he may make.
• Don't make disapproving comments.
• Avoid long explanations. Speak in short sentences.
• Be clear about your decisions and don't defend them.
• Remain calm and open.
• Use positive, non-verbal communication such as smiling and nodding.

• If the patient becomes combative, you should take immediate steps:
— Call for help. Ask your assistance team to remain nearby and explain to them how you're trying to handle the patient.
— Protect yourself and be aware of possible escape routes.
— Don't turn your back on the patient.
— Avoid speaking to the patient in an authoritarian or threatening tone of voice.
— Test your progress in resolving the conflict by moving closer to the patient. If the patient backs away, you should respect his need for space.
— Continue to emphathize with the patient. Try to bargain and reason with him. But you should never make unrealistic promises to him.
— Use restraints if necessary, but only after consulting with a doctor. Ask your co-workers for assistance.
— Document any episodes in your nurse's notes.

Getting a complainer to comply

Dealing with a patient who complains requires ingenuity. Here are a few guidelines to consider:

• Avoid using pat formulas, which demean the patient and can worsen the situation.
• Assign a staff member with good communication skills to the patient.
• Limit the number of staff members working with the patient to improve communication with him.
• Expand the patient's care plan to further communication. Discuss these changes with the staff.
• Have a positive attitude. Feel that you can overcome a patient who complains rather than give in to him.
• Use behavior modification techniques with the guidance of a trained consultant.
• Respect the patient's individuality.

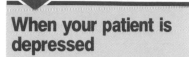

When your patient is depressed

Hospital patients are prone to depression, particularly those with terminal or chronic illness or drug dependencies. Thrust into new surroundings, a patient may fear the loss of control and fear being separated from his family and friends. You can reduce the patient's stress by using certain coping mechanisms and listening techniques.

Terminal prognosis
Patients suffering from a terminal illness such as acquired immunodeficiency syndrome (AIDS) may be depressed and may express thoughts of suicide. How you can help:
• Let the patient talk about his feelings. Listen attentively and reflect his thoughts.
• Give the patient non-verbal support by nodding your head or placing your hand on his shoulder.
• Talk about the patient's depression with his doctor, who will order a psychiatric consultation.
• Alert other nurses on the floor to the patient's moods and alter his care plan if necessary.
• Assess the patient's potential for suicide. Is he preoccupied with death? Does he talk about suicide? Does he discuss various suicide techniques? If so, suggest one-on-one observation.
• When possible, discuss the situation with a psychiatrist or a nurse who specializes in clinical psychiatry.

Debilitating illness
Chronically ill patients such as diabetics suffer bouts of depression as a result of complications caused by their illnesses. A potential amputee, for example, may want to discuss the operation and the changes his body may undergo. How you can help:
• Tell the patient that he seems depressed. This will open the discussion to any feelings of fear and abandonment.
• If you are discussing amputation, let the patient talk about his physical condition and the possibility of his undergoing physical changes.
• Offer emotional support, *not* tranquilizers. Medication is not a substitute for communication.

Drug dependency
A drug-dependent patient can be abrupt and anxious, or quiet and withdrawn. He may also become restless and depressed, and cry often. How you can help:
• Determine if the patient's depression is related to drug withdrawal.
• Determine his potential for suicide. Ask him if he's thinking about hurting himself. If so, does he have a plan? Has he ever attempted suicide? Listen for statements that suggest a feeling of hopelessness.
• Investigate, through appropriate resources, the possibility of the patient entering a drug-treatment program after his discharge from the hospital.

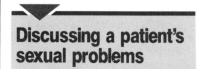

Discussing a patient's sexual problems

Knowing how to talk to a patient about his sexual concerns is crucial. It enables you to identify areas which require immediate treatment. It also shows the patient that you view sexual functioning as important and that you are willing to discuss the subject.

Tell the patient that you need information about his sexual functioning and experiences so that you can provide adequate care. Assure the patient that this information will remain confidential.

Begin your discussion with general information, then move to the specific. For example, start with urinary problems before asking about sexual functioning.

Integrate your questions about sex with other questions relating to the patient's daily routine. This will help him understand that discussing sexual problems or concerns is acceptable. Ask open-ended questions such as, "Did you just notice this problem recently?" rather than, "When did you first notice this problem?"

Avoid using technical terms when possible. You can, however, use slang, depending on the patient's age and your rapport with him.

Don't signal disapproval. If you do, the patient will be less willing to discuss sexual matters. You should end the interview by asking the patient if he has any additional questions or concerns.

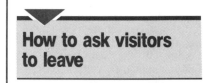

How to ask visitors to leave

Visitors can be a burden or a blessing, depending on the circumstances. How to determine this is difficult, but here are a few key questions to ask yourself:

Is the patient undergoing an intimate or invasive procedure?
The patient may prefer privacy during procedures such as rectal thermometer insertion. Visitors can step into the hallway for a few minutes. If the doctor is performing a medical procedure, he may ask visitors to leave.

If the patient prefers their company—and the doctor agrees to it—one support person can be chosen to stay. Explain where he

Recognizing the stages of grief

Understanding the various stages of grief helps you determine how a terminally ill patient feels about his condition, and whether he has accepted or denied the reality of his illness. Below are the stages of grief a patient will experience. Some occur at the same time, others overlap.

Stage 1: Shock and denial
The patient is overwhelmed by shock and disbelief, rejects reality, and may experience physical reactions such as sweating, pallor, faintness, nausea, and confusion.

Stage 2: Anger
The patient is impatient, uncooperative, bitter, and jealous.

Stage 3: Depression
The patient feels helpless, melancholic, and exhausted. He avoids reality, and may experience physical symptoms, such as weakness and dyspnea.

Stage 4: Acceptance
The patient gradually begins to accept the reality of his illness, becomes contemplative and serene, and is able to discuss his condition.

---

should stand and how he should behave during the procedure. Reassure the other visitors that they can return when the doctor is finished.

Are the visitors interfering with the patient's rest?
Patients who are tired may be reluctant to ask loved ones to leave. You can direct visitors to a waiting area and tell them that they'll be notified as soon as the patient awakens. Or, if the patient prefers, they may remain quietly in the room.

Are the visitors ill?
If a visitor is obviously ill and his presence is not critical, tell him that it would be better for the patient if he remained at home until he's well.

Do the visitors hover?
Hovering is usually a mechanism for coping with a crisis. If the patient is comfortable with the visitor's behavior—and, in fact, finds it reassuring—then there's no problem. Distraught visitors, however, may require special attention from members of the clergy or a social service representative in order to calm them.

Are the visitors disturbing the patient's roommate?
Caution loud or disruptive visitors that unless they behave, they'll have to visit with the patient in a waiting area or leave the hospital altogether. Few visitors will argue about leaving if they feel that you're being fair and that it's in the patient's best interest if they leave.

Before the visitors leave, give them a status report on the patient's condition and, if possible, a time when they can return. If you handle this situation diplomatically, you may actually improve your standing with the patient's family.

How to comfort the dying patient

A terminally ill patient needs you to help ease his feelings of loneliness and separation. You can comfort a dying patient and help him confront his feelings by:
• being honest. Be yourself and answer questions candidly. Don't shy away from discussing the patient's illness. On the other hand, don't offer information on the patient's condition if he has not requested it.
• advocating for him. Occasionally, a doctor will not have answered a patient's questions fully. You'll need to communicate with both the doctor and the patient, relaying the patient's questions to his doctor when necessary.
• acknowledging the patient's feelings. Shock, disbelief, loneliness, anger, and hostility are common reactions among terminally ill patients. Talk with the patient, even if a co-worker has to "cover" for you briefly. You can return the favor.
• fostering the patient's self-image. The dying patient needs to be reassured of his own self-worth. By talking to him, patting him on the back, or touching his shoulder, you give him dignity and self-confidence.
• discussing the patient's care. If the patient is mentally and physically able, include him in discussions concerning his care. Reassure the patient that you will be giving him medication to keep him comfortable. Reassure his family that actual death is usually painless.

Slimming tips for overweight patients

Losing weight is a tough challenge, but keeping the weight off is even harder. The reason is that during the first few weeks of dieting a patient loses fluids. All diets require cutting calories, and over time, if the patient follows a sensible eating and exercise program, his body will also burn fat. But it takes time because fat tissue has a lower metabolic rate than muscle and therefore takes longer to burn.

A patient should see his doctor before starting a weight-loss program and follow this list of tips to help him slim down safely.

Keep a food diary
A patient should keep track of what he eats and when. This way he can keep track of his particular cravings and when hunger usually strikes.

Count calories
How many does the patient need? This will depend on his daily activities, which fall into four basic categories:
• Sedentary (no exercise): Figure 13 calories per pound (cal/lb) of body weight to maintain current weight.
• Mildly active (no sports or regular exercise): 15 cal/lb body weight.
• Moderately active (regular exercise): 20 cal/lb body weight.
• Extremely active: 25 cal/lb body weight.

When a patient has determined how many calories he needs to maintain his weight, he can calculate what he will need to *lose* weight. One pound of body weight equals 3,500 calories. By reducing his calorie intake by 500 calories a day, the patient can lose one pound a week. Women should never drop below 1,200 calories a day.

Exercise regularly
Exercising will help a patient lose weight. Regular aerobic activity — running, swimming, walking, bicycling, and other exercises — burns fat and calories. It also strengthens the heart and muscles.

Eat less fat and more carbohydrates
A patient can eat fatty foods like meat and cheese in moderation, but he should concentrate on eating more complex carbohydrates like whole-grain products and vegetables.

Keep trying
Everyone hits plateaus during a diet. At certain points, a patient will find it hard to lose weight because his body reaches a "set point," a genetically determined threshold of body fat that his metabolism tries to maintain. His body may resist weight loss by altering its metabolic rate. But as he consumes fewer calories and continues to exercise, the weight will come off.

Remember: Food is not a friend
Some people eat for comfort. Compulsive overeating can be treated through counseling or with the help of organizations such as Overeaters Anonymous. Consult the Yellow Pages for details.

Let hunger, not the clock, determine meal times
Overeaters often rely on time rather than appetite to determine their meal schedule. A patient should eat when he needs to eat, but not overindulge.

Choose foods from a sensible diet plan
This includes:
• Fruits and vegetables (4 servings/day). These foods are high in vitamins and fiber.
• Bread and cereal (4 servings/day). Complex carbohydrates such

as grains, enriched breads and cereals provide nutrients and are filling.
• Milk and dairy products (2 servings/day). Use low-fat products to provide calcium and vitamins.
• Meat group (2 servings/day). Beef, poultry, and fish are protein-rich. Choose leaner cuts of beef to reduce fat intake.

Practice smart eating

• Choose low-calorie foods that fill you up, such as multi-grain bread, soups, skim milk, and yogurt.
• Eat a salad before each meal, if possible.
• Watch for hidden calories. Coffee with sugar, cookies, muffins, granola cereals, and candy can put on the pounds.
• Eat at home rather than in restaurants when possible. Restaurant meals, with big portions cooked in fat or oil, can be expensive and fattening.

Debunking fad diets

"Take off 16 pounds in 2 weeks!"
"Melt away ugly bulges forever!"
"Lose weight on watercress!"

The claims of fad diets are everywhere—in bold type in magazine advertisements, screaming from the headlines of tabloids at supermarket checkout stands, in window displays of health-food stores.

As a health educator, it's up to you to set your patients straight, explaining that fad diets are just that—a fad. They usually promise rapid and painless weight loss using a special—and sometimes expensive—formula. You can counter such trendy, quick weight-loss claims by pointing out to the patient why fad diets don't work.
• On a fad diet, you may lose weight quickly, but much of it's

Determining obesity

Obesity, an overabundance of body fat resulting in body weight 20% or more above normal, affects an estimated 25% to 45% of the population in the United States. One way to tell if your patient is clinically obese is to compare his triceps skinfold measurement to this chart.

If his skinfold measurement is equal to or greater than that indicated for his age, consider him clinically obese. *Note:* Use metal calipers, because plastic calipers generally won't have a large enough jaw face to measure an obese patient's skinfold.

Triceps skinfold measurements (millimeters)

Age	Women	Men
18	27	15
19	27	15
20	28	16
21	28	17
22	28	18
23	28	18
24	28	19
25	29	20
26	29	20
27	29	21
28	29	22
29	29	23
30 +	30	23

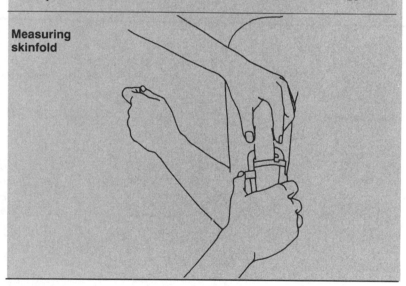

Measuring skinfold

fluid, and you often gain it right back.
• Fat shed on fad diets also returns quickly because the body's metabolic rate and the way it actually burns fat remains unchanged. The only way to burn fat efficiently and keep the weight off is with a sensible diet and exercise program.

• Fad diets often rely on costly gimmicks. A regular, balanced diet program does not. Moreover, "quick" diet programs usually repeat meals—you're always eating grapefruits, for instance—while a more sensible diet program varies what you eat and includes meat, fish, chicken, vegetables, and grains.

Determining body frame type

To determine your patient's body frame type, use the graph below to compare his wrist measurement with his height. This comparison will give you the patient's body frame type.

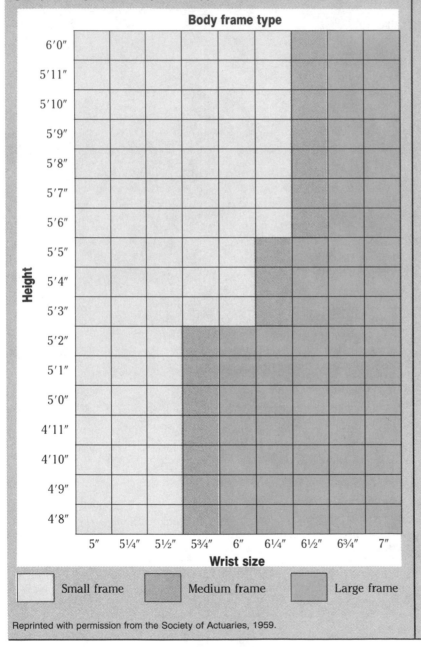

Reprinted with permission from the Society of Actuaries, 1959.

Body frames

Depending on your patient's body frame, you may classify him as an ectomorph, a mesomorph, or an endomorph. Below is a list of the characteristics for each of these classifications, which applies to both males and females.

Ectomorph
• Small, slender body that appears weak
• High proportion of skin and bones
• Long arms and legs
• Slender, delicate bone structure
• Stringy muscles
• Subcutaneous tissue
• Slightly developed abdominal viscera

Mesomorph
• Athletic appearance
• Well-developed muscles
• High proportion of muscle
• Prominent body joints, particularly at the shoulders and hips
• Massive, muscular chest (in males); chest more prominent than abdomen
• Flat stomach
• General hardness and ruggedness in all regions (especially in males)

Endomorph
• Large body type with short arms and legs
• High proportion of fat
• Arms and legs appear to taper from proximal to distal
• Abdominal mass dominates body section in males (females may be proportioned somewhat differently)
• Large abdominal viscera overhangs pelvis
• General roundness, with soft contours in all regions

Assessing body weight

To assess your patient's weight accurately, you must know his height and body frame type. Using the charts below, find the ideal weight for his height and body frame type. Then, compare this range with what he actually weighs. If he falls within this range, consider his body weight normal. If he is above or below this range, consider him underweight or overweight.

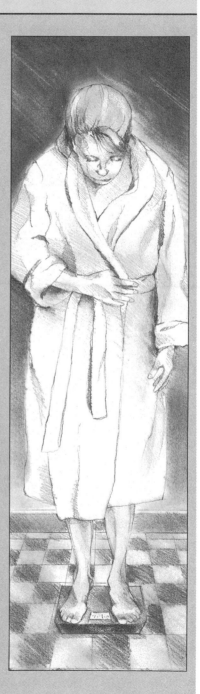

Weights for women age 25 and over

Height	Weight		
	Small frame	**Medium frame**	**Large frame**
4'8"	92-98	96-107	104-119
4'9"	94-101	98-110	106-122
4'10"	96-104	101-113	109-125
4'11"	99-107	104-116	112-128
5'0"	102-110	107-119	115-131
5'1"	105-113	110-122	118-134
5'2"	108-116	113-126	121-138
5'3"	111-119	116-130	125-142
5'4"	114-123	120-135	129-146
5'5"	118-127	124-139	133-150
5'6"	122-131	128-143	137-154
5'7"	126-135	132-147	141-158
5'8"	130-140	136-151	145-163
5'9"	134-144	140-155	149-168
5'10"	138-148	144-159	153-173

Weights for men age 25 and over

Height	Weight		
	Small frame	**Medium frame**	**Large frame**
5'1"	112-120	118-129	126-141
5'2"	115-123	121-133	129-144
5'3"	118-126	124-136	132-148
5'4"	121-129	127-139	135-152
5'5"	124-133	130-143	138-156
5'6"	128-137	134-147	142-161
5'7"	132-141	138-152	147-166
5'8"	136-145	142-156	151-170
5'9"	140-150	146-160	155-174
5'10"	144-154	150-165	159-179
5'11"	148-158	154-170	164-184
6'0"	152-162	158-175	168-189
6'1"	156-167	162-180	173-194
6'2"	160-171	167-185	178-199
6'3"	164-175	172-190	182-204

Reprinted with permission from Metropolitan Life Insurance Company. Based on Society of Actuaries data, 1959.

Recommended dietary allowances in the United States[a]

	Infants (both sexes)		Children (both sexes)			Males	
Age	0 to 6 mos.	6 to 12 mos.	1 to 3	4 to 6	7 to 10	11 to 14	15 to 18
Weight	13 lb 6 kg	20 lb 9 kg	29 lb 13 kg	44 lb 20 kg	62 lb 28 kg	99 lb 45 kg	145 lb 66 kg
Height	24 in 60 cm	28 in 71 cm	35 in 90 cm	44 in 112 cm	52 in 132 cm	62 in 157 cm	69 in 176 cm
Protein (g)	13	14	16	24	28	45	59
Fat-soluble vitamins							
Vitamin A (mg RE)[b]	375	375	400	500	700	1,000	1,000
Vitamin D (μg)[c]	7.5	10	10	10	10	10	10
Vitamin E (α TE)[d]	3	4	6	7	7	10	10
Vitamin K (μg)	5	10	15	20	30	45	65
Water-soluble vitamins							
Vitamin C (mg)	30	35	40	45	45	50	60
Thiamine (mg)	0.3	0.4	0.7	0.9	1.0	1.3	1.5
Riboflavin (mg)	0.4	0.5	0.8	1.1	1.2	1.5	1.8
Niacin (mg NE)[e]	5	6	9	12	13	17	20
Vitamin B_6 (mg)	0.3	0.6	1.0	1.1	1.4	1.7	2.0
Folate (μg)[f]	25	35	50	75	100	150	200
Vitamin B_{12} (μg)[g]	0.3	0.5	0.7	1.0	1.4	2.0	2.0
Minerals							
Calcium (mg)	400	600	800	800	800	1,200	1,200
Phosphorus (mg)	300	500	800	800	800	1,200	1,200
Magnesium (mg)	40	60	80	120	170	270	400
Iron (mg)[h]	6	10	10	10	10	12	12
Zinc (mg)	5	5	10	10	10	15	15
Iodine (μg)	40	50	70	90	120	150	150
Selenium (μg)	10	15	20	20	30	40	50

[a]The allowances are intended to provide for individual variations among most normal persons as they live in the United States under usual environmental stresses. Diets should be based on a variety of common foods in order to provide other nutrients for which human requirements have been well defined.
[b]Retinol equivalents. 1 Retinol equivalent = 1 mcg retinol or 6 mcg beta carotene.
[c]As cholecalciferol. 10 mcg cholecalciferol = 400 IU vitamin D.
[d]Alpha tocopherol equivalents (Alpha TE). 1 mg d-Alpha-tocopherol = 1 Alpha TE.
[e]1 NE (niacin equivalent) is equal to 1 mg of niacin or 60 mg of dietary tryptophan.
[f]The folacin allowances refer to dietary sources as determined by *Lactobacillus casei* assay after treatment with enzymes ("conjugases") to make polyglutamyl forms of the vitamin available to the test organism.

			Females					Pregnant	Lactating	
19 to 24	25 to 50	51+	11 to 14	15 to 18	19 to 24	25 to 50	51+		1st 6 mos.	2nd 6 mos.
160 lb 72 kg	174 lb 79 kg	170 lb 77 kg	101 lb 46 kg	120 lb 55 kg	128 lb 58 kg	138 lb 63 kg	143 lb 65 kg	—	—	
70 in 177 cm	70 in 176 cm	68 in 173 cm	62 in 157 cm	64 in 163 cm	63 in 160 cm	—	—	—		
58	63	63	46	44	46	50	50	60	65	62
1,000	1,000	1,000	800	800	800	800	800	800	1,300	1,200
10	5	5	10	10	10	5	5	10	10	10
10	10	10	8	8	8	8	8	10	12	11
70	80	80	45	55	60	65	65	65	65	65
60	60	60	50	60	60	60	60	70	95	90
1.5	1.5	1.2	1.1	1.1	1.1	1.1	1.0	1.5	1.6	1.6
1.7	1.7	1.4	1.3	1.3	1.3	1.3	1.2	1.6	1.8	1.7
19	19	15	15	15	15	15	13	17	20	20
2.0	2.0	2.0	1.4	1.5	1.6	1.6	1.6	2.2	2.1	2.1
200	200	200	150	180	180	180	180	400	280	260
2.0	2.0	2.0	2.0	2.0	2.0	2.0	2.0	2.2	2.6	2.6
1,200	800	800	1,200	1,200	1,200	800	800	1,200	1,200	1,200
1,200	800	800	1,200	1,200	1,200	800	800	1,200	1,200	1,200
350	350	350	280	300	280	280	280	320	355	340
10	10	10	15	15	15	15	10	30	15	15
15	15	15	12	12	12	12	12	15	19	16
150	150	150	150	150	150	150	150	175	200	200
70	70	70	45	50	55	55	55	65	75	75

gThe RDA for vitamin B_{12} in infants is based on average concentration of the vitamin in human milk. The allowances after weaning are based on energy intake (as recommended by the American Academy of Pediatrics) and consideration of other factors such as intestinal absorption.

hThe increased requirements during pregnancy cannot be met by the iron content of habitual American diets nor by the existing iron stores of many women; therefore, the use of 30 to 60 mg of supplemental iron is recommended. Iron needs during lactation are not substantially different from those of nonpregnant women, but continued supplementation of the mother for 2 to 3 months after parturition is advisable in order to replenish stores depleted by pregnancy.

Recommended dietary allowances in Canada[a,b]

	Infants (both sexes)				Children (both sexes)			Males				
Age	0 to 2 months	3 to 5	6 to 8	9 to 11	1	2 to 3	4 to 6	7 to 9	10 to 12	13 to 15	16 to 18	19 to 24
Protein (g/day)[c]	11[h]	14[h]	17	18	19	22	26	30	38	50	55	58
Fat-soluble vitamins												
Vitamin A (RE/day)[d]	400	400	400	400	400	400	500	700	800	900	1,000	1,000
Vitamin D (μg/day)[e]	10	10	10	10[a]	10	5	5	2.5	2.5	2.5	2.5	2.5
Vitamin E (mg/day)[f]	3	3	3	3	3	4	5	7	8	9	10	10
Water-soluble vitamins												
Vitamin C (mg/day)	20	20	20	20	20	20	25	35	40	50	55	60
Folacin (μg/day)[g]	50	50	50	55	65	80	90	125	170	150	185	210
Vitamin B_{12} (μg/day)	0.3	0.3	0.3	0.3	0.3	0.4	0.5	0.8	1.0	1.5	1.9	2.0
Minerals												
Calcium (mg/day)	350	350	400	400	500	500	600	700	900	1,100	900	800
Magnesium (mg/day)	30	40	50	50	55	70	90	110	150	210	250	240
Iron (mg/day)	0.4[i]	5	7	7	6	6	6	7	10	12	10	8
Iodine (μg/day)	25	35	40	45	55	65	85	110	125	160	160	160
Zinc (mg/day)	2[j]	3	3	3	4	4	5	6	7	9	9	9

[a]Recommended intakes of energy and of certain nutrients are not listed in this table because of the nature of the variables upon which they are based. The figures for energy are estimates of average requirements for expected patterns of activity. For nutrients not shown, the following amounts are recommended: thiamine, 0.4 mg/1,000 kcal (0.48 mg/5,000 kj); riboflavin, 0.5 mg/1,000 kcal (0.6 mg/5,000 kj); niacin, 7.2 NE/1,000 kcal (8.6 NE/5,000 kj); vitamin B_6, 15 μg, as pyridoxine, per gram of protein; phosphorus, same as calcium.

[b]Recommended intakes during periods of growth are taken as appropriate for individuals representative of the mid-point in each age group. All recommended intakes are designed to cover individual variations in essentially all of a healthy population subsisting upon a variety of common foods available in Canada.

[c]The primary units are grams per kilogram of body weight. The figures shown here are only examples.

[d]One retinol equivalent (RE) corresponds to the biological activity of 1 μg of retinol, 6 μg of β-carotene or 12 μg of other carotenes.

		Females								Pregnant (additional)			Lactating (additional)
50 to 74	75+	7 to 9	10 to 12	13 to 15	16 to 18	19 to 24	25 to 49	50 to 74	75+	1st trimester	2nd	3rd	
60	57	30	40	42	43	43	44	47	47	15	20	25	20
1,000	1,000	700	800	800	800	800	800	800	800	100	100	100	400
2.5	2.5	2.5	2.5	2.5	2.5	2.5	2.5	2.5	2.5	2.5	2.5	2.5	2.5
7	6	6	7	7	7	7	6	6	5	2	2	2	3
60	60	30	40	45	45	45	45	45	45	0	20	20	30
220	205	125	180	145	160	175	175	190	190	305	305	305	120
2.0	2.0	0.8	1.0	1.5	1.9	2.0	2.0	2.0	2.0	1.0	1.0	1.0	0.5
800	800	700	1,000	800	700	700	700	800	800	500	500	500	500
250	230	110	160	200	215	200	200	210	220	15	20	25	80
8	8	7	10	13	14	14	14k	7	7	6	6	6	0
160	160	95	110	160	160	160	160	160	160	25	25	25	50
9	9	6	7	8	8	8	8	8	8	0	1	2	6

[e]Expressed as cholecalciferol or ergocalciferol.
[f]Expressed as d-α-tocopherol equivalents, relative to which β- and γ-tocopherol and α-tocotrienol have activities of 0.5, 0.1, and 0.3 respectively.
[g]The folacin allowances refer to dietary sources as determined by *Lactobacillus casei* assay after treatment with enzymes ("conjugases") to make polyglutamyl forms of the vitamin available to the test organism.
[h]Assumption that the protein is from breast milk or is of the same biological value as that of breast milk and that between 3 and 9 months adjustment for the quality of the protein is made.
[i]Based on the assumption that breast milk is the source of iron for the first 2 months.
[j]Based on the assumption that breast milk is the source of zinc for the first 2 months.
[k]After menopause the recommended intake is 7 mg/day.

Walking to health

One of the best ways to strengthen the heart is by walking. In fact, walking is now a favorite pastime in America in part because, unlike running, it's not stressful to the knees or lower back. Below is a sample exercise program. But before starting, do some stretching exercises to limber muscles and prevent strain.

The calf stretch is done by placing both hands on a wall, about shoulder height. Step with one foot toward the wall and lean against it, keeping the palms flat on the wall and the feet flat on the floor. Push against the wall until there is a pull. Don't bounce. This stretch should be done slowly and smoothly. For the shoulder stretch, clasp both hands over the head and pull the shoulders backward.

Week	Warm up	Exercise	Cool down	Total time
1	Stretch 2 min. Walk slowly 3 min.	Walk briskly 5 min.	Walk slowly 3 min. Stretch 2 min.	15 min.
2	Stretch 2 min. Walk slowly 3 min.	Walk briskly 7 min.	Walk slowly 3 min. Stretch 2 min.	17 min.
3	Stretch 2 min. Walk slowly 3 min.	Walk briskly 9 min.	Walk slowly 3 min. Stretch 2 min.	19 min.
4	Stretch 2 min. Walk slowly 3 min.	Walk briskly 11 min.	Walk slowly 3 min. Stretch 2 min.	21 min.
5	Stretch 2 min. Walk slowly 3 min.	Walk briskly 13 min.	Walk slowly 3 min. Stretch 2 min.	23 min.
6	Stretch 2 min. Walk slowly 3 min.	Walk briskly 15 min.	Walk slowly 3 min. Stretch 2 min.	25 min.
7	Stretch 2 min. Walk slowly 3 min.	Walk briskly 18 min.	Walk slowly 3 min. Stretch 2 min.	28 min.
8	Stretch 2 min. Walk slowly 5 min.	Walk briskly 20 min.	Walk slowly 5 min. Stretch 2 min.	34 min.
9	Stretch 2 min. Walk slowly 5 min.	Walk briskly 23 min.	Walk slowly 5 min. Stretch 2 min.	37 min.
10	Stretch 2 min. Walk slowly 5 min.	Walk briskly 26 min.	Walk slowly 5 min. Stretch 2 min.	40 min.
11	Stretch 2 min. Walk slowly 5 min.	Walk briskly 28 min.	Walk slowly 5 min. Stretch 2 min.	42 min.
12 and after	Stretch 2 min. Walk slowly 5 min.	Walk briskly 30 min.	Walk slowly 5 min. Stretch 2 min.	44 min.

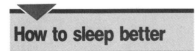

How to sleep better

Here are some tips for your patient to improve his sleep and make his nights more restful:

• Exercise regularly. Activity will tire him out by bedtime.
• Establish a bedtime routine. Performing the same activities each night will put him in a restful mood.
• Engage in soothing activities, such as reading or listening to music just before bedtime.
• Take a tepid bath to relax before going to bed. Or practice the relaxation techniques suggested in *Managing stress*.
• Take any prescribed pain medications 30 minutes before bedtime.

Calf stretch

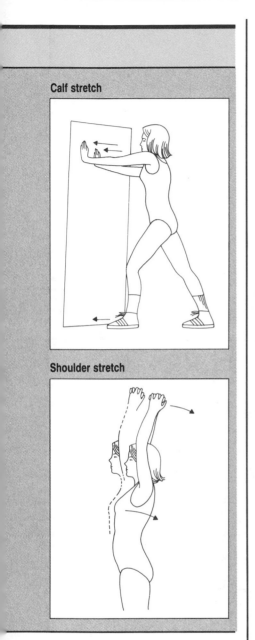

Shoulder stretch

• Use clean, wrinkle-free bedding and wear comfortable nightclothes for better comfort.
• Drink a glass of warm milk, wine, brandy, or beer before bedtime if not prohibited by his doctor.

What to avoid
• Going to bed with worries. If possible, the patient should try to resolve his problems before bedtime.
• Engaging in strenuous physical activity before going to bed.
• Overeating before bedtime. A large meal can keep a patient awake. So can beverages containing caffeine or excessive amounts of alcohol.
• Being mentally stimulated before bed. Studying for an exam or balancing a checkbook doesn't induce restful thoughts.
• Taking diuretic medications that will interrupt his sleep.

Managing stress

Various techniques can help a patient learn to handle stress better, and in doing so, help him prevent illness and mental fatigue. Some of these techniques, such as meditation and exercise, can be incorporated into a daily routine. Others, such as deep-breathing and self-hypnosis, are useful when the patient finds himself in stressful situations.

Breathe deeply
When a patient feels anxious, he takes short breaths, which may cause him to hyperventilate. To avoid this, the patient should take several deep breaths, which will calm him down and help him relax in tense situations.

Repeat a slogan
The patient should tell himself to "calm down," that "this will pass." He should repeat these words while taking deep breaths. Not only will this technique help him collect his thoughts, it will also give him constant positive reinforcement.

Meditate
The patient can learn meditation from an instructor, who will teach him the proper sitting and breathing techniques. But in the meantime, he can follow the four basic steps to meditation:
• Find a quiet, comfortable room.
• Choose a word he can repeat to himself to help tune out his surroundings.
• Let himself relax and think calming thoughts.
• Sit comfortably.

Use mental imagery
The patient should relieve stress by relaxing every part of his body, beginning at his toes and working upward, while imagining pleasant thoughts.

Practice self-hypnosis
An instructor can teach the patient how to put himself into a relaxed, passive state of mind.

Massage
A patient doesn't need a professional to help relieve back and neck pains (see *Relieving back pain,* page 276, for techniques).

Exercise frequently
The many benefits of exercise regularly include a relaxed, healthy state of mind. Exercise releases endorphins, which can relieve anger and stress. Exercise will also improve a patient's sleeping patterns, release tension, lower his blood pressure, and control his weight.

Take vacations
One of your patient's priorities should be taking regular rest intervals in order to reduce stress and to regenerate. A patient shouldn't feel that he has to put his vacation time to definite use. The point of taking time off is to let go and relax.

Relieving back pain

You can help ease a patient's back pain by teaching her about good posture. The following guidelines help the patient stand, sit, and lie properly, prevent back pain, and also provide the exercise to strengthen her back.

Standing correctly
This will strengthen the patient's abdominal and buttock muscles, which support the back. To stand correctly, she should draw an imaginary line from her ear through the tip of her shoulder, the middle of her hip, the back of her knee, and the front of her ankle. This mental exercise will help the patient stand properly, will correct arching or stooping her back, and will help prevent sagging in her abdominal muscles.

The patient should also follow this simple exercise. She should lean against a wall with her knees slightly bent; then tighten her abdominal and buttock muscles to tilt her pelvis back and flatten her lower back. Holding this position, she should ease up the wall until she's standing. The patient should try to maintain this posture during daily activities, periodically leaning against a wall to check her progress.

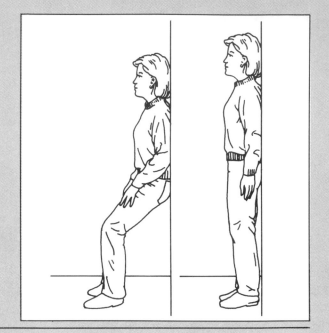

Sitting correctly
The patient should sit with her neck and back in as straight a line as possible, without slumping or thrusting her neck and head forward. Straight, hard chairs cultivate good posture.

She can relieve strain by sitting forward in her chair, tightening her abdominal muscles to flatten her back, and crossing her legs. She can correct swayback, a form of curvature of the spine, by using a footrest to bring her knees higher than her hips.

She can alleviate back strain when driving by positioning the seat close to the pedals. She should tighten the seat belt and use a hard backrest to flatten her lower back.

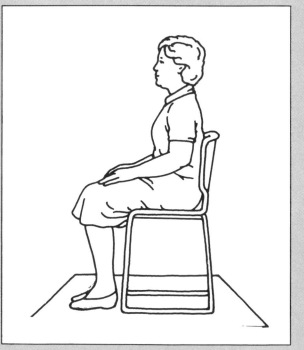

Exercising the back (performed in bed)

Tell the patient to lie on her back with her knees bent and a pillow supporting her neck. Bring one knee up to her chest, then lower it slowly, straightening her leg. Repeat with each leg 10 times. Then bring both knees up to her chest. Tell the patient to tighten her ab-

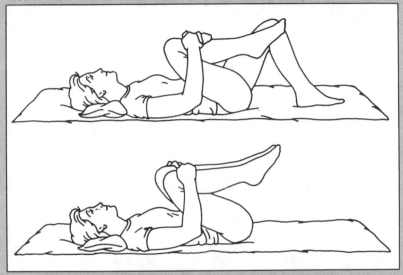

dominal muscles and press her back flat against the mattress. She should hold this position for 20 seconds, then lower her knees slowly. Repeat 5 times. To finish, clasp both knees to her chest and gently rock back and forth, but not side to side.

Periodically, during the day, she should roll her shoulders forward and backward and turn her head slowly from side to side. She should touch her left ear to her left shoulder, then repeat this on the right side. She should raise and lower both her shoulders as far as possible. She should also pull in and tighten her abdominal muscles, then count to 8 while holding her breath, then relax slowly. She should gradually increase the count and practice breathing normally with her abdominal muscles tightened while sitting, standing, and walking.

Lying correctly

A firm mattress or supporting bed board relieves back strain. The patient should avoid using high pillows or sleeping on his back or stomach. These positions exagger- ate swayback and cause neck and shoulder strain. Instead, the patient should lie on his side with his knees bent and a pillow between his knees to flatten his back.

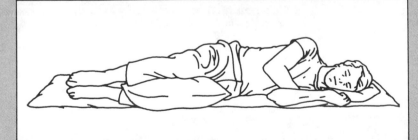

The patient should:
• Keep his neck and back as straight as possible at all times.
• Cross his legs during prolonged sitting.
• Use a footrest during prolonged standing.
• Bend from the hips and knees, not the waist.
• Wear shoes with moderately high heels.
• Hold heavy objects close to his body.
• Turn and face any object he wishes to lift.

The patient should not:
• Carry unbalanced loads.
• Lift heavy objects above his waist.
• Try to move heavy furniture.
• Sit on sofa chairs or deep couches.
• Strain to open windows or doors.

Rating sports

The ideal sport is one that strengthens the heart, builds muscles, enhances flexibility, and is relatively injury-free, while being inexpensive and easy to do. Below is a list of popular sports with assigned values, from 1 to 10, for their aerobic benefit, muscle development, and flexibility. There are also liability ratings, from 0 to −7, for each sport's special injury hazards, expense, and access. Total point values are: 19-23 excellent, 13-18 good, 7-12 fair.

Activity	Aerobic benefit	Muscle development	Flexibility rating	Injury hazard
Badminton	7	6	8	0
Baseball	3	3	4	−1: The most severe injuries are prevented by wearing a batting helmet.
Basketball	9	7	6	−2: High-speed collisions seem inevitable.
Bicycling	9	8	4	−5: Traffic accidents are a big problem. Otherwise, injuries are from wheel spokes and spills.
Football	7	9	5	−7: Even the best-conditioned athletes suffer injuries ranging from pulled muscles to broken bones and more serious damage.
Handball	9	7	8	0
Ice skating	9	7	7	−2: Rough ice and inexperience cause sprains and fractures. Skate blades frequently cause serious cuts.
Jogging	10	7	4	−1: Jogging alongside other kinds of traffic has caused fatalities. Joggers also suffer foot and knee injuries.
Racquetball	9	7	8	−1: A racquetball ball is about the same size as the human eye. Goggles are essential.
Rowing	10	10	6	0
Skiing (cross-country)	10	9	7	−2: Heavy exertion—not an activity for asthmatics and the older population. Most injuries are on downhill runs.
Soccer	9	6	5	0
Squash	9	7	8	0: Eye protection is recommended.
Swimming	10	7	8	0
Table tennis	5	5	7	0
Tennis	8	7	6	0
Volleyball	7	6	8	−1: Finger injuries are common.

Access	Expense	Comments	Total rating
−2	0	Indoor courts are recommended because of the wind factor.	19
−2	0	When the pitcher is doing a good job, everyone else is usually standing around.	7
−2	0	An excellent conditioning sport, but taller players have a definite advantage.	18
−2	−1	A lot of bicycles, unfortunately, are gathering dust in garages, their owners reluctant to take them out for fear they'll be stolen.	13
−2	−2	Even in "touch" football, you can expect to get hurt and should play with protective gear.	10
−3	−1	If you wear goggles when you play, your worst injury will be no more than a bruised palm.	20
−4	0	Long-distance skating is the skater's equivalent to jogging.	17
−1	0	Jogging isn't the only aerobic activity, as its press notices sometimes suggest, but it's one of the best.	19
−3	−1	A fast-paced sport that has grown in popularity in the last 10 years.	19
−2	−1	Not accessible for most people, but the experience and the exercise are worth the extra trouble.	23
2	1	Nordic skiing has finally reached the same level of popularity as downhill skiing.	21
−2	0	Of all outdoor team sports, soccer ranks first in aerobic effect.	18
−3	−1	Squash facilities do not exist in all areas.	20
−2	0	Finding a place to swim can sometimes present a problem.	23
−1	−1	If played with skill, table tennis—a great standby for rainy days— can be fast and exciting.	15
−3	−2	Play singles for the best training. Even poor players get good exercise chasing down loose balls.	16
−2	0	With a portable net, volleyball can be played on any reasonably even surface.	18

Signs of pregnancy: Presumptive, probable, and positive

Diagnosis of pregnancy depends on *presumptive* signs and symptoms (those you or your patient recognize); *probable* signs and symptoms (evidence of pregnancy you find during the physical examination); and *positive* signs (confirming diagnostic indications usually not apparent until the fourth month of pregnancy).

Presumptive signs
• Amenorrhea
• Nausea, with or without vomiting
• Frequent urination
• Breast changes
• Discoloration of vaginal mucosa
• Increased skin pigmentation and abdominal striae
• Fatigue
• Quickening

Probable signs
• Uterine enlargement
• Softening of uterine isthmus (Hegar's sign)
• Changes in shape of uterus
• Softening of cervix (Goodell's sign)
• Upper vagina and cervix purplish or bluish (Chadwick's sign)
• Braxton Hicks contractions
• Palpation of fetal parts
• Positive pregnancy test results for human chorionic gonadotropin (HCG) in urine or serum

Positive signs
• Identification of fetal heart sounds
• Palpation of active fetal movements
• Identification of fetal skeleton by radiography or ultrasonography

Assessing the pregnant patient

Conduct a complete review of systems to determine if your patient has any other health disorders. Ask her if she has any of the following signs and symptoms, which may result from the physiologic changes of pregnancy.

Metabolic
Weight changes and fatigue common early in pregnancy, possibly because of a fall in metabolic rate.

Skin
Pruritus, a common skin complaint whose cause is unknown, may be localized to abdomen or vulva or spread over the body.

Ears
Impaired hearing caused by blocked eustachian tubes.

Nose
Altered smell and nasal stuffiness, from mucosal hyperemia.

Mouth
Increased gingival bleeding when brushing the teeth.

Cardiovascular system
Uterine pressure may inhibit venous return and reduce cardiac output, causing faintness and dizziness when in a supine position.

Respiratory system
Hyperventilation resulting from increased progesterone levels.

GI system
Relaxed smooth muscles cause nausea, vomiting, heartburn, flatulence, constipation, hemorrhoids.

Reproductive system
Breast tenderness, engorgement; vaginal discharge, itching.

Musculoskeletal system
Backaches common, possibly due to kyphosis and slouching caused by enlarging breasts and lumbar lordosis.

▼
Understanding normal changes of pregnancy

Gestational age	Normal changes of pregnancy
First trimester	
Weeks 1 to 4	• Amenorrhea occurs; breast changes begin • Immunologic pregnancy tests become positive: radioimmunoassay test is positive a few days after implantation; urine human chorionic gonadotropin (HCG) test is positive 10 to 14 days after occurrence of amenorrhea • Nausea and vomiting begin between the fourth and sixth weeks
Weeks 5 to 8	• Goodell's sign occurs (softening of cervix) • Ladin's sign occurs (softening of uterine isthmus) • Hegar's sign occurs (softening of lower uterine segment) • Chadwick's sign appears (purple-blue vagina and cervix) • McDonald's sign occurs (easy flexion of the fundus over the cervix) • Cervical mucus plug forms; uterine shape changes from pear to globular • Urinary frequency and urgency occur
Weeks 9 to 12	• Fetal heartbeat is detected using ultrasonic stethoscope • Nausea, vomiting, and urinary frequency and urgency lessen • By 12 weeks, uterus is palpable just above symphysis pubis
Second trimester	
Weeks 13 to 17	• Mother gains approximately 10 to 12 lb (4.5 to 5.4 kg) during second trimester • Uterine souffle is heard on auscultation • Mother's heartbeat increases approximately 10 beats/minute between 14 and 30 weeks • By the 16th week, mother's thyroid gland enlarges by approximately 25%, and the uterine fundus is palpable halfway between the symphysis and umbilicus • Fetal movements, or quickening, occur between 16 and 20 weeks
Weeks 18 to 22	• Uterine fundus is palpable just below umbilicus • Fetal heartbeat is heard with fetoscope at 20 weeks' gestation • Fetal rebound or ballottement is possible
Weeks 23 to 27	• Umbilicus appears level with abdominal skin; striae gravidarum are usually apparent • Uterine fundus is palpable at umbilicus • Shape of uterus changes from globular to ovoid • Braxton Hicks contractions start
Third trimester	
Weeks 28 to 31	• Mother gains approximately 8 to 10 lb (3.6 to 4.5 kg) in third trimester • Uterine fundus is halfway between umbilicus and xiphoid process • Fetal outline is palpable • Fetus is very mobile and may be found in any position
Weeks 32 to 35	• Mother may experience heartburn and shortness of breath • Striae gravidarum become more evident • Uterine fundus is palpable just below the xiphoid process • Braxton Hicks contractions start to increase in frequency and intensity
Weeks 36 to 40	• Umbilicus protrudes • Ankle edema is evident; urinary frequency recurs • Engagement, or lightening, occurs • Mucus plug is expelled; cervical effacement and dilation begin

Evaluating gestational age by measuring fundal height

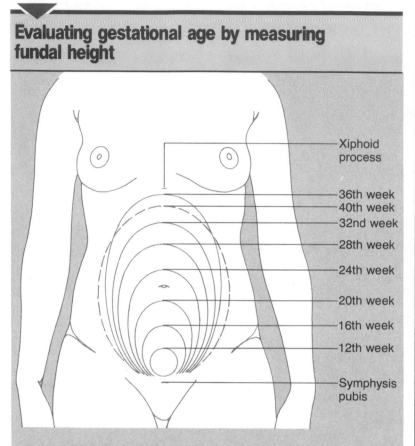

- Xiphoid process
- 36th week
- 40th week
- 32nd week
- 28th week
- 24th week
- 20th week
- 16th week
- 12th week
- Symphysis pubis

By estimating your patient's uterine size, you can evaluate the fetus's gestational age. How? By measuring fundal height. Between the 18th and 32nd weeks of pregnancy, the fundal height in centimeters equals the fetus's gestational age in weeks. For example, if your patient is at 24 weeks' gestation, her fundal height should be about 24 cm. Remember, though, that fundal height measurements taken late in pregnancy may not be accurate because fetal weight variations can distort your reading.

To measure fundal height, follow these steps. With your patient lying flat, place the end of a tape measure at the level of her symphysis pubis. Stretch the tape to the top of the uterine fundus. Record this measurement. Another method of determining fundal height involves using three landmarks: the symphysis pubis, the umbilicus, and the xiphoid process. At 16 weeks, the fundus can be found halfway between the symphysis pubis and the umbilicus. At 20 to 22 weeks, the fundus is at the umbilicus. At 36 weeks, the fundus is at the xiphoid process.

Choose one method of determining fundal height and use it consistently throughout the patient's pregnancy. Depending on your clinical setting, you may measure with calipers. Other factors, such as a patient's full bladder, amniotic fluid volume, obesity, or tension, can affect fundal height measurement.

Characteristics of high-risk pregnancy

A pregnancy is classified as high risk when the neonate or the mother is in danger of disability or death because of maternal, paternal, fetal, or neonatal history, or intrapartal complications.

Not all high-risk factors are equally hazardous to the mother and the neonate. Some may require only careful observation. Others require both observation and medical intervention.

Remember, it's not just the number, presence, or absence of risk factors that suggest a high-risk situation, but the combination of factors and the response of family members that's important.

Here is a checklist of risk factors that can affect a pregnancy:

Maternal risk factors

Demographic factors
- Age > 35 or < 19
- Weight < 100 lb or 20% over the ideal body weight
- Height < 5'
- Education
- History of inherited disorders
- Occupation

Socioeconomic factors
- Unemployed or low income
- Poor housing
- Unwed, especially adolescent
- Nutritional deprivation
- Exposure to hazardous environment
- Lack of support system

Habits
- Smoking during pregnancy
- Regular alcohol intake
- Drug use or abuse

Past medical history
- Cardiac or pulmonary disease
- Diabetes or thyroid disease
- Seizure disorder

- Chronic renal disease or chronic urinary tract infection
- Chronic hypertension
- Exposure to infections, including toxoplasmosis, cytomegalovirus, rubella, or chicken pox
- Major emotional disorder
- Cancer
- Surgery during pregnancy
- Blood type — Rh sensitization or ABO incompatability

Past obstetric history
- Previous infertility
- Less than 3 months between pregnancies
- More than seven pregnancies
- Previous stillbirth, neonatal death, or miscarriage(s)
- Previous premature labor, prolonged labor, low-birth-weight infant
- Previous cesarean birth or mid-forceps delivery
- Problems during pregnancy: bleeding in first trimester, placenta previa, abruptio placentae, pregnancy-induced hypertension, hydramnios, premature rupture of membranes
- Previous genital tract anomaly

Current obstetric status
- Precipitous delivery
- Prolonged labor
- Abnormal fetal presentation: breach, footling, shoulder, brow, or face
- Prolapsed umbilical cord
- Intrapartal drugs
- Multiple birth
- Late or no prenatal care
- Rh sensitization
- Cephalopelvic disproportion
- Polyhydramnios
- Placenta previa
- Abruptio placentae
- Postmaturity
- Maternal anemia

Paternal risk factors
- Age > 40 or < 19
- Blood type (may lead to Rh- or ABO-incompatibility problems)
- Positive family history of genetic disorder or chronic illness

Identifying danger signs in pregnancy

Certain signs and symptoms may indicate that the mother's health and the course of her pregnancy are being threatened. If your patient reports any of the following, notify the doctor immediately.

Sign or symptom	Possible cause
Dyspnea	• Impending cardiac decompensation, premature separation of the placenta, excessive amniotic fluid accumulation, or pulmonary embolus
Persistent or recurring headache	• Pregnancy-induced hypertension
Persistent nausea and vomiting	• Hyperemesis gravidarum or systemic infection
Vision changes (flashing lights, dots before eyes, dimming or blurring of vision)	• Pregnancy-induced hypertension
Dizziness when not supine	• Hypoglycemia, anemia, or cardiac dysrhythmias
Abdominal pain	• Ectopic pregnancy, abruptio placentae, or uterine rupture
Edema of the face and hands	• Pregnancy-induced hypertension
Cessation of fetal movement	• Fetal death
Vaginal bleeding	• Placenta previa, abruptio placentae, or spontaneous abortion
Sudden escape of fluid from the vagina	• Premature rupture of membranes

- Street drug usage, such as cocaine, heroin, or marijuana
- Alcohol consumption
- Exposure to hazardous environmental conditions, such as toxic gases, chemicals, or radiation

Neonatal risk factors
- Multiple birth
- Low Apgar scores
- Respiratory depression
- Cardiac depression

- Small (< 10th percentile) or large (> 90th percentile) for gestational age
- Bleeding
- Meconium staining of the newborn or amniotic fluid
- Foul-smelling amniotic fluid
- Abnormal appearance or weight of placenta
- Prematurity (< 37 weeks)
- Postmaturity (≥ 42 weeks)
- Hydrocephalus or microcephalus
- Obvious congenital anomaly
- Infant not accepted by parent(s)

Caring for the teenage mother

Teenage pregnancy brings with it a whole set of special concerns. Because up to 70% of pregnant adolescents don't receive adequate prenatal care, they're likely to develop specific problems. What's more, the complications go beyond the physical. The pregnant adolescent often feels guilty, confused, and afraid. The pregnancy affects not only her, but also her family and friends, the father of the child, and, possibly, his family. Your understanding of this complex situation is essential for good nursing care.

Facts and figures
• In the United States, an estimated 1 million adolescents become pregnant every year.
• Adolescents account for one-third of all abortions performed in the United States.
• As a general rule, the younger the mother, the greater the health risk for both her and the infant.
• Pregnant adolescents are more likely to develop complications such as poor weight gain during pregnancy, premature labor, pregnancy-induced hypertension, abruptio placentae, and pre-eclampsia.
• The infant born to an adolescent mother is more likely to have a low birth weight and a higher neonatal mortality. He may be predisposed to injury at birth, possible retardation, or other neurologic defects. He may also have an increased risk for childhood illnesses.
• Some of the above complications are related to the pregnant adolescent's physical immaturity, rapid growth, interest in fad diets, and generally poor nutrition. Other complications may stem from the adolescent denying her condition,

or not knowing the early signs of pregnancy, and waiting too long to get prenatal care.

Nursing care
The pregnant adolescent requires the same prenatal care as a pregnant adult, but she also needs psychological support and close observation for signs of complications. Since you may be the first health care professional the pregnant adolescent encounters, it's up to you to get her to follow sound medical advice without being judgmental, condescending, or threatening.
• Emphasize the importance of keeping to a prescribed diet, getting plenty of rest, and taking prescribed medication and iron supplements.
• Encourage the patient to ask questions and express her feelings about the pregnancy. Answer her questions fully.
• Try to help the pregnant adolescent identify her own strengths and various support systems for coping with pregnancy, birth, and parenting.
• Prepare the patient—and her partner, if she has one—for the physical and psychological processes of labor and birth. Encourage her to attend prenatal classes; educational films, hospital tours, and role-playing techniques will be of help to her.
• Following the birth, encourage the patient to set realistic goals for the future. If she chooses to put the child up for adoption, make sure she understands her legal rights and responsibilities. Note her progression through the grieving process; if she seems unable to deal with her grief, arrange for follow-up after her hospital stay. In the meantime, let her care for the infant as she desires.
• If the patient decides to raise the infant, help her make the transition from pregnancy to parenthood during the postpartum period. Facilitate bonding. Help her

establish a realistic plan for the care of the child, returning to school or work, and relating to the infant's father.
• In the event of stillbirth or death of the neonate, help the patient through the grieving process.
• Before the patient is discharged, provide her with information on contraception.

Administering drugs to a pregnant patient

Almost every drug administered to a pregnant patient crosses the placenta and enters the fetal circulation. This doesn't necessarily mean the drug is harmful to the fetus, but you should nevertheless be cautious about administering drugs to a pregnant patient.
• Before administering any drug to a patient of childbearing age, ask her the date of her last menstrual period and whether she could possibly be pregnant.
• Avoid administering all drugs except those essential to maintaining the pregnancy or the mother's health. Be particularly cautious during the first and third trimesters, when the fetus is most vulnerable. Strongly advise the patient to avoid all self-prescribed drugs during the first trimester, when fetal organs are differentiating.
• To minimize harmful effects on the fetus, administer the safest possible drug in the lowest possible dose.
• Apply topical drugs cautiously. Many topically applied drugs can be absorbed in amounts large enough to harm the fetus.
• As a precaution, remind the pregnant patient to check with her doctor before taking any drug, even a seemingly harmless over-the-counter medication.

Protecting the fetus

The more a pregnant patient knows about substances and behaviors, the better she can protect her own and the fetus's well-being. Your guidance can be invaluable, especially during the early stages of pregnancy.

Abused drugs
You should warn a pregnant patient about the use of street drugs, which can cause intrauterine growth retardation and predispose the fetus to other complications. These include amphetamines, barbiturates, cocaine, heroin, lysergic acid diethylamide (LSD) and other hallucinogens, marijuana, and phencyclidine (PCP).

The use of crack cocaine, in particular, is on the rise, and an alarming number of infants are crack addicts at birth because their mothers use the drug.

If you have reason to believe your pregnant patient is abusing drugs, arrange to have her meet with a hospital social worker for counseling.

Alcohol
Up to 50% of women who drink excessively during pregnancy give birth to affected infants. Over 80% of these infants have *fetal alcohol syndrome* with signs and symptoms including a small head with mild to moderate mental retardation and a wide range of facial, skeletal, cardiac, kidney, and external genital malformations.

Even as little as 2 to 3 tablespoons of alcohol a day may increase the risk of prematurity and decreased birth weight. Advise a pregnant patient to avoid drinking alcohol completely.

Cigarettes
Cigarette smoking during pregnancy increases the risk of spontaneous abortion, premature delivery, low birth weight, stillbirth, or death within the first month of life.

A heavy smoker is almost twice as likely to have a spontaneous abortion as a nonsmoker. Advise the patient to stop smoking.

Caffeine
A pregnant patient should use caffeine cautiously. Recommend that she drink decaffeinated coffee, herbal teas, and caffeine-free soft drinks. She should also avoid foods like chocolate, which contain caffeine.

Radiation
Ionizing high radiation is harmful to a fetus. An exposure of over 25 rads during the first trimester will produce congenital malformations.

Routine diagnostic X-rays involving the chest, kidneys, gallbladder, and GI tract expose the fetus to 1 to 3 rads for each examination. This low-dosage exposure doesn't seem to harm the fetus; nevertheless, advise your patient to avoid unnecessary exposure during her pregnancy.

If your patient needs X-rays, remind her to tell the X-ray technician she's pregnant so that he can take special precautions.

Chemicals
Most chemicals in large enough quantities can be harmful to a developing fetus, so you should caution a pregnant patient about unnecessary exposure to chemical agents. To date, most cases of toxicity have involved high-level exposure, usually related to occupation.

If a patient thinks her occupation could be harmful to her pregnancy (for instance, if she works in a photography lab, where chemicals are used regularly), she should discuss her concerns with her doctor.

Nutrition
Remind your patient that proper nutrition is essential for both herself and her infant. Pregnancy is no time to diet. The patient should eat well-balanced meals, lots of fresh fruits and vegetables, and take an iron supplement. She should stay away from processed foods and junk food.

If the expectant mother is a vegetarian, she should be sure to get enough protein. She should also take iron pills and vitamin C, as well as additional daily supplements if she doesn't drink milk.

Exercise and sports
A healthy woman who has exercised regularly before becoming pregnant should be able to continue her exercise program, with modifications as her pregnancy progresses.

In general, a pregnant woman should avoid exercising in hot, humid weather. She should avoid contact sports like basketball and volleyball, where trauma to the abdomen could occur. She should stop exercising before she becomes overtired or dehydrated, and should not exercise if she's at risk of premature labor or has any vaginal bleeding.

Traveling
A healthy pregnant woman can travel without risk. However, she should always consider the mode of transportation, the stage of her pregnancy, and the length of the trip. In the eighth and ninth months of pregnancy, it's probably a good idea not to do any long-distance traveling.

High temperatures
First trimester exposure to a fever of 104° F (40° C) or higher for 1 day or more, prolonged hot baths, or sauna baths can have harmful effects on the fetus. Advise your patient to limit hot baths or avoid them completely. Tell her that if she has a fever, she should call her doctor immediately.

Understanding fetal growth and development

At fertilization, fetal growth and development begin. The complete process takes 40 weeks.

1 month
At the end of the first month, the embryo has a definite form. The head and trunk are apparent, and the tiny buds that will become the arms and legs are discernible. The cardiovascular system has begun to function, and the umbilical cord is visible in its most primitive form.

1 month (10 times actual size)

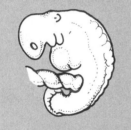

2 months
In the second month, the embryo (called a fetus from the seventh week on) grows to 1″ (2.5 cm) in length and weighs ⅓ oz (9 g). The head and facial features develop as the eyes, ears, nose, lips, tongue, and tooth buds form. The arms and legs also take shape, with the elbows, forearms, hands, fingers, thighs, knees, ankles, and toes becoming visible. Although the gender of the fetus is not yet discernible, all external genitalia are present. Cardiovascular function is complete, and the umbilical cord has a definite form. At the end of 2 months, the fetus resembles a full-term infant except for size.

2 months (actual size)

3 months
During the third month, the fetus grows to 3″ (7.6 cm) in length and weighs 1 oz (28 g). Teeth and bones begin to appear, and the kidneys start to function. Although the mother can't yet feel its activity, the fetus is moving. It opens its mouth to swallow, grasps with its fully developed hands and, even though its lungs are not functioning, it prepares for breathing by inhaling and exhaling. At the end of the first trimester, its gender is distinguishable.

3 months (actual size)

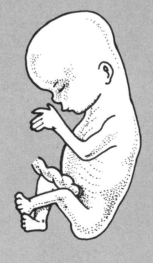

4 to 9 months
In the remaining 6 months, fetal growth continues as internal and external structures develop at a rapid rate. In the third trimester, the fetus stores fats and minerals it will need to live outside the womb. At birth, the average full-term fetus measures 20″ (51 cm) and weighs 7 to 7½ lbs (3 to 3.5 kg).

9 months (⅓ actual size)

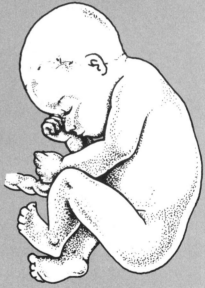

Evaluating fetal well-being

Test	Description	Uses and indications
Pelvic ultrasonography	An ultrasonic transducer, placed on the mother's abdomen, transmits high-frequency sound waves. These pass through the abdominal wall, deflect off the fetus, bounce back to the transducer, and are translated into a visual image on a monitoring screen.	• Early diagnosis of pregnancy • Biparietal diameter measurement • Placental localization • Discovery of placental anomalies • Intrauterine device detection • Identification of multiple gestation • Fetal position and presentation • Discovery of fetal anomalies • Demonstration of hydramnios and oligohydramnios • Discovery of fetal death • Detection of incomplete or missed abortion • Observation of fetal cardiac activity and breathing movements
Estriol measurement	The placenta converts fetal adrenal precursors to estriol, which enters the mother's blood and urine in measurable amounts. For correct interpretation of estriol values, serial measurements should be performed. In general, rising estriol levels are a positive indicator of fetal well-being; falling levels are a negative indicator. Chronically low estriol levels may indicate intrauterine growth retardation.	• Evaluation of placental function and fetal well-being • Performed especially in situations involving high-risk conditions, such as maternal diabetes or hypertensive diseases, postmature pregnancy, intrauterine growth retardation syndrome, poor obstetric history, or late antepartal care
Amniocentesis	A sample of amniotic fluid is aspirated for diagnostic tests, which are indicative of fetal well-being. After an adequate pocket of amniotic fluid is localized with sonography, a needle is inserted into the patient's abdomen, through the uterus, and into the amniotic sac to aspirate a sample of the amniotic fluid.	• Assessment of fetal maturity, especially with premature labor or when planning a cesarean section of a patient with a questionable estimated date of confinement • Biochemical monitoring of fetal well-being, especially in an Rh-isoimmunized pregnancy or when other fetal hemolytic disease is suspected • Prenatal diagnosis of genetic disorders, especially if maternal age is advanced (over 35 years), or a history of chromosomal abnormalities in previous pregnancies exists in parents or close family members
Chorionic villi sampling	This is an experimental prenatal test that may someday replace amniocentesis for quick, safe assessment of fetal well-being. The doctor checks the placement of the patient's uterus bimanually, then inserts a Grave's speculum into the patient and swabs the cervix with antiseptic solution. A catheter is then directed through the cannula to the chorionic villi, finger-like projections surrounding the embryonic membrane. Suction is applied to the catheter to remove tissue from the villi, which is examined and cultured for further tests.	• Early detection of fetal abnormalities • Discovery of chromosomal and biochemical disorders • Detection of up to 200 diseases prenatally

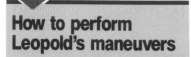

How to perform Leopold's maneuvers

Performing the four Leopold's maneuvers helps you determine fetal presentation and position, which is useful information for accurate transducer placement for monitoring the fetus.

First maneuver
To determine whether the fetus's head or buttocks occupies the fundus, face the mother and palpate the upper abdomen with both hands. If the fetus is in the vertex position—left occipito-anterior—you'll feel an irregularly shaped, soft part: the fetus's buttocks. If the fetus is in the breech position, you'll feel a hard, round, movable fetal part: the fetus's head.

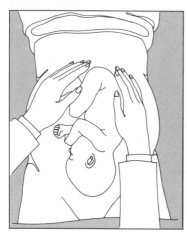

Second maneuver
To locate the fetal back, palpate both sides of the abdomen separately. To palpate the right side of the abdomen, apply deep but gentle pressure with the palm of your right hand while steadying the uterus with your left hand. Repeat for the left side, using your left hand to palpate and your right hand to steady the uterus. On one side you should

feel a smooth, hard surface offering resistance: the fetus's back. On the other side of the abdomen, expect to feel some irregular knobs or lumps: the fetus's hands, feet, elbows, and knees. If the fetus is in the breech position, its back will be more difficult, if not impossible, to find.

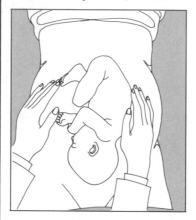

Third maneuver
To determine which fetal part lies over the inlet, spread the thumb and fingers of your dominant hand and gently grasp the lower portion of the abdomen just above the symphysis pubis. If the fetus is in the vertex position, you should feel a hard fetal part: the head. If the fetus is in the breech position, expect to feel a soft part: the fetus's buttocks. This maneuver confirms the findings of the first maneuver.

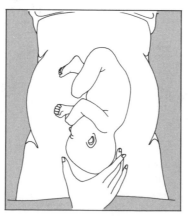

Fourth maneuver
To assess fetal descent into the pelvis, turn and face the mother's feet, then palpate both sides of the lower abdomen, moving toward the pubis. If the fetus is in the vertex position and you feel its head, then the head isn't engaged in the pelvic inlet. If you have difficulty feeling the head, it's probably engaged. If the fetus is in the breech position and you feel its hips, the buttocks probably aren't engaged in the pelvic inlet. If you have difficulty feeling the hips, the buttocks are probably engaged.

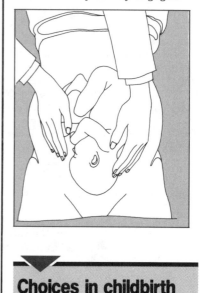

Choices in childbirth

Parents today frequently want to control the circumstances of their child's birth, from the method of delivery, to where the delivery takes place, to who delivers the neonate. It's your responsibility, while preparing the patient for labor and delivery, to explain to her the various options in childbirth.

Natural childbirth
Women with normal, low-risk pregnancies have a range of delivery methods from which to choose. Of all natural childbirth methods, the *Lamaze method* is

Using the Apgar scoring system

To help assess a neonate's condition, use the Apgar scoring system. Make your observations within 1 minute of the neonate's delivery, then again within 5 minutes. Notify the doctor of your findings and document them on the neonate's chart.

A neonate with a score of 10 is considered to be in the best possible condition. A score of 7 to 9 is considered adequate and requires no treatment. A score of 4 to 6 requires close observation and intervention, such as suctioning. A score below 4 necessitates immediate intervention and further evaluation.

SIGN	0	1	2	Rating	
				1 min	5 min
Heart rate	Not detectable	Below 100	Over 100		
Respiratory effort	Absent	Slow, irregular	Good, crying		
Muscle tone	Flaccid	Some flexion of extremities	Active motion		
Reflex irritability (response to flick on sole)	No response	Grimace, slow motion	Cry		
Color	Blue, pale	Body pink, extremities blue	Completely pink		
			TOTAL		

the most familiar. Both parents are taught to recognize and understand the pregnant body and its processes and to deliver a healthy baby without medication and with minimal aid from hospital personnel. The mother learns exercises to tone up her body and prepare it for birth. The father participates as coach, timer, and observer.

The *LeBoyer method* emphasizes the neonate's transition from the womb to life. There are no bright lights or loud noises (LeBoyer believed these frightened the newborn); instead, the neonate is gradually introduced to his new environment by continuing the sensations he felt while in the uterus.

Nurse-midwifery
Nurse-midwives are available for home, hospital, or family center births. They provide parents with both preparation and specialized service. The nurse-midwife works with the family throughout the pregnancy.

Rather than joining the parents during the last stage of the labor process, the general practice in other prepared birthing methods, the nurse-midwife joins the parents early in the labor process.

Birth centers
Family Centered Maternity Care (FCMC) combines professional care, prepared delivery, and shared family experience. Family maternity centers seek to bring the comforts of home into the delivery and postdelivery settings. The father can be at the mother's side during delivery and has unlimited visiting privileges after the birth. The newborn rooms with the mother, and older children are allowed to visit them.

Assessing the neonate

You should inspect the neonate from head to toe. Begin by observing the pulse and respiratory rates while the neonate sleeps. Use a radiant warmer or take other precautions, such as exposing only those areas of the neonate being assessed, to ensure thermoregulation.

Respirations and pulse rate
Immediately after the neonate's birth, assess respirations. The normal irregular and shallow respiratory rate ranges from 30 to 60 breaths/minute. Brief (15 seconds) apnea, also called periodic breathing, occurs characteristically. The chest and abdomen should rise simultaneously with respiration.

Auscultated breath sounds are bronchial and loud.

Next evaluate the pulse rate and heart sounds. The pulse rate changes and usually follows a pattern similar to the respiratory rate. Auscultated apically with a stethoscope for a full minute, normal pulse rate is 120 to 160 beats/minute, increasing to 180 beats/minute during crying and motor activity. During deep sleep, the pulse rate may drop to 100 beats/minute. If the heartbeat is slower, report it to the doctor. Neonatal heart sounds have a higher pitch, shorter duration, and greater intensity than adult heart sounds.

General appearance
Assess overall skin color. Is the neonate jaundiced (yellow), pale, cyanotic (blue), or ruddy? To determine muscle tone and level of consciousness, observe position and motor activity. Is the neonate crying? What type of cry? Is it high-pitched, weak, or lusty? Is the neonate moving all extremities? Are movements symmetrical? Continue these observations throughout the assessment.

Weight ranges from 5 lb, 8 oz to 8 lb, 13 oz (2,500 to 4,000 g). To weigh the neonate, calibrate the scale at zero, drape a protective covering on the weighing platform, and place the unclothed neonate on it. Weigh at the same time each day. A neonate may lose up to 10% of birth weight within the first 3 or 4 days of life. Length assessment usually accompanies weight assessment. Measure the neonate from crown to heel. The normal range is 18″ to 22″ (45.7 to 55.8 cm).

Skin and hair
Observe the skin for color and condition. A large amount of vernix caseosa (a gray-white, cheese-like, protective skin covering) is normally seen immediately after birth, diminishing after several days. Vernix residues cling to the

neck and groin creases and to the genital region. Skin tones range from pink in Caucasian neonates to creamy tan in darker-skinned, Black, Hispanic, or Asian neonates. Acrocyanosis (blue and red discoloration), resulting from sluggish peripheral circulation or from chilling, commonly appears during the first 24 hours. Also, when the neonate is cold, mottling (a patchy, purplish skin discoloration) may appear. Milia, white papules caused by accumulated sebum in the sebaceous glands, frequently occur across the nose, cheeks, and chin. These disappear within 2 to 3 weeks.

Note the type and amount of hair. The full-term neonate should have some head hair, but the amount varies. Lanugo (downy fetal hair) normally covers the face, shoulders, and back.

Head
Within a couple of hours of the neonate's birth, measure the head circumference at its greatest diameter, usually the occipitofrontal circumference. The normal size range is about 12¾″ to 14½″ (32.3 to 36.8 cm).

Next, palpate, inspect, and measure the fontanels. The diamond-shaped anterior fontanel normally measures 1⅛″ to 1⅝″ (3 to 4 cm) long and ¾″ to 1⅛″ (2 to 3 cm) wide and may enlarge as molding resolves. The triangle-shaped posterior fontanel may be closed at

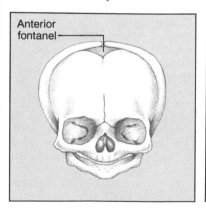

Anterior fontanel

birth (from molding) but can remain palpable for about 3 months. The anterior fontanel is flat and should remain open for about 18 months.

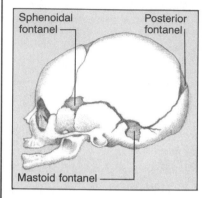

Sphenoidal fontanel

Posterior fontanel

Mastoid fontanel

Inspect the face for overall appearance and symmetry. Features should be appropriately placed and proportionate. Structures, muscle tone, and expression should be symmetrical.

Eyes, symmetrically sized and shaped, should be framed by eyebrows and eyelashes. Eyeballs should be round and firm. Watch for the neonate to focus momentarily, follow an object to the midline, and face toward a speaking voice. Nystagmus (involuntary oscillating eye movements) and strabismus (crossed eyes) are common in the first 2 to 3 months. Because of immature lacrimal glands, tears or discharge may appear. Occasionally, an exudate or swelling results from prophylactic drugs used to prevent ophthalmia neonatorum (neonatal conjunctivitis).

Check the ears for proper placement. The pinnas should intercept an imaginary line from the outer canthus of the eyes. Palpate for cartilage in the pinnas and confirm hearing by eliciting the neonatal startle response to a sudden loud noise.

The nose should be midline, usually flat and broad. Some mucus may appear but no drainage. Because a neonate is an obligatory nose breather, check nostril patency by occluding one nostril at a time and observe for respiratory distress signs, such as sternal retraction.

Chest
Measure the chest at the nipple line. The average chest circumference is 12" to 13" (30 to 33 cm) or ¾" (2 cm) to 1½" (4 cm) less than the head circumference.

Palpate the normally rounded chest for signs of fracture, such as asymmetrical movement and crepitus. The nipples are normally symmetrical and measure less than ½" (1.25 cm) in diameter in a full-term neonate. Because of maternal estrogen in utero, breast engorgement may occur.

Abdomen
Inspect, auscultate, and palpate the abdomen, which should be rounded, dome-shaped, and soft with no masses. Bowel sounds should exist 1 to 2 hours after birth. Meconium (the thick, sticky, green or black first stool) should pass within the first 24 to 48 hours, indicating an intact and functioning GI tract.

The umbilical stump falls midline at the lower abdomen. The umbilical cord—at birth moist, soft, and creamy white—should be securely clamped, nonbleeding, and free of signs of infection. It should remain dry and odorless. Then it progressively shrinks, turns black, and detaches in approximately 2 weeks.

Back
To inspect the back, turn the neonate to a prone position with the head to the side to prevent occluding the nostrils. Look first for a straight spine and planar alignment of shoulders, scapulae, and iliac crests; then palpate the spine. It should be intact, without indentations or dimpling.

Extremities
Note positions and movements of the arms and legs. The neonate usually assumes a position reflecting its normal position in utero. Motor activity should include a full range of motion with all four extremities moving spontaneously and equally. Often the fist is clenched with the thumb under the fingers. Fingernails and toenails should extend slightly beyond the tips of the fingers and toes. The legs should be equally long with comparable gluteal folds. Because the lateral muscles are more developed than the medial

Testing neonatal reflexes

You should assess several reflexes to help determine whether a neonate's muscular system is intact. Keep in mind that gestational age and neonatal muscle tone can alter the reflex responses, and that some reflexes are not as age-specific as others.

Reflex	Eliciting the reflex	Normal response
Sucking or rooting	Touch neonate's lip, cheek, or corner of mouth	Neonate will turn head toward stimulation and open mouth; suckling activity will be noted
Extrusion	Touch or depress tongue	Neonate will force tongue outward
Tonic neck or "fencing"	Turn head of supine neonate from midline to one side	Extremities will extend on side toward which neonate is turned; opposite extremities will reflex
Palmar grasp	Apply pressure to palm of hand	Neonate's fingers will curl around examiner's finger
Plantar grasp	Apply pressure to base of toes	Neonate's toes will curl downward
Moro or "startle"	Produce a sudden stimulus, such as a hand clap, when neonate is lying quietly	Neonate will draw up legs and bring arms up in an embracing motion; extremity movements should be symmetrical
Stepping or "walking"	Hold neonate vertically; allow soles of feet to touch table surface	Neonate will step, simulating walking

muscles, the legs should appear bowed.

Test hip joint stability by using Ortolani's maneuver. With the neonate supine, flex the hips and knees at right angles; abduct them until the lateral aspects of the knees touch the examination table; next, bring the knees together, keeping the hips and knees flexed, and attempt to rotate the hips clockwise and counterclockwise to evaluate symmetry of movement. You may hear and feel a click or popping sound if the joint is unstable.

Anus and genitalia
Take the neonate's temperature rectally to assess anal patency in either sex.

In the male neonate, palpate the two pendulous and wrinkled scrotal sacs for evidence of a testis in each. Then observe that the prepuce (the foreskin, which does not retract easily) covers the glans penis and that the urinary meatus appears as a slit at the penile tip.

In the female neonate, the external genitalia usually look edematous and hyperpigmented. The labia majora dominate and cover the labia minora. The clitoris, also edematous, is noticeable. A grayish white mucus discharge (smegma), which is normal, or a blood-tinged discharge (pseudomenstruation), caused by maternal hormones in utero, may be present. The urinary meatus, positioned beneath the clitoris, is difficult to see.

Assess urination in both sexes. Because the fetal kidneys function, the neonate commonly voids within 24 hours of birth. Urine voided in the first few days may be scant and infrequent (2 to 6 times daily); however, as dietary intake increases, the frequency of daily voidings also increases (15 to 20 times daily).

Performing postpartum assessment

Most mothers and their new infants leave the hospital a day or two after delivery, both of them healthy and happy. But there's always a chance of complications such as uterine or episiotomy infections, breast abscesses, phlebitis, and others. That's why, even if you don't work in the maternity unit, you should know how to perform a postpartum assessment.

Breasts
The first 2 days after giving birth, a mother has a tingling sensation in her breasts. They secrete colostrum, the precursor of breast milk that appears on about the third day. The breasts become engorged the second day after delivery because of lymph and venous stasis. They're temporarily full, tender, and uncomfortable until the milk supply is ready. To maintain supply, the breasts need to be stimulated by a nursing infant, a breast pump, or manual expression.

Whether the mother is nursing or not, she should wear a snug bra for support. A nursing mother should wear the bra until her milk supply is established. A mother who isn't nursing should wear it until lactation stops.

To assess her breasts, have the mother lie down and remove her bra. Palpate both breasts for engorgement or nodules. Inspect her nipples for pressure, soreness, cracks, or fissures.

Uterus
Next, identify the location of your patient's uterus. In the first 24 hours after birth, the uterus should be midline or near the umbilicus and should feel firm. Expect the uterus to be large in a woman who's had several pregnancies or large babies.

The uterus descends below the umbilicus about a centimeter each day after delivery. On the third postpartum day, it should be 2 cm below the umbilicus. Record its location as U-2, U-3, and so on.

The top of the uterus, also called the fundus, should remain very firm. If it becomes soft, the uterine muscles probably aren't contracting properly or the uterus has retained placental fragments. Both conditions predispose the patient to hemorrhage. Gently massage the uterus to help the muscles contract and expel placental fragments.

Bladder
Your patient may urinate a lot the first few days after giving birth. At least 200 ml each time the patient voids is satisfactory. When her bladder is empty, you shouldn't be able to palpate it over the symphysis pubis. Be alert for signs of infection, including infrequent or insufficient voiding, discomfort, burning, or foul-smelling urine.

Also note urinary frequency, dysuria, or urine retention. These may occur if the patient has perineal edema, lacerations, or had a long labor during which she couldn't void regularly.

When the bladder is full, the uterus can't contract. It pushes up toward the right and vaginal bleeding increases. Careful assessment helps you identify urinary problems so you can intervene.

Bowels
The first bowel movement usually occurs on the second postpartum day. Because of early discharge from the hospital, however, many women leave without having had a bowel movement.

An abdomen that feels soft, isn't distended, and has bowel sounds usually indicates that the patient isn't constipated. But if the patient is constipated, the doctor may order a stool softener, enema, or suppository to stimulate intestinal activity. (Enemas and suppositories are contraindicated if the patient has rectal sphincter lacerations.)

Lochia

The first 3 days after a woman gives birth, her lochia (vaginal discharge) is dark red and may contain small clots; this is called *lochia rubra.* From the fourth through the tenth day, she has *lochia serosa,* which is thinner and brown to pink. From the tenth day through the third or fourth week after birth, *lochia alba,* a yellowish white discharge, is present.

Lochia has a definite musky scent, but if it starts to smell foul the patient might have an infection. Lochia is an excellent medium for bacterial growth, so make sure the patient changes perineal pads frequently. Assess the type and amount of lochia and the presence of clots larger than a quarter. A woman who delivered 4 days before examination would normally have a little lochia serosa with few, if any, clots.

Episiotomy

Although some women deliver without an episiotomy, most do not. In some cases, the episiotomy or perineal lacerations extend into surrounding tissue.

The episiotomy may be midline in the center of the perineum, or outward and downward from the vagina at a left or right angle.

To assess the episiotomy, position the patient on her affected side. For example, a woman with a right mesiolateral episiotomy should lie on her right side. Have her flex her left leg at the knee and draw it up toward her waist. (With a midline episiotomy, position her on either side.) Use a goosenecked lamp or flashlight to provide adequate lighting during the assessment. Stand behind the woman and gently lift her top buttock upward to expose the perineum. Inspect the episiotomy for

irritation, ecchymosis, tenderness, or edema. Also assess for hemorrhoids.

A white line the length of the episiotomy is a sign of infection, as is swelling or discharge. Severe, intractable pain, perineal discoloration, and ecchymosis indicate a perineal hematoma, a potentially dangerous condition. Apply ice to the hematoma to relieve discomfort and reduce edema. Document your actions and notify the doctor.

By the second postpartum day, the patient should obtain relief of episiotomy pain from warm sitz baths, topical anesthetics or steroid-based ointments, and mild analgesics.

Homans' sign

Superficial or deep vein thrombophlebitis is sometimes a complication of childbirth. It's caused by hypercoagulability of the blood in pregnancy, severe anemia, pelvic infection, traumatic delivery, or obesity. A patient with a history of thrombophlebitis is at special risk. Getting the patient up and around soon after delivery reduces the incidence of thrombophlebitis.

To assess your patient for this complication, position her legs flat on the bed. Place your left hand on the top of her knee and gently flex her foot toward her ankle. Repeat the test on the other leg. If she experiences calf pain when you flex either foot, the Homans' sign is positive and further assessment is needed. Also check your patient's legs for tenderness, nodular or warm areas, discoloration, or varicosities.

Emotional status

To determine your patient's emotional status, consider the classic phases most new mothers pass through. The first is "taking in," the time immediately after delivery when the patient needs sleep, depends on others for nurturing and food, and relives the events surrounding the birth.

As the patient regains control over her bodily functions during the next few days, she will be "taking hold" and becoming preoccupied with the present. She'll be particularly concerned about her health, the baby's condition, and her ability to care for him. She'll show her independence by caring for herself and learning to care for her newborn.

The next phase, "letting go," comes later, when the patient reestablishes relationships with other people.

Nurturing and listening to the mother are important during the taking-in phase. The taking-hold phase is a good time for patient teaching, since the mother is especially ready for learning. Unfortunately, the mother may already be at home. At this time, she may also feel vulnerable and experience mood swings, insomnia, irritability, and crying episodes. This period of "baby blues," usually temporary, is caused by hormonal changes, role redefinition, discomfort, and fatigue.

When a woman is readmitted to the hospital for a complication of childbirth, she's apt to be in this taking-hold phase, so the separation from her baby and family is a crisis for her. You can help relieve the crisis by being a sensitive listener and by arranging for her to see and care for her newborn. If she chooses to breast-feed, support her decision and obtain a breast pump for her to use every 3 to 4 hours. Consider her need for information and her readiness to learn. Tell her about her progress, explain any diagnostic and therapeutic measures, and include her in setting goals.

Finally, monitor the patient's emotional status. Note how she interacts with her family, her level of independence, her sleep and rest patterns, her mood swings, irritability, or crying.

13 When your patient is a child

The hospitalized child: Helping him cope with his fears

When a child is treated with kindness and respect, he copes with the stress of hospitalization remarkably well. Your sensitive nursing care can help a child adapt to the hospital environment and prevent long-term emotional effects. Follow these guidelines:

Provide one-to-one nursing care
If possible, you or another nurse, a nurse's aide, or any other staff member should serve as the child's special friend, calling him by his first name or nickname, to make him feel at ease throughout his hospital stay.

You or another staff member should play with him and be available for support during any stressful treatment procedure, especially if the child's parents aren't present.

Teach the child
Assess the child's understanding of his illness and treatment by asking him why he thinks he's in the hospital. Then use his responses to plan patient teaching and to assess his need for emotional support.

Schedule teaching sessions for times when the child will be rested and alert. Don't prolong these sessions beyond the child's attention span.

Use group-teaching techniques when possible. This will save you time and also provide peer-group support for each child.

Be consistent and honest
Foster the child's trust with consistent behavior and honest communication. Tell him you'll warn him before you do anything that will hurt him, and then keep your promise. This way, he won't feel he must be on guard all the time.

Communicate carefully
Choose your words carefully, especially if your patient is a preschooler. A child this age thinks in literal terms and in terms of his own experience. For example, if you tell him that he'll be "put to sleep" for surgery, he may think of the old family dog who never returned from the veterinarian.

If you tell him that surgery will occur when he's asleep, he may be reluctant to fall asleep at night, fearing that something awful will happen to him if he does. Emphasize that anesthesia is a special sleep he'll experience only when the doctor gives him a special medicine, and that the doctor will wake him up when the surgery is over.

Question the child about his understanding of treatments and procedures. Suppose he asks you, for example, "How does the doctor take out my tonsils?" Reply by saying, "How do *you* think he does it?" Listen carefully to his explanation; in addition to revealing the depth of his understanding, you can discover his unique fears and fantasies.

Let the child express himself
Provide the child with opportunities to display his feelings of fear, anger, or frustration, and don't show disapproval.

During periods of illness, a child may regress. Help the parents recognize the child's behavior as a reaction to stress and allow the child to depend on you, making him feel loved and cared for.

Prepare the child for treatments
Describe the events and sensations he'll experience during treatments, including surgery. But avoid being too specific because he may get upset if events don't happen exactly as you predicted.

Prepare the child for any unexpected event by asking him to try and remember anything that happened to him that was different from what he expected. Then you can discuss it with him later.

Important: Tell the child about painful or unpleasant aspects of his treatment last. Otherwise, he may get overanxious and fail to listen to the rest of your explanation. Perform all painful or upsetting procedures in the treatment room—not the child's hospital room, which should be a safe haven for him.

Let the child choose, if possible
Give the child a sense of control. For example, he can't choose whether or not to have an injection, but you can ask him if he'd like another minute to get ready.

Ask another child to help you prepare a newcomer for an unpleasant procedure. For instance, if the new patient is afraid of an injection, a more experienced child may be able to reassure him that it's not so bad.

Allow the child playtime
Build playtime into your daily routine. This encourages the child to associate you with comfort and fun, not just pain, and gives you a chance to learn more about him.

Use play therapy to explain procedures to him and help him work through his emotions. For example, before changing his dressings, you might bandage the head of his teddy bear or other toy, to show him what you're going to do.

Play provides clues to how well the child is adjusting to his illness and treatment. It also helps him work through his feelings. For instance, violent play suggests anger or fear; drawings that distort body parts suggest a poor self-image and fear of mutilation.

If the child seems unusually disturbed, consult with a child psychologist or a specially trained social worker. Tell the child that no one will be mad if he cries. Remain supportive of the child regardless of how he behaves.

Assessing the pediatric patient

Ask the parents of the child if he has complained of—or they have been aware of—any of the following problems.

Eyes
Vision difficulties, problem with tearing, crossed eyes

Ears
Hearing difficulties, earaches

Nose
Nosebleeds, sinus infections

Throat
Sore throats (streptococcal), pneumonia, colds (more than four in a year)

Cardiovascular system
Coloring (bluish), fatigue

Respiratory system
Breathing difficulties, shortness of breath, frequent exhaustion

GI system
Changes in bowel habits, diarrhea, constipation, bleeding, pain, vomiting

Renal system
Frequency of urination, pain, bleeding on urination; straight urinary flow in males

Female reproductive system
Menstrual cycle onset

Nervous system
Headaches, convulsions, fainting spells, tremors, twitches, blackouts, dizziness

Musculoskeletal system
Painful joints, redness around joints, swelling, sprains, broken bones, coordination difficulties

Surveying the child's daily activities

To learn about a child's activities of daily living (ADLs), you'll probably want to interview his parents instead of the child himself. Here are questions you should ask to compile an ADL survey for a child:

Diet and elimination
• How is the child's appetite?
• Is he on a formula? What type?
• When are his usual mealtimes?
• Does he eat with the family?
• Does someone help him eat?
• Does he use utensils?
• Does he have any difficulty eating? What sort?
• What are his favorite foods and beverages?
• Does he snack? What does he usually eat for a snack?
• Does he take daily vitamins?
• Is he toilet-trained? At what age did he learn?
• What are his usual bowel habits?
• Does he wet the bed?

Sleep
• What is his normal amount of sleep? From when to when?
• Does he take naps?
• Does he have a routine before going to sleep (drinking a bottle, playing, being read to)?
• Does he sleep alone?
• What is his favorite sleeping position?
• Does he have any sleeping problems? Does he have nightmares?
• Is he tired during the day?

Exercise and recreation
• Does he have any special exercises he performs regularly?
• Does his schedule include play?
• Does he participate in sports?
• How much time does he get for recreation each day?
• Does he have a group of friends with whom he plays?
• What are his favorite games?

How four psychoanalysts view development

Freud's theory

Oral stage
(age 0 to 18 months)
• Uses mouth as source of satisfaction
• *Passive phase:* is helpless, narcissistic, and egocentric. Operates on pleasure principle, feels omnipotent, wants to satisfy hunger, sucking, and the need to feel secure
• *Active phase:* bites as a mode of pleasure, experiments and associates continuously, exhibits sensory discrimination, differentiates between mental images and reality, differentiates between others, discovers self

Anal stage
(age 1½ to 3)
• Learns muscular control of urination and defecation (toilet-training period)
• Exhibits increasing self-control (walks, talks, dresses, and undresses)
• Asserts independence by learning to say no (negativism)
• Delays gratification until proper time (reality principle)
• Begins ego and superego development
• Engages in parallel play

Phallic stage
(age 3 to 6)
• Focuses libidinal energy on genitalia
• Learns sexual identity
• Experiences internalization of superego
• Engages in sibling rivalry
• Manipulates parents
• Experiences refinement of intellectual and motor activities
• Increases socialization and associative play

Latency stage
(age 6 to 12)
• Enters quiet stage: sexual development lies dormant; emotional tension eases
• Experiences normal homosexual phase: boys join gangs and girls form cliques
• Increases intellectual capacity
• Starts school
• Identifies with teachers and peers
• Weakens home ties
• Recognizes authority figures outside home (hero worship)

Genital stage
(age 12 to young adult)
• Develops secondary sex characteristics and experiences reawakened sex drives
• Exhibits increased concern over physical appearance
• Strives toward independence
• Exhibits sexual maturity
• Identifies member of opposite sex as love object
• Matures intellectually
• Plans future
• Experiences identity crisis

Sullivan's theory

Infancy stage
(age 0 to 18 months)
• Uses mouth as source of satisfaction; sucks, bites, spits out objects introduced by others; cries, babbles, and coos to call attention to self
• Biological needs are met, experiences feelings of contentment and fulfillment (satisfaction response)
• Perceives others' feelings as his own immediate feelings (empathic observation)
• Feels he's master of all he surveys (autistic invention)

• Experiments, explores, and manipulates to acquaint self with environment

Childhood stage
(age 1½ to 6)
• Has capacity for communicating through speech
• Uses language as tool to communicate wishes and needs
• Uses bowel control to manipulate parents by giving or withholding a part of self (feces)
• Experiences emerging concept of self and integrates it with appraisals of significant persons
• Knows that postponement of own wishes may bring satisfaction
• Begins to understand limits to experimentation, exploration, and manipulation
• Becomes more aggressive
• Uses play and curiosity to explore environment
• Uses masturbation and exhibitionism to get acquainted with self and others
• Demonstrates beginning ability to think abstractly
• Experiences beginning need for peer association

Juvenile stage
(age 6 to 9)
• Forms satisfactory relationships with peers
• Begins to assign more value to peer norms
• Competes, experiments, explores, and manipulates
• Cooperates and compromises
• Demonstrates capacity to love
• Distinguishes fantasy from reality
• Exerts internal control over behavior

Preadolescent stage
(age 9 to 12)
• Relates to friend of same sex (chum relationship)
• Participates in and derives satisfaction from group accomplishment
• Shows signs of rebellion — restlessness, hostility, and irritability
• Assumes less responsibility for own actions
• Moves from egocentricity to a fuller social state
• Experiments, explores, and manipulates
• Seeks peer confirmation of reality (consensual validation)

Early adolescent stage
(age 12 to 14)
• Experiences physiologic changes
• Rebels to gain independence
• Fantasizes and overidentifies with heroes
• Discovers and begins relationships with opposite sex
• Demonstrates higher anxiety levels in most interpersonal relationships

Late adolescent stage
(age 14 to 21)
• Establishes an enduring intimate relationship
• Experiences a stabilized self-concept
• Attains physical maturity
• Uses logic and abstract concepts

Adult stage
(age 21 and older)
• Assumes responsibility relevant to station in life
• Maintains balance and involvement between self, family, and community
• Develops creativity further
• Reaffirms values

Erikson's theory

Orosensory stage
(age 0 to 12 months)
• Develops basic attitudes of trust versus mistrust (through mother's reaction to infant needs)
• Uses mouth as source of satisfaction and means of dealing with anxiety-producing situations

Anal-muscular stage
(age 1 to 3)
• Focuses on development of basic attitudes of autonomy versus shame and doubt
• Learns limits of ability to affect the environment by direct manipulation
• Exerts self-control and willpower

Genitolocomotor stage
(age 3 to 6)
• Experiences development of basic attitudes of initiative versus guilt
• Learns limits of ability to affect the environment through assertiveness
• Explores the world through senses, thoughts, and imagination
• Demonstrates direction and purpose through activities
• Engages in first real social contacts through cooperative play
• Develops conscience

Latency stage
(age 6 to 12)
• Experiences development of basic attitudes of industry versus inferiority
• Creates, develops, and manipulates
• Initiates and completes tasks
• Understands rules and regulations
• Displays competence and productivity

Puberty and adolescent stage
(age 12 to 18)
• Experiences development of basic attitudes of identity versus role diffusion
• Integrates life experiences
• Seeks partner of opposite sex
• Begins to establish identity and place in society

Young adulthood stage
(age 18 to 25)
• Experiences development of basic attitudes of intimacy versus isolation
• Wants to develop an intimate relationship with another adult

Adult stage
(age 25 to 45)
• Experiences development of basic attitudes of generativity versus stagnation
• Wants to establish and maintain a family
• Displays a marked degree of creativity
• Adjusts to middle-age circumstances
• Reevaluates life's accomplishments and goals

Maturity stage
(age 45 and older)
• Experiences development of basic attitudes of ego integrity versus despair
• Accepts life-style as meaningful and fulfilling
• Remains optimistic
• Continues personal growth
• Adjusts to limitations
• Adjusts to retirement
• Adjusts to reorganized family patterns
• Adjusts to losses
• Accepts death with serenity

(continued)

How four psychoanalysts view development *(continued)*

Piaget's theory

Sensorimotor stage
(age 0 to 12 months)
• Experiences preverbal intellectual development
• Learns relationships with external objects
• Develops physically and experiences gradual increase in thought and language ability

Preoperational stage
(age 2 to 7)
• Learns to use symbols and language
• Learns to imitate and play
• Displays egocentricity
• Endows objects with power and ability (animistic thinking)

Concrete operations stage
(age 7 to 11)
• Deals with visible concrete objects and relationships
• Experiences increased intellectual and conceptual development; uses logic and reasoning
• Becomes more socialized and rule-conscious

Formal operations stage
(age 11 to 15)
• Develops true abstract thought
• Formulates hypotheses and applies logical tests
• Exhibits imaginative thinking and explores ideas about own experiences (conceptual independence)

Adapted from Kreigh and Perko, *Psychiatric and Mental Health Nursing*, 1979. Reprinted with permission of Reston Publishing Co., a Prentice-Hall Co., Reston, Va.

Understanding the child's psychological development

Infant and toddler

Age and minor problems
• *Crying:* A normal activity (but may provoke child abuse; observe parents for angry reaction to crying).
• *Self-comforting measures:* Infant sucks finger, thumb, or pacifier; clings to favorite toy or blanket; masturbates.

Normal variations
• *Hair-pulling, head-banging, body-rocking:* Signs of mild or serious anxiety.
• *Temper tantrums:* Common, usually benign (overreaction to the tantrums may create long-term problems).
• *Colic:* Probably caused by incomplete myelinization of the nervous system; usually ends by fourth month.
• *Toilet training:* May turn into a battle between parents and children.

Severe problems
• *Autism:* Infant can't relate to other people but may demonstrate attachment to inanimate objects.
• *Failure to thrive:* Infant doesn't grow, shows minimal development, and is unresponsive and lethargic. Although this problem may result from an organic cause, it characteristically results from lack of love and contact with surroundings. Failure to thrive is a serious, even life-threatening problem.
• *Anaclitic depression:* Infant ignores adults and surroundings, sleeps poorly, and proves more susceptible to infections. Expressionless, the infant seems unaware of his surroundings approximately 3 months after signs and symptoms appear. Occurs in infants with strong maternal attachment who are separated from their mothers between the 10th and 12th month.
• *Indiscriminate attachment:* Infant appears starved for affection. For instance, the infant will willingly go to an examiner even after parents leave and exhibit no separation anxiety. This problem indicates poor attachment.
• *Extreme emotions:* Infant exhibits fear and anger; requires further evaluation.

Preschooler

Age and minor problems
• Nightmares, sleep-walking, sleep-talking: Preschooler wakes up frightened after 2 or 3 hours of sleep, usually able to recall the dream. The dream may represent the child's attempts to deal with monstrous feelings or a daytime problem.
• *Nose-picking, masturbating:* If excessive, may indicate high stress.
• *Stuttering:* Usually outgrown; long-term stuttering may result from overattention to the child's speech.

Normal variations
• *Encopresis:* May indicate psychological problems or organic disease. Encopresis begins after years of bowel control. It also occurs during the daytime.

• *Bruxism (teeth-grinding):* Possibly related to daytime tension. This problem may also begin at toddler or school-age stage.
• *Extreme emotions:* Especially anger, fear, anxiety, shyness, or antisocial behavior. In a preschooler, this problem requires further evaluation.
• *Enuresis:* May be normal, but persistent enuresis may require treatment.

Severe problems
• *Hyperactivity:* Preschooler displays short attention span, low frustration tolerance, and frequent emotional outbursts. Typically, this problem peaks during late preschool and early school years, and should subside during adolescence.
• *Accident-prone behavior:* Preschooler displays impulsiveness, hyperactivity, restlessness, immaturity, and resentment of authority. This behavior is more prevalent in boys.
• *Hair-pulling:* Preschooler has obvious bald patches, indicating severe stress.

School-age child

Age and minor problems
Normal developmental occurrences seldom appear as signs of problems.

Normal variations
• *Cheating:* May reflect child's view of adult culture or indicate attempt to handle poor self-image.

• *Lying:* Similar to cheating. Pathologic lying may indicate serious coping problems.
• *Fighting:* May result from lack of self-control or imitating adult behavior; may indicate deep-seated feelings of hostility or unhappiness.
• *Scatology:* Common, may be an attempt to irritate adults or be part of a group.
• *Psychosomatic signs and symptoms:* Headache, upset stomach, vomiting, and occasionally, psychogenic cough. These signs and symptoms may result from stress.
• *Enuresis:* May result from or cause psychological problems.

Severe problems
• *School phobia:* Child fears school and refuses to attend; problem relates to mother's ambivalent feelings toward separation from child.
• *Learning disabilities:* May be related to intelligence or to emotional or perceptual problems. They require further evaluation and treatment.
• *Schizophrenia:* Child loses interest in surroundings; exhibits blank expression and poor appearance and hygiene; becomes withdrawn and isolated; and develops special preoccupation, phobia, and anxiety. A child gradually becomes schizophrenic.

Adolescent

Age and minor problems
• *Peer-group behavior:* Compliance with previous standards; represents normal behavior.

• *Dating and social life:* Emphasis on social life represents normal development.

Normal variations
• *Conflict with parents:* Common sources of disagreements include driving the car, dating, smoking, homework habits, choice of friends.
• *Sexual experimentation:* Fear of being unattractive, homosexual, oversexed, or undersexed. Problems and confusion commonly occur during search for sexual identity.

Severe problems
• *Severe acting out:* Adolescent uses behavior to express unconscious emotions, including sexual acting out, delinquency, running away, social withdrawal, and failure in school.
• *Depression:* May be accompanied by suicidal thoughts or actions.
• *Substance abuse:* Indicates poor adjustment. Alcohol abuse occurs most commonly, but such drugs as marijuana, cocaine, crack, hallucinogens, sedatives, stimulants, and analgesics are also abused.
• *Hysteria:* Occurs occasionally; most common in girls.
• *Anorexia nervosa:* Adolescent shows excessive weight loss; could be fatal.
• *Obesity:* May result from or cause psychological problems.
• *Pregnancy:* May be a symptom of a psychological problem, such as rebellion against parents. Pregnancy may also represent a need to escape from an unpleasant home situation.

How vital signs change during childhood

When you check the blood pressure and monitor the temperature of a child, you should interpret vital signs by the standards appropriate for his age. Pulse and respiratory rates decrease as a child gets older, whereas blood pressure gradually increases with age.

Age	Pulse	Respirations	Systolic blood pressure
Neonate	125	64-70	
1 year	120	35-40	
2 years	110	31-35	96
4 years	100	26-31	96
6 years	100	23-26	96-98
8 years	90	21-23	104
10 years	90	21	110
12 years	85-90	21	115
14 years	80-85	21-22	118-120
16 years	75-80	20	120-124

How body proportions change

The Stratz chart at right shows how the size of a person's head changes in proportion to other areas of his body. During maturation, total head size decreases proportionately and the face elongates. Keep these changes in mind when evaluating the neurologic development of your pediatric patient.

Adapted from Robbins, W.J., et al., *Growth.* New Haven, Conn.: Yale University Press, 1928, with permission of the publisher.

When children should be immunized

Before immunization, ask the parent if the child receives corticosteroids or other drugs that depress the immune response, or if he's had a recent febrile illness. Obtain a history of allergies, especially to antibiotics, eggs, or feathers, and of past reactions to immunization. *After immunization*, tell the parents to watch for and report a severe reaction. Give them a record of their child's immunizations.

Usually, childhood immunizations are given on a fixed schedule, as follows:

Age	Immunization
2 months	First dose: diphtheria/tetanus/pertussis (DPT) vaccine, polio vaccine
4 months	Second dose: DPT vaccine, polio vaccine
6 months	Third dose: DPT vaccine, polio vaccine
15 months	Measles, mumps, and rubella vaccine
18 months	DPT vaccine booster, polio vaccine booster
18 months to 5 years	*Haemophilus influenzae B* vaccine
4 to 6 years	DPT vaccine booster, polio vaccine booster

When teeth typically erupt

Primary dentition

Maxillary
A Central incisor: 8 to 12 months
B Lateral incisor: 10 to 12 months
C Cuspid: 18 to 24 months
D First molar: 12 to 15 months
E Second molar: 24 to 30 months

Mandibular
F Central incisor: 5 to 9 months
G Lateral incisor: 12 to 15 months
H Cuspid: 18 to 24 months
I First molar: 12 to 15 months
J Second molar: 24 to 30 months

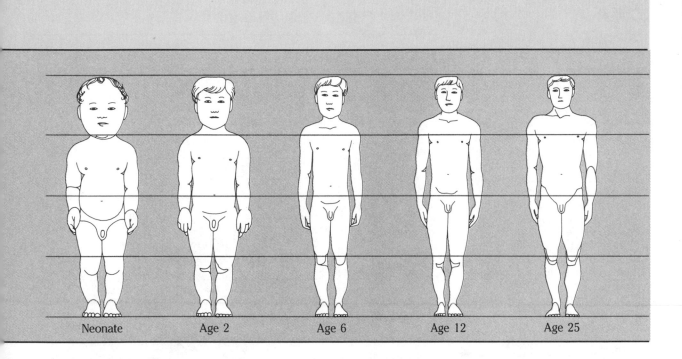

| Neonate | Age 2 | Age 6 | Age 12 | Age 25 |

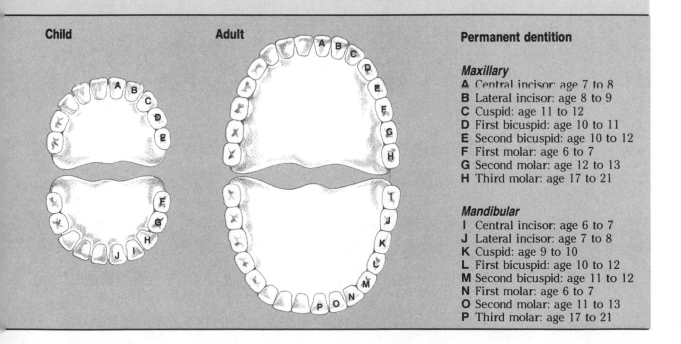

Child   **Adult**

Permanent dentition

Maxillary
A Central incisor: age 7 to 8
B Lateral incisor: age 8 to 9
C Cuspid: age 11 to 12
D First bicuspid: age 10 to 11
E Second bicuspid: age 10 to 12
F First molar: age 6 to 7
G Second molar: age 12 to 13
H Third molar: age 17 to 21

Mandibular
I Central incisor: age 6 to 7
J Lateral incisor: age 7 to 8
K Cuspid: age 9 to 10
L First bicuspid: age 10 to 12
M Second bicuspid: age 11 to 12
N First molar: age 6 to 7
O Second molar: age 11 to 13
P Third molar: age 17 to 21

Childhood undernourishment

Undernourishment can impair normal growth and development in a child, affect his body function, and have other long-term effects. During the prenatal period and the first 9 months of life, undernutrition can cause permanent retardation. Clues to undernourishment in a child include listlessness, apathy, pallor, dental caries, and decreased resistance to infections. Other factors include:
• Parents' neglect or abuse
• Illnesses that impair digestion, absorption, or nutrient utilization
• Increased demand for nutrients due to growth
• Stress in a child due to trauma, surgery, or emotional upset.

Childhood obesity

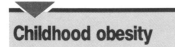

Obesity can affect children of all ages, including infants, causing psychological problems and foreshadowing adult obesity. Because it's less responsive to therapy than adult obesity, early detection and treatment are imperative. Obesity standards in children are the same as in adults: a weight-to-height ratio greater than 120% and a triceps skinfold measurement indicating obesity. Other factors include:
• Inactivity or chronic illnesses that impair mobility
• Overfeeding, common in bottle-fed infants or when parents use food as a pacifier or insist that their child clean his plate
• Genetic predisposition to obesity, although children may become obese imitating their obese parents' eating patterns
• Metabolic, endocrine, or neurologic abnormalities (rare).

Using pediatric growth grids

When performing a dietary pediatric assessment, you should include a growth grid. Correlate both the child's height and weight with his age. Consider the child's growth normal if he falls between the 5th and 95th percentiles; consider his growth abnormal if he falls below the 5th or

Boys: Ages 2 to 18 physical growth percentiles

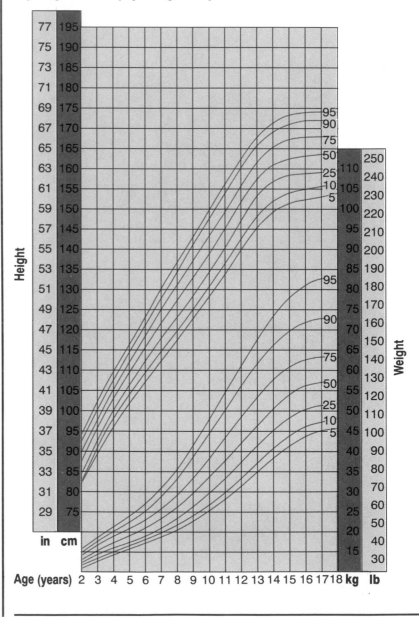

above the 95th percentile. Also consider abnormal any sharp, sudden deviation from the child's usual percentile. Abnormal results indicate the need for further evaluation.

Girls: Ages 2 to 18 physical growth percentiles

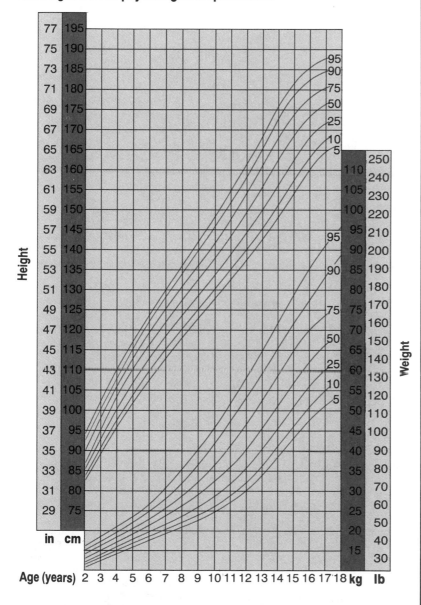

Experts say that about one out of every ten children with burns or soft tissue, head, or bone injuries may be a victim of abuse. Whether you work in an emergency department (ED), a doctor's office, or a pediatric unit, consider the possibility of child abuse when you see such injuries.

Whenever the parents' explanation doesn't seem to fit the child's injuries, investigate further, asking yourself the following questions.

How does the child react to touch?

If you put your hand on his shoulder and he ducks or flinches, he probably associates touch with pain. Typically, an abused child isn't hugged often, so he doesn't associate touch with affection.

Does the child willingly part company with his parents?

Normally, when he must undergo a painful procedure like having a wound sutured, even an older child will cling to his parents. A child who walks away without hesitation may be eager for escape.

Is the child's reaction bravery or a conditioned response?

If the child undergoes a painful procedure without reacting, he's either extremely ill or used to pain. An abusive parent who observes such passive behavior may say something like, "He knows better than to cry."

How do the parents feel about the injury?

Most parents will blame themselves—at least partly—for their child's accidental injuries. Abusive parents, on the other hand, may say something like, "I don't know why he's so bad. He never does what I tell him," rationalizing that if their child hadn't misbehaved, he wouldn't have had to be punished.

Does the child have old injuries that his parents can't explain?
Most toddlers have bruised shins, but when there are bruises above the waist, ask the parents about them. Note any suspicious marks on the skin. Are the marks on the child's back really ant bites, as the parents claim, or are they cigarette burns? Are the teeth marks really from his brother? Adult bite marks are surprisingly small.

Do the parents allow the child to answer the questions you ask him?
Most parents will urge their child to "Tell the nurse what happened." Abusive parents often try to direct the child's response, saying something like, "Tell the nurse how your brother hit you" or "Tell the nurse how you fell off your bike." Parents who won't allow the child to speak at all may fear what he'll say.

How does the child respond to questions?
An abused child may be vague about how he was injured, or tell different stories to different people. When asked directly about specific injuries, he may answer evasively or not at all. Sometimes he'll minimize or try to hide his injuries.

What do the parents expect from the child?
Frequently, abusive parents have unreasonable expectations and demand complete obedience. They may, for example, expect a 5-year-old to sit quietly for an hour, or a 2-year-old to control his bowels when he's under stress or in pain.

How does the child relate to his parents?
Does he seem afraid or look guilty when they enter the room? Does he look to them for support? If his parents have been abusing him, he'll probably feel guilty about their having to bring him in for medical care.

How do the parents interact with each other?
Do they support and comfort each other? Or do they argue and blame each other for the incident? One of them may accuse the other of mistreating or abusing the child.

How do the parents react to authority figures?
If a policeman happens to be in the ED, note the parents' reaction. Do they seem furtive or try to hide their faces? Also note their reaction when you mention the child welfare agency. Most parents will be a little defensive. Hostile or paranoid behavior is a clue that they're afraid you suspect child abuse.

Caring for the abused child

When you suspect that a child is the victim of abuse, you should take certain steps immediately.

Tend to the child's physical needs first
• Tell the doctor that you suspect the child has been abused and ask him to order a total-body X-ray. If the doctor resists, talk directly to the radiologist, who can do it on his own authority. Don't hesitate in taking this action into your own hands, but inform your supervisor of the situation.
• If you suspect the child has been forced to ingest drugs or alcohol, have the doctor order toxicology studies of the child's blood and urine.
• If the child is severely bruised, get the doctor to order a blood coagulation profile.
• If X-rays or other studies suggest the child has been abused, talk to the doctor about confronting the parents, offering to help him do this. If a parent admits to abusing the child and appears to want help, supply the address and telephone number of a local group, such as the Child Abuse Prevention Effort, and encourage the parent to call.
• Arrange to have an agency caseworker or law enforcement official photograph the child's injuries (if you aren't legally permitted to take the photos yourself). In states that don't grant you the right to photograph, the examining doctor has the responsibility of authorizing photographs.

Ease the child's emotional pain
• Often, an abused child feels guilty. He sees his parents' abuse as punishment for his own bad behavior. Try to make the child understand that it isn't his fault.
• Ease the child's concern that his parents are in trouble because of him. If he keeps asking for them, talk to the caseworker about the possibility of their visiting him. Never mention the police to the child.
• If the child wants to talk about his experiences, listen quietly, ask open-ended questions, and remain nonjudgmental. Reassure him that he isn't responsible for what's happened. (When you're alone, record his comments on his chart; document only what he said and how he behaved, not your interpretations.)
• As the child relaxes, he may regress and even become disruptive. If you have to discipline him, stay calm and matter-of-fact. You want him to learn that discipline is not synonymous with pain.

• Finally, if you do have dealings with the child's parents, resist the temptation to show anger. Treat them with understanding, remembering that they, too, need your help.

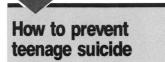

How to prevent teenage suicide

When pressure mounts, an adolescent may not be able to handle it and may try to take his life. Three simple actions could stop him: recognizing the clues he'll give, talking to him, and listening to him.

Recognizing the clues
• Verbal clues like "Nothing will matter where I'm going" or "They'll be better off without me"
• A dramatic shift in academic performance
• Changes in social behavior
• Excessive use of drugs or alcohol
• Changes in daily behavior and living patterns
• Extreme fatigue
• Boredom
• Decreased appetite
• Preoccupation and inability to concentrate
• Overt signs of mental illness, such as hallucinations, delusions, talking to himself
• Giving away treasured possessions
• Truancy
• Failure to communicate with family and school personnel
• Isolation and morose behavior
• Insomnia
• Lack of a sufficient father-son relationship, possibly because of death, divorce, or the father's preoccupation with career
• A difficult mother-daughter relationship, especially if a strong father figure is absent

• Pregnancy
• Excessive smoking
• Violent behavior
• Apparent "accidental" self-poisoning, especially if the behavior is repeated.
    Consider these clues to be cries for help. Don't be afraid to explore the teenager's feelings.

Taking action
Once you've determined that the patient *is* serious about suicide, take action to help him:
• Listen to what he is saying and try to fully understand him. Repeat his statements, using your own words.
• Evaluate the seriousness of the situation. If he has a specific plan, he's probably more serious than someone who's vague about his method.
• Evaluate the intensity of his emotional disturbance. An adolescent who's been depressed and then becomes agitated and restless is at especially high risk. But remember, an adolescent can be very upset and not be suicidal.
• Take everything he says seriously. He might be speaking in a low-key manner, but inside he may be seething.
• Ask him directly whether he's thought of suicide. You won't plant the idea by asking.
• Don't be fooled if he says the crisis has passed. He may feel an initial sense of relief after talking to you, but the same thoughts will probably recur. Be sure to follow through.
• Be affirmative and supportive. Let him know you'll do everything you can to prevent him from taking his life.
• Act specifically. Do something tangible. Arrange to see him later, and make sure he has someone else to depend on.
• Ask for assistance and consultation. Use community resources such as a crisis center or suicide prevention hotline.
• Involve the family. If you've been

able to glean a motive, talk about it privately with family members. If they've been pressuring him too heavily to succeed in school, for example, ask them to praise him in some other area where he's excelled. Ask them also to confront the issue of pressuring him.
• Meet with the adolescent and his family. Let him talk about his feelings, even if his problems stem from his relationship with his family.
• In all your dealings with a suicidal adolescent, do everything possible to preserve his sense of dignity and self-worth.

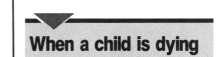

When a child is dying

Caring for a dying child is one of the most difficult challenges you can face. Making rules that apply to all dying children and their survivors is impossible because no two children, two families, or two nurses are alike. Some general recommendations can, however, help you in this difficult task.

The nurse's role
Defining your role in caring for a dying child is critical. Try to distinguish between your own problems and the child's problems in dealing with his terminal condition.

Act as the child's advocate and informant. Although you work as a colleague with the doctor, the family, and other professionals, the parents and doctor are primarily responsible for keeping the child informed of his condition. Avoid becoming a crusader for the child's rights, even when you feel the child should know more than he does.
    Nurses, particularly pediatric nurses, often have a special rapport with children. On the other

hand, they may have difficulty establishing the same rapport with the parents. Remember that the child needs all parties, so don't alienate the doctor or the parents. Work as an advocate and a catalyst, not an adversary.

Respect your own needs. Caring for a dying child requires that you distance yourself emotionally. Be as open, warm, and giving as you can, but also consider your professional duties, your responsibilities to other patients, and your personal life. Some days, you'll have a lot to give; other days, you'll have very little. Try not to feel guilty about the days when you feel you've fallen short. And don't give in to the desire to be "supernurse" at the expense of your family and friends.

Understand and respect the grieving process. Everyone, including the entire health care team and the dying child, will grieve in their own way. Respect your own feelings and allow for the grieving of others around you, no matter how it manifests itself.

Anyone who works with the dying needs someone to whom they can vent their feelings and frustrations. If you can't find a companion at work, you need to find one at home.

More and more pediatric wards and intensive care units sponsor wakes or memorial services when a patient widely known and deeply loved dies. This gives all levels of staff a chance to share time and vent feelings that, if left unspoken, could result in widespread depression and psychosomatic illness.

Know when you reach your emotional limits. Because of guilt and loyalty, pediatric nurses often resist being transferred or taking breaks. But even the strongest nurse should take a break occasionally, to preserve her sense of balance and thus serve as a

model for younger, less-experienced nurses.

If your hospital has a policy that allows such breaks, take advantage of it. A short leave of absence will help you do your job better and keep you from reaching the point where you'll have to leave work permanently.

The child's needs

A dying child needs communication more than anything else. Not just verbal exchanges, but touching, hugging, teasing, lap-sitting. He needs someone to be near him, to play games with him, to be warm and loving in conduct, tone, posture, and mood.

Read the child's signals. Don't be unduly surprised by displaced anger, fear of isolation, depression, hysteria, or bargaining for life with nurses and doctors. Some children feel guilty about dying and causing so much trouble. Some greet the prospect of death and the end of suffering with relief and acceptance.

In routine verbal exchanges, you may mistake what a child is trying to say. But when he's unable or unwilling to talk, he'll resort to a host of conscious or unconscious signals. Assess each child carefully; listen, watch, and share with others.

Be accepting and nonjudgmental. Try to create an atmosphere in which the child can be himself. You don't have to be explainer, protector, caretaker, problem-solver, and final authority. But you do have to be a good listener.

Let the child talk about whatever he wants, including sickness and death. If he won't talk, a tender, supportive presence may encourage him to communicate in other ways. It's better to allow a child to despair openly than to give him little real support, and let him suffer alone.

Respond to the child from the child within you. Children don't make speeches. They don't beat a subject to death. They don't find brutally frank answers inappropriate. They aren't baffled by questions as answers, and they can spot a phony. Don't give a child false hope or refer him to a parent or doctor you know won't be honest with him. By responding to him from the child within yourself, you can enter his world without losing dignity or propriety.

Share secrets. Often, a child with uncommunicative parents deals with issues important to him by discussing them with playmates, siblings, and teachers—anyone other than his parents. If a child wants to talk to you in confidence about his illness, let him. Your secret conversations won't usurp the parents' authority.

Respect the maturity the child often gains during a lengthy illness. Treating a chronically ill patient as a typical child underestimates his capacity. The ups and downs, the disappointments and the many losses he experiences prepare him to face death in a manner others can hardly comprehend.

Some families deal with a dying child by indulging him, constantly giving him presents. But pampering a child through a final illness only makes him feel lonely and unloved. A tired and desperate family can't always see what's happening. But a perceptive nurse can see it at once, and may be able to help the child and his family preserve their love.

The grieving family

Nothing in life seems to affect parents more deeply than the death of a child. Their grief is often beyond comprehension, and usually nothing you can say or do will console them. But here are some measures that may provide comfort.

Give careful attention to both parents and siblings. Don't look at the family as a unit, but as individuals, each one with specific questions and needs. Listen considerately, but don't feel you have to supply them with easy or final answers.

Don't take sides. Even if you have favorites within a family, avoid the futile, defeating practice of entering the fray. Family members have to work through their grief themselves.

When a child dies, parents become obsessed with a host of questions about genes, family heritage, parental adequacy. Too often, the death of a child results in the death of a marriage. Though grieving yourself, you can become a ready confidant to every family member.

Give them privacy. Most relatives need privacy to work through the shock and disorganization following a sudden death. Most hospitals are stingy with space for intimate and profound grief. But you can offer the grief-stricken family an acceptance and openness that makes them forget time and space. Touching is appropriate for some; closeness for most. You can help soothe them by simply being there.

If the family blames the hospital, try to accept their criticisms quietly rather than defending yourself. Quarreling will just make the situation worse. Your tolerance could help them get beyond their confusion, hurt, and helplessness, so that they can start the healing process.

Be understanding when families finish grieving before the actual death. During a child's long illness, the family may come to terms with their having to say good-bye. You may be able to discuss the day when the child will be gone, when only memories and love remain.

When death finally comes, the family may feel relief that the pain and struggle have ended. Many parents can barely admit such a seemingly inappropriate reaction even to themselves, let alone to you. You can help them avoid guilt if you let them know their response is normal.

When a child dies suddenly: Easing the parents' pain

What do you say to the parents of a child who's just died or is dying? There's probably not much you can say that will make a difference, but try to communicate with compassion.

When a child is near death
• Prepare the family for what they'll see before you take them into the child's room. Explain the need for the machines, tubes, needles and anything else. Clean and bandage the child before the family sees him. Show the family members where they can safely touch the child.
• Refer to the child by name. This shows the parents that you care.
• Let the parents watch you caring for the child if they want to.
• Show the parents that the child is special to you, that you're not just doing your job.
• Try to anticipate the parents' questions. When answering them, avoid complicated terminology.
• Be truthful. Tell them what you know and be honest about what you don't know. Give them specifics such as blood pressure, temperature, and pulse measurements.
• Let the parents participate in the child's care as much as possible.

Later, they'll need to feel they helped.
• Reassure the parents that everything possible is being done to help the child.
• Let the parents be with the child at the moment of death if they want to. Some parents will want to hold the child while he's dying.

After a child dies
• Give emotional support to both the father and the mother when breaking the news. Don't assume that the father needs less support.
• Understand that parents may not accept news of the child's death at first. Be patient and remember, denial is a form of emotional protection. Because of the stress they're experiencing, the parents may want you to repeat an explanation.
• Tell the parents what they should do next. They'll be shocked and confused and will need guidance.
• Don't rush away from the parents after breaking the news. If you can't handle the situation, get someone who can.
• Put your hand on the parent's arm, or keep your arm around him or her. Touching is a basic form of communication.
• Remember, the two things that concern parents most are whether the child suffered and whether he was afraid. Be prepared to answer these questions honestly.
• Allow parents as much time as they need with the child. This experience is vital to their healing process.
• Express your personal frustration and pain at the loss of the child.
• Ask the parents about organ donation. Assure them that their child's body will be treated with respect.
• Go to the child's funeral if possible. Parents will appreciate this more than you can imagine.

14 When your patient is elderly

Improving communication with elderly patients

In your relationship with an elderly patient, be caring and genuine. Remember, he's a human being with the same needs and feelings as everyone else. Treat the elderly patient with warmth, but temper your nurturing with respect, communicating with him as an equal.

Here are some pointers:

Know your patient
• Begin by exploring your patient's value system so you can understand his background and his decision-making process. This will help you develop an effective nursing care plan.
• Keep in mind that your patient has the same needs for shelter and safety, belonging, self-esteem, and self-actualization as any other person. Aging brings on change, and an elderly patient may have difficulty meeting his own needs, which can in turn lead to illness and depression.
• Never give an elderly patient too much information too rapidly. Instead, wait until he has finished processing earlier verbal or visual stimuli. Ask for feedback as you go along.
• Write down important information, or tie it into a conversation about something your patient already knows. Otherwise, he may forget it quickly.

Show respect
• Never use "baby talk."
• Always call your patient by his formal name—"Mr. Smith," for example. Don't use his first name unless he asks you to, and don't use terms like "Gramps."
• Avoid using words like "senior citizen" and "oldster."
• Let the patient speak for himself and control his own life as much as possible. Remember, for example, that he has the right to refuse medication.

Be subtle
• Speak in a normal tone of voice, using a medium to low pitch, and don't shout. (In fact, the hearing-impaired usually lose the ability to hear loud, high-frequency sounds.)
• Always face your patient so he can watch what you're saying. Multiple stimuli, both verbal and visual, help him retain information.
• If you're a woman, wear bright lipstick or gloss so the patient can follow your lip movements more easily. If you're a male nurse, avoid wearing a heavy mustache and beard.
• If the patient has poor vision, identify yourself by touching him on the arm and telling him who you are.
• When you give written instructions, use nonglare paper, and write or print information in large black or red letters, using a broad felt-tip pen. Read the information to the patient and ask for feedback.
• Communicate through touch, but do so carefully. Your patient may consider a pat on the shoulder condescending. So instead, clasp his hand while you talk. If you've become close to the patient, you can even hug him.
• Speak directly to the patient when discussing his care. Never "talk through" him to someone else, as if he weren't there.

Protect your patient
• Guard him against the depersonalizing rounds made by doctors and nurses with their student entourages. Remind them that the person in bed is a human being, not some organism hooked up to high-tech equipment.
• Performing several activities too close together will deplete the patient's energy.

• Whenever possible, do things at the patient's pace, not your own. An elderly person is slow because his reaction time increases with age. Being considerate can improve your patient's self-esteem, and the extra time you spend with him, even doing ordinary tasks, can fulfill his social needs.

Assessing an elderly patient: Areas to cover

Certain disorders commonly affect elderly people. When assessing your patient, note the following signs, which could be pathologic:

Skin
Delayed wound healing, change in texture

Nails
Brittleness, clubbing, pitting

Head
Facial pain or numbness

Eyes
Diplopia, tunnel vision, halo effect, glaucoma, cataracts

Ears
Excessive wax formation

Nose
Epistaxis, allergic rhinitis

Mouth and throat
Sore tongue, problems with teeth or gums, bleeding gums at night, hoarseness

Neck
Pain, swelling, restricted range of motion

Respiratory system
Tuberculosis, difficulty or painful breathing, excessive cough producing excessive or blood-streaked sputum

Breasts
Discharge, change in contour, change in nipples, gynecomastia, lumps

Cardiovascular system
Chest pain on exertion, orthopnea, cyanosis, syncope, fatigue, murmur, leg cramps, varicosities, coldness or numbness of extremities, hypertension, myocardial infarction

Surveying an elderly patient's daily activities

Use general questions to discover an elderly patient's activities of daily living (ADLs) and whether he has any problems perfoming them. An elderly patient may also have personal concerns, such as financial worries or transportation problems, which affect his daily routines. Structure your questions as outlined here.

Diet and elimination
• What do you eat on a typical day?
• Do you feel hungry between meals?
• Do you prepare your own meals?
• With whom do you eat?
• What types of food do you enjoy most?
• Do you have any specific problems eating?
• Have you noted any change in your sense of taste?
• Do you snack? When are your snack times? What do you have for a snack?
• What are your usual bowel habits? Have you noticed any changes in them?

Exercise and sleep
• Do you take daily walks?
• Do you do your own housework?
• Do you have any difficulty moving about?
• Has your doctor restricted your exercise or suggested a special exercise program?
• What time do you go to bed at night?
• What time do you wake up?
• Do you follow a routine that helps you sleep?
• Do you sleep soundly or wake often?
• Do you take a nap during the day? How often and for how long?

Recreation
• Do you belong to any social groups, such as senior citizen clubs or church groups?
• What do you enjoy doing in your leisure time?
• How many hours a day do you watch television?
• Do you share leisure time with your family?

Tobacco and alcohol
• Do you use tobacco? If so, do you smoke cigarettes, cigars, or a pipe? How long have you smoked? How much do you smoke each day? If you quit smoking, when did you quit?
• Do you drink alcohol? How often do you drink? Do you drink with friends or alone? How much do you normally drink? Has your drinking increased recently?

Personal concerns
• Do you wear dentures? Are they a hindrance when eating or talking?
• Do you wear glasses? Do you have any problems with your vision when wearing your glasses?
• Do you hear those around you without difficulty? Does poor hearing hinder any of your activities?
• What is your source of income?
• Do you shop for your own groceries? If not, who does this for you?

GI system
Difficulty swallowing, epigastric pain, abdominal pain, intolerance to certain foods, increased thirst, dysphagia, change in bowel habits, rectal bleeding

Renal and urologic systems
Flank pain, dysuria, polyuria, nocturia, incontinence, enuresis, hematuria, renal or bladder infections or stones

Male reproductive system
Hernia, testicular pain, prostatic problems

Female reproductive system
Postmenopausal problems (bleeding, hot flashes, painful intercourse)

Endocrine
Goiter, tumor

Musculoskeletal system
Pain, joint swelling, crepitus, restricted joint movement, arthritis, gout, rheumatism, lumbago, amputations

Nervous system
Memory loss, loss of consciousness, nervousness, nightmares, insomnia, changes in emotional state, tremors, muscle weakness, paralysis, aphasia, speech difficulty, pain or numbness

Recognizing neurologic changes in elderly patients

During the neurologic examination of an elderly patient, you may find several sensory alterations. Note the following cranial nerves that may be affected by aging, and the alterations produced.

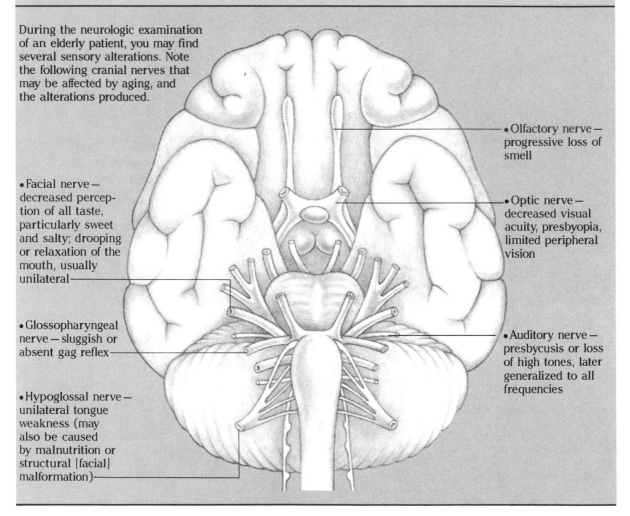

• Facial nerve— decreased perception of all taste, particularly sweet and salty; drooping or relaxation of the mouth, usually unilateral

• Glossopharyngeal nerve—sluggish or absent gag reflex

• Hypoglossal nerve— unilateral tongue weakness (may also be caused by malnutrition or structural [facial] malformation)

• Olfactory nerve— progressive loss of smell

• Optic nerve— decreased visual acuity, presbyopia, limited peripheral vision

• Auditory nerve— presbycusis or loss of high tones, later generalized to all frequencies

Recognizing and reporting elder abuse

Elder abuse is estimated to involve from 3% to 20% of the elderly population, depending on the type of abuse. You're most likely to see incidences of elder abuse if you work in the emergency department. But every nurse should be aware of this growing problem. Here are some important facts you should know:
• Those who abuse the elderly include related caregivers (including spouses), paid caregivers who work in the elder's home or in a boarding home, and caregivers who work in long-term and acute care facilities.
• Elder abuse includes both acts of omission and acts of commission, or neglect. It commonly takes one of the following forms: physical abuse (including sexual), psychological abuse, financial or material exploitation, health-related abuse (neglect), environmental abuse, and human rights violations.
• Although you may detect all of the forms of abuse listed above, you'll most commonly see elderly patients with severely neglected health problems. Typically, you'll see conditions such as dehydration, malnutrition, poor hygiene, untreated skin problems (often pressure sores), and untreated bowel and bladder problems (fecal impactions and urine retention).
• You should suspect elder abuse whenever you see severe, unexplained deterioration; unexplained or implausibly explained injuries; conditions for which treatment has been delayed; families reluctant to expend the elder's resources for health care; family members who are unusually concerned or not at all concerned about the elder's condition; and elders who appear extremely fearful or suspicious.

• You should report elder abuse in accordance with the law, which varies from state to state. You should know the law in your state as well as your institution's procedure for reporting elder abuse. You should also be prepared to make appropriate referrals to social service agencies and to local adult protective services.

Getting elderly patients to comply with drug therapy

Elderly people often do not cooperate when it comes to drug therapy. Their ability to follow a prescribed regimen can be affected by forgetfulness, transportation problems, not understanding instructions, and the cost of medication. Assess your patient's potential for noncompliance by asking the following questions:

Is the patient taking more than one drug?
Multiple daily doses of different drugs can be confusing or inconvenient.

Is the patient suffering from more than one illness?
If so, the patient may be receiving different drugs that counteract or heighten the effects of each other or increase risks to the patient's health.

Is the patient responding to the therapy?
If not, the patient may be taking the drug less often than he should and may not be refilling his prescription. Aging often impairs drug metabolism and excretion, and the patient may be decreasing the dosage to avoid discomfort or other possible adverse effects.

Hormonal changes in elderly patients

Use this chart as a guide to hormonal changes in elderly patients.

Hormone	Serum concentration
Growth hormone	No change
Thyroid-stimulating hormone	No change
Thyroxine	No change
Triiodothyronine	Decreases
Parathyroid hormone	Decreases
Cortisol	No change
Adrenal androgens	Decreases
Aldosterone	Decreases
Insulin	No change
Glucagon	No change

Is the patient living alone?
If so, the patient may not have the transportation to get to his health care appointments or to pick up his prescriptions. And he may not have anyone to explain how or when to take his medication.

How you can help
• Discuss the problem with the patient, his family, and his health care team. They may have suggestions.
• Review medication instructions. Stress the importance of taking the correct dosage on schedule.
• Make sure the drugs are clearly labeled. Suggest to the patient that he attach prescription labels to the outside of tinted containers for

Reviewing medication aids for elderly patients

Approximately one-third of elderly patients fail to comply with their prescribed drug therapies. Here are some medication aids that could help your patient:

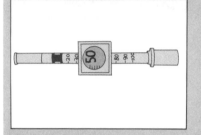

Scale magnifier
Purpose: To help a vision-impaired diabetic patient read syringe markings and independently fill his own syringe.
Description: Plastic magnifier snaps onto syringe barrel.
Special considerations: May not be appropriate for an arthritic patient, who may have difficulty attaching the device.

Syringe filling device
Purpose: To measure insulin doses precisely (especially for a patient with vision impairment).
Description: Plastic device designed for use with a disposable U-100 syringe and an insulin bottle. The device is set to accommodate the syringe's width; then the plunger is positioned at the point determined by the dose and the stop is tightened. When set, the patient can draw up the precise dose ordered for each injection.
Special considerations: Not for mixed or variable doses of insulin.

Settings must be checked and adjusted when syringe size or type is changed.

Screws may become loose after repeated use of device; instruct the patient to regularly check them.

Needle can be contaminated easily.

easy reading, or request clear bottles, unless contraindicated.

Patients with failing eyesight should consult their pharmacists for special packaging. Write dosage instructions and the medication schedule on a separate piece of paper and tape a sample tablet or capsule to it so the patient, his family, or visiting nurse can consult it if they have any questions.
• Suggest he label empty jars, extra prescription bottles, or envelopes with the time of day or days of the week he's supposed to take medication. He should use a separate container for each time, filling them each morning with the correct dose of each medication.

(Some drugs deteriorate when exposed to light; check with the pharmacist before removing drugs from their original containers.)
• Have him make a medication calendar on which he writes the names of the drugs he needs to take each day. Tell him to put a check mark next to the name of the drug after he takes each dose.
• Show him how to make a chart listing the name of each drug, what it's for, what it looks like, directions, precautions or adverse reactions, and the time of day to take it. Have him hang the chart near his medicine cabinet.
• Tell him to set an alarm clock or have a relative or friend remind

him when to take his medication.
• Check container caps. If the patient has arthritis or Parkinson's disease, he may prefer standard caps to child-proof caps for prescription refills providing, of course, that youngsters have no access to the containers.
• Analyze the patient's eating habits. If he tends to skip meals, he may also be missing the medication that is supposed to be taken with these meals. Plan a realistic medication schedule, then contact a social service program, such as Meals On Wheels, for further help.
• Consider the patient's finances. If he is on a fixed income, he may try to make his medication last

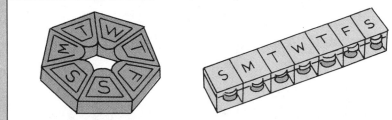

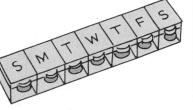

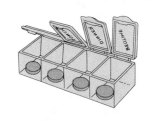

Seven-day pill reminder
Purpose: To help the patient remember if he has taken all the tablets and capsules prescribed for each day of the week.
Description: Both plastic devices shown here have seven medication compartments, marked with the initials for each day of the week (in both braille and roman letters).
Special considerations: Family

members or visiting nurse must remember to fill the device with ordered medications at the beginning of each week.

Not appropriate for large numbers of tablets and capsules, or tablets and capsules that must be taken at specific times each day.

Useful if patient takes a medication every other day, rather than daily.

One-day pill reminder
Purpose: To help the patient determine if he's taken all the medications prescribed for a single day.
Description: Plastic device with four medication compartments marked breakfast, lunch, dinner, and bedtime. The initial letter of each word is also marked in braille on each compartment.
Special considerations: Family member or visiting nurse must fill device with ordered medications each day. Not appropriate for large numbers of tablets or capsules.

longer. Stress the importance of following the doctor's orders exactly. If necessary, refer the patient to a social service representative for financial aid information.

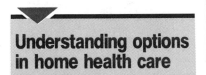

Understanding options in home health care

What do you say to a patient who asks about home health care? Do you know what alternatives are available, and which one will best suit his needs? You should be familiar with these specialty groups and what they provide:

Home health care agencies
Traditionally, these agencies provide Medicare-reimbursed services: they're certified—and in some cases licensed—by the government. Because of the Medicare connection, they provide intermittent care (2 or 3 hours a day, 1 to 3 days a week) rather than custodial or continuous care. Their services include visits by RNs, LPNs, home health aides, social workers, and physical, occupational, and speech therapists.

Service hours are usually 9 to 5, Monday through Friday. Many agencies provide care or at least take emergency calls on weekends. Check for specifics with agencies in your area.

Some hospitals have their own home health care agency, which is usually Medicare-reimbursed. These agencies enjoy the built-in advantage of quick access to medical records, progressive technology, and different departmental services and resources. Ideally, they provide the best system for continuity of care, depending on communication between the hospital and the agency while the patient is in and out of the hospital.

Home health care services
Services (as opposed to agencies) are private corporations that aren't Medicare-certified. They can provide almost any level of nursing care around the clock.

Recognizing drugs deleterious to elderly patients

Classification	Possible effects
CNS depressants and other psychotropic drugs	
secobarbital (Seconal), phenobarbital (Luminal, Eskabarb), and other barbiturates	• Bizarre perceptual disturbances, delusions, thought disorders, panic, memory disorders
chlorpromazine (Thorazine, Chlorprom), thioridazine (Mellaril), and other phenothiazines; haloperidol (Haldol)	• Hypotension impairs mental ability; possibly leads to syncope if blood pressure drops too low for adequate cerebral perfusion
amitriptyline (Elavil), imipramine (Tofranil), and other tricyclic antidepressants	• Hypotension from phenothiazines is common and serious; dosage is adjusted for elderly patients.
chlordiazepoxide (Librium), diazepam (Valium), flurazepam (Dalmane), and other benzodiazepines	
alcohol intake alone, or with any of these central nervous system (CNS) depressants (lethal dose of barbiturates drops almost 50% when taken with alcohol)	
Analgesics	
salicylates and other nonnarcotic analgesics	• Bizarre perceptual disturbances, delusions, thought disorders, panic, memory disorders
narcotic analgesics such as hydromorphone hydrochloride (Dilaudid)	
propoxyphene hydrochloride (Darvon)	
Antihypertensive drugs	
guanethidine sulfate (Ismelin), reserpine (Serpasil), methyldopa (Aldomet), and other sympatholytics	• Hypotension impairs mental ability; may lead to syncope if blood pressure drops too low for adequate cerebral perfusion
Anticholinergic or atropine-like drugs and other GI drugs	
atropine, scopolamine (included in many nonprescription sleep-producing preparations), and other belladonna alkaloids	• Disorientation, delusions, recent memory impairment, agitation, confusion (cimetidine)
antiparkinson agents such as diphenhydramine (Benadryl), trihexyphenidyl (Artane), benztropine mesylate (Cogentin)	
propantheline bromide (Pro-Banthine)	
cimetidine (Tagamet)	

Some states have laws that require licensure for private home health services as well as Medicare-certified agencies. The Joint Commission on Accreditation of Healthcare Organizations is working on home health care standards, but the fact remains that in some states there are still no guidelines or requirements for private home health care services. So you and your patient should inquire about the necessary basics: nursing assessments, care plans, nursing notes, regular updating of doctors' orders, supervision of employees, careful hiring procedures, and pertinent qualifications of administrative and supervisory staff.

Some private insurers cover limited aspects of private home

care (skilled nursing, but not home health aide or custodial care). However, private care costs are deductible from federal income taxes, just like medications or prescribed equipment.

Hospice

Hospice teams vary from community to community, in terms of services, eligibility, charges or donations, the extent of actual hands-on nursing care, and the supplies they provide. Most require a full-time caregiver in the home and stipulate that the patient be within 6 months to a year of expected death.

Ideally, hospice care teams work closely with the local American Cancer Society to avoid duplication of effort and to promote continuity and comprehensiveness of care. Trained hospice volunteers are on call 24 hours a day.

Be knowledgeable about the philosophy and services of hospice in your area before you explain the concept to your patient. Be tolerant, too, if the patient or family is in the denial stage and refuses or rejects the concept of hospice.

Registries

Registries have been in existence for decades, but are usually licensed as employment agencies, not home health care agencies. Registry nurses are independent contractors. They're totally responsible for nursing care and should be licensed by the state. They set their fees with the patient and collect them, giving a percentage to the registry.

Registry nurses provide skilled nursing care, but are not supervised and may not be adequately covered by insurance (liability, bonding, workers' compensation, unemployment). The patient, as the employer, could be responsible for these concerns, so warn him to ask whether the registry nurse is insured before he signs any agreement.

Pharmaceutical home health care

These companies specialize in high-tech home care, especially total parenteral nutrition, I.V. antibiotic therapy, enteral feeding solutions, and chronic pain control.

They employ pharmacists and RNs to visit patients at home, bringing with them solutions, supplies and equipment. They monitor the patient's status, keep the doctor informed of the patient's progress, and give the patient and his family instructions and support in home therapy.

An increasing number of Medicare home health care agencies and private home health care services have expanded to high-tech care in the home, including I.V. therapy, ventilator care, and newborn phototherapy. Talk to your patients and their families before giving a referral. If they can make their own arrangements, encourage them to do so.

Before you give *any* information about a patient to an agency or service, check your hospital's policy. You may need a signed release from the patient and consent from his doctor first.

15 Improving patient-teaching skills

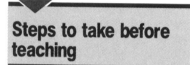

Steps to take before teaching

Before you begin teaching, you'll need to take four important steps to set the stage for your instruction. Going through these steps, you may discover other areas for teaching based on what your patient and his family want to learn. If so, you'll need to reassess the patient or modify your teaching standards to create the best possible teaching plan. The steps to take for beginning instruction are:

Set teaching standards
• What does the patient need to learn?
• What does the health care team want the patient to learn?
• When does teaching need to take place?

Collect data
• What do interviews with the patient and his family tell you about learning needs, goals, and responses?
• What does the patient's chart reveal?
• What information can other members of the health care team provide?

Evaluate data
• What does the patient want to learn?
• Do his goals conflict with those of his family or the health care team?
• Are there any barriers to learning?
• Are there any factors that can promote learning?

Establish a teaching diagnosis
• What is the patient ready, willing, and able to learn?
• Do the patient, family, and health care team confirm your findings?
• Do you need to set new teaching standards?

What to assess before teaching

You can teach faster, easier, and more effectively if you first determine what your patient knows, what he needs to know, if he's willing to learn, and if he's capable of being taught. So before you teach, assess the following factors in your patient:

• Current emotional state
• Stage of adaptation to illness
• Emotional maturity
• Developmental stage

• Self-image
• Learning goals—and those of his family
• Health beliefs
• Sociocultural background
• Religious beliefs
• Physical condition
• Intellectual state
• Learning style
• Socioeconomic status
• Family support system and the availability of support groups.

Is your patient ready to learn?

A patient goes through stages in adapting to his illness. By recognizing which stage the patient is in, you can avoid trying to teach him something he's not ready to learn.

Stage 1: Disbelief

Patient's thoughts
• "There's nothing wrong with me."
• "This can't be happening to me!"

Patient's actions
• Denies seriousness of illness, disregards restrictions
• Ignores attempts to teach him self-care

Stage 2: Developing awareness

Patient's thoughts
• "Why me?"
• "If only I'd been more careful, maybe I wouldn't have gotten sick."

Patient's actions
• Places blame for illness on self or others
• Strikes out at others to relieve pent-up hostilities

Stage 3: Reorganization

Patient's thoughts
• "How does my family see me now?"
• "I'm beginning to see how my life is changing."

Patient's actions
• Avoids discussing his condition or changes with family
• Asks more questions about his condition

Stage 4: Resolution

Patient's thoughts
• "I see how my life has changed."
• "Other people with my condition seem to get along all right."

Patient's actions
• Seeks out others with same condition
• May express emotions more openly

Stage 5: Identity change

Patient's thoughts
• "I've changed."

• "My life is going to be different from now on."

Patient's actions
• Actively seeks out information about his condition
• Attempts greater independence

Stage 6: Successful adaptation

Patient's thoughts
• "I accept the way my life has changed."
• "I want to make each moment count."

Patient's actions
• Complies with health care regimen
• Freely discusses his condition with family

Modifying teaching approaches by developmental stage

Stage of development	Typical behavior during hospitalization	Teaching approaches
Infant	*Under 7 months:* • Responds well to nurse • Allows parents to leave *Over 7 months:* • Anxious and unhappy • Clings to parents and cries when they leave	• Teach the parents to participate in their infant's care. • Handle the infant gently and speak in a soft, friendly tone of voice. • Use a security toy or pacifier to reduce the infant's anxiety and elicit cooperation.
Toddler	• Commonly experiences separation anxiety • May show anger by crying, shaking crib • Rejects nurse's attention • May become apathetic, crying intermittently or continuously • May reject parents and respond to nurse	• Teach the parents to participate in their child's care. • Give the child simple, direct, and honest explanations just before treatment or surgery. • Use puppets or coloring books to explain procedures. • Let the child play with equipment to reduce anxiety. • Let the child make appropriate choices, such as choosing the side of the body for an injection.
Preschooler	• Experiences separation anxiety; may panic or throw tantrums, especially when parents leave • Often regresses (enuresis) • Commonly shows eating and sleeping disturbances	• Teach the parents to participate in their child's care. • Use simple, neutral words to describe procedures and surgery to the child. • Encourage the child to fantasize to help plan his responses to possible situations.

(continued)

Modifying teaching approaches by developmental stage *(continued)*

Stage of development	Typical behavior during hospitalization	Teaching approaches
Preschooler *(continued)*		• Use body outlines or dolls to show anatomic sites and procedures. • Let the child handle equipment before a procedure. • Use play therapy as an emotional outlet and a way to test the child's sense of reality.
School-age child	• May have insomnia, nightmares, enuresis due to anxiety about the unknown • Alternately conforms to adult standards and rebels against them	• Use body outlines and models to explain body mechanisms and procedures. • Explain logically why a procedure is necessary. • Describe the sensations to anticipate during a procedure. • Encourage the child's active participation in learning. • Praise the child for cooperating with a procedure.
Adolescent	• Fluctuates in willingness to participate in care because of need for both independence and approval • Shows concern about how procedure or surgery may affect appearance	• Ask the patient if he wants his parents present during teaching sessions and procedures. • Give scientific explanations, using body diagrams, models, or videotapes. • Encourage the patient to verbalize his feelings or express them through artwork or writing. • Offer praise appropriately.
Adult	• Directs and participates in his own care • Complies with hospital regulations • Freely asks questions when he has concerns or uncertainties • Demonstrates continued interest in personal roles • Shows concern for family and economic results of hospitalization	• Negotiate learning goals with the patient. • Include family members in teaching. • Use problem-centered teaching. • Provide for immediate application of learning. • Let the patient test his own ideas, take risks, and be creative. Allow him to evaluate his actions and change his behavior. • Use the patient's past experiences as a learning resource.
Older adult	• Demonstrates anxiety over new procedures or a change in routine • Often forgets new material or ideas or takes a long time to make decisions • Maintains interest in personal matters • Asks for instructions to be repeated • Participates in care and decision making • Requires frequent rest periods	• Negotiate learning goals with the patient. • Include family members in teaching. • Schedule frequent, short teaching sessions (15 minutes maximum) at times of peak energy. • Avoid holding sessions after the patient has bathed, ambulated, or taken medications that affect learning ability. • Check for memory deficit by asking for verbal feedback. • Present one idea at a time. • Use simple sentences, concrete examples, and reminders such as calendars or pillboxes. • Speak slowly and distinctly in a conversational tone. • Use large-print materials and equipment with oversized numbers. Avoid using teaching materials printed on glossy paper.

Reviewing religious beliefs and practices

A patient's religion can affect his willingness to learn by influencing his attitudes toward illness and traditional medicine. Try to determine the nature and strength of your patient's religious beliefs.

Does he, like many Christian Scientists who shun traditional medical treatment, believe a person can cure illness by altering his thought processes? What role does religion play in the patient's daily routine? Does his religion prohibit him from eating certain foods? If it does, he may resist learning about dietary changes that conflict with his beliefs.

By trying to accommodate a patient's religious beliefs and practices in your teaching plan, you can increase his willingness to learn and comply.

Religion	Birth and death rituals	Dietary restrictions	Practices in health crisis
Adventist (Advent Christian Church, Seventh-Day Adventist, Church of God)	None (baptism of adults only)	Alcohol, coffee, tea, narcotics, and stimulants prohibited; in many groups, meat prohibited also	Communion and baptism performed. Some members believe in divine healing, anointing with oil, and prayer. Some regard Saturday as Sabbath.
Baptist (27 different groups)	At birth, none (baptism of believers only); before death, counseling by clergy and prayer	Alcohol prohibited; in some groups, coffee and tea prohibited also	Some believe in healing by laying on of hands. Resistance to medical therapy occasionally approved.
Church of Christ	None (baptism at age 8 or older)	Alcohol discouraged	Communion, anointing with oil, laying on of hands, and counseling by minister.
Church of Christ, Scientist (Christian Scientist)	At birth, none; before death, counseling by Christian Science practitioner	Alcohol, coffee, and tobacco prohibited	Many members refuse all treatment, including drugs, biopsies, physical examination, and transfusions. Vaccination only when required by law. Alteration of thoughts believed to cure illness. Hypnotism and psychotherapy prohibited. (Christian Science nursing homes honor these beliefs.)
Church of Jesus Christ of Latter-day Saints (Mormon)	At birth, none (baptism at age 8 or older); before death, baptism and gospel preaching	Alcohol, tobacco, tea and coffee prohibited; meat intake limited	Divine healing through the laying on of hands; communion on Sunday; some members may refuse treatment. Many wear special undergarment.
Eastern Orthodox Churches (Albanian, Bulgarian, Cypriot, Czechoslovakian, Egyptian, Greek, Polish, Romanian, Russian, Syrian, Turkish)	At birth, baptism and confirmation; before death, last rites. For members of the Russian Orthodox Church, arms are crossed after death, fingers are set in cross, and unembalmed body is clothed in natural fiber	For members of the Russian Orthodox Church and usually the Greek Orthodox Church, no meat or dairy products on Wednesdays, Fridays, and during Lent	Anointing of the sick. For members of the Russian Orthodox Church, cross necklace replaced immediately after surgery and no shaving of male patients except in preparation for surgery. For members of the Greek Orthodox Church, communion and Sacrament of Holy Unction.

(continued)

Reviewing religious beliefs and practices *(continued)*

Religion	Birth and death rituals	Dietary restrictions	Practices in health crisis
Episcopalian	At birth, baptism; before death, occasional last rites	For some members, abstention from meat on Friday, fasting before communion	Communion, prayer, and counseling by minister.
Islam (Muslim)	If abortion occurs before 130 days, fetus treated as discarded tissue; after 130 days, as a human being. Before death, confession of sins with family present; after death, only relatives or friends may touch the body	Pork prohibited; daylight fasting during ninth month of Islamic calendar	Faith healing for the patient's morale only; conservative members reject medical therapy.
Jehovah's Witnesses	None	Abstention from foods to which blood has been added	Generally, no blood transfusion; may require court order for emergency transfusion.
Judaism	Ritual circumcision after birth; burial of dead fetus; ritual washing of dead; burial (including organs and other body tissues) occurs as soon as possible; no autopsy	For Orthodox and Conservative Jews, kosher dietary laws (for example, pork and shellfish prohibited); for Reform Jews, usually no restrictions	Donation or transplantation of organs requires rabbinical consultation. For Orthodox and Conservative Jews, medical procedures may be prohibited on Sabbath—from sundown Friday to sundown Saturday—and on special holidays.
Lutheran	Baptism usually performed 6 to 8 weeks after birth	None	Communion, prayer, and counseling by minister.
Orthodox Presbyterian	Infant baptism; scripture reading and prayer before death	None	Communion, prayer, and counseling by minister.
Pentecostal (Assembly of God, Foursquare Church)	None (baptism only after age of accountability)	Abstention from alcohol, tobacco, meat slaughtered by strangling, food to which blood has been added, and sometimes pork	Divine healing through prayer, anointing with oil, and laying on of hands.
Roman Catholic	Infant baptism, including baptism of aborted fetus without sign of clinical death (tissue necrosis); before death, anointing of the sick	Fasting or abstention from meat on Ash Wednesday and on Fridays during Lent; this practice usually waived for the hospitalized	Burial of major amputated limb (sometimes) in consecrated ground; donation or transplantation of organs allowed if benefit to recipient is proportional to the donor's potential harm.
United Methodist	None (baptism of children and adults only)	None	Communion before surgery or similar crisis; donation of body parts encouraged.

Six ways to polish your teaching skills

Effective and timely instruction can improve a patient's understanding of his condition and the prospects for his compliance with treatment.

To improve your teaching skills, use these tips:
• Expand your knowledge base by reading professional publications, attending in-service and continuing-education programs, and maintaining a broad range of professional contacts.
• Ask your institution's staff development department to schedule in-service classes that can benefit your entire unit. Then follow up with conferences on your unit for more detailed discussions about what you've learned.
• If you're not up to date on a subject you have to teach, ask the staff development department to supply the names of specialists in that area. Then call one for an appointment.
• Observe more experienced nurses while they're teaching patients. What makes their teaching effective? What kind of rapport do they have with their patients? How do they reach difficult-to-teach patients? Which of their methods could you use effectively?
• If you have a patient who's unusually difficult to teach, ask a colleague or a nursing consultant to teach him while you observe.
• Ask a colleague you consider an especially good teacher to sit in while you teach. Ask her to review your teaching tools and techniques and offer pointers for your next teaching session. If you're uncomfortable having a third person present while you teach, try role-playing beforehand. This can smooth out any rough edges in your presentation and help put you at ease for the actual session.

Setting priorities for teaching

Teaching patients what they need to know often seems impractical: there's too much to cover and not enough time. If you find yourself hard-pressed for time, try this method:
• List the patient's learning needs.
• Rank his needs: most important, next most important, and so on.
• Write your "teaching-to-be-done" list based on this ranking.

This should help you distinguish the patient's *learning* needs from his *nursing care* needs. It also helps organize your time and can help redirect your actions after an interruption.

To simplify the task of ranking the patient's learning needs, classify them as:
• *immediate* or *long-range*
• *survival* (life-dependent) or *related to well-being* (nice to know but not essential)
• *specific* (related to the patient's disorder or treatment) or *general* (teaching that's done for every patient).

After you've classified the patient's learning needs, establish priorities. An immediate survival need, like teaching him the warning signs of adrenal crisis, would take top priority.

Teaching timesavers

Consider these techniques to save time when teaching patients:
• Before you begin teaching, have the patient review written materials, audiocassettes, or videotapes to gain a basic understanding of his disorder.

• Use diagrams, charts, and other visual aids in your teaching sessions to speed comprehension.
• Rely on support staff to augment your teaching. For example, have the dietitian discuss meal plans with your patient, the respiratory technician explain spirometry, and the physical therapist teach crutch walking.
• If the patient's family will be participating in his care at home, schedule your teaching sessions during their visits.
• Teach the patient while you're providing routine nursing care. Let his questions guide your teaching.
• If you're teaching a short-stay patient and a home health nurse has been selected for him, you may want to emphasize the major points in your teaching and leave the minor points for the home health nurse.
• Document your teaching to avoid duplication of instruction.
• Document a patient's repeated resistance to teaching, then move on to teach another patient.
• Give the patient preprinted information and instructions to take home, rather than write new ones yourself.
• Once you've developed a teaching plan for a specific disorder, keep it filed for reuse or adaptation.
• Constantly evaluate your teaching to find the methods that work best for you. Then use those methods.

Saving staff time

To save time for your colleagues, suggest implementing timesaving programs that have worked in other institutions:
• Use group-teaching sessions for patients with similar needs, such as diabetes, hypertension, cardiac rehabilitation, and postnatal care.
• For same-day surgery patients, add a nurse to the preadmission testing staff and make preoperative and postoperative teaching that nurse's responsibility.

Group teaching: Setting the stage for success

When teaching a group, you'll want to enhance the learning process by helping the patients develop a group identity and a feeling of cohesiveness. Here are some useful techniques:

Shape the environment
• Hold the meeting at a round table or arrange chairs in a circle. This increases interaction by making participants feel equal to each other and to the teacher.
• Limit the group to five to seven patients to allow maximum personal exchange and discussion.
• Check the temperature and lighting of the meeting room to make sure neither causes discomfort or distraction.
• Serve coffee, tea, or cold drinks

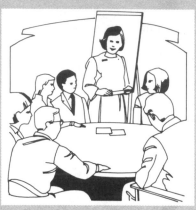

to keep the atmosphere informal and relaxed.

Initiate discussion and maintain an overview
• Introduce yourself.

• Ask patients to introduce themselves and to share a bit of personal information.
• Explain the meeting's purpose.
• Invite the group to identify the meeting's goals and set the ground rules.
• Encourage everyone's participation, but also allow anyone who isn't comfortable or doesn't wish to join in to leave.
• Use a light rein, but keep the group close to the agreed-upon areas for discussion.
• Act as a resource, providing information and clarification when necessary.
• Summarize at the end of the discussion, and lead the group to agree on what has been learned.

Giving your patients feedback

Patient teaching requires two-way communication: You teach, the patient tells or shows you what he's learned, and you point out his successes as well as areas that need improvement.

Be helpful
Present alternatives, don't dictate rules. Avoid using absolutes like "always" and "never."

Focus on the patient's behavior, not his progress or personality, and make sure you discuss *current* behavior, not past.

Always begin by giving positive feedback to reinforce desired behavior. Then discuss the points he

still needs to master. If you talk about the negatives first, you'll put the patient on the defensive and he may be unwilling to listen to whatever else you have to say.

Be prompt
Give the patient feedback as soon as possible after you observe behavior. The more comfortable a patient becomes with an undesirable behavior or attitude, the more difficulty he'll have changing it.

Be specific
Offer specific suggestions for improvement along with an explanation. If the patient understands why something needs to be done, he'll remember more easily to do it—and do it correctly.

Make sure the patient understands what you're telling him. If he's perfecting a technique, have

him repeat it at once, so you can check his efforts. If he's working on changing his attitude, ask him to rephrase what you have told him in order to see if he's really listening. Look for other clues, like facial expressions and offhand remarks to you or others.

Be practical
Comment on situations the patient can change, not those beyond his control. For instance, if your colostomy patient has limited finances, don't emphasize the advantages of using expensive disposable equipment.

Be flexible
The patient, not you, should dictate the pace. Keep in mind his needs, his abilities, and the amount of information he can absorb.

Improving your discharge teaching

It's important that you teach your patient to continue his care after he's been discharged from the hospital. Base your discharge teaching on what the patient demonstrates he can do, documenting what you've taught the patient, and what he's learned. You can use this checklist for almost every patient:

Appointments
• Schedules appointment with his doctor
• States when he should make an appointment
• Has appointment with other health care worker (nurse, physical therapist, occupational therapist), if needed
• States reasons for calling his doctor or nurse before the scheduled appointment—for example, bleeding, swelling, increased pain, signs of infection, or other complications

Activity
• States recommendations—for example, increase walking to 1 mile within 2 weeks

• Discusses limitations on positioning, weight-bearing, lifting, or stair-climbing
• Demonstrates prescribed exercises

Diet
• Describes diet he will follow after discharge
• Has copy of his diet
• Explains reason for his diet
• Names person to call with questions about his diet
• Lists suggestions or restrictions on fluid intake, including what he should or shouldn't drink, and how much

Medications
States for each medication he must take:
• Its name
• The proper dose
• How often he must take it
• When he takes it (before or after meals)
• Why he takes it
• Special precautions and adverse reactions to recognize or to report to doctor
• Whether a prescription is needed

Special treatment, procedures, and dressings
• Demonstrates he or a caregiver can perform necessary treatments, procedures, or dressing changes

• Has printed explanation, if needed
• Has the necessary equipment, supplies, and dressings, or knows where to obtain these items
• Lists alternative supplies (disposable or permanent, for purchase or lease, small or large)
• Explains the equipment's use in the treatment or procedure
• Describes how to dispose of soiled dressings

Assistance needs
• Has referral to home care services, if needed
• Lists available community resources (for example, American Cancer Society chapter; stroke, laryngectomy, or ostomy club; hot lines; support groups)
• Has printed information about appropriate community resources

Leaving the hospital
• Has appropriate clothing, including footwear, for the season and for his altered physical condition
• States check-out time
• Explains how the bill will be handled
• Names who will go to the billing office
• Tells how he will leave (by car, cab, or ambulance)

IV PROFESSIONAL DEVELOPMENT

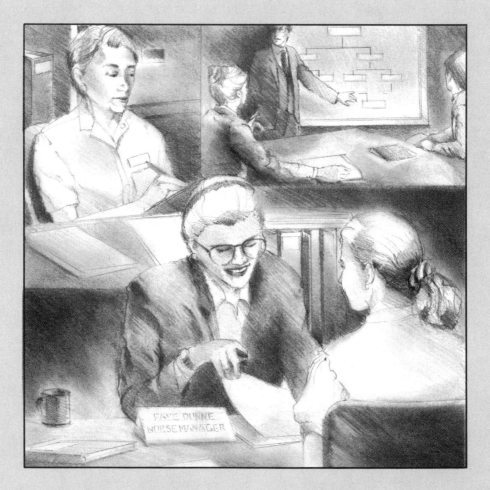

16 Making sound educational choices

What nurses' titles mean

A nursing career can take many turns, but it typically begins with considering educational requirements and various job duties. Here is a run-down of titles, what they mean, their educational requirements, and the duties that usually go along with them.

Registered nurse

A registered nurse (RN) has completed study at a nursing school accredited by the National League for Nursing and has passed the State Board Test Pool Examination. (In Canada, an RN has passed an examination administered by the Canadian Nurses' Association Testing Service.)

An RN spends most of her time in direct patient care. She delegates certain responsibilities to other staff members and coordinates the services of other health care personnel, including nutritionists, pharmacists, psychologists, respiratory therapists, and physical and occupational therapists.

Most RNs practice in hospitals, but there are many other opportunities in private homes, industry, schools, clinics, health maintenance organizations, nursing homes, and nursing care centers.

Nurse practitioner

A nurse practitioner usually has a master's degree and clinical experience beyond her basic nursing education. She can take health histories, perform physical assessments, offer guidance and counseling, and treat minor illnesses with the consultation of a doctor. She usually works in an ambulatory or non-hospital setting.

Clinical nurse specialist

A clinical nurse specialist usually has a master's degree. She is an expert in a particular area of nursing and practices in either a hospital or a community setting.

Nurse anesthetist

A nurse anesthetist is an RN with advanced training from an accredited program for nurse anesthetists. She manages the anesthetic care of the patient during surgery.

Certified nurse-midwife

A nurse-midwife is educated in both nursing and midwifery, and is certified by the American College of Midwives. Her responsibilities include supervising pregnancy, labor, delivery, and postpartum care. A nurse-midwife can practice in a hospital, clinic, maternity home, or a private home.

Licensed practical nurse

A licensed practical nurse (LPN), sometimes called a licensed vocational nurse (in Canada, a nursing assistant), is trained in basic nursing techniques and direct patient care, and practices under the supervision of an RN or a doctor.

An LPN's training usually lasts 1 year. She works in hospitals, clinics, private homes, sanitariums, and similar institutions, often caring for convalescent patients, patients with long-term illnesses, and new mothers and their babies.

Nurse's aide

Nurse's aides are typically, but not always, high school graduates. They're usually trained after being hired. Some institutions combine on-the-job training, under the close supervision of RNs or LPNs, with classroom instruction.

Most nurse's aides work in hospitals, but some work in nursing homes and other health care institutions. Their duties vary, depending on the institution, but their responsibilities can range from cleaning patients' rooms and other household tasks to assisting in patient care.

Comparing nursing programs

Nursing diploma
• Prepares hospital staff nurse
• Affiliated primarily with hospitals, but may be associated with a college for supporting course work
• Requires high school diploma or equivalent, and for most schools, college entrance examination
• Runs 3 years—27 to 36 school months

Associate degree in nursing
• Combines nursing and sciences with some general education to prepare hospital staff nurse
• Affiliated primarily with community or junior colleges; some, with 4-year college
• Requires high school diploma or equivalent and, for most schools, college entrance examination
• Runs 2 years—18 to 21 school months

Bachelor of science degree in nursing
• Combines liberal arts and general education with nursing courses to prepare nurse who can function in various nursing roles and health care settings
• Affiliated with colleges and universities
• Requires high school diploma or equivalent and college entrance examination; may require prerequisite courses before admission to nursing major
• Runs 4 to 5 years

Master's degree in nursing
• Prepares nurses to assume increased accountability and leadership in administration and specialized areas of clinical practice
• Most require graduation from National League for Nursing-accredited bachelor's program with a major in nursing, RN licensure,

Evaluating a BSN program

To decide if a bachelor of science degree in nursing (BSN) program is right for you, ask yourself the following questions to help you decide if a particular program meets your requirements.

The program's philosophy and goals
• Do they match mine?
• Do the course descriptions meet my needs?
• Do the courses spark my interest?

Accreditation
• Does the institution have National League for Nursing (NLN) accreditation? Does it have regional accreditation?
• Is accreditation full or provisional, or pending?
• Has the institution been awarded accreditation?

Admissions policy
• Can I get credit for past education and experience?
• Does the school use its own examinations or accept results of standardized ones, like American College Test and College Level Examination Program? (Challenge policies for course credit vary with each school, so know the policy of the school you're considering.)

Program cost
• What does the tuition cost?
• What's the deadline for payment?
• If the school is state-run, do out-of-state students pay more?
• How much are laboratory fees, challenge fees, travel-related costs?
• How much will it cost to have my college credits evaluated?

• How much will required books and clinical supplies, such as a stethoscope and scissors, cost?
• Does the school offer financial aid? Are work-study programs available? (Don't let a school's higher tuition scare you off until you've examined your financial options.)

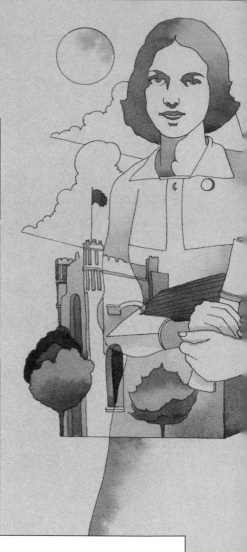

Program credits
• How many total credits do I need to graduate?
• How many of those credits do I have to earn in residence or through the particular school?

Program content
• What's the emphasis in nursing and clinical courses?
• Can the work setting be used for clinical learning?
• Can I select the clinical area which interests me?
• Is the program's course material something I've already learned?

Program completion
• How long will it take me to complete the program?
• Are courses offered frequently or at convenient times, so that I can meet the program requirements comfortably?
• Can I study part-time?
• Can I meet any of the program requirements off campus, through correspondence or independent study?

School and faculty reputation
• What degrees do the faculty members and the program director have?
• What do present and former students think about the school and the faculty? Are students' names available for reference?
• Are the administration and faculty responsive to the needs of adult students?
• What voice do the students have in the governing process?
• Can students in nontraditional programs participate in policy-making procedures?
• What's the ratio of teachers to students in theory courses? In clinical courses?

satisfactory grade-point average and satisfactory scores on Graduate Record Examination or Miller Analogies Test, or both
• Most programs require a specific amount of full-time study, but part-time study, work-study, evening, and weekend programs are becoming increasingly available. Full-time master's degree programs run a minimum of 2 years

Doctoral degrees
• Can be a springboard to greater career success and personal enrichment, whether the nurse's strength or preference is in clinical practice, research and teaching, or administration
• Strengthens competency by increasing knowledge and developing problem-solving abilities
• Gives greater opportunity to participate in policymaking
• The Doctor of Philosophy (PhD) program emphasizes research and creative scholarship, while the Doctor of Nursing Science (DNS or DNSc) emphasizes advanced clinical practice with integration of research to improve nursing care; the Doctor of Nursing (ND) prepares you for entry-level practice in a hospital setting as part of a multidisciplinary health care team

Preparing for the licensure examination

Taking the 2-day national licensure examination is a nerve-racking experience. The following suggestions can help you improve your performance and increase your chances of passing.

The night before the exam
• Assemble the materials you'll need as specified in your instruction booklet.
• Get a good night's sleep. Don't stay up all night trying to learn

new material.
• Avoid using stimulants or depressants. They may affect your ability to think clearly during the test.
• Approach the test with confidence, determined to do your best. Think positively. Concentrate on what you *do* know, not on what you think you *don't* know.

The day of the exam
• Eat a good breakfast.
• Allow yourself ample time to get to the testing site, park, and locate the proper room.
• Choose a location in the testing room away from friends, where you're least likely to be distracted.

During the exam
• Read the directions carefully, so you'll know how to proceed.
• Review the scoring rules. Since points are not subtracted for guessing, it's to your advantage to guess when you don't know the answer to a question.
• Make maximum use of the allotted time: determine the total number of questions, then estimate how much time you'll have for each one.
• Answer the practice questions to get a feel for the testing process.

Using your time wisely
• Start at the beginning of the test, check the time periodically, and maintain a good rate of progression. Don't spend too much time on any one question. If there's time left at the end, go back to any questions about which you were uncertain.
• Try to answer all the questions. If you don't know an answer, leave it and go back to it later.
• On multiple-choice questions, first eliminate the answers you know are wrong. Then decide among the ones that are left. If you're not sure of an answer, pencil in your guess and go back to it later if you have time.

Reading and understanding the questions
• Read each question carefully. Determine exactly what the question is asking; sometimes details are extraneous.
• Mentally underline important factors, paying attention to key terms and phrases.
• Be alert. Watch for questions that ask which answers are *not* correct, or that say, "All the following are correct *except...* "
• When a series of questions is preceded by a clinical situation, refer to the situation for information. The questions will test your ability to analyze a situation and apply your nursing knowledge.

Selecting an answer
• Don't look for a pattern in the answer key. There is none.
• Evaluate the possible answers in relation to the question, not the other answers.
• When several alternatives are correct, choose the answer that is broader, more general. When several alternatives look equally correct, compare them. Ask yourself what the difference is between them and choose the better one.
• Recognize answers that are obviously different from what is logically right, such as an answer given in grams when other choices are given in milligrams.
• Be wary of possible answers that contain specific qualifiers, like *always* and *never*. Remember, however, that some qualifiers are correct; some situations are true only when a qualifier is added.

Continuing education for RN, LPN, and LVN relicensure: Where it's mandatory, how it works

In the states listed below, continuing education (CE) courses are required for license renewal. In other states, however, continuing education is voluntary. If you have any questions regarding changes in procedures or requirements for relicensure, contact your state board of nursing or approval body.

State	Contact hour requirements	Approval body	Special considerations
California	• 30 hours, every 2 years	• For registered nurses (RNs) and licensed vocational nurses (LVNs): California Board of Registered Nursing 1030 N. 13th St. Sacramento, CA 95814 • For LVNs only: Board of Vocational Nurses and Psychiatric Technician Examiners 1020 N St. Room 406 Sacramento, CA 95814	• 3 hours course-related clinical practice = 1 contact hour • Approval of nonapproved offerings not possible
Colorado	• 20 hours, every 2 years	• Any of over 20 credentialing agencies approved by Colorado Board of Nursing	• No more than 5 hours home study per licensing period • Approval of nonapproved offerings not possible

How to evaluate a continuing education program

To evaluate a continuing education (CE) program, you have to first determine what your CE needs are and identify what exactly you want from a CE program. You'll have to decide what aspects of nursing practice you need to learn in order to perform your job competently. For example, if you're beginning work in a critical care unit, you may need to learn more about managing arterial lines.

Then, prior to enrolling in a CE program, you should ask yourself the following questions:
• Is it a program in which I will earn CE units (CEUs), or just an orientation to my institution?
• What are the prerequisites, if any? For example, do I have to work in a clinical specialty area to attend a program on that topic?

• Am I released from on-duty work to attend these programs, or do I have to attend them before or after work?
• Do I have to pay for the program or will my employer pay for it?
• Does my employer require me to earn a given number of CEUs? Is CE tied to the employee evaluation process?
• If I attend an in-house CE program, am I then expected to file a report or hold a conference to discuss the program with my co-workers?

Documentation requirements	Requirements for maintaining license elsewhere	Those exempt from licensure	Continuing education requirements for reactivation of license
• Complete an application renewal statement listing each offering by title, date, provider number, and contact hours earned • Keep attendance certificates or grade slips from academic courses for at least 4 years	• Take academic courses or participate in CE offerings approved by: national nursing, medical, and hospital associations; regional specialty groups; other state boards of nursing; or nurses' associations whose offerings meet California standards	• New graduates (for first renewal) • Nurses overseas at least 1 year • Nurses totally disabled or with a totally disabled dependent for at least 1 year • Federal RNs, military RNs, and LVNs working out of state	• Same as to renew
• Fill out license renewal notices listing CE courses	• Meet Colorado requirements; take courses approved by credentialing agency	• Inactive nurses	• Same as to renew

(continued)

Continuing education for RN, LPN, and LVN relicensure: Where it's mandatory, how it works *(continued)*

State	Contact hour requirements	Approval body	Special considerations
Florida	• 24 hours, every 2 years, earned by 3/31 of renewal year	• Florida Board of Nursing 111 E. Coastline Dr. Jacksonville, FL 32202	• Monitoring by random audit every 2 years
Iowa	• 45 hours, every 3 years	• Iowa Board of Nursing 1223 E. Court Des Moines, IA 50319	• All can be earned through home study • Approval of nonapproved offerings possible only for out-of-state offerings
Kansas	• 30 hours, every 2 years	• Kansas State Board of Nursing 900 S.W. Jackson Suite 551S Topeka, KS 66601	• No more than 20% of required contact hours may be earned through home study • For approval of nonapproved offerings, fill out board's approval and nonapproval courses form before CE offering begins; submit to board of review

Documentation requirements	Requirements for maintaining license elsewhere	Those exempt from licensure	Continuing education requirements for reactivation of license
• In state: For academic courses, send official transcript with license number to board; for board-approved offerings, the provider will forward proof of attendance to the board • Out of state: For academic courses, send official transcript with license number to board; for offerings, send a copy of attendance certificate, and (if not included on certificate) a brochure or other program literature that specifies the accrediting organization	• Participate in an accredited CE offering	• New graduates (for first renewal) • Military personnel • Inactive nurses	• If inactive since 1987, 33 contact hours needed • If inactive since 1989, 24 contact hours needed
• Complete CE report form and send to board with renewal application • Keep attendance certificates and transcripts for at least 4 years	• Take academic courses or participate in out-of-state Iowa-approved offerings; if the other state has mandatory CE, meet that state's requirements; develop an individualized plan with that state board	• Residents of another mandatory CE state who meet that state's requirements • Active-duty military members • Overseas government employees • Some mentally and physically disabled nurses • Inactive nurses *Note: Licensees must apply for an exemption each year*	• 15 contact hours earned within 1 year prior to reactivation
• Submit an *Individual Nurse Participant Record Form* within 4 weeks after participation: if in state, get form from the instructor with his signature; if out of state, get form from the board • When renewing license, list offerings by titles, provider number, date, location, and contact hours earned	• Participate in offerings approved by the American Nurses' Association (ANA) or the National Federation of LPNs; for other offerings, contact board before attending	• Inactive nurses	• Same as renewal requirements for year in which nurse applies for reactivation • Different fee • Different application

(continued)

Continuing education for RN, LPN, and LVN relicensure:
Where it's mandatory, how it works *(continued)*

State	Contact hour requirements	Approval body	Special considerations
Kentucky	•30 hours, every 2 years	•Kentucky Board of Nursing 4010 Dupont Circle Suite 430 Louisville, KY 40207	•All requirements can be met through home study •Staff development activities, but no in-service education, accepted •2 hours of planned, supervised clinical practice designed to meet educational objectives = 1 contact hour
Massachu-setts	•For RNs: 15 hours, every 2 years, earned by 12/31 of year before renewal •No requirements for LPNs	•Massachusetts Board of Registration in Nursing 100 Cambridge St. Room 1509 Boston, MA 02202	•All requirements can be met through home study •Nursing offerings must include a qualified licensed nurse as a planner or instructor •For approval of nonapproved offerings, complete and submit board's approval and nonapproval courses form, 60 days before or 30 days after completing the offering
Minnesota	•For RNs: 30 hours, every 2 years •If licensed in another state, 15 hours for first registration renewal •No requirements for LPNs	•No prior approval necessary. Nurse must evaluate program to make sure it meets criteria established by: Minnesota Board of Nursing 2700 University Ave. W #108 St. Paul, MN 55414	•All requirements can be met through home study •Successful demonstration of skill required
Nebraska	•75 hours in last 5 years; or 200 practice hours and 20 contact hours or in-service education in last 5 years •Graduation from an approved nursing program	•No prior approval necessary. Nurse must evaluate program to make sure it meets criteria in board's CE manual: Nebraska State Board of Nursing P.O. Box 95007 Lincoln, NE 68509	•No limit on contact hours, but courses must be nursing-related •Courses must have an evaluation device, such as a final test •No more than 20% of contact hours can be earned through home study

Documentation requirements	Requirements for maintaining license elsewhere	Those exempt from licensure	Continuing education requirements for reactivation of license
• Send transcripts, a copy of attendance certificates with a description of the offering, and the provider's seal or signature with renewal application	• Participate in CE offerings approved by National League for Nursing (NLN); State Board of Nursing; Continuing Education Approval and Recognition Program (CEARP); the National Federation of LPNs; the National Association for Practical Nurse Education and Service; or ANA-approved agencies	• New graduates (for first renewal) • Inactive nurses	• 30 contact hours; if inactive for more than 5 years, also complete a refresher course
• Complete statement on renewal application, listing offerings by title, provider, provider number, date, and contact hours earned	• Participate in CE offerings approved by the ANA, NLN, or National Federation of LPNs; offerings of other state-approved providers, or approved academic nursing programs; for all other offerings, follow regular approval procedures	• New graduates (for first renewal) • Inactive nurses	• Same as to renew license, earned within the 12 months preceding application for reactivation; if inactive for more than 5 years, also complete a refresher course
• When renewing license, complete a board-provided *Evidence Form* • Keep records for 2 years after renewal period ends	• Same as in state	• Only inactive nurses, but new graduates can obtain credit for course work completed within 2 years before licensure	• If less than 2 years since expiration, 30 contact hours needed before applying for reactivation
• Complete and send CE form with license renewal notice	• Meet Nebraska requirements; make sure courses meet criteria in Nebraska's CE manual	• None	• Same as to renew

(continued)

Continuing education for RN, LPN, and LVN relicensure:
Where it's mandatory, how it works (continued)

State	Contact hour requirements	Approval body	Special considerations
Nevada	•30 hours, every 2 years	•Nevada Board of Nursing 1135 Terminal Way Suite 209 Reno, NV 89502 •Can also be authorized by an ANA-accredited approver	•No more than 10 hours can be earned through home study •Courses given by an accredited college or university need not be approved •For approval of nonapproved offerings, send all required information for board review with license renewal form; no guarantee of approval
New Mexico	•30 hours, every 2 years	•New Mexico Nurses' Association 525 San Pedro N.E. Suite 100 Albuquerque, NM 87108 •Can be authorized by an approver accredited by the ANA or recognized by the board	•For approval of nonapproved offerings, complete a New Mexico Nurses' Association approval form before participating in offering •All can be earned through home study if approved
Texas	•20 hours, every 2 years	•Pending	•Pending

What do nurses' name-tag initials stand for?

You may be puzzled by all the initials that appear on nurses' name tags, but they usually indicate that a nurse is certified in a specific area of practice. Here's a guide to initials you're most likely to encounter.

C	Certified
CARN	Certified Addictions Registered Nurse
CCRN	Critical Care Registered Nurse
CDE	Certified Diabetes Educator
CEN	Certified Emergency Nurse
CETN	Certified Enterostomal Therapy Nurse
CGC	Certified Gastrointestinal Clinician
CHN	Certified Hemodialysis Nurse or Community Health Nurse
CIC	Certified Infection Control
CNA	Certified Nursing Administration
CNAA	Certified Nursing Administration, Advanced
CNM	Certified Nurse Midwife
CNOR	Certified Nurse Operating Room

Documentation requirements	Requirements for maintaining license elsewhere	Those exempt from licensure	Continuing education requirements for reactivation of license
• Send a board-provided form with renewal application • Keep grade slips, transcripts, and attendance certificates at least 4 years	• Take academic courses; or participate in ANA or ANA-accredited offerings, or home-study courses	• Inactive nurses (however, the board is asking for a legislative change to exempt new graduates for the first renewal)	• 30 hours in the preceding 2 years (or as negotiated with board) • Renewal application must include copies of certificate of CE, plus fee
• Send an association-provided notarized form with renewal application	• Participate in offerings approved by organizations listed under *Approval body* column at left	• Inactive nurses	• If inactive for less than 5 years, and reactivated in first year of licensure biennium, meet CE requirements by time of renewal; if reactivated in second year of biennium, meet CE requirements by time of second renewal • If inactive for 5 years or more, also complete a refresher course
• Pending	• Pending	• Pending	• Pending

CNRN Certified Neuro-surgical Registered Nurse	**CPNA** Certified Pediatric Nurse Associate	**CS** Clinical Specialist
CNSN Certified Nutrition Support Nurse	**CPNP** Certified Pediatric Nurse Practitioner	**CSN** Certified School Nurse
COHN Certified Occupational Health Nurse	**CRNA** Certified Registered Nurse Anesthetist	**CURN** Certified Urological Registered Nurse
CPAN Certified Post-Anesthesia Nurse	**CRNI** Certified Registered Nurse Intravenous	**OCN** Oncology Certified Nurse
CPN Certified Pediatric Nurse	**CRRN** Certified Rehabilitation Registered Nurse	**RN,C** Registered Nurse, Certified

Learning about national certification programs

If you've decided to specialize in a particular area of nursing, you should explore the requirements for becoming certified. Certification is a prerequisite in certain clinical areas, such as anesthesia, but isn't mandatory in other areas. The advantage of being certified is that, based on predetermined standards, you're qualified to practice nursing within that specialized area. Below is a selection of organizations and the certifications they govern.

Organization	Type of certification and purpose	Eligibility
American Association of Critical Care Nurses (AACN) Certification Corporation	Critical Care Registered Nurse (CCRN); recognizes nurse's expertise in critical care	Experience required
American Board of Occupational Health Nurses	Certified Occupational Health Nurse (COHN); recognizes nurse's expertise in occupational health practice	Experience required
Association of Operating Room Nurses (AORN) National Certification Board	Certified Nurse, Operating Room (CNOR); recognizes nurse's expertise in operating room practice	Experience required
Board of Nephrology Examiners, Nurses, and Technicians	Community Health Nurse (CHN); recognizes nurse's expertise in nephrology care	Experience required
American Board of Neurosurgical Nursing	Certified Neurosurgical Registered Nurse (CNRN); recognizes nurse's expertise in neuro-surgical care	Experience required
Council on Certification of Nurse Anesthetists	Certified Registered Nurse Anesthetist (CRNA); recognizes nurse's ability to perform as a nurse-anesthetist	Education required
American College of Nurse-Midwives, Division of Examiners	Certified Nurse Midwife (CNM); permits nurse to practice as nurse-midwife	Education required
American Nurses' Association; Division on Medical/Surgical Nursing Practice, Gerontological Nursing Practice, Community-Health Nursing Practice, Maternal and Child Health Nursing Practice, and Psychiatric and Mental Health Nursing Practice	Registered Nurse Certified (RN,C), Registered Nurse, Clinical Specialist (RN,CS), Certified Nursing Administration (CNA), and Certified Nursing Administration, Advanced (CNAA); recognizes nurse's competence in specific areas	Education or experience required
Emergency Department Nurses Association	Certified Emergency Nurse (CEN); recognizes nurse's competency in emergency nursing care	Experience required
Nurses' Association of the American College of Obstetricians and Gynecologists (NAACOG) Certification Corporation	Registered Nurse Certified (RN,C); recognizes nurse's expertise in obstetric or gynecologic care	Education or experience required
National Board of Pediatric Nurse Practitioners and Associates	Certified Pediatric Nurse Associate (CPNA), Certified Pediatric Nurse Practitioner (CPNP); recognizes nurse's competency in pediatric care	Education required

Certification process	Certifica-tion term	Certification maintenance
Multiple choice question (MCQ) examination: 4 hours, given twice a year	3 years	Reexamination or 100 points in CEARP program during 3-year certification period
MCQ examination: given once a year	4 years	Continuing education, 60 hours during 5-year certification period
MCQ examination: 4 hours, given once a year	5 years	Reexamination
MCQ examination: given if at least 25 people request	6 years	Reexamination or 30 contact hours within 2 years combined with clinical experience
MCQ examination: 4 hours, given once a year	5 years	Reexamination
MCQ examination: 4 hours, given twice a year	2 years	Active practice and continuing education
Essay examination: 6 hours, given as requested	Indefinite	Not determined
MCQ examination: given twice a year	5 years	Reexamination or continuing education
MCQ examination: 4 hours, given twice a year	4 years	Not determined
MCQ examination: 3 to 4 hours, given once a year	3 years	Reexamination or 45 contact hours in 3-year certification period
MCQ examination: 1 day, given once a year	6 years	Reexamination or three self-assessment exercises within 5 years

17 Getting the right job

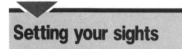

Setting your sights

Before you begin looking for a job, you should give some thought to your long-term career goals. What kinds of things do you enjoy doing? What do you feel you're especially good at? What do you feel you're *not* particularly good at? Where do you see yourself 1, 5, 10 years from now?

Answering these types of questions is not easy. It demands your being completely honest with yourself, while being realistic about your abilities and your professional ambitions. But a few hours spent examining your goals will be well worth the time and can help you discover exactly what kind of work you'll find satisfying now and in the future. Start by taking inventory of your skills.

People skills
Do you interact well with other people? Are you understanding and patient? Do friends come to you for advice? If so, you might consider a job in psychiatric, pediatric, or emergency department nursing, which require an ability to relate well to other people. You might also consider becoming a patient representative.

Communication skills
Are you adept at relaying information to others? Are you confident about speaking in public? Do you have a talent for writing? If you combine these skills with a knack for problem-solving, a management job — head nurse, supervisor, nursing director, or team leader — could be perfect for you.

If you're a good teacher, you could become a lecturer in an occupational health setting. Or you could go into patient education. If writing is your strong suit, you might consider journalism or consulting work.

Analytical skills
Are you good with numbers? Are you adept at reading statistics? Do you prefer paperwork to bedside nursing? Do you enjoy working with computers? If you have these skills, then you could be a perfect candidate for a job in utilization review.

Combined with your clinical background, these skills qualify you to evaluate charts and make decisions about discharging patients. Other areas that require these kinds of skills include management, laboratory research, consulting or accrediting work, and hospital equipment assessment.

Other skills and interests
Do you enjoy working alone? Do you prefer to concentrate on one task at a time? If the answer to these questions is yes, then you should consider private-duty nursing or home health care.

Do you have good telephone and interpersonal skills? Do you like taking care of clerical and business matters? Would you prefer to work regular hours instead of nights shifts and weekends? Do you enjoy teaching preventive medicine? If you answer "yes" to these questions, maybe you'd be happy working in a doctor's office or in an outpatient clinic.

Do you like to handle several tasks at once? Do you enjoy hands-on patient care? Do you also have good communication skills? If you do, a position as a staff nurse could be perfect for you.

Do you like crisis-oriented procedures such as trauma and one-on-one nursing care? Do you like to work with a team? Why not look into critical care, flight, or emergency nursing?

Are you adept at using electronic equipment? If you are, consider becoming an intensive care unit nurse, a nurse consultant for a product manufacturer, or a medical equipment salesperson.

Considering opportunities outside the hospital

The list below details the responsibilities of nurses working in four alternative settings: schools, industries, communities, and businesses.

School nurse

- Provides nursing care for sick or injured students
- Gives first aid in emergencies
- Gives students medications (when authorized by the school doctor)
- Helps school doctor give routine examinations
- Gives annual screening tests — for example, vision, hearing, and scoliosis tests — and refers students for further testing or treatment, when appropriate
- Counsels parents and students
- Meets with teachers and other staff members about health problems and health education programs
- Enforces state immunization policies for school-age children
- Visits sick or injured students at home, when necessary
- Helps identify and meet special needs of handicapped students

Occupational health nurse

- Provides nursing care for sick or injured employees and counsels employees on health matters
- Gives first aid in emergencies
- Performs medical screening tests or helps doctor perform them
- Refers sick or injured employees for appropriate treatment
- Meets with employer regarding health-related issues
- Develops and maintains employee medical records
- Maintains records for government agencies, such as workers' compensation agencies, the Occupational Safety and Health Administration, and state or federal labor and health departments
- Alerts employer to potential health and safety hazards

Community health nurse

- Provides nursing care for community patients, visiting sick or injured persons in their homes
- Refers patients for treatment, when appropriate
- Coordinates patient care services with patient, family, and health care staff
- Supervises home health aides and other community health workers
- Assists in agency planning by helping to define and set priorities
- Works with other professionals to identify and evaluate threats to community health, such as communicable diseases
- Works with private-sector community health workers, such as visiting nurses
- Works as a public school nurse, when needed

Nursing case coordinator for insurance company

- Screens new patients, reviewing records and insurance claims
- Helps assess an insurance claim by talking to the patient, his doctor, his family, and his employer
- Helps design patient care plans, including medical, nursing, social service, and payment goals
- Monitors the patient's progress and prognosis by talking to the patient and his doctors
- Helps coordinate medical, rehabilitation, and other services to improve the insured patient's physical condition so he can return to work
- Supervises other nursing case reviewers
- Develops and maintains insurance company records

Should you practice as an independent contractor?

Thousands of nurses in the United States, including nurse practitioners and private-duty nurses, have chosen to become independent contractors. These nurses work directly for patients or patients' families, and bill the patients or third-party insurers on a fee-for-service basis.

If you're considering practicing as an independent-contractor, you'll want to weigh the pluses and minuses.

The pluses
• You can schedule your work hours to suit your life-style.
• You can put your nursing philosophy into practice by independently planning each patient's nursing care.
• You'll be relatively free from institutional politics and bureaucracy.
• You can negotiate your own contract with each patient and set your own fee for nursing services.
• You may improve your working relationship with other professionals because you'll assume a more prestigious role in the health care community.
• You'll keep more of the money you make, because tax laws favor self-employment.
• You can tailor your benefits package to your own personal needs.
• You can become more involved in the total care of your patient.

The minuses
• You'll lose the security that continuous employment provides.
• You may experience strained working relationships with professionals who feel threatened by

your autonomy and status.
• You'll have to compete for work with other nurses working as independent contractors.
• Your patients may sometimes be admitted to hospitals or other health care institutions where you don't have privileges.
• You'll have to deal with unclear legal definitions of your practice.
• You'll have to educate yourself about the financial and legal aspects of running a business.
• You'll have to deal with getting patients to pay their bills.

Starting your own business: Do you have what it takes?

Going into business for yourself can be a great idea. But you need a strong support network and an even stronger self-image, and you'll have to plan ahead. Before you make any moves, consider the following questions:
• Do you know how to operate on a shoestring budget? Can you get the necessary capital to start a service business? Are you willing to ask relatives and friends for the money if you have to?
• Can you offer a service or product people can't get easily elsewhere? Can you provide it better, cheaper, and faster than your competition?
• If you're marketing yourself—for example, if you're thinking of doing consulting or educational service work—are you convinced you're one of the best?
• Can you promote yourself? Introduce yourself to strangers? List your accomplishments and attributes without hesitation or qualification?
• Can you move quickly to respond to changing trends?
• Can you work well on your own?

Will you able to spend a lot of time alone, developing the product or service, writing marketing copy, addressing envelopes, completing invoices, or just waiting for the phone to ring? Will you miss your coffee-break buddies, office parties, the shoulders to cry on?
• Are you able to set priorities and budget your time? If you work at home, can you resist the temptation to sleep in, watch a favorite TV show, or whip up something special for dinner just because you're there?
• Do you have the skills to be your own staff? Are you willing to type, file, answer the phone, label envelopes, mail invoices, keep records, and project a budget—at least until you can afford to hire someone else to perform these tasks?
• If you don't know how to use a personal computer, are you willing buy one and learn how?
• Do you know how much money you'll need? Can you compute cash flow projections and conduct budget analyses to figure out when you'll break even? Do you know that charging too little for your product or service will bankrupt you, and that charging too much may put you out of the market?

Is it time to change jobs?

Changing jobs is a fact of life for nurses. The annual turnover rates are as high as 50% in some hospitals. But before you make definite plans to change jobs, take a careful look at your current position to get a clear idea of the advantages and disadvantages of your present job. Ask yourself the following questions:

• Does my job offer me career mobility? Where can I go? How can I grow?

• Is the job challenging?

• Am I given recognition for a job well done? Am I encouraged to speak up? Are my opinions considered important?

• Is my job compatible with my life-style?

• Does the job provide me with support and friendships I'd hesitate to leave?

• Are my fringe benefits good? (Consider tuition reimbursement, organizational memberships, retirement contributions, dental insurance, and free health care.)

• Is my salary competitive with the salaries of similar jobs at other institutions?

• Am I being paid in proportion to my skills and responsibilities?

• Has my salary kept pace with the cost of living?

• Do I like my current geographic location, or would I rather live somewhere else?

When you've taken inventory of your current job, think about what you'd want in your "dream job":

• Do I want accountability, responsibility, and authority in patient care?

• Do I want a fast pace? A slow one?

• What kinds of people do I want to work with?

• If I could have any job in the world, what would I choose?

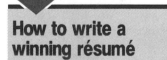

How to write a winning résumé

A well-written, neatly typed résumé is essential in getting the job you want. It's often the first impression potential employers receive of you and is often a key to your future contact with them.

Knowing what you want before changing jobs

Before changing jobs, be sure you know what you're looking for. Ask yourself the following questions: Which job factors are important to me? And of those, which are more important than others?

These same questions were posed to 581 nurses. Below are their answers, listed in the order of job factors they considered most important. To determine what's important to you, take the test yourself.

Check the factors you consider important and put them in order, from most important to least important. This will give you a definite sense of what's important to you in a new job.

Percentage of RNs who consider these job factors important

Reputation of hospital	98%	Personal safety	94%
Salary	98%	Type of hospital	86%
Shift and scheduling policies	97%	Number of specialty units	77%
Nurse-to-patient ratio	96%	Hospital size	76%
Educational benefits	95%	City hospital	66%
Fringe benefits	95%	Rural hospital	53%
Continuing-education assistance	94%	Internship program	51%
Advancement opportunities	94%	Social and recreational opportunities	36%

Therefore, you need to compose your résumé carefully, briefly summarizing your qualifications and experience, so a prospective employer will want to learn more about you and will invite you for an interview.

Certain basic components should be included in every résumé, but you'll have to decide what other information to include, how to organize the information, and what writing style to use.

Common formats

The two most common résumé formats are the chronological format and the achievement-oriented format. The chronological format, presenting a person's education and work history in reverse chronological order, is used more frequently. An achievement-oriented résumé presents a person's most impressive achievement first, followed by other achievements in descending order of importance.

Standard components

You should always include the following information in a résumé:

Identifying data. Every résumé should contain your full name (no nicknames), address, and the telephone number where you may be reached. (Make sure that you're available at the number you give or that someone will politely and accurately take your messages.)

Other information, like your age, marital status, and number of de-

How to write a winning cover letter

You should include a cover letter when you're responding to an employment advertisement or sending your résumé to the personnel office of an institution where you'd like to work. The letter should be concise, well-written and neatly typed, explaining why you wish to apply for a job. Hopefully, along with your résumé, it will convince a prospective employer to grant you an interview.

Follow this example to prepare your cover letter correctly:

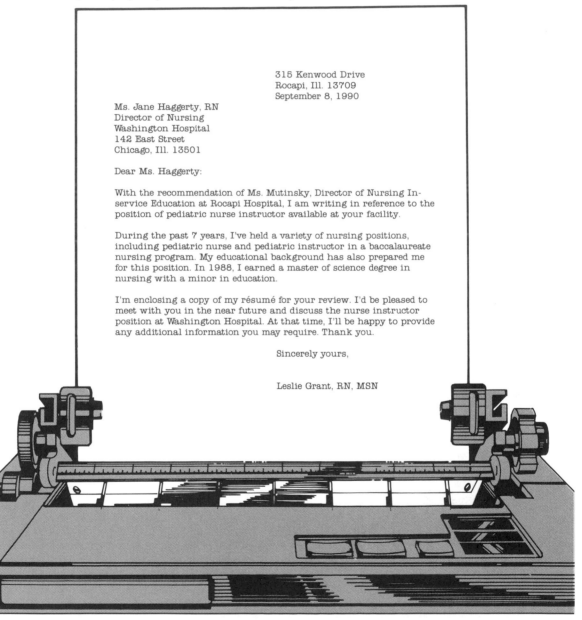

315 Kenwood Drive
Rocapi, Ill. 13709
September 8, 1990

Ms. Jane Haggerty, RN
Director of Nursing
Washington Hospital
142 East Street
Chicago, Ill. 13501

Dear Ms. Haggerty:

With the recommendation of Ms. Mutinsky, Director of Nursing In-service Education at Rocapi Hospital, I am writing in reference to the position of pediatric nurse instructor available at your facility.

During the past 7 years, I've held a variety of nursing positions, including pediatric nurse and pediatric instructor in a baccalaureate nursing program. My educational background has also prepared me for this position. In 1988, I earned a master of science degree in nursing with a minor in education.

I'm enclosing a copy of my résumé for your review. I'd be pleased to meet with you in the near future and discuss the nurse instructor position at Washington Hospital. At that time, I'll be happy to provide any additional information you may require. Thank you.

Sincerely yours,

Leslie Grant, RN, MSN

pendents, may be included, but it's not required. If you consider it an invasion of your privacy, then leave it out.

Educational qualifications. This section should begin with credentials related to your highest level of education, followed by the others in reverse chronological order.

Explain any degrees or credentials that have only local or regional significance. Include information about your continuing education, too. (You may want to spell this out in detail in another section of your résumé.)

The following examples show how you can briefly describe your educational experiences:
• "Diploma in Nursing, Tunley Hospital, 9/81 to 6/84.

"This 3-year, NLN-accredited school of nursing gave me the opportunity to learn in a large medical center affiliated with a local college. The psychiatric rotation was made available through the state mental health center. During this time I was active as an officer in the Student-Nurse Association.
• "B.S. in Nursing, Wenczel University, 9/85 to 6/89.

"This NLN-accredited baccalaureate program included clinical experiences at numerous hospitals and public health agencies. I was able to take a clinical elective in the coronary care unit for 5 weeks. My extracurricular activities included work on the university newspaper."
• "A.D. in Nursing, Pearl Ridge Community College, 9/88 to 6/90.

"This NLN-accredited, 2-year program included practice in two hospitals and a mental health center. The 5-week pediatric rotation took place in the local children's hospital. I graduated with honors from the school and received a recognition award from the pediatric nursing staff."

You'll have to decide whether to include information related to your educational record: your professional license or registration number, certificates you've earned, your class rank or standing.

Be sure to highlight certificates, such as the cardiopulmonary resuscitation certificate awarded by the Red Cross, and specialty certificates, given by the American Nurses' Association and the American Association of Critical Care Nurses — all very desirable credentials to have.

Do *not* include your state-board test results or school grades, although these may be discussed in the interview.

Employment background. Present your employment history in reverse chronological order on your résumé. Put your most recent or current position first, the one before that next, and so on. Be specific about your title. A charge nurse and a unit manager, or an assistant nursing director and a nursing supervisor, may or may not be synonymous in various parts of the country.

Don't forget to write "charge nurse duties" after "staff nurse" if taking charge was part of your job. To give your résumé that winning edge, you may want to describe, in a short paragraph, the major responsibilities each job involved. The following examples show how to highlight these jobs.
• "Staff Nurse, Emergency Room, Jonesville Hospital, 9/86 to 10/90.

"As a staff nurse in this trauma center emergency department, I was often assigned triage duty. I also developed written instructions for patients who were sent home with casts or sutures. In addition, I specialized in intervening with parents who were suspected of child abuse."
• "Staff Nurse, Medical Floor, Captree Hospital, 8/84 to 10/89.

"As a staff nurse on this 36-bed oncology and cardiovascular floor, I became comfortable in caring for adults with chronic disorders in these areas. I often had charge

duty and would delegate responsibilities to five or six other nursing-staff members. I instructed all the new employees on our unit in our discharge planning procedure."
• "Nurse Technician, Surgical Floor, Homeport Hospital, summer 1990.

"The technician position included nursing-aide duties and expanded responsibilities for patient care under an RN's guidance. On the surgical floor, I worked with the enterostomal therapist, teaching ostomy patients."

Information in this section of your résumé can vary in format, depending on how much you want to say. Decide, for example, whether you'll list, or list and describe, your previous jobs and whether you'll give your reasons for leaving those jobs. (This information is not required, although you may be asked about it in an employment interview.)

As a general rule, don't include your present salary, your salary history, or the salary you're looking for in your résumé. Salary negotiating is more appropriate during an interview.

Professional activities. The final section of your résumé focuses on your professional affiliations. Your memberships reflect your interest in various organizations and your support for their work toward improving the profession.

These memberships may also reflect your interest in maintaining your own competence, because many of these organizations are known for providing continuing education for their members.

Membership in health-related organizations that aren't specifically nursing organizations, such as heart, cancer, or arthritis associations, shows that you support research and public education.

Besides professional memberships, include volunteer work, committee work, offices you've held, and any honors you've received, such as certificates of recognition or attendance.

Also list honors you've received from educational institutions, community groups, your church, and your fellow nurses, which shows that others respect you.

List any professional articles or books you've published and any research you've done. Publishing books and articles reflects concern for your profession and an ability to communicate.

Other items to consider including
Although every résumé should contain the standard components discussed above, a winning résumé may include information considered optional, which may be what grabs an employer's attention. Optional information that can enhance your résumé includes dates of professional licensure or certification, references, continuing-education activities, and personal hobbies or interests.

References. Under this heading, you should state, "Available upon request." But have the list handy when you go to an interview, so you can give it to your prospective employer if he asks for it.

Include the names, addresses, titles, and telephone numbers of individuals who can personally endorse your professional and personal qualifications. Contact these individuals in advance to get permission to use their names—and their assurance that they not only can recommend you but also have time to write a reference.

Keep the list short, preferably four to six people. Two or three of your references should be professional people who have worked with you. The others should be personal references, people who can attest to your being mature, responsible, and trustworthy.

You might also include as references a previous supervisor, a school instructor, and professional colleagues. Sometimes a prospective employer will ask you to contact your references to request that they send him letters of recommendation.

Continuing-education activities. You can also add a list of your continuing-education experience to your résumé. Consider organizing these activities by topic to enhance your background. For example:
- Clinical Workshop on ECGs, State University, 6/85.
- Interpreting Laboratory Studies, In-service training, 9/87.
- Management Workshops, Time Management and Delegating for Nurse Managers, 7/90.
- Staffing Patterns, Belair College, 11/90.

Personal activities. Some search committees consider how well-rounded a person is, so you may want to include hobbies, volunteer work, and church or political activities in your résumé.

When you're making decisions about what to put in or leave out, try putting yourself in the place of the person who'll be reading your résumé. What information would make the best impression?

Overcoming the job interview jitters

For many people, a job interview can be a painful experience filled with awkward moments. But it doesn't have to be. A few guidelines can help you overcome any awkwardness.

The preliminaries
In order to feel composed and confident at a job interview, you have to do a lot of preparation.

Before any interview, take these steps:
- Respond to an employer's advertisement by sending a cover letter and your résumé to the prospective employer.
- In the letter, ask for a personal appointment with the director of nursing or whoever is in charge of hiring.
- Practice the interview. Rehearse the answers to foreseeable questions about your education, your nursing experience, why you want to change jobs or why you left your previous job, your duties in your last job, and your nursing philosophy.
- Be prompt on the day of the interview. You should arrive 10 minutes ahead of the scheduled time, if possible.
- Look your best for the interview. Dress conservatively, and make sure you're neatly groomed.

The interview: What to do
When you walk into the interviewer's office, follow these tips:
- Stand until the interviewer invites you to sit.
- Place any personal belongings beside you on the floor.
- Address the interviewer as Ms. or Mr. unless you're asked to use a first name.
- Don't slouch or fidget. Sit upright and be attentive.
- Don't chew gum or smoke cigarettes.
- Answer the interviewer's questions with confidence.

What to ask the interviewer
When the interviewer finishes questioning you, then it's your turn to ask questions. To evaluate the job and the hospital, ask about the following:
- Patient care assignments
- Staffing policies
- Advancement opportunities
- Continuing education
- Salary
- Working conditions and work shifts
- Employee benefits

How to answer an interviewer's questions

Expect certain questions to be asked at nearly every job interview. Prepare yourself by reading over the following commonly asked questions and noting the suggestions on how to answer them.

Why are you interested in this position?

You might begin by praising the institution's fine reputation, its philosophy of nursing, and its high regard for nurses. Be sure to talk specifically about the job you're applying for, the things about the position that attract you, as well as the opportunities the job presents for future advancement. Don't talk about money and fringe benefits, no matter how important they are to you. That's not really what the interview is about at this point.

What don't you like about your present job?

No matter how unhappy you are in your present job, don't complain about the management, the policies, the work load—don't complain about anything. You should accentuate the positive things the new job offers that the old job can't—for example, the opportunity to make a bigger contribution to patient care.

What kind of people do you feel uncomfortable working with?

Don't criticize your colleagues or supervisors at your present job. Instead, you should tell the interviewer that you don't like working with people who are uncooperative and uncommunicative.

What are your strengths and weaknesses?

Don't brag, but don't be modest, either. You should talk about two or three of your strongest points, giving the interviewer examples of how you've used those strengths. Rather than point out specific weaknesses, talk about areas that you're trying to improve upon or perfect.

Why did you become a nurse?

This is a very personal question. If you have a story to tell that will help you answer it, by all means tell it. Talk about things you've experienced since becoming a nurse that have reinforced your decision.

What do you want to be doing 5 years from now?

If you have specific plans, you should mention them. If you don't, give the interviewer a general answer: for example, that you'd like to move into management. Don't say you don't know what you want to do, because the interviewer may think you're unfocused and that you don't really care about your career.

Tell me about yourself

The interviewer wants to hear about your professional, not your personal life. You should give her a brief summary of your career, detailing a few of the highlights.

What an interviewer can and can't ask

During a job interview, you'll be asked many questions, most of which you can expect to be fair and appropriate. Some questions, however, are inappropriate or even prohibited by law. If you're asked such a question, don't feel obligated to answer it. You can discreetly refuse to answer or turn the conversation to another subject.

Legal questions	Illegal questions
• Have you ever worked for this company under a different name?	• What is your maiden name? Is the name on your application your real name?
• Where do you live? How long have you lived there?	• Where were you born? Where were your relatives born?
• Are you 18 years of age or older?	• How old are you? What is your birth date?
• Are you a citizen of the United States? If not, are you authorized to work in the U.S.? Can you verify your U.S. citizenship or your right to work in the United States?	• What is your native language? How did you learn to read, write, or speak a foreign language?
• What languages do you speak and write fluently?	• What is your religion?
• Do you belong to any organization which you consider relevant to your ability to perform this job?	• Are you married? What are your living arrangements?
• Have you ever been convicted of a criminal offense other than minor traffic violations?	• Do you have any children or plan to have children in the future?
	• Have you ever been arrested?

Also mention your clinical preferences and your long-term goals. Refer back to your strengths, relating them to the job for which you're applying.

What do you like least about nursing?

It's all right to mention one or two things that bother you, but don't go into a litany of grievances. On the other hand, don't sound smug by saying "Nothing."

What are your hobbies and interests?

Now is the time to go into your personal life a bit. Talk about community and volunteer work you've done, and talk about your family. You might also mention activities your participate in that make you a better nurse, for example, a sport that keeps you in shape. But be selective. Don't go overboard and tell the interviewer more than she could possibly want to know about you.

What can you contribute to this job?

Your personality and experience are what count here. You should tell the interviewer what you have that others don't, whether it's a technical skill, excellent rapport with patients, a knack for solving problems, or an ability to get along with colleagues. Try to make yourself stand out from the crowd.

What position interests you the most?

Don't answer this question by giving the interviewer job titles. Instead, talk about the skills you want to use, the patients you want to care for, and the future work you want to do.

Weighing the extras: Understanding fringe benefits

Fringe benefits—the "extras" a prospective employer offers in addition to the standard wage and benefits package—may not be central to your decision to take or turn down a particular job. But if you're weighing two job offers that are otherwise equally attractive, fringe benefits might tip the scales. The following chart lists some common and less common benefits, their basic features, and questions you should ask about each.

Benefit	Basic features	Questions to ask
Relocation and moving expenses	Employer reimbursements paid either when you move or periodically during your first year	Must you promise to work a specific period of time to receive this benefit?
Free housing	Free housing—for example, in a hotel—usually limited to 60 days	Will employer help you find suitable, permanent housing, or are you on your own?
Subsidized housing	Subsidized housing—in which you share the cost—usually for more than 60 days	Must you promise to work a specific period of time for this benefit?
Employer-sponsored credit union (CU)	Accounts similar to those offered by savings and loans or thrift institutions, but with higher interest rates on savings accounts and lower interest rates on loans. Some CUs will make automatic deductions from your payroll check. Some also offer checking accounts.	Do you have to be a CU member for a specific period of time—for example, 1 year—before you can obtain a loan? Does the CU have an annual membership fee? Is the CU's location convenient for you?
On-site child care center	Supervised day-care center	Is this service free? Does the center have any age restrictions for the children? (For example, does it only allow children between ages 3 and 6?) What are the center's hours of operation?

Keeping score of your interviews

Chances are you'll talk with a number of interviewers before deciding on the position that's right for you. While you're making the rounds, try to keep track of the working conditions at each job, the career opportunities, the salary, and the fringe benefits. This won't be easy. But to help you, use the following scorecard to rate the positions you investigate. Give each job opportunity a plus (+) or minus (−) for each question. When you've concluded your interviewing, add up the scores for each one, and compare the totals. The one with the highest score is probably the right one for you.

Scorecard	Hospital			
1. Were you given a written description of the responsibilities for the nursing position?				
2. Will you be responsible for a reasonable number of patients?				
3. Does the position offer opportunities for administrative and clinical advancement?				
4. Is the chain of command such that you'll report to a nursing administrator (for example, the director of nursing), or to a nonnursing administrator?				
5. Does the institution specify standards of nursing practice?				
6. Will you receive what sounds like adequate orientation for the position?				
7. Is the policy for department transfers fair?				
8. Is adequate professional liability insurance provided?				
9. Is the starting salary for the position acceptable?				
10. Are there shift and weekend differentials?				
11. Is shift rotation or floating required?				
12. Is the benefits package (health, life, and disability insurance, vacations, and holidays) good?				
13. Are there other benefits such as pharmacy discounts and child care services?				
14. Does the institution offer continuing education?				
15. Is there tuition reimbursement for continuing-education courses at colleges and universities?				
16. Are there special benefits for working weekends or holidays?				
17. Is flexible scheduling available (for example, work 3 days, off 3 days)?				
18. Does the area offer adequate and acceptable housing accommodations?				
19. Is subsidized housing available?				
20. Is transportation to and from work provided for all shifts?				
21. Are there patrolled parking facilities and escort services for late-night shifts?				
Total				

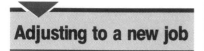

Adjusting to a new job

Whether you're fresh out of school and starting your first job, or you're an experienced nurse who's just changed positions, you're likely to feel nervous and uncomfortable. But these feelings don't last long. Here are some tips to help you adjust as quickly as possible:

When it's your first job after graduation
• Make the most of orientation, carefully observing procedures and volunteering to help with as many of them as possible. Learn by doing.
• Read policy manuals and review protocols for different procedures and treatments.
• Try to find an experienced staff member who's willing to act as your mentor. Make her your role model.
• Learn the role of a practicing nurse, which is very different from that of a student nurse. You'll have to handle a full patient load, cope with emergencies, and make decisions about patient care.
• Form support systems with co-workers and peers. Share the good times and the bad by trading stories about problems and mis-

takes. Try to develop good working relationships not just with nurses, but with your other colleagues as well.
• Keep learning. Attend nursing association meetings, read care plans, research clinical topics in the library. Study patients' charts, listen to the doctors when they make their rounds, and keep up to date on medications.
• Manage your time by learning to set priorities. If you have a hard time fitting everything in, analyze the areas where you have problems, then develop a timetable to help you accomplish all your tasks.
• Learn to cope with stress. Realize that everyone experiences stressful situations on the job and try to decide in advance how you'll deal with them. If you handle something badly, don't be too hard on yourself; instead, try to learn from the experience.
• Take care of your health. Make time for yourself and don't become overworked. Try not to make too many other major changes in your life, at least for the first few months on the job. Take your mind off your work with a hobby you enjoy.
• Be patient. Remember, adjusting to any new experience takes time. Soon, you'll be competent and self-assured in your role as a practicing nurse.

When you're an experienced nurse at a new job
• Accept the fact that your level of performance may drop at first. An unfamiliar environment often reduces effectiveness. If you don't fight the situation, it will pass quickly and you'll regain your old level of competence. Remember, no one expects you to be perfect right from the start.
• Don't brag about your last job to compensate for feelings of inadequacy in your new one. Just pitch in, work hard, and show you're willing to learn. This will earn you the respect of your colleagues.
• Don't try too hard to please. It's only natural to want your new co-workers to accept you. But your best bet is simply to be yourself, be businesslike, and be professional.
• Don't let the pressure get you down. Chances are you'll be so busy during your first few weeks on the job that you won't have time to reflect on whether you've made the right decision in taking the position. If you find yourself having doubts, remember your long-term goals and the reasons why you chose this job in the first place; this should help get you through this period of adjustment.

18 Managing your career

How to make better decisions

Decision making is like any other skill. The more you do it, the better you become at it. Follow these guidelines the next time you have to make an important decision.

Define the problem
Begin by carefully assessing what you're up against. Prepare a list of the problems you need to solve, starting with the most pressing and working your way down to those with the lowest priority. Then focus on one problem at a time, even if some of them overlap.

Consider your overall goal
After you've defined a problem, consider it in relationship to your overall goal. If your problem is the suctioning of a patient with copious secretions, remind yourself that your overall goal is to maintain a patent airway. Suctioning is just one way to achieve that goal. This simple example illustrates how considering your overall goal can expand your thinking and help you evaluate a problem within a larger context.

To help you relate a problem to your overall goal, try reducing the problem and goal to one clear statement. For example: "When caring for the patient with copious secretions, I must see that he maintains a patent airway." The clarity of such a statement will help you decide how to solve the problem.

Identify your options
List every possible solution you can think of. This will give you the luxury to pick and choose. It also has built-in benefits, such as preventing unwelcome surprises and reducing any fears you have of tackling the unknown.

Evaluate your options
By doing this, you can determine which options are considered practical, desirable, and adequate. Once you've weeded out those you think are inappropriate, check the similarities and differences among those options you have left.

Can you combine options? For example, as a patient on the coronary care unit improves, you might identify three options: transferring him to a step-down unit, transferring him to a medical unit, or assigning a senior nursing student with a special interest in cardiac nursing to care for him. In this case, the patient's need for less sophisticated moni-toring and the student's need for clinical experience combine to form the best alternative.

Consider your own values
As you evaluate your options, consider what's important to you. For example, will you put your own needs above the hospital's if you're asked to work overtime? Your values will help you identify priorities. You'll know where you can compromise and where you can't.

Use your resources
Before making a decision, ask for the advice of colleagues whose opinions you respect. If you've already made your decision, try to enlist the support of influential colleagues.

Develop a plan of action
When confronted with a complex problem, you may be tempted to put off making a decision about how to solve it. For instance, starting weekly case conferences may seem monumental. But instead of dragging your feet, tackle the problem by breaking it into smaller parts — subject, people, time, and place. Make decisions in steps. But be sure to set — and meet — deadlines, so you'll learn *not* to procrastinate.

Sort fact from fantasy

How many times have you said, "I wish that..." or "If only..."? Unfortunately, wishing won't do it. But dealing with your problem realistically will. For example, when you assign a nurse to a patient, do so based on your knowledge of her skills, not on the hope that she might be able to handle the case.

When sorting fact from fantasy, also determine what you can and cannot control. A high staff turnover or a doctor who's hard to get along with may be beyond your control. But you *can* control your feelings, attitudes, and expectations.

Reevaluate the decision

No decision is carved in stone. Instead of looking for universal rules to follow, you should consider the individual circumstances. Then determine how and when you'll reevaluate your decision. Remember, you can always change your mind, if necessary.

Improving your communication skills

One of the keys to working well with other people is communication. But chances are you probably don't know whether you're an effective communicator. So here are some techniques to help you evaluate and improve your communication skills:

• Throughout the course of one workday, keep a record of every conversation you have. In those conversations, did you do most of the talking or most of the listening? Which of these *should* you have been doing? Asking yourself these questions will make you more conscious of the proper role you should take in future conversations.

• Prior to an interview or meeting, write down what you expect the outcome to be. Afterward, decide if your expectations were accurate or realistic. What did you do, or not do, to fulfill them? Did others seem to have different expectations? What could you have done to resolve the differences?

• Following the next meeting you attend, take a moment and write down what you considered the major points. Then, ask others who also attended the meeting what exactly they thought the major points were. You may get different responses; if you do, try to figure out why.

• In the course of a conversation

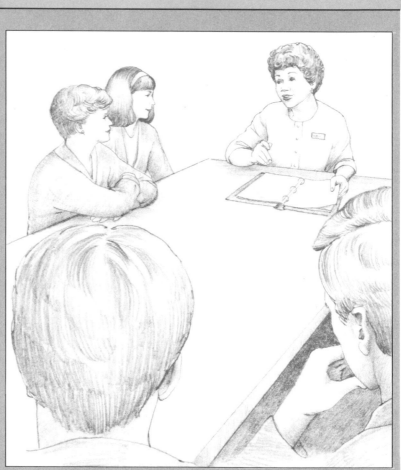

with someone, try to win that person over to your point of view. If you succeed in convincing him that your point of view is right, take a moment afterward and ask him what exactly you said or did that caused him to see things your way.

Overcoming communication barriers

To succeed in your relationships with your coworkers, you need effective communication skills. Otherwise, frequent misunderstandings, poor morale, and low productivity can result. Here are some common barriers to communication and tips on how to avoid or overcome them.

Communication barriers	How they result in miscommunication	How to avoid or overcome them
Being fearful	If you're not honest about your feelings (because they may reveal what you perceive as inadequacies), you may lie about your feelings in order to project the proper image.	Think of someone you're afraid to be honest with and say to her, "I have trouble telling you what I really feel and think about this matter." She'll probably be just as relieved as you are to talk about it.
Not listening	The person who wants to tell you something will not get through to you if you're thinking about something else while she's talking.	Use active listening: concentrate on the speaker's words and restate them to be sure you've heard them correctly. This clarifies communication and shows the speaker that you understand her feelings.
Being defensive	Instead of listening, you may be thinking of ways you can enhance your image, escape punishment, dominate, or win.	Recognize the kind of behavior that makes you defensive. When someone displays that behavior, tell her you're uncomfortable with her message as you're hearing it.
Suppressing feelings	Refusing to recognize your own feelings during a conversation prevents you from taking proper action in the situation.	Learn to analyze your feelings during a conversation, and then to communicate them, such as, "I'm feeling annoyed...happy...afraid."
Not giving feedback	Refusing to communicate your reaction to what someone is saying to you increases the chances of misunderstanding.	Offer feedback in a supportive way. Also, provide feedback as soon as possible after the conversation, so both of you can remember the details. Confine your feedback to your own feelings; don't try to tell her how she feels.
Giving advice	Telling someone what you think she should do makes her defensive, reduces her self-esteem.	Practice active listening, giving the person your time, not your advice or opinions.
Being excessively repetitive	Repetition lulls the person into not listening, because she's heard it before.	Listen to yourself. Say what you want to say once, as clearly as possible, and ask for a specific response.
Being distracted	Being concerned with other matters prevents you from listening effectively, causing you to miss or misunderstand the other person's message.	Concentrate on using active listening techniques. If you can't concentrate, interrupt to deal with the distraction.
Using inappropriate language	Using words unfamiliar or offensive to the other person prevents her from understanding—and sometimes from accepting—your message.	Choose your words carefully, being aware of the situation you're in and the person to whom you're talking.

Using your time more effectively

You probably accomplish a great deal during your busy workday, but you could be even more productive if you managed your time better. Below are some practical methods for managing your time and tips on how to avoid on-the-job time-wasters.

Time-management techniques

To use your time effectively, you have to plan ahead. This includes establishing goals and identifying objectives. You'll need to distinguish between long-term and short-term goals, assigning to them priorities that will help determine the order in which you go about accomplishing them.

Here are several common and successful time-management techniques that can enable you to keep focused on your goals and get the maximum use of your time.

Write a daily to-do list. Each day, compose a list of all the tasks you must perform. Give each item a priority. For example, designate a task you consider critically important an A priority. Use a B priority for moderately important tasks and a C priority for tasks of minimal importance.

Concentrate first on A-priority tasks. Resist the temptation to proceed first with C-priority tasks, which are often fairly straightforward, easily accomplished, and promise a quick return for your effort.

You may feel satisfied crossing C-priority tasks off your to-do list, but it won't help you achieve your more important goals. Remember, when you work on C-priority tasks, you're using valuable time that would be better spent completing tasks with A priorities.

When you find yourself with a few extra minutes, tackle an A-priority task. If you don't have time to complete the task, you can at least do a portion of it. By taking this portion-at-a-time approach, you're breaking down a difficult task into smaller, more manageable tasks.

Establish deadlines. Deadlines provide you with target dates and help you avoid delays. Deadlines become particularly important when you're working toward a goal that involves achieving many objectives along the way.

Concentrate on one task at a time. By doing this, you can complete that task in a minimal amount of time with as little aggravation as possible. This is particularly true when you must suddenly deal with a potential crisis, which automatically becomes an A priority.

Avoid distractions. Distractions interrupt your concentration and rob you of precious time. For example, nurses' stations are notoriously noisy and busy. If the noise there distracts you while you're trying to do your charting, find a quiet place where you can complete the task quickly and more accurately.

Delegate tasks. This takes time initially because you have to know your staff's skills, knowledge, and interests well. But delegating tasks can help you use your time more effectively, so it's worth the initial effort.

When you delegate a task, make sure you clearly assign responsibility, grant authority, and create accountability. You and the staff member to whom you delegate a task must understand the desired outcome and the deadline. Decide, too, how frequently you'll assess a staff member's progress in completing a delegated task.

Avoid postponements. Putting off a task until the last minute can waste time and increase stress. Working under severe stress can increase your mental and physical fatigue, and it may take twice as long to complete a task because you're tired. Similarly, when you're asked to complete a task that's an A priority for your supervisor but a C priority for you, don't waste time complaining. Perform the task competently and as soon as you can.

Make appointments. Arrange appointments to meet with people who are helping you get your work done or achieve your goals. Appointments let each of you know the meeting's purpose. Then you can set aside the necessary time and come prepared. For instance, if you want to talk to your head nurse about your performance appraisal, schedule an appointment with her and tell her what you want to talk about.

Don't answer the telephone. Let the unit's secretary answer the phone, unless she's extremely busy. When you do answer it, usually the call isn't for you, and you'll have to find the person or the information the caller wants. This may not be particularly difficult, but it takes time, *your* time.

Keep a daily time log. To help identify time-wasting activities, keep a daily time log and review it regularly to see how you're spending your time. You don't need an elaborate journal, just a written log of the tasks you perform during the day. Fill in the log at regular intervals, such as every 15 minutes, for a week. Though you don't need to keep a time log for any specific period, the longer you keep it, the more data you'll have to help you identify the activities that waste time.

Activities that waste time: Minimizing their effects
Certain activities eat away at valuable time, forcing you to miss deadlines and creating stress. Here's a list of a nurse's most common time-wasting activities and some tips on how to minimize their effects.

Interruptions. Interruptions are a fact of daily life in nursing. Moreover, most interruptions are part of your job, and some, like a family's requests for information, simply can't be avoided. But if you've identified your goals, you can get back on track after any interruption by asking yourself: "What's the best use of my time right now?" This will help, once you've dealt with the interruption, to refocus your efforts toward your original goals.

Crises. You can't avoid crises, but you can keep them to a minimum by planning—for example, dealing with a doctor assertively now, to avoid a possible crisis later—and by using time-management techniques. When crises do arise, don't panic. Use your skills to confront one task at a time.

Once a crisis has passed, don't forget how you reacted to it. Learn from each crisis by analyzing it and asking yourself: "How and why did this crisis happen? How did I handle it? What can I do to prevent it or a similar crisis from occurring?" Remember, every crisis you can prevent means more time for you.

Socializing with coworkers. Socializing at work wastes considerable amounts of time, so keep it to a minimum. When coworkers want to socialize, politely tell them that you have work to do. Otherwise, you'll come to a day's end and find you haven't accomplished your goals.

Misidentifying the problem. Fostering a problem-solving climate is an excellent time-management technique. But problem solving can become a serious time-waster if you haven't first clearly identified the problem. So be sure to get all the facts before taking action.

Excessive paperwork. Most nurses consider excessive paperwork a significant time-waster. But paperwork is necessary to ensure documentation and continuity of care. You can't avoid paperwork, so don't postpone it. Just do it, and don't waste time complaining about it.

When you have to enter the same information on several different forms, try combining the paperwork to get it done faster. If you have a suggestion on how to alleviate paperwork, confer with your coworkers and supervisors.

Inability to say no. Learn to say no logically, rationally, and tactfully. When you're asked to accept an additional responsibility or to work an extra shift, consider your own—and your patients'—priorities. If you say yes, will you be able to achieve your goals according to the priorities you've established for that particular day? If the answer is no and you decide to refuse the extra work, don't feel guilty.

Initiating change

Change is an ever-present force in nursing, regardless of what position you're in. New technologies, new procedures, and new management ideas are constantly affecting nurses.

The effective nurse anticipates change, initiates it, or takes action to direct it in order to improve patient care and working conditions for herself and her nursing colleagues.

What follows are some practical steps you can take to make change work for you.

Identify the problem correctly
Exactly what is the problem? More change efforts falter at this step than at any other because nurses fail to understand or carefully define the problem they're trying to solve.

Enlist others who want change
Do others share your desire to bring about change? Are they willing to work for it with you? You'll find that some coworkers want change but aren't willing to contribute to the process. Ideally, you should know from the start how much real support you can count on.

You'll be able to help bring about change more easily if you have a support group sharing the work. Recruit those who can present your argument for change persuasively—someone who can write, someone who knows her way around the organization and power structure, and someone who has influence on the right committees. Once you recruit them, keep them enthusiastic and involved.

Gather the facts
Collect data to help you identify the problem or the factors that contribute to the problem, as well as its effects on the staff, the patients, and the patients' families. To gather the data, you'll need to ask yourself the following questions:
• What factors have contributed to this problem?
• What are the financial implications of not resolving the problem? (While you may not have all of the financial data you need for this analysis, you can suggest the general financial implications of not resolving the problem.)

• What effects has this problem had on staff, on patients, and on patients' families?

• Has this problem affected other departments and disciplines as well? If so, how?

• What are the organizational implications of continuing the status quo without resolving this problem?

Find a practical solution

Once you've accurately diagnosed the problem, work with the support group to arrive at a practical solution by brainstorming, and compile a list of the possible solutions that this process yields.

Then examine each solution by asking several questions. What are the risks involved in this solution? Is the solution feasible in terms of cost, time, resources, and potential obstacles? Will it improve staff morale and productivity? Or will it generate resistance?

Finally, choose the best solution from among the ones you've examined.

Know the power structure

To succeed in your plan for change, you must know your institution's power structure and its resources.

Why its power structure? Because the simple fact is you'll never institute lasting change without access to people in positions of power, those ultimately responsible for accepting and implementing new ideas.

Why the institution's resources? Because those with the power to approve your change will want to know what materials or personnel you'll need to implement the change, whether they're presently available or have to be purchased or hired, and the costs involved. You'll be competing for allocations with other individuals and groups, so careful documentation is critical to your strategy.

Plan each step – and choose one course of action

Too many of those who initiate change have good ideas but fail to plan wisely. Develop a course of action, indicating what to do first, second, third, and so on. Then develop alternative plans in case your initial plan doesn't work.

Don't make the mistake of launching several courses of action simultaneously. This will cause confusion, waste energy and resources, and may ultimately fail. Also, pursuing several courses of action at once makes evaluating the effectiveness of any one of them difficult. If your plan of choice doesn't work, then try one of your alternative plans.

A practical point to remember is that when you choose a solution, begin implementing it on a small scale. Remember, you stand the best chance of succeeding if you implement the change in a unit strongly in favor of it and and excited by it.

Choose an effective strategy

Once you've established a plan for change, you need a strategy to implement it. Two of the more common strategies are coercion and cooperation.

Coercion entails using power or authority to force change. To use this strategy, you need position power and reward power. Understandably, this strategy usually breeds resentment and resistance.

Cooperation, the most time-consuming strategy, requires your using interpersonal skills and open communication techniques. The gains secured by cooperation tend to meet the least resistance and last the longest. Build into your plan strategies to decrease resistance. For example, include doctors, not just nurses, in your support group.

Implement your change

To implement the change, make sure everyone involved clearly understands the new procedures. Let it be known, through official channels like the institution's newsletter and by word-of-mouth, when the change has proved successful. Be prepared to iron out any problems that emerge by making adjustments in your plan. Remember, be flexible.

Evaluate the results

Establish evaluation criteria before you initiate the change, as a method for measuring its success. Analyze the change's result by asking the following questions: Was the problem solved? What evidence shows this? Were the best means used to solve the problem?

Make the change last

Take measures to reinforce and maintain the change. Keep the channels of communication open among coworkers to minimize any growing resistance to the change. Continue follow-up measures until the change becomes an established part of the system. Remember, unless the change becomes part of everyday routine, you can lose all that you've accomplished.

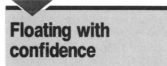

Floating with confidence

Floating to an unfamiliar unit – and sometimes even a familiar one – strikes fear in the hearts of many good nurses. You may worry about using skills you feel are rusty, about leaving work you know and enjoy. To deal with the pressures of floating, follow these tips.

Act professionally

When you float to a new unit, introduce yourself to the charge nurse and tell her your usual clinical responsibilities. Be cooperative and respectful, using a self-assured voice and maintaining eye contact. Show your willingness to work. The charge nurse will realize that you're assertive and able to handle yourself.

As introductions are made and assignments are given, assess the charge nurse as a leader and as a resource person. If she has a laissez-faire approach or isn't available as a resource, ask her to designate a specific nurse to help you. You have a right to request this, for the good of your patients.

If the charge nurse is autocratic or overly direct about responsibilities you're uncomfortable fulfilling, gently but firmly define your capabilities. Reassure her that you plan to stay in touch with her to offer periodic reports about your work. But don't take her need for information personally. After all, you have the authority to care for patients, but she's ultimately accountable for what happens on the unit.

Clarify your assignment, communicate your limits
Find out as much as you can about what's expected of you on the unit and what the usual routine is. When are meals served? Who takes patients to other departments? What are the visiting hours? Get a report on the patients assigned to you and be sure that the assignments are appropriate, never accepting any you're not qualified to handle. If you have any reservations about your assignment, tell the charge nurse and suggest an alternative plan. Remember, making safety your first priority protects both you and your patients.

Get the job done
After you've accepted the assignment, make the best of the situation. Approach coworkers in a spirit of cooperation. Ask someone to familiarize you with the unit layout and procedures. If you find that you have extra time, offer to

help with other patients. Be flexible. Integrate your style of doing things with the way the staff does things on the unit. Use your floating experience to learn new things, to share information, and to test your interpersonal and professional skills.

Evaluate your performance
At the end of the shift, you'll have many thoughts and feelings about the experience. To determine how well you did, consider the dynamics of the situation. What was the atmosphere on the unit? How could you have been better accepted into the work group? What did you need that you didn't get? What was the quality of your patient care?

If the atmosphere was friendly, with supportive leadership and staff, then examine your performance against your usual self-expectations. If the situation was tense, chaotic, hostile, or volatile, don't be as critical.

In difficult situations, set realistic expectations about the quality of your care and your influence on the unit. Accept the limitations imposed by an environment beyond your control, and don't be overly critical if your performance is less than perfect. Use what you learned in the situation to make your next floating experience more satisfying.

Understaffing: What to do about it

If you're a charge nurse and you find that your unit is understaffed, you need a strategy with the long-term goal of minimizing understaffing on your unit before it happens. Be prepared to take problem-solving action to help assure quality health care for your patients and quality working con-

ditions for you and other health care team members. Here's how to go about it.

Rally support
Begin by rallying support from your colleagues. Call a meeting with the unit staff, your supervisor, and the staffing coordinator. List the attendees and take meeting minutes. At the meeting, review a copy of the hospital's staffing standards and policies. Find out if nurses or their support staff are performing nonnursing responsibilities. Then encourage nurses to air their concerns.

Once you've obtained the basic staffing information you need and you've identified basic problems, form a committee to develop and present your request for additional staffing. Assign several committee members to obtain information from other hospitals on their staffing patterns.

Know the numbers
When you're ready to start putting information on paper, remember that management consists predominantly of business people. So you must present your request in their language — numbers. Your task is to show how your staff's available nursing-care hours fall short of the number the administration recommended for adequately meeting patient needs.

Identify patterns in understaffing, too. Does understaffing occur at a certain time of year? On certain shifts? On weekends? If you discover a pattern, try to find the reason for it. For example, is staffing allocated unevenly, with overstaffing on certain days or shifts? Are weekend shifts half-staffed without any supplementation? Does the administration consider staff's vacation days and holidays when drawing up their schedule? Is absenteeism a problem?

Once you've discovered a pattern and determined why it occurs, demonstrate why the short staffing is inadequate. First, list all nursing tasks and procedures. Indicate the time required to complete each task. Then pinpoint the tasks usually left undone and figure out the number of extra staff members you'd need to complete these tasks.

Think ahead

Present your request at the right time. Don't wait until Saturday afternoon to handle weekend staffing problems. Do it during the week. Don't discuss summer shortages in May, June, or July. Anticipate the problems and present your requests during the preceding fall and winter months.

Be prepared for opposing arguments such as, "That doesn't have to be done every day," or, "That's not necessary on the weekend." Refute these comments with several verifiable examples of patient complaints and incidents, accidents and errors, all of which may occur because of understaffing.

Realize the other benefits

Solving staffing problems can have other benefits as well, such as easing your work load, improving working conditions on the unit, stabilizing the nursing staff, and improving patient care.

Remember, too, that failing to deal with poor staffing, or submitting to the administration's decisions, is questionable from a legal standpoint. By identifying problems and attempting to assure standards in patient care, you diminish legal risks on your unit.

If your efforts to get action at the administrative level fail, you do have recourse outside the administration. The medical board at your hospital may agree to review your data. If they agree with your conclusion, the board—a powerful ally—can put additional pressure on the administration.

How to calculate nursing-care hours

When you realize your unit is understaffed, you should bring it to your administrator's attention. But before you do, first figure out how many more nurses you'll need for adequate staffing. To calculate the amount, follow these steps:

1. Get a copy of your hospital's patient classification system, which categorizes patients by the number of nursing-care hours (NCHs) they need each day or each shift. If your hospital doesn't have such a list, draw one up by analyzing the care you give your patients, breaking down that care into distinct tasks, and determining how much time it takes to complete each task. Then, *patient by patient*, take that itemized list and determine how many NCHs each patient needs. Take these totals and divide your patients into classes, as follows:
• Class I patient needs up to 1 NCH per shift
• Class II patient needs between 1 and 2 NCHs per shift
• Class III patient needs between 2 and 3 NCHs per shift

2. Multiply the number of patients in each classification by the greatest number of NCHs they need. This figure will represent the total NCHs your patients require each shift.

$$25 \text{ Class I} \times 1 \text{ hr} = 25 \text{ NCHs}$$
$$20 \text{ Class II} \times 2 \text{ hr} = 40 \text{ NCHs}$$
$$5 \text{ Class III} \times 3 \text{ hr} = 15 \text{ NCHs}$$
$$\text{Total} = 80 \text{ NCHs}$$

3. Divide the per-shift NCHs by 7, the number of NCHs one full-time nurse provides during a shift, allowing for a meal break. This figure represents the minimal number of nurses your unit needs per shift to meet your patients' needs.

$$80 \text{ NCHs} \div 7 = 11.4 \text{ (12 nurses)}$$

Resolving conflicts with your supervisor

Inevitably, you'll disagree with your supervisor at one time or another—over a clinical procedure, a work role, or a personal matter. When this happens, you'll want to resolve the disagreement as amicably as possible. Follow these guidelines:

Know the facts. Frequently, once you gather all the facts, you'll discover that the grounds for disagreement dissolve.

Know what you want to achieve. Focus on your goal once you've identified it. Don't cloud the issue by bringing up other problems.

Choose how and when to discuss the disagreement. What you're disagreeing about dictates your approach. For example, you should discuss a patient-safety disagreement immediately. But you can wait to discuss a disagreement over work rules.

Choose a private place. Never air your disagreement in front of other staff members. Having others around won't give you the "safety in numbers" you might expect, and will probably put your supervisor on the defensive.

Be discreet. Don't discuss your disagreement with other staff members. If you do, your supervisor may hear a distorted version from someone else before you even get a chance to approach her.

Follow the proper channels. Always discuss your disagreement with your immediate supervisor first. Give her the opportunity to resolve the disagreement before you go to a higher authority.

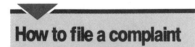

How to file a complaint

Whenever you have a complaint about your job, you should bring it to your supervisor's attention. But make sure you follow your institution's grievance procedure. If your institution doesn't have a grievance procedure, then follow these guidelines:

Meet with your supervisor
• Approach your supervisor and ask to meet privately with her to discuss your complaint. Note the date when you take this step and any subsequent steps.
• If your supervisor puts off your request for a meeting, write up the complaint and submit it to her. Make sure you keep a copy for your records.

• Whether you present your complaint verbally or in writing, make sure it's factual (don't include opinion or hearsay), to the point (don't ramble), specific (don't generalize), and fair (don't attack others).

State your complaint properly
A *properly stated complaint* would be: "I've requested two special days off, at the beginning of October and in the middle of June. You've turned down my requests both times. I haven't received any explanation why my requests were denied. I'd like to discuss this matter with you."
    An *improperly stated complaint* would be: "Why don't you ever grant my requests for days off? I'm constantly amazed at how the rest of the staff always gets what they want. I'd like to know if there's something about me that you don't like. I do my best to please you, but you've obviously chosen to ignore my requests. I demand to know why."

Wait for your supervisor to respond
• You should give your supervisor time to respond to your complaint. Wait several days before approaching her again.
• If your supervisor still fails to respond or doesn't give you a satisfactory answer, tell her you intend to go to a higher authority with your complaint. This will give her one final opportunity to take action.
• If your supervisor still fails to take any action, you should then make an appointment with a higher authority. The higher authority will want to review your complaint and the record you've kept of how you've handled the situation. She may invite your supervisor to come to the meeting with you so the issue is confronted openly.

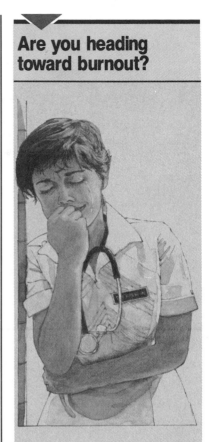

Are you heading toward burnout?

Do you feel you're constantly under a great deal of stress? That you're on the way to burning out? If you're not sure, decide how many of the following statements apply to you. More than two "yes" answers means you're at risk and that you need to improve your ability to handle stress.

• I'm always exhausted.
• I can't get much sleep.
• I can't seem to relax.
• I'm becoming more cynical.
• I'm often impatient and irritable.
• I feel unappreciated.
• I don't seem to care about my job any more.
• I don't feel well much of the time.
• I often feel depressed.
• I feel overburdened with work.

How to measure your stress level

You may not be aware of just how harmful stress can be. To measure the amount of stress you've experienced in the past 24 hours, take the following test. It lists the 20 work situations, rated by staff nurses in a survey, as those they considered the most stressful. Each work situation has been assigned a stress value. Check those you've experienced, total up their stress values, interpreting your score using the scale at the end of the test.

Stressful work situation	Experienced in past 24 hours	
Assuming responsibilities you're not trained to handle	_____	67
Working with unqualified personnel	_____	64
Dealing with nonsupportive supervisors or administrators	_____	61
Working with an insufficient staff	_____	58
Caring for a patient who's having a cardiac arrest	_____	55
Experiencing conflict with coworkers	_____	52
Dealing with a dying patient's family	_____	49
Caring for a dying patient	_____	46
Working with broken or faulty equipment	_____	44
Working with inadequate supplies	_____	42
Working an inconvenient shift or schedule	_____	38
Assuming responsibilities without thanks or recognition	_____	36
Dealing with a difficult doctor	_____	34
Trying to communicate with a bureaucracy	_____	31
Discharging a patient unprepared for discharge	_____	28
Caring for a seriously ill patient	_____	25
Spending long periods of time on paperwork or telephone duties	_____	22
Having a problem over salary or promotion	_____	19
Working with a demanding or noncompliant patient	_____	16
Coordinating supplemental personnel	_____	13
	Your total _____	**Total possible score 800**

The higher your score, the more stress you've experienced in the past 24 hours. You can estimate your present stress level as follows:

0-133 You're under minimal stress, not enough to cause you many problems.

134-266 You're under moderate stress. This is the highest level of stress you should permit yourself on a day-to-day basis.

267-532 You're experiencing high-level stress. You have trouble relaxing, and you become annoyed easily. Do what you can to reduce the stress you're experiencing at work: try relaxation techniques, exercise, and pursuing outside interests to relieve your stress.

533-800 You're under extreme stress. Get help quickly. You're a prime candidate for burnout and serious physical or emotional problems if you let this level of stress continue.

Minimizing stress by working more efficiently

Stress can make your work more difficult and less enjoyable. Your job will always involve some degree of stress, but you can manage it better if you learn to work more efficiently. This chart shows how you can plan ahead to minimize the effects of stress on the job.

You're working inefficiently when:	You're working more efficiently when:
• You rush around searching for needed supplies.	• You keep bedside units and crash carts fully stocked with supplies.
• You must call a doctor twice because you weren't organized or concentrating the first time you spoke to him, so you forgot important information.	• You write down what you plan to report before you telephone a doctor. • You read the doctor your notes. • You write down orders the doctor gives you and read them back to him. • You document that you repeated the orders and that the doctor confirmed them.
• You allow demanding activities to pile up until you're too tired to do them efficiently.	• You plan to do the most demanding activities when you're most alert during the shift. • You alternate tasks you like and dislike.
• You try to keep track of all routine tasks without writing anything down.	• You develop checklists to simplify keeping track of routine tasks.
• You use narrative charting on multiple charting forms.	• You use checklists and flowcharts for charting as often as possible.
• You document at shift's end.	• You document when you complete one task before you go on to the next.
• You react strongly to annoyances and cause hurt feelings.	• You take time to cool off when you're angry so you won't say something you'll regret.
• You focus on a problem's difficulty.	• You focus on ways to solve the problem.
• You complain to coworkers when a problem develops.	• You talk to the person who can solve the problem.
• You complain to coworkers that patients demand too much.	• You make expectations and limits clear to patients.
• You delay decisions.	• You make decisions and act on them.
• You do the work that inefficient nurses have overlooked.	• You challenge others' inefficient work habits constructively.
• You do float nurses' work as well as your own.	• You orient float nurses to your unit and offer to help them when they need it.
• You work longer hours and more overtime.	• You pace yourself to get your work finished in the allotted time.
• You skip exercise because you're too tired and rushed.	• You exercise regularly to relieve tension.

Controlling stress by listening to yourself

Certain psychological factors can increase job-related stress by making problems seem bigger than they really are. To make matters worse, recognizing these psychological factors within ourselves is difficult because we've grown so used to the quirks in our personalities that we're often blind to them.

The following list of psychological distortions, with examples of each, will help you recognize whether you have these same tendencies, which you can then try to eliminate because they only cause you added stress.

Filtering

Selectively eliminating some details of a conversation or event to find fault with yourself.

Example: You've just finished a detailed care plan for a difficult patient when your supervisor compliments you and says, "I wish you'd write care plans like that for all your patients." You bristle and say to yourself, "She's always criticizing me. Nothing I do is good enough."

Internalizing

Blaming yourself for every problem, feeling that everyone at work depends on you, and feeling guilty for not doing work you think is expected of you.

Example: As you check a despondent patient at the end of your shift, he accuses you of not spending enough time with him. You've worked hard to apportion your time to all your patients, but driving home, you think, "He's right. I should've talked to him more about his problems."

Externalizing

Blaming only others for your problems, never yourself.

Example: Your supervisor asks you to work a couple of hours overtime to help care for an obese cardiac patient whose condition has deteriorated. When you get home, your family is angry because you didn't call to say you'd be late. You think, "It's all her fault. This never would happen if she'd staff properly."

Overgeneralizing

Thinking in absolute terms and exaggerating, drawing a broad conclusion from a shred of evidence.

Example: Your supervisor asks you to float to an intensive care unit. You set the rate on a monitor incorrectly and have to write an incident report. You tell your supervisor, "I'll never accept a float assignment again."

Polarizing

Thinking in extremes, seeing everything in black and white, with no gray areas.

Example: A postoperative renal patient on your unit puts on his call light several times a day. Even though you know he's in pain, you remark to a friend, "He complains all the time about nothing."

Using "shoulds"

Using inflexible rules about how you and others should act, disallowing any deviation from the rules.

Example: You firmly believe that patients should cooperate with their care. So when Mr. Boughton refuses to take his medication, you become angry and delay answering his call light each time he rings it that afternoon. You think, "Why should I work so hard when he won't cooperate?"

Needing to be right

Thinking that you're always right, that anyone who disagrees with you is wrong.

Example: "I've been catheterizing patients since before you were born," you tell a new graduate nurse, who wants to show you a new technique. "I don't need a new technique."

Transferring to another unit to relieve stress

Sometimes the only way you can relieve the relentless stress of a particular job is to transfer to another unit. To do this properly, follow these steps:

• Put your request for transfer in writing, specifying the unit and shift you want. Then briefly list your reasons for requesting the transfer, keeping the tone of the request positive. Make three copies of the request, keeping one for yourself.

• Tell your current supervisor about your request and give her a copy. Maintain rapport with her, even though you hope to leave.

• Make an appointment with the person who initiates transfers in your hospital, and give her your request personally. Explain why you want to transfer—for example, that you want new or different challenges.

• Follow up on your request in a few weeks to show the supervisor in charge of transfers that you're serious about your decision.

• If you get approval, don't expect the transfer immediately. You may have to wait for an opening or for management to find a replacement for you on your current unit.

Directory of professional organizations

International

International Council of Nurses and the Florence Nightingale International Foundation
3 Place Jean-Marteau
CH-1201 Geneva, Switzerland

Pan American Health Organization
WHO Regional Office for the Americas
525 23rd St., NW
Washington, D.C. 20037
(202) 861-3200

People to People Health Foundation (Project Hope)
Millwood, Va. 22646
(703) 837-2100

World Health Organization
Avenue Appia
CH-1211 Geneva 27, Switzerland
(022) 791-21-11

Canada

National organization

Canadian Nurses Association
50 The Driveway
Ottawa, Ont. K2P 1E2
(613) 237-2133

Provincial professional associations/Boards of Nursing

Alberta
Alberta Association of Registered Nurses
11620 168th St.
Edmonton, Alta. T5M 4A6
(403) 426-0160

Alberta Association of Registered Nursing Assistants
17410 107th Ave.
Edmonton, Alta. T5S 1E9
(403) 483-8126

British Columbia
Registered Nurses' Association of British Columbia
2855 Arbutus St.
Vancouver, B.C. V6J 3Y8
(604) 736-7331

British Columbia Council of Licensed Practical Nurses
3405 Willingdon Ave.
Burnaby, B.C. V5G 3H4
(604) 660-5750

Manitoba
Manitoba Association of Registered Nurses
647 Broadway Ave.
Winnipeg, Man. R3C 0X2
(204) 774-3477

Manitoba Association of Licensed Practical Nurses
1-130 Marion
Winnipeg, Man. R2H 0T4
(204) 222-6743

New Brunswick
New Brunswick Association of Registered Nurses
231 Saunders St.
Fredericton, N.B. E3B 1N6
(506) 454-5591

Association of New Brunswick Registered Nursing Assistants
39 Coventry Crescent
Fredericton, N.B. E3B 4P4
(506) 454-0747

Newfoundland
Association of Registered Nurses of Newfoundland
55 Miltary Rd., P.O. Box 6116
St. John's, N.F. A1C 5X8
(709) 753-6040

Northwest Territory
Northwest Territory Registered Nurses' Association
Box 2757
Yellowknife, N.W.T. X0E 1H0
(403) 873-2745

Nova Scotia
Registered Nurses' Association of Nova Scotia
6035 Coburg Rd.
Halifax, N.S. B3H 1Y8
(902) 423-6156

Nova Scotia Board of Registration for Nursing Assistants
5614 Fenwick St.
Halifax, N.S. B3H 1P9
(902) 423-8517

Ontario
College of Nurses of Ontario
101 Davenport Rd.
Toronto, Ont. M5R 3P1
(416) 486-5460

Registered Nurses' Association of Ontario
33 Price St.
Toronto, Ont. M4W 1Z2
(416) 923-3523

Prince Edward Island
Association of Nurses of Prince Edward Island
P.O. Box 1838
Charlottetown, P.E.I. C1A 7N5
(902) 892-6322

(continued)

Directory of professional organizations (continued)

Prince Edward Island Licensed Nursing Assistants Association
P.O. Box 1253
Charlottetown, P.E.I. C1A 7M8
(902) 566-1512

Quebec
Order of Nurses of Quebec
4200 Dorchester Blvd. W.
Montreal, Que. H3Z 1V4
(514) 935-2501

Professional Alliance of Quebec Nurses Aides
132 Blvd. Labelle, Rm. 220
Rosemere, Que. J7A 2H1
(514) 437-1511

Saskatchewan
Saskatchewan Registered Nurses' Association
2066 Retallack St.
Regina, Sak. S4T 2K2
(306) 527-4643

Yukon Territory
There are no associations for nurses in the Yukon.

United States

National organizations

Alpha Tau Delta National Fraternity for Professional Nurses
5207 Mesada St.
Alta Loma, Calif. 91701
(714) 980-3536

American Academy of Ambulatory Nursing Administration
Box 56, N. Woodbury Rd.
Pitman, N.J. 08071
(609) 582-9617

American Association of Colleges of Nursing
1 Dupont Circle, Suite 530
Washington, D.C. 20036
(202) 463-6930

American Association of Critical-Care Nurses
One Civic Plaza
Newport Beach, Calif. 92660
(714) 644-9310

American Association of Nephrology Nurses and Technicians
Box 56, N. Woodbury Rd.
Pitman, N.J. 08071
(609) 589-2187

American Association of Neuroscience Nurses
218 N. Jefferson St. #204
Chicago, Ill. 60606
(708) 993-0043

American Association of Nurse Anesthetists
216 Higgins Rd.
Park Ridge, Ill. 60068
(708) 692-7050

American Association of Occupational Health Nurses
50 Lenox Pointe
Altanta, Ga. 30324
(404) 262-1162

American Cancer Society
1599 Clifton Rd.
Atlanta, Ga. 30329
(404) 320-3333

American College of Nurse-Midwives
1522 K St., NW, Suite 1120
Washington, D.C. 20005
(202) 347-5445

American Heart Association
7320 Greenville Ave.
Dallas, Tex. 75231
(214) 373-6300

American Holistic Nurses' Association
5 W. Hargett St.
Raleigh, N.C. 27601
(919) 821-0071

American Hospital Association Division of Nursing
840 N. Lake Shore Dr.
Chicago, Ill. 60611
(708) 280-6000

American Nurses' Association
2420 Pershing Rd.
Kansas City, Mo. 64108
(816) 474-5720

American Public Health Association
1015 15th St., NW
Washington, D.C. 20005
(202) 789-5600

American Red Cross
17th & D St., NW
Washington, D.C. 20006
(202) 737-8300

American Society for Nursing Service Administrators, American Hospital Association
840 N. Lake Shore Dr.
Chicago, Ill. 60611
(708) 280-6000

American Urological Association Allied
6845 Lake Shore Dr.
P.O. Box 9397
Raytown, Mo. 64133
(816) 358-3317

Directory of professional organizations *(continued)*

Association for the Care of Children's Health
3615 Wisconsin Ave., NW
Washington, D.C. 20016
(202) 244-1801

Association of Operating Room Nurses
10170 E. Mississippi Ave.
Denver, Colo. 80231
(303) 755-6300

Association of Pediatric Oncology Nurses
c/o Georgina Bru
6728 Old McLean Village
McLean, Va. 22101
(703) 556-9222

Association for Practitioners in Infection Control
505 E. Hawley St.
Mundelein, Ill. 60060
(708) 949-6052

Association of Rehabilitation Nurses
2506 Gross Point Rd.
Evanston, Ill. 60201
(708) 475-7300

Emergency Nurses Association
230 E. Ohio, #600
Chicago, Ill. 60611
(708) 649-0297

Catholic Health Association of the United States
4455 Woodson Rd.
St. Louis, Mo. 63134
(314) 427-2500

Federation for Accessible Nursing Education and Licensure
2033 Sixth Ave., #804
Seattle, Wash. 98122
(206) 441-6020

National Association for Practical Nurse Education and Service
1400 Spring St., Suite 310
Silver Spring, Md. 20910
(301) 588-2491

National Association of Hispanic Nurses
2300 W. Commerce, Suite 304
San Antonio, Tex. 78207
(512) 226-9743

National Association for Healthcare Recruitment
P.O. Box 5769
Akron, Ohio 44372
(216) 867-3088

National Association of Orthopaedic Nurses, Inc.
Box 56, N. Woodbury Rd.
Pitman, N.J. 08071
(609) 582-0111

National Association of Pediatric Nurse Associates and Practitioners
1000 Maplewood Dr., #104
Maple Shade, N.J. 08052
(609) 667-1773

National Association of School Nurses
Lamplighter Lane
Box 1300
Scarborough, Me. 04074
(207) 883-2117

National Black Nurses Association, Inc.
P.O. Box 1823
Washington, D.C. 20013
(202) 393-6870

National Council of State Boards of Nursing
625 N. Michigan Ave., Suite 1544
Chicago, Ill. 60611
(708) 787-6555

National Federation of Licensed Practical Nurses, Inc.
P.O. Box 18088
Durham, N.C. 27703
(919) 781-4791

Intravenous Nurses Society
2 Brighton St.
Belmont, Mass. 02178
(617) 489-5205

National League for Nursing
10 Columbus Circle
New York, N.Y. 10019
(212) 582-1022

National Nurses Society on Addictions
2506 Gross Point Rd
Evanston, Ill. 60201
(708) 475-7300

National Student Nurses' Association, Inc.
555 W. 57th St., #1325
New York, N.Y. 10019
(212) 581-2211

Nurses Association of the American College of Obstetricians and Gynecologists
409 12th St., SW
Washington, D.C. 20024
(202) 638-0026

Nurses Christian Fellowship
P.O. Box 7895
Madison, Wis. 53707
(608) 274-9001

Nurses Educational Funds, Inc.
555 W. 57th St.
New York, N.Y. 10019
(212) 581-2211

(continued)

Directory of professional organizations (continued)

Nurses House, Inc.
10 Columbus Circle, #2416
New York, N.Y. 10019
(212) 582-1022

Oncology Nursing Society
1016 Greentree Rd., 3rd floor
Pittsburgh, Pa. 15220
(412) 921-7373

**Sigma Theta Tau
National Honor Society of
Nursing**
1200 Waterway Blvd.
Indianapolis, Ind. 46202
(317) 634-8171

**The Society for Nursing
History**
Nursing Education Dept.
Box 150
Teachers College
Columbia University
New York, N.Y. 10027
(212) 678-3421

Regional organizations

Midwest Alliance in Nursing
Nursing Education Dept.
Box 150
Teachers College
Columbia University
New York, N.Y. 10027
(212) 678-3421

**New England Board of Higher
Education**
45 Temple Pl.
Boston, Mass. 02111
(617) 770-7300

**Southern Regional Education
Board**
1340 Spring St., NW
Atlanta, Ga. 30309
(404) 875-9211

**Western Interstate Commission
for Higher Education**
P.O. Drawer P
Boulder, Colo. 80302
(303) 497-0224

State professional associations

**Alabama State Nurses
Association**
360 N. Hull St.
Montgomery, Ala. 36104
(205) 262-8321

Alaska Nurses Association
237 E. 3rd Ave.
Anchorage, Alaska 99501
(907) 274-0827

Arizona Nurses Association
1850 E. Southern Ave.
Tempe, Ariz. 85282
(602) 831-0404

**Arkansas State Nurses
Association**
117 S. Cedar
Little Rock, Ark. 72205
(501) 664-5853

California Nurses Association
1855 Folsom St., Rm. 670
San Francisco, Calif. 94103
(415) 864-4141

Colorado Nurses Association
5453 E. Evans Place
Denver, Colo. 80222
(303) 757-7484

Connecticut Nurses Association
1 Prestige Dr.
Meriden, Conn. 06450
(203) 238-1208

Delaware Nurses Association
2634 Capitol Trail, Suite C
Newark, Del. 19711
(302) 368-2233

**District of Columbia Nurses
Association**
5100 Wisconsin Ave., NW
Suite 306
Washington, D.C. 20016
(202) 244-2705

Florida Nurses Association
Box 536985
Orlando, Fla. 32853
(305) 896-3261

Georgia Nurses Association
1362 W. Peachtree St., NW
Atlanta, Ga. 30309
(404) 876-4624

Hawaii Nurses Association
677 Ala Moana #1014
Honolulu, Hawaii 96813
(808) 531-1628

Idaho Nurses Association
200 N. 4th St., Suite 20
Boise, Idaho 83706
(208) 345-0500

Illinois Nurses Association
20 N. Wacker Dr., Suite 2520
Chicago, Ill. 60606
(708) 236-9708

**Indiana State Nurses
Association**
2915 N. High School Rd.
Indianapolis, Ind. 46224
(317) 299-4575

Iowa Nurses Association
100 Court Ave.
Des Moines, Iowa 50309
(515) 282-9169

**Kansas State Nurses
Association**
820 Quincy St., Rm. 520
Topeka, Kan. 66612
(913) 233-8638

Directory of professional organizations *(continued)*

Kentucky Nurses Association
1400 S. 1st St.
Louisville, Ky. 40201
(502) 637-2546

Louisiana State Nurses Association
712 Transcontinental Dr.
Metairie, La. 70004
(504) 889-1030

Maine State Nurses Association
P.O. Box 2240
Augusta, Me. 04330
(207) 622-1057

Maryland Nurses Association
5820 Southwestern Blvd.
Baltimore, Md. 21227
(301) 242-7300

Massachusetts Nurses Association
340 Turnpike St.
Canton, Mass. 02021
(617) 821-4625

Michigan Nurses Association
120 Spartan Ave.
East Lansing, Mich. 48823
(517) 337-1653

Minnesota Nurses Association
1295 Bandana Blvd., N
St. Paul, Minn. 55108
(612) 646-4807

Mississippi Nurses Association
135 Bounds St., Suite 100
Jackson, Miss. 39206
(601) 982-9182

Missouri Nurses Association
206 E. Dunklin St.
P.O. Box 325
Jefferson City, Mo. 65102
(314) 636-4623

Montana Nurses Association
P.O. Box 5718
715 Getchell
Helena, Mont. 59604
(406) 442-6710

Nebraska Nurses Association
941 O St., Suite 707-711
Lincoln, Neb. 68508
(402) 475-3859

Nevada Nurses Association
3660 Baker Lane
Reno, Nev. 89509
(702) 825-3555

New Hampshire Nurses Association
48 West St.
Concord, N.H. 03301
(603) 225-3783

New Jersey State Nurses Association
320 W. State St.
Trenton, N.J. 08618
(609) 392-4884

New Mexico Nurses Association
525 San Pedro, NE, Suite 100
Albuquerque, N.M. 87108
(505) 268-7744

New York State Nurses Association
2113 Western Ave.
Guilderland, N.Y. 12084
(518) 456-5371

North Carolina Nurses Association
Box 12025
Raleigh, N.C. 27605
(919) 821-4250

North Dakota State Nurses Association
212 N. 4th St.
Bismarck, N.D. 58501
(701) 223-1385

Ohio Nurses Association
4000 E. Main St.
P.O. Box 13169
Columbus, Ohio 43213
(614) 237-5414

Oklahoma Nurses Association
6414 N. Santa Fe, Suite A
Oklahoma City, Okla. 73116
(405) 840-3476

Oregon Nurses Association
9700 S.W. Capitol Hwy., Suite 200
Portland, Ore. 97219
(503) 293-0011

Pennsylvania Nurses Association
2578 Interstate Dr.
Harrisburg, Pa. 17105
(717) 657-1222

Puerto Rico Board of Nurse Examiners
Office of Regulation and Certification of Health Professionals
Call Box 10200
Santurce, P.R. 00908
(809) 725-7506

Rhode Island State Nurses Association
345 Blackstone Blvd.
H.C. Hall Bldg. (South)
Providence, R.I. 02906
(401) 421-9703

South Carolina Nurses Association
1821 Gadsden St.
Columbia, S.C. 29201
(803) 252-4781

(continued)

Directory of professional organizations (continued)

South Dakota Nurses Association
1505 S. Minnesota, Suite 6
Sioux Falls, S.D. 57105
(605) 338-1401

Tennessee Nurses Association
1720 West End Bldg., Suite 400
Nashville, Tenn. 37203
(615) 329-2511

Texas Nurses Association
314 Highland Mall Blvd.,
Suite 504
Austin, Tex. 78752
(512) 452-0645

Utah Nurses Association
1058 E. 9th South
Salt Lake City, Utah 84105
(801) 322-3439

Vermont State Nurses Association
500 Dorset St.
S. Burlington, Vt. 05403
(802) 864-9390

Virginia Nurses Association
1311 High Point Ave.
Richmond, Va. 23230
(804) 353-7311

Washington State Nurses Association
83 King St.
Seattle, Wash. 98104
(206) 622-3613

West Virginia Nurses Association
2 Players Club Dr.
P.O. Box 1946
W. Charleston, W. Va. 25301
(304) 342-1169

Wisconsin Nurses Association
6117 Monona Dr.
Madison, Wis. 53716
(608) 221-0383

Wyoming Nurses Association
Majestic Bldg., Rm. 305
1603 Capitol Ave.
Cheyenne, Wyo. 82001
(307) 635-3955

Boards of Nursing

Alabama
State Board of Nursing
500 East Blvd., Suite 203
Montgomery, Ala. 36117
(205) 261-4060

Alaska
Board of Nursing Licensing
Division of Occupational Licensing
P.O. Box D-LIC
Juneau, Alaska 99811
(907) 465-2544

Arizona
State Board of Nursing
5050 N. 19th Ave., Suite 103
Phoenix, Ariz. 85015
(602) 255-5092

Arkansas
State Board of Nursing
1123 S. University Ave., Suite 800
Little Rock, Ark. 77204
(501) 371-2751

California
Board of Registered Nursing
1030 13th St.
Sacramento, Calif. 95814
(916) 322-3350

Board of Vocational Nurse & Psychiatric Technician Examiners
1020 N St.
Sacramento, Calif. 95814
(916) 445-0793

Colorado
State Board of Nursing
1560 Broadway, Suite 670
Denver, Colo. 80202
(303) 894-2430

Connecticut
Department of Health Services, Nurse Licensure
150 Washington St.
Hartford, Conn. 06106
(203) 566-1032

Delaware
Board of Nursing
Margaret O'Neill Bldg.
Federal & Court Sts.
Dover, Del. 19901
(302) 736-4522

District of Columbia
Registered Nurses Examining Board
614 H St., NW, Room 923
Washington, D.C. 20001
(202) 727-7468

Practical Nurses Examining Board
614 H St., NW
Washington, D.C. 20001
(202) 727-7468

Florida
Board of Nursing
111 E. Coastline Dr.
Jacksonville, Fla. 32202
(904) 359-6331

Georgia
Board of Nursing
166 Pryor St., SW
Atlanta, Ga. 30303
(404) 656-3943

Directory of professional organizations (continued)

**Georgia Board of Licensed
Practical Nurses**
166 Pryor St., SW
Atlanta, Ga. 30303
(404) 656-3943

**Hawaii
Board of Nursing**
P.O. Box 3469
Honolulu, Hawaii 96801
(808) 548-4100

**Idaho
State Board of Nursing**
500 S. 10th St., Suite 102
Boise, Idaho 83720
(208) 334-3110

**Illinois
Department of Professional
Registration**
320 W. Washington St.
Springfield, Ill. 62786
(217) 785-0800

**Indiana
State Board of Nursing
Health Professions Bureau**
P.O. Box 82067
Indianapolis, Ind. 46282
(317) 232-2960

**Iowa
Board of Nursing**
1223 E. Court
Des Moines, Iowa 50319
(515) 281-3255

**Kansas
State Board of Nursing**
900 S.W. Jackson, Suite 551 S.
Topeka, Kan. 66601
(913) 296-4929

**Kentucky
Board of Nursing Education
and Nurse Registration**
4010 Dupont Circle
Louisville, Ky. 40207
(502) 897-5143

**Louisiana
State Board of Nursing**
150 Baronne St.
New Orleans, La. 70112
(504) 568-5464

**State Board of Practical Nurse
Examiners**
1440 Canal St., Suite 2010
New Orleans, La. 70112
(504) 568-6480

**Maine
State Board of Nursing**
295 Water St.
Augusta, Me. 04330
(207) 289-5324

**Maryland
Board of Nursing**
201 W. Preston St.
Baltimore, Md. 21201
(301) 225-5880

**Massachusetts
Board of Registration in
Nursing**
100 Cambridge St., Room 1519
Boston, Mass. 02202
(617) 727-9961

**Michigan
Board of Nursing**
P.O. Box 30018
905 Southland
Lansing, Mich. 48909
(517) 373-1600

**Minnesota
Board of Nursing**
2700 University Ave. W. #108
St. Paul, Minn. 55414
(612) 642-0567

**Mississippi
Board of Nursing**
239 Lamar St., Suite 401
Jackson, Miss. 39206
(601) 354-7349

Missouri
3523 N. Ten Mile Dr.
Box 656
Jefferson City, Mo. 65102-0656
(314) 751-2334

**Montana
Board of Nursing**
1424 9th Ave.
Helena, Mont. 59620
(406) 444-4279

**Nebraska
State Board of Nursing**
P.O. Box 95007
Department of Health
Lincoln, Neb. 68509
(402) 471-2115

**Nevada
Board of Nursing**
1135 Terminal Way
Reno, Nev. 89502
(702) 786-2778

**New Hampshire
Board of Nursing Education
Division of Public Health**
6 Hazen Way
Concord, N.H. 03301
(603) 271-2323

**New Jersey
Board of Nursing**
1100 Raymond Blvd.
Newark, N.J. 07102
(201) 648-2490

(continued)

Directory of professional organizations *(continued)*

New Mexico
Board of Nursing
4125 Carlisle, NE
Albuquerque, N.M. 87107
(505) 841-6524

New York
Board for Nursing
State Education Department
Cultural Education Center
Albany, N.Y. 12230
(518) 474-3843

North Carolina
Board of Nursing
Box 2129
Raleigh, N.C. 27602
(919) 828-0740

North Dakota
Board of Nursing
919 S. 7th St.
Bismarck, N.D. 58504
(701) 224-2974

Ohio
Board of Nursing
77 S. High St.
Columbus, Ohio 43215
(614) 466-3947

Oklahoma
**Board of Nurse Registration
and Nursing Education**
2915 Classen Blvd., Suite 524
Oklahoma City, Okla. 73106
(405) 525-2076

Oregon
Board of Nursing
1400 S.W. 5th Ave.
Portland, Ore. 97201
(503) 229-5653

Pennsylvania
Board of Nursing
Box 2649
Harrisburg, Pa. 17105
(717) 783-7142

Rhode Island
**Board of Nurse Registration
and Nursing Education**
Cannon Health Building
75 Davis St.
Providence, R.I. 02908
(401) 277-2827

South Carolina
Board of Nursing
1777 St. Julian Place, Suite 102
Columbia, S.C. 29204
(803) 737-6594

South Dakota
Board of Nursing
304 S. Phillips Ave.
Sioux Falls, S.D. 57102
(605) 335-4973

Tennessee
Board of Nursing
283 Plus Park Blvd.
Nashville, Tenn. 37217
(605) 367-6232

Texas
Board of Nurse Examiners
P.O. Box 140466
Austin, Tex. 78752
(512) 835-4880

Utah
**Board of Nursing
Division of Professional
Licensing**
160 E. 300 South
P.O. Box 45802
Salt Lake City, Utah 84110
(801) 530-6733

Vermont
Board of Nursing
26 Terrace St.
Montpelier, Vt. 05602
(802) 828-2363

Virginia
Board of Nursing
1601 Rolling Hills Dr.
Richmond, Va. 23269
(804) 662-9909

Washington
**Board of Nursing
Division of Professional
Licensing**
Box 9649
Olympia, Wash. 98504
(206) 753-2206

West Virginia
Board of Nurse Examiners
Embleton Bldg.
922 Quarrier St.
Charleston, W. Va. 25301
(304) 348-3596

Wisconsin
Board of Nursing
P.O. Box 8936
Madison, Wis. 53708
(608) 266-3735

Wyoming
Board of Nursing
2301 Central Ave.
Cheyenne, Wyo. 82002
(307) 777-7601

19 Steering clear of legal pitfalls

Six everyday situations that can trigger lawsuits

Do you overlook potential legal hazards in everyday nursing situations?

The following examples of nursing liability, based on actual court decisions, show how deviating from accepted standards can harm a patient and result in lawsuits. By being aware of how certain common situations can cause you legal entanglements, you can avoid making similar mistakes.

Failure to assess a patient properly or take an adequate history

When a man traveling between cities began having chest pain and numbness in his left shoulder and arm, he and his companion stopped at a small hospital for help. The nurse on duty in the emergency department (ED) advised him to continue on to a bigger hospital 24 miles away. She failed to perform a physical assessment or obtain a formal history. On his way to the other hospital, the man had a massive myocardial infarction and died.

Clearly, the nurse failed to assess her patient accurately. Her mistake may have cost the patient his life and resulted in a landmark decision that established a nurse's independent relationship with her patient.

The court held the nurse responsible and accountable for her omissions, stating that she had failed to meet her duty to protect the patient from harm.

Failure to observe patients closely and take appropriate precautions

An elderly senile patient with a history of falling down was left in bed with the side rails down. She fell out of bed and hurt herself.

Another patient, an alert 28-year-old, was instructed by a nurse to call for help before getting out of bed. After the nurse left the room, the patient got herself out of bed and fell.

In the first case, the nurse was found liable for failing to raise the side rails. When a patient is at clear risk for injury, the nurse must take extra measures to protect her.

In the second case, the nurse was not held liable for the patient's injuries. Her patient, a competent adult, had received appropriate instructions and chose to ignore them. In such circumstances, a court will hold the patient responsible for her own actions.

Failure to document pertinent information or communicate it to the doctor

A mother took her two sons to an ED with head and chest rashes and high fevers. The mother gave the nurse an accurate history, which included the recent removal of two ticks from one of the boys.

The nurse didn't tell the doctor about the ticks or record the information in the chart. The doctor diagnosed measles in both boys and sent them home.

Two days later, one of the boys died of Rocky Mountain spotted fever, which is transmitted by ticks.

Neither the hospital nor the doctor was held responsible for the boy's death. But the nurse's omission was found to be a contributing cause of death.

Failure to perform nursing procedures correctly

A nurse administered an intramuscular injection in the wrong quadrant of a patient's buttocks. He later developed footdrop from sciatic nerve damage.

In this case, both the nurse and the hospital were found negligent. The law expects a nurse to administer drugs and treatments without injuring patients by following set standards of care. (Drug-related errors are the most common source of negligence claims against nurses.)

Seven leading causes of malpractice suits against nurses

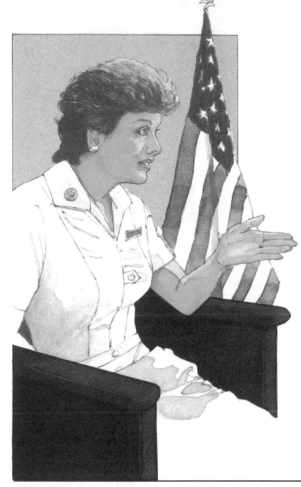

A study, conducted by a Pennsylvania insurance company, found the leading causes of malpractice suits against nurses to be:

1. Medications
- Incorrect medications and dosages
- Injury from injections

2. Obstetrics and related care
- Nursing error or negligence causing injury during delivery
- Delay in notifying doctor causing injury
- Failure to monitor neonate's condition
- Failure to provide proper neonatal care

3. Patient falls
- Side rails left down
- Medicated patients left unattended
- Injury caused when moving or turning patient
- Patient left unattended on stretcher or examining table

4. Surgery and related care
- Foreign object left in patient
- Failure to monitor patient in recovery room
- Negligent postoperative care

5. I.V.s, catheters, and tubes
- Infiltration
- Negligence causing emboli
- Improper insertion causing injury

6. Record-keeping
- Inaccuracy, or failure to record information
- Failure to communicate with doctor
- Breach of confidentiality

7. Personal liability
- Injury to insured's property

The hospital's liability was established under the legal doctrine *respondeat superior,* which holds an employer responsible for an employee's errors.

Failure to report known or suspected deviations from accepted practice
While delivering a patient's baby, an obstetrician made an incision in the patient's cervix to relieve a constrictive band of muscle. After delivery, he failed to suture the incision.

The patient was sent to the postpartum unit for care and observation. The patient's nurse, noticing that the patient was bleeding heavily, called the obstetrician three times. He assured the nurse that the bleeding was normal. Within two hours, the patient went into shock and died.

Even though the nurse contacted the patient's doctor, the court held the nurse negligent for failing to intervene further. The courts expect nurses to exercise professional, *independent* judgment and to object when a doctor's orders are inappropriate. In this case, the nurse should have reported the facts to her manager or the unit's medical director, insisting that the patient receive proper care.

Failure to ensure removal of all foreign objects left in the patient's body

During a cholecystectomy, the surgical team accidentally left a sponge in the patient's body. When the sponge was discovered later, the patient needed another operation to remove it.

When the court awarded damages, both the surgeon and the nurse paid. At one time, the surgeon would have been fully responsible under the "captain of the ship" doctrine. Today, all members of the surgical team are responsible for their actions.

▼

Preventing malpractice claims

The best way to protect yourself against a malpractice claim is to practice preventive nursing. First, take a close look at yourself to be sure your practice is competent and up to date. Then, look at your work setting to make sure you're thoroughly familiar with your unit and the hospital's policies and procedures. Here's how to begin.

Know yourself

Identify your strengths and weaknesses. When you identify a weakness, try to improve upon it by taking a continuing education course or by asking a coworker for help or advice. Don't be afraid to discuss your weaknesses with your supervisor, either.

Don't accept responsibilities for which you're not prepared. For example, if you haven't worked in pediatrics for 10 years, accepting an assignment to a pediatric unit without orientation only increases your chances of making an error. If you do make an error, claiming you weren't familiar with the unit's procedures won't protect you against liability.

As a professional, you shouldn't accept a position if you can't perform as a reasonable, prudent nurse would *in that setting*. Courts may, however, be more lenient about working in emergency settings, such as a fire or flood. But simply being told "We need you here today" does *not* constitute an emergency.

Evaluate your assignment

You may be assigned to help out on a specialized unit, which is reasonable, as long as you're assigned duties you can perform competently and as long as the experienced nurse on the unit assumes responsibility for the specialized duties. Assigning you to perform total patient care on the unit is unsafe because you don't have the skills to plan and deliver that care.

For example, if you're assigned to coronary care, you could monitor the I.V. lines, take vital signs, and report your observations to the coronary care nurse. She'll check the monitors, administer the medications, and make decisions. This arrangement fragments the patient's care, however, so it's not appropriate as a permanent solution to a staffing problem.

Follow hospital policies and procedures

You have a responsibility to be familiar with the policies and procedures of the hospital where you work. If the policies and procedures are sound, and you follow them carefully, they can protect you against a malpractice claim.

The medication procedure may involve checking all medication cards against a central Kardex. If you do this and the Kardex is in error, you may not be liable for a resulting medication error, because you followed all appropriate procedures and acted responsibly.

The person who made the original error, however, would be liable. But if you didn't follow the procedure, you might also be liable because you didn't do your part to prevent the error.

Keep policies and procedures up to date

As nursing changes, so should the hospital's policies and procedures. As a professional, you're responsible for maintaining up-to-date procedures.

For instance, do you have written policies on dealing with emergency situations? "We've always done it this way" isn't an adequate substitute for a clearly written, officially accepted policy.

If administrators are reluctant to make policy changes based on one nurse's suggestion, join with colleagues to present the legal implications.

Document accurately

From a legal standpoint, documented care is as important as the actual care. If a procedure wasn't documented, the courts assume it wasn't performed. Documentation of observations, decisions, and actions is considered much more solid evidence than oral testimony.

Therefore, accurate and complete documentation is crucial to prevent litigation. It also protects you from becoming liable for someone else's error by showing that you did everything you could to prevent harm.

Because problem-oriented medical records provide less detailed information, they're considered less helpful in defense against litigation. But any system of charting and record-keeping can provide adequate documentation of care.

If you identify something that needs to be documented but you can't find a provision for it within your system, work to have the system revised. Bring it to the attention of the committee that reviews charting policies, along with a plan for new procedures.

Better still, serve on the committee yourself. Finally, consult with the hospital's attorney to be sure the new plan for record-keeping is legally sound and professionally useful.

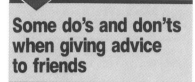

Some do's and don'ts when giving advice to friends

You're assuming legal risks whenever you give health care advice to your friends. In the courts' view, even a casual conversation can sometimes establish a nurse-patient relationship, making you liable for the consequences of your advice. To minimize your legal risks, keep in mind these do's and don'ts:

Do
• Find out if your professional liability insurance, or your employer's, provides you with off-the-job coverage.
• Know whether your state's nurse practice act discusses giving advice to friends.
• Give advice only within the confines of your nurse practice act, education, and experience.
• Make sure the advice you give is up to date. Remember, you'll be judged on current nursing standards if your advice results in a lawsuit.

Don't
• Speculate about your friends' illnesses or ailments.
• Suggest that friends change or ignore their doctors' orders.
• Give your friends any advice about medical care.
• Offer any advice that, if wrong, could result in serious or permanent injury.

Avoiding problematic abbreviations

Every hospital is required by the Joint Commission on Accreditation of Health Care Organizations to develop a list of approved abbreviations for staff use. But certain abbreviations should *never* be used because they're easily misunderstood. Here's a list of abbreviations to avoid.

Abbreviation	Intended meaning	Example
Apothecary symbols	dram	*Elixophyline 3T t.i.d.*
	minim	*TR opium 10 ℳ*
AU	*auris uterque* (each ear)	*Colymycin gtts ⅲ au t.id.*
D/C	discharge discontinue	*D/c meds: Digoxin 0.25 mg Lasix 40 mg*
Drug names		
MTX	methotrexate	
CPZ	Compazine (prochlorperazine)	
HCl	hydrochloric acid	
DIG	digoxin	
MVI	multivitamins *without* fat-soluble vitamins	
HCTZ	hydrochlorothiazide	
ARA-A	vidarabine	
μg	microgram	*Vit B₁₂ 1 mg IM now*
o.d.	once daily	*KCl 15 meq OD*
OJ	orange juice	*Lugol's sol'n gtts X̄ in OJ*
t/d	once daily	*Diabinese 250 mg t.i.d.*
per os	orally	*Lugol's sol'n gtts X̄ per os*
q.d.	every day	*Digoxin 0.25 mg q.d.*
qn	nightly or at bedtime	*Librium 10 mg qh*
q.o.d	every other day	*Digoxin 0.25 mg q.o.d.*
sub q	subcutaneous	*Heparin 5000 units sub q 2 hrs before surgery*
U or u	unit	*NPH 6u now sub q NPH 4u now sub q*

Misinterpretation	Correction
Not understood or misread.	Use the metric system.
Has been mistaken for OU (*oculus uterque* — each eye).	Don't use this abbreviation.
Patients' medications have been prematurely discontinued when D/C, intended to mean "discharge," was misinterpreted as "discontinue," when followed by list of drugs.	Write out "discharge" and "discontinue."
Mustargen (mechlorethamine HCl) chlorpromazine potassium choride ("H" misinterpreted as "K") digitoxin multivitamins *with* fat-soluble vitamins hydrocortisone (HCT) cytarabine (ARA-C)	Use the complete spelling for drug names.
When handwritten, this can easily be mistaken for "mg."	Use mcg.
Frequently misinterpreted as "right eye" (OD — *oculus dexter*), so that oral medication is administered in a patient's right eye.	Don't abbreviate "daily"; write it out.
Mistaken for "OD" (*oculus dexter* — right eye) or "OS" (*oculus sinister* — left eye). Medications that were meant to be diluted in orange juice and given orally have been given in a patient's right or left eye.	Write out "orange juice."
Mistaken as "t.i.d."	Write it out.
The "os" can be mistaken for left eye.	Use "P.O." or "by mouth" or "orally."
The period after the "q" has sometimes been mistaken for an "i," and the drug has been given q.i.d. rather than daily.	Write it out.
Misinterpreted as "every hour" when poorly written.	Use "hs" or "nightly."
Misinterpreted as "daily" or "q.i.d." if the "o" is poorly written.	Use "q other day" or "every other day."
The "q" has been mistaken for "every." In the example, a prophylactic heparin dose meant to be given 2 hours before surgery was given every 2 hours before surgery.	Use "subcut." or write out "subcutaneous."
Seen as a zero or a four (4), causing a tenfold or greater overdose.	"Unit" has no acceptable abbreviation. Write it out.

A strategy for minimizing your legal risks

To minimize the chances that a patient will sue you after an incident and to protect yourself and the hospital if he does, follow the "three Rs" of risk-management strategy: rapport, record, and report.

Maintain a rapport with the patient

Answer his questions honestly. Don't offer any explanation if you weren't personally involved in the incident. Instead, refer him to someone who can supply answers. If you try to answer his questions without direct knowledge of the incident, inconsistencies could arise and the patient could interpret these as a cover-up.

Don't offer any explanation if doing so might make you visibly nervous. Ask your supervisor, hospital patient-relations specialist, or an administrator for advice on how to answer the patient. If you still feel uncomfortable, have one of them talk to the patient, but still try to maintain rapport.

Don't blame anyone for the incident. If you feel someone was at fault, tell your charge nurse or supervisor, not the patient.

If an incident necessarily changes the way you care for the patient, tell the patient about it and clearly explain the reasons for the change.

Record the incident in the medical record

Remember, truthfulness is the best protection against lawsuits. If you try to cover up or play down an incident, you could end up in far more serious trouble than if you report it objectively.

Never write in the medical record that an incident report has been completed. An incident report is not clinical information: it's an administrative tool.

Report every incident

Some nurses think incident reports are more trouble than they're worth. Furthermore, they feel that these reports are a dangerous admission of guilt, which simply isn't true.

Incident reports are important because:

• They jog memories. A considerable amount of time may pass between when an incident actually occurs and when it comes to court. A nurse can't trust her memory to recall all the pertinent details, but she can trust an incident report.

• Incident reports help administrators act quickly to change the policy or procedure that seems to be responsible for the incident. An administrator can also act quickly to talk with families and offer assistance, an explanation, or other support. Sometimes helpful communication with an injured patient and his family can soothe a family's anger and prevent a lawsuit.

• Incident reports provide the information hospitals need to decide whether restitution should be made. When a patient is injured instead of being helped during his hospital stay, the hospital sometimes decides that it has a moral obligation to compensate the patient. In fact, this moral obligation is another reason (besides protection against having to pay damages awarded in a lawsuit) why hospitals carry professional liability insurance.

• Finally, incident reporting will become increasingly important as health care consumers become more aware of their rights. A long period may elapse between an incident and subsequent court proceedings, and documentation may be the only objective proof of what actually happened.

Filing an incident report

Despite the best training and the best intentions, unfortunate incidents do occur, and it's your legal duty—whether you're a registered nurse, a licensed practical nurse, a licensed vocational nurse, a staff nurse, or a nurse manager—to report any incident of which you have first-hand knowledge.

An incident report serves two main purposes. The first purpose is to inform hospital administration of the incident so that they can consider changes that will help prevent similar incidents from occurring in the future. The second purpose is to alert the administration and the hospital's insurance company to the possibility of liability claims and the need for further investigation.

Failure to report an incident could lead to your dismissal and also expose you to personal liability for malpractice, especially if your failure to report the incident causes injury to a patient.

When to file a report

In most hospitals and other health care institutions, you must file an incident report when any of the following occur:
• Patient injuries
• Patient complaints
• Medication errors
• Injuries to employees and visitors.

What to include

An incident report should include only the following:
• The identities of the patient and any witnesses
• Information about what happened and the consequences for the patient (you should supply enough information so that the hospital administration can decide whether the matter needs further investigation)

Tips for better documentation

If you're ever involved in a malpractice case, what you documented, how you documented it, and what you didn't document will heavily influence the outcome. Here are some tips on how to document so that in case of a lawsuit, your records work for you, not against you.

- Use the appropriate form, and document in ink.
- Record the patient's name and identification number on every page of his chart, to avoid any possible confusion.
- Record the complete date and time of each entry. Be specific, avoiding general terms and vague expressions that could be interpreted in different ways.
- Use standard abbreviations only.
- Use a medical term only if you're sure of its meaning.
- Document symptoms by using the patient's own words.
- Document any nursing action you take in response to a patient's problem, for example: "8 p.m.—medicated for incision pain." Be sure to include the medication route and site.
- Document the patient's response to medications and other treatment.

- Document safeguards you use to protect the patient. For example: "raised side rails" or "applied safety belts."
- Should any incident occur, document it in two places: once in your progress report, and again in an incident report.
- Document each observation. Failure to document observations will produce gaps in the patient's records, suggesting that you neglected the patient.
- Document procedures only after you've performed them, never in advance.
- Write on every line. Don't insert notes between lines or leave empty spaces for someone else to insert a note.
- Sign every entry.
- Document an omission as a new entry. Never back-date or add to previously written entries.
- Draw a thin line through an error. Never erase one.
- Document only your own care, never someone else's.

- Any other facts that you think are relevant.

What not to include

Other information should never be entered in an incident report because it could seriously hinder the defense in any lawsuit arising from the incident. This includes:
- Mention of events that were not actually seen by the reporter (such as something another employee said happened)
- Opinions (such as the reporter's opinion of the patient's prognosis)
- Conclusions or assumptions (such as what caused the incident)
- Suggestions of who was responsible for causing the incident
- Suggestions to prevent the incident from happening again.

When to question a doctor's orders

Do you always assume the doctor is right and follow his orders even if they seem vague or medically inappropriate? If you do, you could be jeopardizing your nursing career.

Your responsibility as a nurse is to question *any* dubious order you receive. Some types of orders may actually be detrimental to your patient's health—and legally dangerous for you. Here are four types of orders you must always question:

Ambiguous orders
Follow your hospital's policy for clarifying any orders that are

vague or have more than one possible interpretation, and make sure you document your actions. If your hospital doesn't have a policy covering this type of situation, contact the prescribing doctor and always document your actions. Then ask your nursing administration for a step-by-step policy to follow in this situation, so that if it happens again, you'll know exactly what to do.

Inappropriate orders
A change in your patient's condition may mean that a standing order is no longer appropriate. When this occurs, delay treatment until you've contacted the doctor and clarified the situation. Again, you should follow your hospital's policy for clarifying the order.

Note: If you're an inexperienced nurse, clarify all standing orders by contacting the prescribing doctor for guidance. Or tell your supervisor you're uncertain about following the order, and let her decide whether to delegate the responsibility to a more experienced nurse.

If after you carry out the order the treatment is affecting the patient adversely, discontinue it. Then report all unfavorable signs and symptoms to the patient's doctor.

You should resume treatment only after you've discussed the situation with the doctor and clarified his orders.

Any order a patient questions

A doctor can change his orders at any time, even when you're off duty, and a patient may know something about his prescribed care that no one has told you. If a patient protests a procedure, medication dosage, or medication route, claiming that it's different from the usual or that it's been changed, give him the benefit of the doubt. Question the doctor's orders, following your hospital's policy, if one exists.

Telephone orders

Whenever a doctor gives you an order by telephone, document all the details. Follow your hospital's policy to the letter. If your hospital has no formal policy, document your conversation and subsequent actions as follows:

• Write down the date and time of the call and the doctor's name, and describe the patient's condition and other circumstances that prompted the call.

• Review the patient's condition in detail with the doctor.

• Write down his orders as you listen.

• Read the orders back to him to be sure you've recorded them accurately.

• Document the fact that you've read the orders back to the doctor and he has confirmed them.

Where nurse practitioners can prescribe drugs

The laws concerning the privileges of nurse practitioners (NPs) to prescribe drugs vary from state to state. In a given state, a specific law may authorize NPs to prescribe or, more often, may formulate regulations to include prescribing privileges within the scope of nursing as defined by the state's nurse practice act. NPs now have such privileges in 20 states, with enabling legislation pending in several more. This table shows how prescribing by NPs is regulated by the various states.

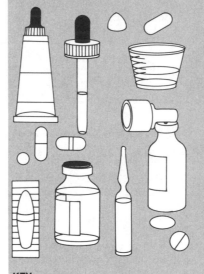

KEY

ANP = adult nurse practitioner
FNP = family nurse practitioner
GNP = geriatric nurse practitioner
NM = nurse-midwife
NNP = neonatal nurse practitioner
NP = nurse practitioner
O-G NP = obstetric-gynecologic nurse practitioner
PNA/P = pediatric nurse associate or practitioner
SNP = school nurse practitioner

State	Date of law
Alaska	1979
Arizona	1982
California	1987
Idaho	1971
Maine	1977
Maryland	1981
Massachusetts	1984
Michigan	1980
Mississippi	1980
Nevada	1983
New Hampshire	1983
New Mexico	1978
North Carolina	1975
Oregon	1979
Pennsylvania	1977
South Dakota	1979
Tennessee	1980 (revised 1985)
Utah	1983
Vermont	1983
Washington	1979

Approval body	Eligible nurses
Board of Nursing	Advanced NP (NM, PNA, FNP, ANP, O-G NP, NNP, SNP)
Board of Nursing	Registered NP (NM, PNA, FNP, ANP, O-G NP, NNP, SNP)
Board of Nursing (which notifies Board of Pharmacy)	NP
Board of Nursing (unless NP is new to state; then State Medical Board required)	NP
Board of Medicine	NP
Written agreement between doctor and nurse, approved by Board of Nursing	NP
Department of Public Health	NPs in long-term care facilities
Prescribing protocols filed with Board of Nursing	RN
Prescribing protocols filed with Board of Nursing	NP (NM, PNP, FNP, ANP, O-G NP, family planning NP, primary care NP)
Boards of Nursing and Pharmacy	NP
Prescribing protocols filed with Board of Nursing	Lack of implementing rules makes law inoperative
Prescribing protocols filed with Board of Nursing	NP (PNP, FNP, ANP, O-G NP, SNP, GNP, college health NP, women's health care NP)
Board of Medicine	Nurses performing medical procedures
Board of Nursing	NP
Prescribing protocols filed with Board of Nursing	Lack of implementing rules makes law inoperative
Board of Nursing; medical and osteopathic examiners	NP (certified in specialty)
Board of Nursing	NP (certified in specialty)
Board of Prescription Practices (an independent board of NPs, MDs, and pharmacists)	NP with prescription practice license
Prescribing protocols filed with Board of Nursing	NP (CNM, PNP, FNP, ANP, O-G NP, CRNA, clinical specialist in psychiatric and mental health nursing)
Board of Nursing	Advanced NP (ARNP)

Distinguishing between types of malpractice insurance

Professional liability insurance can protect you at the time a patient claims the malpractice occurs (occurrence policy) or when he brings a lawsuit for damages (claims-made policy).

Occurrence policy
This type of policy, considered your best protection, guards you against an error of omission or commission occurring during a policy period, regardless of when, after the policy ends, the patient makes a claim against you. Remember, a malpractice claim doesn't necessarily have to be filed during the same year in which the incident occurred. State laws govern the amount of time an injured person has to file a claim.

Claims-made policy
This type of policy protects you only against claims made against you during the policy period. A claims-made policy is cheaper than an occurrence policy because the insurance company is at risk only for the duration of the policy.

However, you can purchase an extended-reporting endorsement, or tail coverage, which in effect turns your claims-made policy into an occurrence policy.

When you're comparing the features of different policies, check for these options:
• Coverage when nurses under your supervision are negligent
• Coverage for misuse of equipment
• Coverage for errors in reporting or recording care
• Coverage for failure to teach patients properly

• Coverage for errors in administering medication
• Coverage in case the hospital sues you
• Coverage for professional services you perform outside your employment setting.

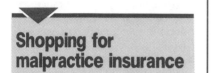

Shopping for malpractice insurance

The terms used in a malpractice insurance policy can make your head spin. Use the following questions and answers as a guide, whether you're buying personal insurance or reviewing your employer's policy.

What should my malpractice insurance cover and how much will it cost?
All malpractice insurance policies cover professional liability. Some also cover personal liability, medical payments, assault-related bodily injury, and property damage.

The amount of coverage varies, as does your premium. For example, depending on your specialty, a policy costing about $70 a year may provide up to $1 million for each incident (single-occurrence limit) and up to $2 million per year (the maximum annual protection).

When you secure a policy, watch for an "excess coverage clause" or "other insurance clause" indicating that your coverage begins only after other insurance has been exhausted.

What will the insurance company do if I'm sued?
Most policies state that the company has the duty to defend you in any suit payable under the terms of the policy, even if the charges against you are groundless, false, or fraudulent.

This includes investigating, evaluating, negotiating, and communicating with all parties, especially with you. If the company breaches its duty by not settling the claim within policy limits, you can sue the company for bad faith.

The policy may also state that the company will investigate and settle claims as it sees fit. Some policies specify that the company must get your agreement before settling. If so, you can't unreasonably withhold consent to settle or you may lose your coverage. Also, if you withhold your consent and a jury awards a verdict that exceeds the settlement offer, the company might not pay the difference.

How are terms defined?
Definitions of terms can vary from policy to policy. If your policy includes any restrictive definitions, you won't be covered for any actions outside of those guidelines. So, for the best protection, seek the broadest definitions possible and ask the agent for examples of actions that the company hasn't covered.

Be sure your policy covers your nursing role, whether you're a student, a graduate nurse, or a working nurse with advanced education and specialized skills.

How long is a policy in effect?
Insurance is an annual contract that can be renewed or canceled each year. The policy usually specifies how it can be canceled — in writing by either you or the company. Some contracts require 30 days' notice for cancellation. If the company is canceling the policy, you'll probably be given at least 10 days' notice.

What are exclusions?
Exclusions specify areas not covered, for example: "This policy does not apply to nurse anesthetists or nurse-midwives" or

"...does not apply to injury arising out of performance by the insured of a criminal act."

What happens if I'm involved in an incident?
Follow the conditions of your policy. You may be required to give written notice to the company of any claim or circumstances likely to result in a claim against you. Include your name and information about the time, place, and circumstances surrounding the incident, such as the names and addresses of the injured and witnesses. Another condition may be that you immediately forward to the company any demands, notices, or summonses you receive.

You have a duty to cooperate with the company when it requests your help in making settlements, conducting the suit, or enforcing the terms of the contract. You may also have to attend hearings and help provide evidence.

Most insurance contracts prohibit you, except at your own cost, from voluntarily making payments, assuming obligations, or incurring expenses. The contract generally provides that unless you've fully complied with the terms of the policy, you can't take action against the insurance company.

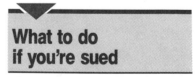

What to do if you're sued

As you expand your nursing expertise and take on more patient care responsibilities, you'll also be accepting greater legal risks. To protect yourself, you need to keep abreast of changes in the laws that affect nursing, while continuing to practice within the limits prescribed in your nurse practice act.

Despite taking these precautions, you may find yourself being sued one day, in which case you should follow these recommendations, which apply throughout the United States and Canada.

If you're insured

• If you're covered by your employer's insurance, you should immediately contact your employer's legal services administrators. They will tell you how to proceed.

• If you have your own professional liability insurance, your policy will tell you whom to notify and how much time you have to do it. Telephone the representative immediately and tell him you've been sued.

Document the date and time, the representative's name and his instructions. Then hand-deliver the lawsuit papers to him, getting a signed and dated receipt for them. Or send them by certified mail with a return receipt requested, so you're assured of a signed receipt.

• If you don't contact the appropriate representative within the specified time, the insurance company can refuse to cover you.

• When you notify your insurance company that you've been sued, the company will first consider whether it must cover you at all. Your company does this by checking for any policy violations you may have committed—for example, giving late notice of the lawsuit, giving false information on your insurance application, or failing to pay a premium on time.

• If the company is sure you've committed such a violation, it will use this violation as a policy defense and can simply refuse to cover you.

• If the company thinks you've committed such a violation but isn't sure it has the evidence to support a policy defense, it will probably send you a letter by certified mail informing you that the company may not have to defend

you, but stating that it will do so while reserving the right to deny coverage later, withdraw from the case, or take other actions. Meanwhile, the company will seek a declaration of its rights from the court.

• If the court decides the company doesn't have to defend you, the company will withdraw from the case. Usually, an insurance company takes this action only after careful consideration, because it may provide the insured nurse with grounds for suing the company.

If you receive such a letter, find a malpractice attorney to defend you in the lawsuit against you and advise you in your dealings with the insurance company. If your case against the insurance company is sound, he may suggest that you sue them.

• If your insurance company doesn't assert a policy defense, your company representative will select and retain an attorney or a law firm specializing in medical malpractice cases as your attorney of record in the lawsuit. Once the attorney's designated as your attorney of record, he is legally bound to do all that's necessary to defend you.

• Your employer will almost certainly be named as a codefendant in the lawsuit. But even if this isn't the case, you should notify your employer that you're being sued. Your insurance company may try to involve your employer as a defendant.

If you're not insured

• If you don't have insurance, don't even consider trying to defend yourself. Find an attorney who's experienced in medical malpractice; the case will be complex and the opposition will be composed of experienced attorneys.

• Make appointments with a few attorneys who seem qualified to defend you. When you meet with each one, ask how long he thinks

Finding an attorney

What happens if a patient sues you and you don't have an attorney?

If the patient sues you and the hospital where you work, then the hospital's insurance company will handle the case, supplying an attorney to defend you as the hospital's employee.

If the patient sues only you, then you're on your own. The first thing you should do is see your professional liability agent. Most often your insurance company will appoint an attorney to defend you.

If you don't have insurance, or you're not satisfied with the attorney the insurance company provides, or the company uses a policy defense and doesn't cover you, try to find an attorney using the following methods.

• If you work in a hospital with a legal services department, find out if the hospital will provide you with an attorney or refer you to one.

• If you have a relative or a friend who is an attorney or a judge, ask him for a referral.

• If you're a member of a professional association, the association may be able to refer you to an attorney.

• If none of these situations applies to you, contact your local bar association, listed in the Yellow Pages, for a referral. Try to find an attorney who's experienced in medical malpractice cases.

• Before you hire anyone to defend you, ask other health care professionals if they've heard of the attorney you're thinking of using, and go by his reputation.

the lawsuit will take and how much money he'll charge. Also, try to get a feel for the attorney's understanding of the issues in your case. Then choose one as your attorney of record. Do this as soon as possible.

What your attorney will do

• Your attorney will file the appropriate legal documents in response to the papers you were served. He'll ask you for help in preparing your defense. He should give you a chance to present your position in detail. Remember, all such discussions between you and your attorney are privileged. This means that your attorney can't disclose this information without your permission.

• Your attorney will also obtain complete copies of the pertinent medical records and any other documents you and he feel are important to your defense. In addition, he'll use discovery devices to uncover every pertinent detail about the case against you. These discovery devices are legal procedures for obtaining information.

• Some discovery devices your attorney may use include an interrogatory (questions written to the other party that require answers under oath), a deposition (oral cross-examination of the other party, under oath and before a court reporter), and a defense medical examination (a medical examination of the injured party by a doctor selected by your attorney or by your insurance company).

• The plaintiff-patient's attorney will also use discovery devices, so you may have to answer interrogatories and appear for a deposition as well. Your attorney will carefully prepare you for these procedures.

• Your attorney will also prepare you to testify at the trial. He'll tell you how to dress and how to act. Remember, he wants to win the case, too, so do what he tells you.

• Your failure to cooperate with an attorney provided by an insurance company can be used as a policy defense. This doesn't mean you must say or do anything he asks. If you feel you must contradict him, you have the right to state your position and to protect your professional reputation in court. If you feel he is asking you to do or say things that aren't in your best interest, tell him so.

• You have the right to change attorneys at any time. If you believe an attorney selected by your insurance company is more interested in protecting the company than in protecting you, discuss the problem with a company representative. Then, if you still feel that he isn't defending you properly, hire your own attorney. If this happens, you may have grounds for suing the insurance company and the company-appointed attorney.

Before your case goes to trial

• Study the copies of the medical records. Examine the complete medical chart, including nurses' notes, laboratory reports, and doctors' orders. On a separate sheet of paper, make appropriate notes on key entries or omissions. But don't make any changes on the records. Such an action will destroy your case by undermining your credibility.

• Create your own legal file. Ask your attorney to send you copies of all documents and correspondence pertaining to the case. Try to maintain a file that's as complete as your attorney's. If you receive a document you don't understand, ask your attorney to explain it.

• If the hospital or clinic where you work asks you to fill out an incident report, consult with your attorney before doing so. Usually, these incident reports can't be used as evidence, but they may influence future prospective employers. So have your attorney

help you fill out the report, because your career may be at stake.

• Limit talk about the case. Don't try to placate the person suing you by calling him and discussing the case. Your chances of talking him into dropping his lawsuit are very slim, and every word you say to him can be used against you in court.

• Don't discuss the lawsuit with anyone except your attorney. This will help prevent information leaks that could compromise your case. To protect your professional reputation, don't even mention to your colleagues that you've been sued.

• Ask your attorney about the legal devices you can use to protect your property. Many states have homestead laws that permit you to protect a substantial part of the equity in your house, as well as other property, from any judgment against you. Such protection is essential if you don't have insurance or if damages exceed your insurance, and you'll be glad you have it if you lose the case and the damages awarded do exceed your insurance coverage.

Your day in court

• While your attorney prepares your defense, he'll also explore whether it's desirable to try and reach an out-of-court settlement. If he decides such a settlement is in your best interest, he'll try to achieve a settlement in the period before your trial date.

• If your case does go to trial, you'll participate in selecting the jury. During this selection process, attorneys for both sides will question prospective jurors, and your attorney will ask your opinion on their suitability.

Either attorney may reject a small number of prospective jurors without any reason. You, the plaintiff, or either attorney are allowed to reject an unlimited number of jurors for specific reasons.

• To help prepare you to testify at

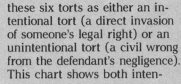

Understanding tort claims

Like all health care professionals, you're vulnerable to lawsuits.
If a patient feels your nursing
care is inappropriate, he might
file a lawsuit, claiming one of six
torts. The law classifies each of
these six torts as either an in-
tentional tort (a direct invasion
of someone's legal right) or an
unintentional tort (a civil wrong
from the defendant's negligence).
This chart shows both inten-
tional and unintentional torts
and examples of improper
nursing actions that could lead a
patient to use each claim in a
lawsuit.

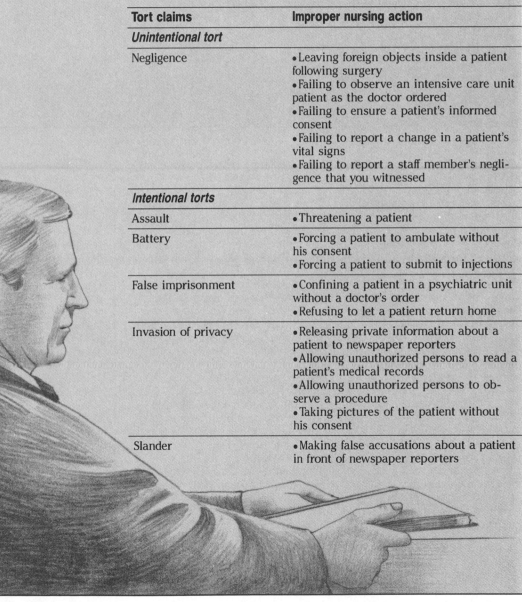

Tort claims	Improper nursing action
Unintentional tort	
Negligence	• Leaving foreign objects inside a patient following surgery • Failing to observe an intensive care unit patient as the doctor ordered • Failing to ensure a patient's informed consent • Failing to report a change in a patient's vital signs • Failing to report a staff member's negligence that you witnessed
Intentional torts	
Assault	• Threatening a patient
Battery	• Forcing a patient to ambulate without his consent • Forcing a patient to submit to injections
False imprisonment	• Confining a patient in a psychiatric unit without a doctor's order • Refusing to let a patient return home
Invasion of privacy	• Releasing private information about a patient to newspaper reporters • Allowing unauthorized persons to read a patient's medical records • Allowing unauthorized persons to observe a procedure • Taking pictures of the patient without his consent
Slander	• Making false accusations about a patient in front of newspaper reporters

Defending against malpractice charges

At some point in your career, a patient who was injured while in your care may sue you. If your attorney can establish one of the following defenses, the court will either dismiss the charges against you or reduce the amount of any damages.

Defense
Lack of proof

Rationale
Does the plaintiff have legally sufficient proof that your actions caused his injuries? If he doesn't, the court will dismiss the case against you.

Defense
Contributory negligence

Rationale
Did the plaintiff, through carelessness, contribute to his injury? If he did, some states permit the court to charge the plaintiff with failing to meet the standards of a reasonably prudent patient, barring him from recovering any damages.

---

the trial, your attorney will ask you to review the complete medical record, your interrogatory answers, and your deposition. In addition, you should review the entire legal file you've been keeping, to make sure you understand all aspects of the case before the trial begins.

• The trial may last several days and, in some cases, even several weeks. After all the witnesses have given their testimony, the jury—not the judge—will decide if you're liable. If the jury finds you liable, it will also assess damages against you.

Protecting your professional reputation

• During the trial, project a positive attitude at all times, suggesting you feel confident about the trial's outcome.

• You should never disparage the plaintiff inside or outside the courtroom. Characterizing him as a gold digger, for instance, will only serve to generate bad feelings that may interfere with the settlement. You won't want to speak to him during the trial, but

if you do, you should always be polite and dignified.

• Losing a malpractice lawsuit can jeopardize your future in nursing. Prospective employers (as well as prospective insurers) will want to know if you've ever lost a nursing malpractice lawsuit or if you've ever been a defendant in one.

If you have, you'll probably find job hunting more difficult than it used to be. You'll also pay an increased insurance premium, and you may find that some insurance companies will simply refuse to cover you.

Looking ahead

Recently, some state legislatures have reformed their laws to limit the number of malpractice lawsuits and their impact. For instance, some legislatures have limited the time allowed for filing suit by amending their states' statutes of limitations.

Others have limited the amount a jury can award to a plaintiff. In addition, the increasing use of arbitration procedures is helping reduce the number of these lawsuits that go to trial.

What to expect at a deposition

A deposition takes place after a lawsuit has been filed against you. In this legal procedure, the attorney for the person suing you questions you in the presence of your attorney and a court reporter. The deposition enables both parties to review each other's case and see if one is stronger than the other. Because most malpractice cases are settled out of court, the deposition is crucial.

Before the deposition

Before the deposition, review all medical records in the case, which may help you recall important facts. During the actual deposition, the plaintiff's attorney has the right to inspect and copy any material you bring with you to aid your memory. So you should show any such material to your attorney for his inspection and approval *prior* to the deposition.

Defense	Defense	Defense
Comparative negligence	Assumption of risk	Borrowed servant doctrine
Rationale	**Rationale**	**Rationale**
A few states permit the court to apportion liability, thereby barring the plaintiff from recovering some, but not all, of the damages he claims.	Did the plaintiff understand the risk involved in the treatment, procedure, or action that allegedly caused his injury? Did he give proper informed consent and therefore voluntarily expose himself to that risk? If he did, the court may rule that the plaintiff assumed the risk, knowingly disregarding the danger and relieving you of liability.	Were you working under the direct supervision of a doctor, such as one in an emergency department? If you were, the court may rule that the doctor is liable for your negligence.

During the deposition

Your attorney will probably advise you to respond to all questions with simple answers and not to volunteer or elaborate on any information. If you have any doubts when responding to the other attorney's questions, avoid absolute answers.

Memory fades with time, and even with the aid of medical records you won't be expected to recall the details of actual conversations that took place some time ago. If the case goes to court, however, you'll be held accountable for the answers you gave at the deposition.

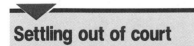

Settling out of court

Malpractice attorneys estimate that only 10% of all malpractice lawsuits actually go to court. Of those cases that go to court, only 10% actually end with a final judgment. The vast majority of malpractice lawsuits are settled out of court.

If you're ever involved in a malpractice lawsuit, there's a good chance that with your help your attorney will settle the case out of court. When you discuss settlement with him, remember these points:

Know the terms of your policy

If you're covered by professional liability insurance, the terms of your policy will determine whether you, your attorney, or the insurance company can control the settlement. Most policies do not permit the nurse to settle a case without the consent of the insurance company.

In fact, many policies, especially those provided by employers, permit the insurance company to settle *without the consent* of the individual nurse involved.

You should review your policy to determine your settlement rights. If the policy isn't clear on this point, call the insurance administrator of your hospital or the insurance company, and ask for clarification.

Provide information

Offer your insurance company's representative and your attorney all the information you can about the case. They will then be able to evaluate your liabilities and the plaintiff's liabilities, and determine the best settlement with the plaintiff.

As an attending nurse, you may be in the best position to provide crucial observations concerning the patient's state of mind — often the basis of a successful settlement.

Avoid further expenses

Remember, if you settle your case out of court, it doesn't mean that you're admitting any wrongdoing. The law regards settlement as a compromise between two parties to end a lawsuit and avoid further expense. In other words, you may choose to pay a settlement rather than incur possibly greater expenses (both financial and emotional) by defending your innocence at a trial.

Statutes of limitations: A state-by-state rundown

In the United States, state laws specify the duration within which a person may file a medical malpractice charge. In Canada, each province has its own statute of limitations. This chart details the statute of limitations in all 50 states and the District of Columbia.

State	Time from occurrence	Time from discovery
Alabama	2 years	6 months
Alaska	2 years	Applicable only to minors
Arizona	3 years	3 years
Arkansas	2 years	1 year
California	1 year	1 year
Colorado	Not applicable	2 years
Connecticut	2 years	2 years
Delaware	2 years	2 years
District of Columbia	Not applicable	3 years
Florida	2 years	2 years
Georgia	2 years	2 years
Hawaii	Not applicable	2 years
Idaho	2 years	1 year (applies only to foreign object lawsuits)
Illinois	Not applicable	2 years
Indiana	2 years	Not applicable
Iowa	Not applicable	2 years
Kansas	2 years	2 years
Kentucky	Not applicable	1 year
Louisiana	1 year	1 year
Maine	2 years	Not applicable
Maryland	5 years	3 years
Massachusetts	3 years	3 years
Michigan	2 years (for doctors) 3 years (for nurses)	2 years (for doctors) 3 years (for nurses)
Minnesota	2 years	2 years

Statutes of limitations: A state-by-state rundown (continued)

State	Time from occurrence	Time from discovery
Mississippi	Not applicable	2 years
Missouri	2 years	2 years
Montana	2 years	2 years
Nebraska	2 years	2 years
Nevada	4 years	2 years
New Hampshire	2 years	Uncertain
New Jersey	Not applicable	2 years
New Mexico	3 years	Not applicable
New York	30 months	30 months
North Carolina	3 years	1 year
North Dakota	Not applicable	2 years
Ohio	Not applicable	1 year
Oklahoma	Not applicable	2 years
Oregon	Not applicable	2 years
Pennsylvania	Not applicable	2 years
Rhode Island	3 years	1 year
South Carolina	3 years	3 years
South Dakota	2 years	Not applicable
Tennessee	1 year	1 year
Texas	2 years	2 years (applies only to limited circumstances)
Utah	Not applicable	2 years
Vermont	3 years	2 years
Virginia	2 years	Not applicable
Washington	3 years	1 year
West Virginia	2 years	2 years
Wisconsin	3 years	1 year
Wyoming	2 years	6 months

Understanding the legal process

Being named as a defendant in a malpractice lawsuit can be confusing as well as stressful. The antidote is knowing what to expect.

This chart summarizes the basic legal process from complaint to appeal. If you're ever involved in a lawsuit, your attorney will explain the specific procedures that your case requires.

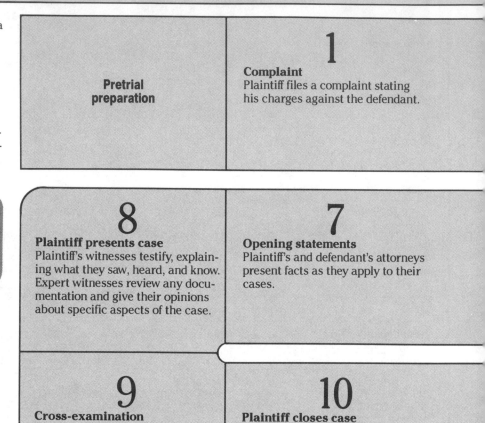

Pretrial preparation

1
Complaint
Plaintiff files a complaint stating his charges against the defendant.

8
Plaintiff presents case
Plaintiff's witnesses testify, explaining what they saw, heard, and know. Expert witnesses review any documentation and give their opinions about specific aspects of the case.

7
Opening statements
Plaintiff's and defendant's attorneys present facts as they apply to their cases.

9
Cross-examination
Defendant's attorney questions plaintiff's witnesses.

10
Plaintiff closes case
Defendant's attorney may make a motion to dismiss the case, claiming plaintiff's evidence is insufficient.

18
Appeal (optional)
Attorneys review transcripts. The party against whom the court ruled may appeal if he feels the judge didn't interpret the law properly, instruct the jury properly, or conduct the trial properly.

17
Verdict
Jury announces verdict before judge and both parties.

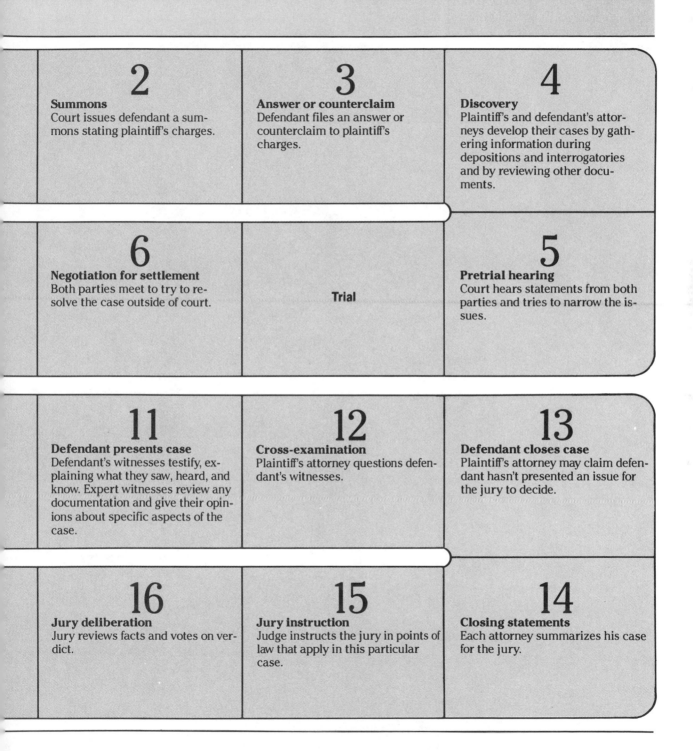

2
Summons
Court issues defendant a summons stating plaintiff's charges.

3
Answer or counterclaim
Defendant files an answer or counterclaim to plaintiff's charges.

4
Discovery
Plaintiff's and defendant's attorneys develop their cases by gathering information during depositions and interrogatories and by reviewing other documents.

6
Negotiation for settlement
Both parties meet to try to resolve the case outside of court.

Trial

5
Pretrial hearing
Court hears statements from both parties and tries to narrow the issues.

11
Defendant presents case
Defendant's witnesses testify, explaining what they saw, heard, and know. Expert witnesses review any documentation and give their opinions about specific aspects of the case.

12
Cross-examination
Plaintiff's attorney questions defendant's witnesses.

13
Defendant closes case
Plaintiff's attorney may claim defendant hasn't presented an issue for the jury to decide.

16
Jury deliberation
Jury reviews facts and votes on verdict.

15
Jury instruction
Judge instructs the jury in points of law that apply in this particular case.

14
Closing statements
Each attorney summarizes his case for the jury.

Index

i refers to an illustration; t refers to a table.

i refers to an illustration; t refers to a table.

i refers to an illustration; t refers to a table.

i refers to an illustration; t refers to a table.

i refers to an illustration; t refers to a table.

i refers to an illustration; t refers to a table.

i refers to an illustration; t refers to a table.

i refers to an illustration; t refers to a table.

i refers to an illustration; t refers to a table.